HEALTH AND HUMAN DEVELOPMENT

ALTERNATIVE MEDICINE RESEARCH YEARBOOK 2012

HEALTH AND HUMAN DEVELOPMENT

JOAV MERRICK – SERIES EDITOR –

NATIONAL INSTITUTE OF CHILD HEALTH AND HUMAN DEVELOPMENT, MINISTRY OF SOCIAL AFFAIRS, JERUSALEM, ISRAEL

Adolescent Behavior Research: International Perspectives
Joav Merrick and Hatim A. Omar (Editors)
2007. ISBN: 1-60021-649-8

Complementary Medicine Systems: Comparison and Integration
Karl W. Kratky
2008. ISBN: 978-1-60456-475-4

Pain in Children and Youth
P. Schofield and J. Merrick (Editors)
2008. ISBN: 978-1-60456-951-3

Obesity and Adolescence: A Public Health Concern
Hatim A Omar, Donald E. Greydanus; Dilip R. Patel and Joav Merrick (Editors)
2009. ISBN: 978-1-60692-821-9

Poverty and Children: A Public Health Concern
Alexis Lieberman, and Joav Merrick (Editors)
2009. ISBN: 978-1-60741-140-6

Living on the Edge: The Mythical, Spiritual, and Philosophical Roots of Social Marginality
Joseph Goodbread
2009. ISBN: 978-1-60741-162-8

Social and Cultural Psychiatry Experience from the Caribbean Region
Hari D. Maharajh and Joav Merrick (Editors)
2011. ISBN: 978-1-61668-506-5

Challenges in Adolescent Health: An Australian Perspective
David Bennett, Susan Towns and Elizabeth Elliott and Joav Merrick (Editors)
2009. ISBN: 978-1-60741-616-6

Children and Pain
P. Schofield and J. Merrick (Editors)
2009. ISBN: 978-1-60876-020-6

Alcohol-Related Cognitive Disorders: Research and Clinical Perspectives
Leo Sher, Isack Kandel and Joav Merrick (Editors)
2009. ISBN: 978-1-60741-730-9

Bone and Brain Metastases: Advances in Research and Treatment
Arjun Sahgal, Edward Chow and Joav Merrick (Editors)
2010. ISBN: 978-1-61668-365-8

Chance Action and Therapy: The Playful Way of Changing
Uri Wernik
2010. ISBN: 978-1-60876-393-1

International Aspects of Child Abuse and Neglect
Howard Dubowitz and Joav Merrick (Editors)
2010. ISBN: 978-1-61122-049-0

Behavioral Pediatrics, 3rd Edition
Donald E. Greydanus, Dilip R. Patel, Helen D. Pratt and Joseph L. Calles Jr. (Editors)
2011. ISBN: 978-1-60692-702-1

Advances in Environmental Health Effects of Toxigenic Mold and Mycotoxins
Ebere Cyril Anyanwu
2011. ISBN: 978-1-60741-953-2

**Rural Child Health:
International Aspects**
Erica Bell and Joav Merrick (Editors)
2011. ISBN: 978-1-60876-357-3

**Principles of Holistic Psychiatry:
A Textbook on Holistic Medicine for
Mental Disorders**
Soren Ventegodt and Joav Merrick
2011. ISBN: 978-1-61761-940-3

**International Aspects of Child Abuse
and Neglect**
*Howard Dubowitz
and Joav Merrick (Editors)*
2011. ISBN: 978-1-60876-703-8

**Positive Youth Development:
Evaluation and Future Directions
in a Chinese Context**
*Daniel T.L. Shek, Hing Keung Ma
and Joav Merrick (Editors)*
2011. ISBN: 978-1-60876-830-1

Alternative Medicine Yearbook 2009
Joav Merrick (Editor)
2011. ISBN: 978-1-61668-910-0

**Understanding Eating Disorders:
Integrating Culture,
Psychology and Biology**
*Yael Latzer, Joav Merrick
and Daniel Stein (Editors)*
2011. ISBN: 978-1-61728-298-0

**Advanced Cancer, Pain
and Quality of Life**
Edward Chow and Joav Merrick (Editors)
2011. ISBN: 978-1-61668-207-1

**Positive Youth Development:
Implementation of a Youth Program
in a Chinese Context**
*Daniel T.L Shek, Hing Keung Ma
and Joav Merrick (Editors)*
2011. ISBN: 978-1-61668-230-9

**Environment, Mood Disorders and
Suicide**
*Teodor T. Postolache
and Joav Merrick (Editors)*
2011. ISBN: 978-1-61668-505-8

**Chance Action and Therapy:
The Playful Way of Changing**
Uri Wernik
2011. ISBN: 978-1-61122-987-5

Public Health Yearbook 2009
Joav Merrick (Editor)
2011. ISBN: 978-1-61668-911-7

**Child Health and Human Development
Yearbook 2009**
Joav Merrick (Editor)
2011. ISBN: 978-1-61668-912-4

Narratives and Meanings of Migration
Julia Mirsky
2011. ISBN: 978-1-61761-103-2

**Self-Management and
the Health Care Consumer**
Peter William Harvey
2011. ISBN: 978-1-61761-796-6

Sexology from a Holistic Point of View
Soren Ventegodt and Joav Merrick
2011. ISBN: 978-1-61761-859-8

**Clinical Aspects of Psychopharmacology
in Childhood and Adolescence**
*D. E. Greydanus, J. L. Calles Jr., D. P. Patel,
A. Nazeer and J. Merrick (Editors)*
2011. ISBN: 978-1-61122-135-0

**Drug Abuse in Hong Kong:
Development and Evaluation of
a Prevention Program**
*Daniel TL Shek, Rachel CF Sun
and Joav Merrick (Editors)*
2011. ISBN: 978-1-61324-491-3

Climate Change and Rural Child Health
*Erica Bell, Bastian M. Seidel
and Joav Merrick (Editors)*
2011. ISBN: 978-1-61122-640-9

**Rural Medical Education:
Practical Strategies**
*Erica Bell and Craig Zimitat
and Joav Merrick (Editors)*
2011. ISBN: 978-1-61122-649-2

**Understanding Eating Disorders:
Integrating Culture,
Psychology and Biology**
*Yael Latzer, Joav Merrick and Daniel Stein
(Editors)*
2011. ISBN: 978-1-61470-976-3

**Positive Youth Development: Evaluation
and Future Directions
in a Chinese Context**
*Daniel T. L. Shek, Hing Keung Ma and Joav
Merrick (Editors)*
2011. ISBN: 978-1-62100-175-1

**The Dance of Sleeping and Eating
among Adolescents: Normal and
Pathological Perspectives**
Yael Latzer and Orna Tzischinsky (Editors)
2011. ISBN: 978-1-61209-710-7

**Child and Adolescent
Health Yearbook 2009**
Joav Merrick (Editor)
2012. ISBN: 978-1-61668-913-1

**Applied Public Health: Examining
Multifaceted Social or Ecological
Problems and Child Maltreatment**
John R. Lutzker and Joav Merrick (Editors)
2012. ISBN: 978-1-62081-356-0

**Adolescence and Chronic Illness.
A Public Health Concern**
*Hatim Omar, Donald E. Greydanus,
Dilip R. Patel and Joav Merrick (Editors)*
2012. ISBN: 978-1-60876-628-4

**Translational Research for
Primary Healthcare**
*Erica Bell, Gert P. Westert
and Joav Merrick (Editors)*
2012. ISBN: 978-1-61324-647-4

**Child and Adolescent Health
Yearbook 2010**
Joav Merrick (Editor)
2012. ISBN: 978-1-61209-788-6

**Child Health and Human Development
Yearbook 2010**
Joav Merrick (Editor)
2012. ISBN: 8-1-61209-789-3

Public Health Yearbook 2010
Joav Merrick (Editor
2012. ISBN: 978-1-61209-971-2

**The Astonishing Brain and Holistic
Consciousness: Neuroscience
and Vedanta Perspectives**
Vinod D. Deshmukh
2012. ISBN: Vinod D. Deshmukh

**Treatment and Recovery
of Eating Disorders**
Daniel Stein and Yael Latzer (Editors)
2012. ISBN: 978-1-61470-259-7

Randomized Clinical Trials and Placebo: Can You Trust the Drugs Are Working and Safe?
Søren Ventegodt and Joav Merrick
2012. ISBN: 978-1-61470-067-8

Alternative Medicine Yearbook 2010
Joav Merrick (Editor)
2012. ISBN: 978-1-62100-132-4

Building Community Capacity: Minority and Immigrant Populations
Rosemary M Caron and Joav Merrick (Editors)
2012. ISBN: 978-1-62081-022-4

Human Immunodeficiency Virus (HIV) Research: Social Science Aspects
Hugh Klein and Joav Merrick (Editors)
2012. ISBN: 978-1-62081-293-8

AIDS and Tuberculosis: Public Health Aspects
Daniel Chemtob and Joav Merrick (Editors)
2012. ISBN: 978-1-62081-382-9

Public Health Yearbook 2011
Joav Merrick (Editor)
2012. ISBN: 978-1-62081-433-8

Alternative Medicine Research Yearbook 2011
Joav Merrick (Editor)
2012. ISBN: 978-1-62081-476-5

Textbook on Evidence-Based Holistic Mind-Body Medicine: Basic Principles of Healing in Traditional Hippocratic Medicine
Søren Ventegodt and Joav Merrick
2012. ISBN: 978-1-62257-094-2

Textbook on Evidence-Based Holistic Mind-Body Medicine: Holistic Practice of Traditional Hippocratic Medicine
Søren Ventegodt and Joav Merrick
2012. ISBN: 978-1-62257-105-5

Textbook on Evidence-Based Holistic Mind-Body Medicine: Healing the Mind in Traditional Hippocratic Medicine
Søren Ventegodt and Joav Merrick
2012. ISBN: 978-1-62257-112-3

Textbook on Evidence-Based Holistic Mind-Body Medicine: Sexology and Traditional Hippocratic Medicine
Søren Ventegodt and Joav Merrick
2012. ISBN: 978-1-62257-130-7

Textbook on Evidence-Based Holistic Mind-Body Medicine: Research, Philosophy, Economy and Politics of Traditional Hippocratic Medicine
Søren Ventegodt and Joav Merrick
2012. ISBN: 978-1-62257-140-6

Our Search for Meaning in Life: Quality of Life Philosophy
Soren Ventegodt and Joav Merrick
2012. ISBN: 978-1-61470-494-2

Health and Happiness from Meaningful Work: Research in Quality of Working Life
Soren Ventegodt and Joav Merrick (Editors)
2013. ISBN: 978-1-60692-820-2

Pediatric and Adolescent Sexuality and Gynecology: Principles for the Primary Care Clinician
Hatim A Omar, Donald E. Greydanus, Artemis K., Dilip R. Patel and Joav Merrick (Editors)
2013. ISBN: 978-1-60876-735-9

Conceptualizing Behavior in Health and Social Research: A Practical Guide to Data Analysis
Said Shahtahmasebi and Damon Berridge
2013. ISBN: 978-1-60876-383-2

Adolescence and Sports
Dilip R. Patel, Donald E. Greydanus, Hatim Omar and Joav Merrick (Editors)
2013. ISBN: 978-1-60876-702-1

Living on the Edge: The Mythical, Spiritual, and Philosophical Roots of Social Marginality
Joseph Goodbread
2013. ISBN: 978-1-61122-986-8

Human Development: Biology from a Holistic Point of View
Søren Ventegodt, Tyge Dahl Hermansen and Joav Merrick (Editors)
2013. ISBN: 978-1-61470-441-6

Building Community Capacity: Case Examples from Around the World
Rosemary M. Caron and Joav Merrick (Editors)
2013. ISBN: 978-1-62417-175-8

Managed Care in a Public Setting
Richard Evan Steele
2013. ISBN: 978-1-62417-970-9

Bullying: A Public Health Concern
Jorge C. Srabstein and Joav Merrick (Editors)
2013. ISBN: 978-1-62618-564-7

HEALTH AND HUMAN DEVELOPMENT

ALTERNATIVE MEDICINE RESEARCH YEARBOOK 2012

SØREN VENTEGODT
AND
JOAV MERRICK
EDITORS

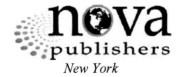

Copyright © 2013 by Nova Science Publishers, Inc.

All rights reserved. No part of this book may be reproduced, stored in a retrieval system or transmitted in any form or by any means: electronic, electrostatic, magnetic, tape, mechanical photocopying, recording or otherwise without the written permission of the Publisher.

For permission to use material from this book please contact us:
Telephone 631-231-7269; Fax 631-231-8175
Web Site: http://www.novapublishers.com

NOTICE TO THE READER

The Publisher has taken reasonable care in the preparation of this book, but makes no expressed or implied warranty of any kind and assumes no responsibility for any errors or omissions. No liability is assumed for incidental or consequential damages in connection with or arising out of information contained in this book. The Publisher shall not be liable for any special, consequential, or exemplary damages resulting, in whole or in part, from the readers' use of, or reliance upon, this material. Any parts of this book based on government reports are so indicated and copyright is claimed for those parts to the extent applicable to compilations of such works.

Independent verification should be sought for any data, advice or recommendations contained in this book. In addition, no responsibility is assumed by the publisher for any injury and/or damage to persons or property arising from any methods, products, instructions, ideas or otherwise contained in this publication.

This publication is designed to provide accurate and authoritative information with regard to the subject matter covered herein. It is sold with the clear understanding that the Publisher is not engaged in rendering legal or any other professional services. If legal or any other expert assistance is required, the services of a competent person should be sought. FROM A DECLARATION OF PARTICIPANTS JOINTLY ADOPTED BY A COMMITTEE OF THE AMERICAN BAR ASSOCIATION AND A COMMITTEE OF PUBLISHERS.

Additional color graphics may be available in the e-book version of this book.

Library of Congress Cataloging-in-Publication Data

ISBN: 978-1-62808-080-3

Published by Nova Science Publishers, Inc. † New York

CONTENTS

Preface		**xiii**
Introduction: Holistic and integrative medicine and challenges *Søren Ventegodt and Joav Merrick*		**xv**
Section one – Changing health paradigm		**1**
Chapter 1	The forum: The people, the place, the process *Jeanne Viall*	**3**
Chapter 2	Consciousness and medicine from the point of view of a family physician *Shadrick Mazaza*	**13**
Chapter 3	Changing the medical paradigm: What does disease look like when we shift our view? *Bernard Brom and Dip Acup*	**21**
Chapter 4	Dimensions of health care and the biomatrix *György Járos*	**33**
Chapter 5	A-causality, consciousness and organisations *Walter Baets*	**43**
Chapter 6	Sustainability and health: Back to the roots and feeding the soil *Jeanne Viall*	**55**
Chapter 7	The science of the art of medicine *Bernard Brom and Dip Acup*	**65**
Chapter 8	On the paradigm of consciousness-based medicine and quality of life as medicine *Søren Ventegodt*	**73**
Chapter 9	The matter-energy-information (MEI) body of the human being *Bernard Brom and Dip Acup*	**85**
Chapter 10	Reflections on a health paradigm *Saadiq Kariem*	**97**
Chapter 11	An integrated approach for HIV disease *Gary Orr*	**103**

x   *Contents*

Chapter 12   The traditional healing system in South Africa   **111**
                  Nhlavana Maseko, Phephsile Maseko and Jeanne Viall

Chapter 13   South African healing villages   **117**
                  Renee Usdin

Chapter 14   Heart matters: The art of healing   **121**
                  Erna Oldenboom

Chapter 15   The third way?   **129**
                  Leslie Pleass

Chapter 16   Conversations: The five star doctor   **137**
                  Saville N Furman

Section two – From sleep to hippocrates   **141**

Chapter 17   Sleep disorders and sleep patterns in adolescents   **143**
                  Donald E Greydanus and Cynthia Feucht

Chapter 18   Adolescence and hypertension   **169**
                  Alfonso D Torres and Donald E Greydanus

Chapter 19   Breath-Meditation: Prana-Dhyana   **185**
                  Vinod D Deshmukh

Chapter 20   Antidiabetic effect of camel milk on alloxane diabetes:
                  Comparison with insulin   **195**
                  Amel Sboui, Touhami Khorchani, Mongi Djegham
                  and Omrane Belhadj

Chapter 21   Transfer of effect of heat shock and drug treatment from
                  one plant to another through water   **203**
                  Sandhimita Mondal, Soma Sukul and Nirmal C Sukul

Chapter 22   The capabilities of new Chinese entrepreneurs in China   **211**
                  Jing Sun, Nicholas Buys and Xinchao Wang

Chapter 23   Mental influencing of the growth of mung bean seedlings:
                  A pilot study   **221**
                  Andrea Leitner, Caroline Weckerle, Wolfgang Matzer
                  and Christiane W Geelhaar

Chapter 24   Gender effects in massage therapy   **229**
                  Thomas Edward Smith, Pamela Valentine
                  and Bruce A Thyer

Chapter 25   A follow-up study on the morphology of isolated rat cortical
                  neurons and information transferred via a "biophoton device"   **237**
                  Dietrich Vastenburg and Sjoerd Pet

Chapter 26   Holistic medicine V: One session healing of rape and
                  incest traumas in a group setting   **245**
                  Søren Ventegodt, Andrew Young and Joav Merrick

Chapter 27	Reflections from a study tour to Hippocrates' Asklepieion on the island of Kos *Søren Ventegodt and Joav Merrick*	**251**

Section three – Life satisfaction   **255**

Chapter 28	Aging and quality of life in Taiwan *Luo Lu*	**257**
Chapter 29	Interplay between mood and physical activity and their effect on life satisfaction in later life *Jessica Jones and Natalie Wakefield*	**271**
Chapter 30	Quality of life in an evolutionary perspective *Bjørn Grinde*	**289**
Chapter 31	Adolescent life satisfaction and well-being *Danilo Garcia and Trevor Archer*	**301**
Chapter 32	The family environment in adolescence as a predictor of life satisfaction *Liisa Martikainen*	**313**
Chapter 33	How people assess present and future quality of life in the elderly from health status information *Maria Teresa Muñoz Sastre* *and Etienne Mullet*	**323**
Chapter 34	Conditions for the dissatisfying effect of reference group income *Chau-Kiu Cheung*	**333**
Chapter 35	Sense of community and income as indicators of life satisfaction *Evie M Muilenburg-Trevino, Megan K Pittman* *and Mary Guilfoyle Holmes*	**351**
Chapter 36	Life satisfaction in Macedonian work organizations *Elisaveta Sardjoska*	**361**
Chapter 37	The transition to cohabitation: The mediating role of self-efficacy between stress management and couple satisfaction *Antonella Roggero, Maria Fernanda Vacirca, Adele Mauri* *and Silvia Ciairano*	**369**

Section four – Positive youth development   **387**

Chapter 38	Spirituality as a positive youth development construct: A conceptual review *Daniel TL Shek*	**389**
Chapter 39	Beliefs in the future as a positive youth development construct: A conceptual review *Rachel CF Sun Daniel TL Shek*	**403**

xii *Contents*

Chapter 40 Cognitive competence as a positive youth development construct:
A conceptual review   417
Rachel CF Sun and Eadaoin KP Hui

Chapter 41 Emotional competence as a positive youth development construct:
A conceptual review   429
Patrick SY Lau and Florence KY Wu

Chapter 42 Self-efficacy as a positive youth development construct:
A conceptual review   443
Sandra KM Tsang, Eadaoin KP Hui and Bella CM Law

Chapter 43 Self-determination as a psychological and positive youth development
construct   455
Eadaoin KP Hui and Sandra KM Tsang

Chapter 44 Positive identity as a positive youth development construct:
A conceptual review   469
Sandra KM Tsang, Eadaoin KP Hui and Bella CM Law

Section five – Acknowledgements   483

Chapter 45 About the editor   485

Chapter 46 About the National Institute of Child Health and Human
Development in Israel   487

Index   491

PREFACE

The field of holistic or integrative medicine needs a scientific approach. We need this kind of medicine - and we even need it to be spiritual to include the depths of human existence - but we need it to be a little less "cosmic" in order to encompass the whole human being. Many important research questions and challenges, empirical as well as theoretical, demand the attention from medical researchers. The field has been too preoccupied with orthomolecular medicine, and dietary supplements without much scientific foundation. Acupuncture needles and other seemingly effective, but strange elements from the traditional medicines, semi-religious procedures of meditation and healing manipulating "energetic dimensions" like "chakras" and "auras" in symbolic ways, and similar approaches have been in the forefront, but not easily compatible with the basic reason and common sense of a modern medical science.

This year book 2012 brings together the work we did over the past year with a broad research agenda on a global basis, addressing questions ranging from a discussion of a changing health paradigm, sleep disorders, Hippocrates, and life satisfaction to positive youth development in Hong Kong. We hope this book will provide you with new knowledge, link research to practice and policy, and help build networks of research collaborations and move science forward in this field.

INTRODUCTION:
HOLISTIC AND INTEGRATIVE MEDICINE AND CHALLENGES

Søren Ventegodt[*], *MD, MMedSci, EU-MSc-CAM*[1,2,3,4,5] *and Joav Merrick, MD, MMedSci, DMSc*[5,6,7,8,9]

[1]Quality of Life Research Center, Copenhagen, Denmark
[2]Research Clinic for Holistic Medicine and
[3]Nordic School of Holistic Medicine, Copenhagen, Denmark
[4]Scandinavian Foundation for Holistic Medicine, Sandvika, Norway
[5]Interuniversity College, Graz, Austria
[6]National Institute of Child Health and Human Development, Jerusalem
[7]Division of Pediatrics, Hadassah Hebrew University Medical Centers, Mt Scopus Campus, Jerusalem
[8]Office of the Medical Director, Health Services, Division for Intellectual and Developmental Disabilities, Ministry of Social Affairs and Social Services, Jerusalem, Israel and
[9]Kentucky Children's Hospital, University of Kentucky, Lexington, US

The field of holistic or integrative medicine needs a scientific approach. We need this kind of medicine - and we even need it to be spiritual to include the depths of human existence - but we need it to be a little less "cosmic" in order to encompass the whole human being. Many important research questions and challenges, empirical as well as theoretical, demand the attention from medical researchers. The field has been too preoccupied with orthomolecular medicine, and dietary supplements without much scientific foundation. Acupuncture needles and other seemingly effective, but strange elements from the traditional medicines, semi-religious procedures of meditation and healing manipulating "energetic dimensions" like "chakras" and "auras" in symbolic ways, and similar approaches has been in

---

[*] Correspondence: Søren Ventegodt, MD, MMedSci, EU-MSc-CAM, Director, Quality of Life Research Center, Frederiksberg Alle 13A, 2tv, DK-1661 Copenhagen V, Denmark. E-mail: ventegodt@livskvalitet.org.

the forefront, but not easily compatible with the basic reason and common sense of a modern medical science.

To encompass the whole human being, a truly holistic medicine needs to include the dimension of consciousness in a scientific way: the subjective experience of the patient and interpretations of the world, her feelings, her hopes and fears, her actual sense of coherence, her level of self-expression or self-actualization and her basic perspective of life.

Within the past decade or two, consciousness has erupted as a legitimate research topic among neurobiologists. Medical scientists are beginning to take notice, become aware and scientific journals, like the Journal of Consciousness Studies are now more often publishing articles from physicians. Needless to say, holistic medicine must equally integrate the influence of personal consciousness on the course, prevention and treatment of disease.

Formidable research challenges loom, however. Many important research questions, empirical as well as theoretical, demand attention from medical researchers. Using conceptual frameworks like quality of life, we have suggested that a patient's quality of life represents a third influence on health beyond the genetic and traumatic factors so far emphasized by mainstream medicine. In our clinical and research efforts, we attempt to specify what a clinician may do to help patients help themselves by mobilizing the vast resources hidden in their subjective worlds, in their hopes and dreams with their will to live.

The field of holistic medicine must be upgraded to fully integrate human consciousness, scientifically as well as philosophically. It appears the new areas of research like psychoneuroimmunology and life mission theory are opening new vistas in medical research concerned with consciousness, wholeness and even spirituality, if this latter term can find a meaning in science.

New directions in health care are called for. We need a new vision of the future of the health care sector in the industrialized countries. Every person has immense potentials for self-healing that we scarcely know how to mobilize. A new holistic medicine must find ways to tackle this key challenge. A health care system that could do that successfully would bring quality of life and health to many people. Are we able to do it and change the health care system over the next hundred years ?

SECTION ONE – CHANGING HEALTH PARADIGM

In: Alternative Medicine Research Yearbook 2012
Editors: Søren Ventegodt and Joav Merrick

ISBN: 978-1-62808-080-3
© 2013 Nova Science Publishers, Inc.

Chapter 1

THE FORUM: THE PEOPLE, THE PLACE, THE PROCESS

*Jeanne Viall, BA**

Freelance journalist, Dennesig, Stellenbosch,
South Africa

ABSTRACT

This presentation discuss a meeting in South Africa in 2010 between 16 international professionals from various backgrounds and countries brought together to brainstorm about the changing paradigm in medicine. The special issue is a result of these discussions and presentations.

Keywords: Health, medicine, integrative medicine, future

INTRODUCTION

What did we expect, bringing together 16 people, leaders in their fields, to discuss the changing paradigm in medicine over four days? Well, we hoped for lively conversation and a sharing of ideas and insights. And we were not disappointed. We were aware that in medicine, as in business and other disciplines, something was shifting, something new was emerging, a new paradigm of medicine. We wanted to get a sense of what this looked like, what its key features were, and its implications for the future of medicine.

Dr Bernard Brom was the initiator and driving force behind this Forum, and I would like to acknowledge his vision here. He has explained his thinking behind the Forum in the editorial and his dictum has long been "the more points of view, the better the view". And so we began organising the Forum bearing in mind we wanted diversity of views.

Rather than a formal lecture-format conference, we wanted to create a space for an open exchange of ideas, and stimulate thinking. We designed the programme to include a mix of

---

* Correspondence: Jeanne Viall, BA, POBox 2229, Dennesig, Stellenbosch, 7601 South Africa. E-mail: jeanne@creatinghealth.co.za.

presentations, brainstorming using the World Café process and some experiential processes. We wanted to share ideas in a relaxed environment where people could speak freely and exchange their ideas in lively debate.

Our Forum was an experiment in what happens when active participation is the focus. For the big group presentations and discussions we decided not to seat people conference style but rather in a large circle. With a group this size it made it possible for everyone to see the others, and participate easily.

THE PEOPLE

Selecting participants was largely Dr Bernard Brom's task. This was the culmination of an idea he had been working on for many years and he knew whom he wanted. These were leading edge thinkers, and we cast the net wide to find people, looking not only for medical doctors, but others who worked in various fields and could share ideas around complexity and sustainability Gathering participants was a journey of surprises. When a person on our list could not make it, others were sought. New avenues opened up, and the programme was adapted to enfold the new. Numbers rose, people emerged we would not have thought of. This was creativity at work, a combined process of planning and allowing. We accepted that the conversation would go the way it was destined to: We were just holding the strings of the warp, while the weft was being handed to us.

Our participants were a lively group of very committed people, and there was seldom a dull moment over the four days. Doctors and experts love to express their opinions, and there were some strong ones. People came from very different spaces in their work lives, with some at the knife-edge of tertiary health care (a paediatric surgeon in a state hospital, a hospital head) and others from the more theoretical world of academia, such as Dr Shadrick Mazaza. Still others like Dr Leslie Pleass, Dr Saville Furman worked in private practice; Dr Renee Usdin in community health care.

PARTICIPANTS AND FACILITATORS

Many of our participants were medical specialists; some were not. We were fortunate to have Professor Walter Baets from the UCT Graduate School of Business; Professor Mark Swilling and Eve Anneke from the Sustainability Institute (although their visit was brief).

Dr Saadiq Kariem, then CEO of Groote Schuur, contributed his years of experience in both public health and politics; Erna Oldenboom brought her experience in Ayurvedic medicine to the Forum. We were honoured by the attendance of Dr Nhlavane Maseko, head of the Traditional Healers Organisation and his daughter Dr Phepsile Maseko, active in the organisation and policy making. Despite his 80 plus years, Dr Maseko was fully present at all the sessions, his sharp mind not missing a thing, his wit ready to interject. Professor György Járos, Dr Gary Orr and Dr Søren Ventegodt came from over the seas.

John Neave and Fiona McKay worked with Dr Brom and myself on planning the programme and helped facilitate the process. Their hard work and humour went a long way to making the event the success it was.

THE PLACE

On the afternoon of 23 April 2010 people began arriving at the Stanford Valley Conference Centre, situated on a farm a few kilometres from the little town of Stanford in South Africa. It was telling to see just how stressed people can be, and a pleasure to watch people slowly unwind in this quiet rural setting.

We chose the Stanford Valley Conference Centre for the four-day residential event. We were generously sponsored by Natural Health Products, and so could include whomever we wished in our group. Being residential, we ate together and spent our evenings together in the charming lounge and dining area, with much jollity and talk. The early birds went for walks.

THE PROGRAM

After months of planning, and anxious moments caused by delayed flights (the Iceland volcano had shown us that no matter how well-planned something is, nature will have its way and final word), everyone gathered. Our introductory session was a brief one, to welcome people and off er a chance for each person to introduce themselves before we retired for supper. It was a lively supper as people started unwinding and getting to know each other.

DAY ONE: THE KNOWN

Our first day was spent exploring "The known". People were asked to share their personal stories, particularly what had influenced them to take the path they had chosen. "There is a good reason why I wanted to hear everyone's story right at the beginning of this Forum," Dr Brom told the group. "It seems to me that when I speak of my passion, what moves me, what inspires me to help others, those who hear me - if they listen with attention and consciousness - open to my viewpoint and then this becomes a dance in which we both participate and share much more than ideas. We bring much more than our bodies to the Forum and my understanding is that we bring much more than our minds as well. So, while points of view are great and very often fruitful, it is the magic of each person and their song that inspires me."

What emerged were the often moving, always interesting stories about the turning points in people's lives - whether it was personal tragedy like the death of a brother, illness as a child, or political circumstances, such as growing up in apartheid South Africa – which led people to choose a life of service to others. For some, like Dr Phepsile and Dr Nhlavane Maseko, there was no choice, they were called to be healers from an early age. "I grew under the feet of my grandfather," said Dr Nhlavane Maseko, "the greatest medicine man in Africa, and my grandmother was a spirit medium."

Dr Shadrick Mazaza then spoke on consciousness, healing and integralism. His submission to this special issues is about paradigm shifts, and he includes a brief history of conventional medicine, the dilemmas and challenges facing modern medicine and current thoughts regarding a new paradigm for health. He concludes with some thoughts on the role of family medicine in an emerging conceptual framework for health in South Africa.

One thing that stayed with me was this: In his talk he said you cannot talk about intergralism without talking about traditional medicine, and told the story of his mother, who when his aunt was ill, was very clear which medicine, traditional or western, she needed. He asked her, "you can tell?" There was no question for her: "Yes," she said. One of his research projects, which resulted in a book, was on Urban African Traditional Healers. "The next paradigm in medicine is going to be personal transformation, and will have to include consciousness, not just for the patient but for doctors."

CAFE CONVERSATIONS

Thus far, the door at one end of the conference room had been closed, with a sign "Café Inside Out". After lunch we opened up our "café", and asked people to make themselves comfortable. We had set out tables for four, covered with blank paper, and a bunch of pens. The World Café process, as developed by Juanita Brown and David Isaacs, is informal and participants are asked to discuss an open-ended question, and then to move to a new table (where one person remains) to carry on the discussion and add new perspectives. After a few rounds, there is feedback.

The idea is to stimulate debate, not necessarily to come up with answers. The World Café process is founded on the assumption that people have the capacity to work together, no matter who they are. The belief behind it is that we humans want to talk together about things that matter to us, and as we talk we are able to access a greater wisdom that is found only in the collective (1). In this process we are looking for collaborative insight, and often the new questions we come up with are as, or more, important than the answers. The idea is to generate insights which help shape the future. People contribute rather than participate, and everyone's contribution is encouraged. People can jot down insights and doodle, using the "table cloths" for this. Cards are then used to write down key insights, and during feedback these may refl ect patterns, themes and deeper questions.

THE CAFE IN PROCESS

In this, the first café, we asked people to ponder the question "What are the limits to what science can discover?" Well, we uncovered a hornet's nest, and discussions proceeded loudly and vigorously. Some comments to emerge were: "What do we mean by science?" "Is there a hard and soft science?" "Can we measure everything?" "Sometimes we may not know what we're measuring." "Are we limited?"

In the discussion that followed participants were reminded that science is a language, and we make choices around which language to use. Every methodology has rules, we choose a methodology according to how we believe the world works. If you do not believe anything, you cannot do research. Researchers need to make their ontological choices clear. At the end we were left with many more questions, of course, and no definitive answers, which was fine by us, although it may have been a bit frustrating for some participants. Questions drive exploration.

DAY TWO: ENTERING THE UNKNOWN

The theme of this day was "entering the unknown" and we started with a guided sound meditation led by Erna Oldenboom together with Walter Baets. It may have seemed a bit unusual to many delegates, but they willingly lay down and let themselves be taken on the journey. Erna Oldenboom has written on heart matters: The art of healing in which she asked us to pay attention to the health of the health professionals themselves, and says: "We need students, future medical doctors, that are able to explain and to recognise in themselves stressful situations, and who are able to listen to their own body language and mental states."

Dr Søren Ventegodt's presentation was on subjective inter-disciplinary science, from head to heart, from mind to wholeness. His input was followed by a practical demonstration of the technique he uses, and then we all had a chance to try it. It was powerful and moving: touch is often taboo, especially in medicine, but through touch powerful feelings are evoked, and major shifts happen. Dr Ventegodt's submission to this special issue is on the paradigm of consiousness-based medicine and quality of life as medicine. He traces the history of the idea that quality of life aff ects health, and writes on the extensive body of research to back it today.

Dr Bernard Brom followed with a presentation on the science of the art of medicine and TDr Nhlavane Maseko and TDr Phepsile Maseko then took us through the many kinds of healers that fall under the umbrella of traditional healing, and asked us to take care when we loosely used the term "sangoma", only one of many, many kinds of healer that practice.

Professor Mark Swilling and Eve Anneke had us thinking about sustainability, and asked us some interesting and challenging questions. We were asked to re-examine sustainability, what it means, and fundamentally question what we mean by development. After the Forum a few of us met to continue this conversation with particular attention paid to health and medicine.

Dr Daniel Sidler gave us his input on the human energy field and does it matter, while Dr Brom further explored the question of energy in his work.

In the afternoon we moved once more to the Inside Out Café, and this time our question was: "How do we investigate the unknown? And how does the unknown communicate with us." This prompted more lively conversations, with questions of how you explore the internal space, how do you get into the heart? What do we mean by the (he)art of medicine? We have so much knowledge, how do we use it in the right way and right places. Do we need more knowledge?

DAY THREE: THE MEDICAL PARADIGM

The third day was dedicated to "the medical paradigm" and Professor György Járos presented his talk on biomatrix and the greater physiology of the human condition. The very nature of the physical universe is activity or action: matter, energy, information (MEI). Everything is part of a living system, and he quoted the Greek (attributed to Heraclitus) ta panta rhei – everything flows. And so for example, he said, it makes no sense looking just at the medical part of HIV/Aids - the drugs - but we also need to look at the processes which feed into each other to see where positive feedback loops are. The "bios" is the totality of life on earth; the

"Matrix" is the mould. The biomatrix allows us to look at something in its totality, the biggest picture, rather than in a reductionistic way. "The new paradigm is interconnection," he said.

Professor Baets followed with his presentation on causality and quantum ontology, which was both stimulating and challenging. On paradigms, he had this to say: You'll never find a new paradigm if you stay within the old paradigm, Einstein would never had found the theory of relativity if he'd stayed in the Newtonian paradigm, although he couldn't prove it for 17 years. "Science doesn't prove, it assumes. With gene therapy there was an assumption it would work, but it was never proved. And that's how science progresses, when someone steps outside the paradigm, and comes up with something which is not standard and accepted in the paradigm," he said. "For me a paradigm is nothing more than a pair of glasses. If I would give you a blue pair and you a rose coloured pair, and told you to look outside and tell me what that tree looks like, you would say it was pink, the other that it was blue and I would say it was green. And we'd all be right. The only thing a paradigm does is that it limits you. It is a window, but you cannot see what is below. I limit myself to what I can see, and that is what we do. "One of the most shocking things I think today is that despite the four big revolutions which have taken place in science over the last century, physics, business, medicine, whatever, is still extremely Newtonian. There is no reason for that other than that we are all afraid to move out of the paradigm. We continue to do what we've done for years." You'll never see the new paradigm if you stay in the old paradigm, he said. "Have you ever seen a PhD which doesn't prove what it sets out to?" asked Professor Baets. "We search where there already is research. Most academic research doesn't go the other way."

When doing research, there are three main ontological (nature of reality) choices we make: Newtonian causality, constructivism (constructed causality) and a-causality. Ontology is the belief in how nature works, the basic functioning of reality. Do I believe the world is Newtonian, or do I believe in the Quantum principle? Paradigms are a matter of choice, and it's not that reality doesn't exist, but rather that everything exists, and it is a matter of making choices. How deeply you want to understand will determine which research methods you want to use, he said. There are also different epistemologies (research methodologies): qualitative, quantitative or first person research (some things are only researchable by introspection).

There are different levels of knowing – among them mathematics, physics, chemistry, biology, noetic science (the nature and potential of consciousness), fractal algebra, energy physics, vibrational chemistry, noetic biology, energy psychology…

What is required is to know there is a limit to how you see things; and be upfront about which level you're operating from. It is not about right and wrong.

A discussion followed, in which Dr Saadiq Kariem, Dr Gary Orr, Dr Saville Furman and Dr Leslie Pleass participated. It was led by Professor Baets. Dr Renee Usdin was to be part of this, but had to leave early due to unforeseen circumstances. She has however contributed a paper South African Healing Villages, documenting an innovative community programme she is involved in. It makes interesting reading, and is a practical example of integrating diff erent models of medicine.

Dr Kariem reiterated that medicine was based in a scientific model paradigm, limited to a particular ontological and epidemiological system. "Therein lies the challenge and the problem," he said. "We have to be pragmatic about the future of the new paradigm. He suggested that since health care is a business, the new way needed to talk to the "bottom line". Dr Orr spoke of his work both in the National Health System in Britain but also in

The forum: The people, the place, the process 9

South Africa with HIV and nutrition using Food State supplements. Work in prisons had showed that nutrition had a profound effect on violence and aggression, but this research had not been acted on. Multiple challenges face any alternative paradigm, he said, such as political ideas and the simplistic basis underlying modern medical science.

Dr Pleass shared a personal journey, as he does in his submission to the document; Dr Furman gave us a delightful look at what it meant to be a family doctor and a "five-star doctor" and what that means in his experience. What emerged from the discussion was that the current medical system is a tightlycontrolled system, and there are a number of political expedients to maintain the status quo. With financial incentives and people in positions of authority with a power base, the system works to keep them in those positions. Medical aids also now determine what doctors can treat and with which drugs, limiting the doctor's choice of treatment.

Professor Baets asked the question: What prevents us from doing things differently now? It is worthwhile to keep asking this question, and this is a conversation which must continue. There is a huge body of research that has been done in the integrative health field, and there was a concern that this was not widely known about. Someone suggested that a home needed to be found for the new paradigm; another that it was beholden on each one in the group to speak about the new paradigm, to connect to a "virtual" body of ideas, to establish a clinical base, to spread the word. One way was to do the work you believe in, do research and become the new, best paradigm. As someone put it: "We are playground participants, and consciousness itself is what is emerging. Are we looking for a place, a space, a home or language or anything else? What is our ethos, what would we like to see?"

The bottom line, people agreed, was: we are searching for good medicine. It was important to have a vision, something greater than the separate parts. Others said they would be taking so much away from the Forum, both in new ideas and practically. TDr Phepsile Maseko said: "We all have the same vision, to see South Africa a better place to be." Our value was serving the community. Our aim was making a long-term diff erence in health.

DAY FOUR: THE EMERGING PARADIGM

Our last day was a short one, with just a morning session. Dr Brom started off with a brief summary: "We have discussed and debated the limits of science, and seen how easy it is to forget the importance of experience. The big view is just bringing the whole human being back into the picture of life and the recognition that the whole is more than the sum of its parts. What kind of guidelines as wise and experienced human beings should we be suggesting as we move forward to develop a model that is more appropriate for health and the management of ill health? "In my life it is important to acknowledge the mystery and all those things that are outside or inside or elsewhere that we also call 'life'; the hidden dimension that has to do with the greater anatomy of human beings, with soul, spirit, the heart, out of which intuition, inspiration and unconditional love arises. And while the logical, thinking mind likes to think it is in control, clearly there is a great deal more going on that is not limited by mind and thought.

"So perhaps in our last conversation together we can bring our heart and mind together and bring forth a vision that can inspire and give direction to a future medicine and at the

10   *Jeanne Viall*

same time acknowledge that medicine needs to be sustainable, practical and dare I say, a more joyful medicine."

Professor Jaros had created a working map of the paradigm shift for us, using the Biomatrix Model, and said he saw it as a map that could accommodate everyone, wherever they are and whatever fi eld of medicine they practice in. "We are all talking a slightly diff erent language – doing diff erent things, but this is like a playground where everyone can come and play – a place for everyone." This was helpful in getting the discussion going.

We soon realised however this meeting was just a first step in our explorations, and that there were many more conversations to be had. We needed much more time to come to a shared vision. Suggestions were for further meetings; a virtual community; the special issue you are reading; research projects; perhaps also collating the vast body of research that has been done. A list of the qualities of the new paradigm was drawn up, and while there was no time to discuss and debate each one, it was agreed that the new paradigm was emerging from the old, from a group of concerned people coming together from a more heart-based place, with new ideas. It was an organic process, and one that saw the limitations of a drug-based approach to disease and recognised the body's inherent healing ability. It was focused on patient-centred healing and was community and society based. It was shift towards a model that integrates new ways of thinking, and moves from treating disease only to supporting and maintaining health.

The meeting ended with a blessing from TDr Maseko, much laughter and a strong sense of community.

AFTERWARDS

Some time has passed since the Forum, and this special issue is now published. What stays with me are a few images from the conference. One was the image of a spring, which Dr Ventegodt used. "We are a spring vibrating with energy – or that's how we should be. We can adjust when we have to, and stretch out, but if sustained over time, we lose that spring, that joyful dynamic state. To heal, we must move back to springiness. We get ill and then have to go into crisis to get better."

Another was the web, the links and connections between all things, between different paradigms, between people, between ideas. I loved the moments of connection, the respect between people.

Our Forum was a very big idea whose time had come, and justice was done to it. I'd like to thank all those who took precious time from their busy schedules (and a public holiday) to take part in what was an unknown quantity. Thanks you for your attention, participation and willingness to engage. I especially like to thank Dr Brom for his vision and energy in making the Forum happen. He is a determined and hard-working man who gets things done.

Thanks to John Neave and Fiona MacKay for keeping the Forum moving, to time, and for taking care of the small things that matter. We chose adventure, love, strength and enthusiasm as the four pillars of the paradigm. Many thanks again to Louis Schutte and Estie Schreiber at SA Natural Heath Products for sponsorship. Also to Solms-Delta for sponsoring the wine; and the staff at Stanford Valley who helped make it happen without hitch, and happily.

REFERENCES

[1] Brown J, Isaacs D. The world café. Shaping our futures through conversations that matter. San Francisco: Berret-Koehler, 2005.

Submitted: May 01, 2011.
Revised: June 01, 2011.
Accepted: June 10, 2011.

In: Alternative Medicine Research Yearbook 2012
Editors: Søren Ventegodt and Joav Merrick

ISBN: 978-1-62808-080-3
© 2013 Nova Science Publishers, Inc.

Chapter 2

CONSCIOUSNESS AND MEDICINE FROM THE POINT OF VIEW OF A FAMILY PHYSICIAN

*Shadrick Mazaza, BSc, MB ChB, MFam MED (UCT), FCFP (SA)**

Oliver Tambo Fellowship Programme, Graduate School of Business,
University of Cape Town, Cape Town, South Africa

ABSTRACT

In this article I reflect on the medical paradigm. First with a historical review of conventional medicine, its perceived shortcomings and what current thoughts are regarding a new paradigm for health. I conclude with some thoughts on the role of family medicine on an emerging conceptual framework for health in South Africa.

Keywords: Medicine, integrative medicine, education

INTRODUCTION

"At this very hour, the world is seething with unrest in its search for not a specialist in this, that or the other, but a specialist in mankind as such, who views man as a combination of spirit, soul and body, and recognition that the interaction of the three is so close that they can never touch one without touching all three."
Alexander Cannon - The invisible influence.

For more than two decades, we have seen an increase in discourse on the state of western medicine in South Africa and throughout the world by academics and the general public. The increase in popularity of complementary and alternative medicine is often offered as evidence of the shortcomings of modern scientific medicine. Kolbe (1) wrote in the South African

---

* Correspondence: Shadrick Mazaza, Senior Lecturer, Oliver Tambo Fellowship Programme, Graduate School of Business, University of Cape Town, Cape Town, South Africa. E-mail: shadrick.mazaza@gsb.uct.ac.za.

Medical Journal an article, where he referred to a 1987 meeting of prominent physicians at Wickenburg, Arizona to discuss what the chairman of that conference, Kerr White, referred to as 'the profession's confused state'. The dialogue was that the teaching and practice of medicine were too narrowly scientific. The humanity of the patient could not be conceptualised within this restricted framework. Both the public and doctors were becoming disenchanted with Flexnerian medicine.

I participated in a recent "Forum for the changing health paradigm" and in this article, I reflect on the medical paradigm. I begin with a historical review of conventional medicine, its perceived shortcomings and what current thoughts are regarding a new paradigm for health. I conclude with some thoughts on the role of family medicine on an emerging conceptual framework for health in South Africa.

PARADIGM SHIFT

Discussion about a "changing paradigm" suggests a paradigm shift, a change from an existing paradigm to an emerging new paradigm. So what exactly do we mean by paradigm shift? Thomas Kuhn (2) described paradigm shift as a change in basic assumptions within the ruling theory of science. This scientific revolution, according to Kuhn, occurs when scientists encounter anomalies, which cannot be explained by the universally accepted paradigm within which scientific progress has hitherto been made. The paradigm, therefore, is not simply the current theory, but the entire worldview in which it exists, and all the implications which come with it.

Our modern biomedicine (biopsychosocial medicine, to be exact) is said to be based on Newtonian physics and it is from this that a new paradigm would shift. This is a paradigm of western cultural evolution.

A brief history of the western cultural world view

Elliott Dacher discussed a move towards a post modern medicine and reminds us of the historical forces that shaped the western cultural worldview (3). Westerners' cultural history can largely be traced to Hellenistic Greece. This was a meeting of the ancient mythological world with the emerging world of rational inquiry giving rise to an extraordinary culture that for a brief period of time sustained a precarious yet highly creative balance between sensory-based and intuitive knowledge – the outer and inner ways of knowing. Dacher goes on to say that the outer way investigating the world and attaining its knowledge through the sensory-based intellectual analysis of what is considered an "objective" pre-given world. In contrast, the inner way uses the first person investigative tools of reflection and meditation to uncover an experiential knowledge of the "lived world", the subjective experience. One of the most important achievements of Hellenistic Greece was the rise of Aesclepian medicine, an amalgam of the rudimentary elements of a scientific medicine interwoven with knowledge of the inner healing capacities.

Several centuries later this union of rational and intuitive knowledge was sundered apart with the rise of the monotheistic Christian mythos. Faith, scripture and external authority replaced rational inquiry and inner exploration as the primary route to knowledge, healing and health. Dacher reminds us of the fact that the rise of a monochromatic perspective in either personal psychology or cultural history always empowers its suppressed counter-balancing force that invariably re-emerges from the shadows, forcing the decline of the previously dominant perspective. This is the manner in which the Christian era and its emphasis on external authority eventually declined, giving way to the Copernican revolution and the modern era with its rational analytic exploration of the outer world, an extraordinary epoch which was to last 500 years and is only now beginning its decline as a dominant perspective. Initiated by Copernicus and completed by Kepler, Galileo and Descartes, this paradigm shift engaged the western world in a compensatory yet equally monotheistic worldview and with it the modern medical paradigm. Dacher suggests an expansion in our way of knowing or else our science and medicine will remain much the same, irrespective of efforts to change it through the addition of more therapies and remedies.

History of conventional (Flexnerian) medicine

Wikipedia (4) describes Flexnerian medicine as the era of modern medical practice that crystallized with the publication of the Flexner Report in 1910 (5). This report criticized the loose standards of medical education that existed in the United States in the 19th century. The report also advocated the establishment of standards that were more strict and better supported by science. The ensuing process led to the establishment of the American Medical Association and the success of conventional modern medicine. These developments however, flourished at the expense of other, discredited schools of medical treatment such as homeopathic medicine.

Thus, the medical profession as we know it today has only existed since the nineteenth century. Before that time, society was served by a variety of healers, only a small proportion of whom were physicians. In the seventeenth and eighteenth centuries, physicians were a small and elite group of learned men, educated in the few universities. They practised in towns among the rich and influential, did not perform surgery or dispense drugs, and did not associate, either professionally or socially, with the craftsmen and tradesmen who administered to the medical needs of poorer and rural people. Surgeons were craftsmen who were trained by apprenticeship; apothecaries were tradesmen, who originally dispensed and sold drugs but who, in response to need, gradually took on the role of medical practitioner. For a long time in America, the graduate physicians maintained their distinctiveness by refusing to practice surgery or dispense drugs. However, the heavy demand for services and the breakdown of old social barriers in the new colonies soon made these aspirations impossible to fulfil. Before long, all practitioners, whether graduates or not, were practising as general practitioners. Thus was the general practitioner born in the eighteenth century America.

In Britain, meanwhile, the same historical process was going on. By the beginning of the nineteenth century, the status of surgeons and apothecaries had risen substantially, and their work had become increasingly medical. Surgical training had been improved, and surgeons took the examination for membership in the Royal College of Surgeons (MRCS) after a combination of apprenticeship and hospital training. In 1815, the Apothecaries Act gave legal recognition to the right of apothecaries in Britain to give medical advice as well as to supply drugs. The act made it compulsory for apothecaries to undergo a five-year apprenticeship and to take courses in anatomy, physiology, the practice of medicine, and materia medica. It also established a qualifying examination, the Licentiate of the Society of Apothecaries (LSA). It soon became customary for practitioners to take the double qualification (LSA and MRCS), and, when an examination in midwifery was added, the graduate was qualified to practice medicine, surgery, and midwifery. The term General practitioner was first used in the Lancet early in the nineteenth century.

By a slow process of response to social demands, surgeons and apothecaries were gradually integrated with physicians to form the modern medical profession.

In Europe and North America, the nineteenth century was the age of the general practitioner. The first half of the twentieth century, however, saw the emergence of the major specialties of medicine. Medical education became increasingly oriented toward laboratory science and the technology of medicine.

DILEMMAS

The "crisis in medicine" that Kolbe (1) described was said to be caused by widespread patient dissatisfaction; doctor disillusionment; spiralling health costs and an outdated concept of disease. The Institute of Noetic Sciences published a collection of essays in a book titled "Consciousness and healing: Integral approach to mind-body medicine" (3) discussing the state of modern medicine and considering the creation of a new, integral perspective. Looking at this from the body-mind perspective, Wilber (6) discussed some of the dilemmas facing conventional medicine which include: doctors being taught not to get involved emotionally with their patients; the "Cartesian dualism" of treating patients as just a body and a machine; patients' non-compliance with what is prescribed to them by doctors and the illusive location of "illness" in the body-mind continuum.

The rising popularity of alternative and complementary therapies (CAM) were discussed and the general view was that in spite legislation to promote CAM and the acceptance of various Universities in the United States to teach complementary medicine, this has had very little impact on the challenges facing medicine. The rise of integrative medicine has largely meant an increase in the tools in the doctor's bag, but has done very little to bring about fundamental change. What is being proposed is a move beyond integrative medicine to what is described as "integral medicine".

INTEGRAL MEDICINE

Wilber (6) puts it thus: "The crucial ingredient in any integral medical practice is not the integral medical bag itself – with all the conventional pills, the orthodox surgery, subtle energy medicine and acupuncture needles- but the holder of that bag". He writes about "integrally informed health-care practitioners" who have opened themselves to an entire spectrum of consciousness. Integral medicine acknowledges the full spectrum of consciousness – body, mind, soul and spirit – and to understand what this means, Ken Wilber's four quadrant model is a useful tool (6).

Wilber's model is a model of evolution of consciousness based on about a dozen principles that guide evolution – orienting generalisations (3). The essence of the model is that there are four dimensions to our human experiences which are Interior subjective and exterior objective for the individual and the collective (see figure 1). Thus the four quadrants are subjective, inter-subjective, objective and inter-objective (see figures 2). In this model it can be seen that scientific modern medicine has reduced the human being to right upper quadrant (objective) domain. An integrally informed medical practitioner is one who is aware of these dimensions of being and consciousness. Consciousness expressed in self, culture and nature. An integral medicine framework integrates subjective and objective, synopsis and synthesis. This post-modern medicine would transcend and include the current scientific medical model and would be neither conventional nor alternative. It would be holistic in that it would include all human dimensions and would accommodate different healing modalities. Perhaps the most important aspect of this model is that the emphasis is on the transformation of the medical practitioner calling for personal transformation of practitioners to become integrally aware doctors.

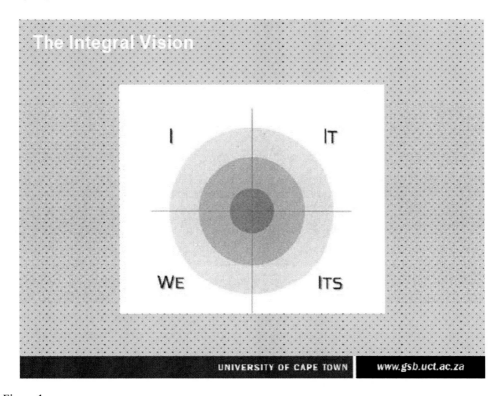

Figure 1.

THE ROLE OF FAMILY MEDICINE

The discipline of family medicine evolved upon the realization that medical graduates left medical schools full of patho-physiology and tools to "fix" diseases. The patient as a whole human being tended to get lost in the process and for doctors entering general practice, it was important to bring the patient back. Central to the discipline of family medicine is the doctor-patient interaction and its therapeutic value. The American Academy of Family Physicians have the slogan: "Doctors who specialise in you" which sums up what the discipline focuses on – whole person and not the body parts other specialist disciplines focus on.

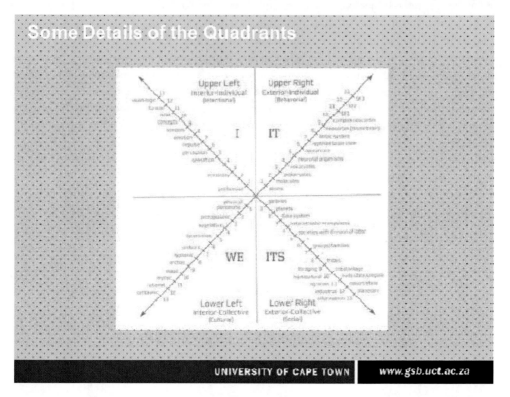

Figure 2.

The three stage assessment in family medicine (compatible with the Wilber model) is clinical, personal and contextual. The clinical diagnosis is an upper right quadrant objective diagnosis of disease; the personal is left lower quadrant cultural aspect while the personal is the left upper quadrant of subjective aspect of health. Family medicine is, therefore the natural home of an emerging integral medicine. The Integral model integrates and transcends the family medicine model. What is required is to introduce consciousness and personal transformation in the training of family physicians to make them integrally aware clinicians. The discipline would also seek to be informed of the essence of African traditional medicine and how the indigenous knowledge can be integrated in the practice of family medicine (7).

CONCLUSION

As the modern cultural paradigm of medicine began to show some serious strains, integrative medicine began to gain popularity, but this has largely emerged as competition to conventional medicine (and more tools in the bag) and has had little impact on the challenges facing modern healthcare. A shift towards an Integral medicine is being suggested which is neither conventional nor alternative but transcending both. This model promises to integrate subjective and objective; body and mind; conventional and alternative; private and public health; ancient and modern wisdom. It is built on consciousness and transformation of medical practitioners producing integrally aware medical practitioners (no one is smart enough to be wrong all the time). Schlitz (3) said: "Integral medicine promotes an approach embedded in the scientific dimension that epitomises the best in modern health care, while equally recognizing that human beings possess emotional, spiritual and relational dimensions that are essential in the diagnosis and treatment of disease and the cultivation of wellness". The approaches would be rigorous in standards of evidence and efficacy. Family medicine is the natural midwife of an emerging integral medicine.

REFERENCES

[1] Kolbe RJ. The crisis in medicine. A response. S Afr Med J 1996;86: 234-5.
[2] Kuhn T. The structure of scientific revolutions. Chicago, IL: Univerty Chicago Press, 1970.
[3] Schlitz MM, Amorok T, Micozzi M, eds. Consciousness and healing. Integral approaches to mind-body medicine. St Louis, MO: Elsevier, 2005.
[4] http://en.wikipedia.org/wiki/Flexnerian-medicine.
[5] Flexner A. Medical education in the United States and Canada. Stanford, CA: Carnegie Foundation Higher Education, 1910.
[6] Wilber K. A theory of everything. Dublin: Gateway, 2000.
[7] Mazaza S. Urban African traditional healers. Germany: Lambert Acad Publ, 2009.

Submitted: May 01, 2011.
Revised: June 15, 2011.
Accepted: June 24, 2011.

In: Alternative Medicine Research Yearbook 2012   ISBN: 978-1-62808-080-3
Editors: Søren Ventegodt and Joav Merrick   © 2013 Nova Science Publishers, Inc.

Chapter 3

CHANGING THE MEDICAL PARADIGM: WHAT DOES DISEASE LOOK LIKE WHEN WE SHIFT OUR VIEW?

Bernard Brom, MB ChB (UCT), CEDH (France) and Dip Acup[*]
Private practice, Dennesig, Stellenbosch, South Africa

ABSTRACT

Modern medical science tends to be equated with the philosophy of reductionism. Reductionism is the belief that complex data can be reduced to seemingly equivalent simple ones. Only phenomena that can be measured and quantified are of any importance. Any theory is a limited understanding. It is now clear that science cannot know absolute truth and therefore what is known is not true, only a theory about possibilities. It is really useful to know this because it will allow a constantly creative approach to the problem that each person presents with. Life itself is too big for the human mind to encompass and comprehend in its entirety. Integrative medicine is an attempt to combine both the reductionistic and holistic approach so that a better working relationship can exist between the doctor and the patient. It means being open-minded to outcomes, to the needs of the patient and to the dictum "do no harm". The incidence of iatrogenic disease (doctor induced disease) needs to be addressed and can no longer be ignored. Practitioners need to know the parts and how they function together, creating a unique body-mind profile; they need to know the techniques available for supporting health and how to respond in a creative way to these possibilities. Only then can the art and science of medicine, the Yin and the Yang which were never separate, participate in a creative dance and allow the new paradigm of medicine to emerge.

Keywords: Medicine, integrative medicine, alternative medicine

---

[*] Correspondence: Bernard Brom, MB ChB (UCT), CEDH (France), Dip Acup, POBox 2229, Dennesig, Stellenbosch, 7601 South Africa. E-mail: bernard@creatinghealth.co.za.

INTRODUCTION

"A major challenge for medicine in the 21st century will be to move toward a thorough understanding of physiological mechanisms that underlie disease rather than simply labelling later-stage effects with the names of diseases"

Jones and Bland (1)

Wanting to change the medical paradigm suggests that perhaps there is something wrong with the present way of practising medicine. At the same time many believe that if the present approach is only inadequate, all that is required is better diagnostic equipment and techniques, better drugs and less invasive surgery, more science and more evidence based medicine (EBM), and that we are indeed well on the way to getting there. That is not, however, what we mean.

EBM is in fact the end of the old paradigm and on its own will not resolve the dilemma of ill health or help to create a new era of health and quality of life. The guardians of the conventional paradigm as indicated by Thomas Kuhn will resist this change and defend their viewpoint. There is a consensus amongst many practitioners around the world that a very fundamental shift in focus needs to happen, and more of the same won't be enough to meet the needs of an aging population in the developed world, on one hand, and diseases of poverty in the developing world. Both require better health and not just better treatment of disease.

In this article I will address some of these issues and hopefully point the way forward to a more inclusive, holistic and creative medicine.

A short history of modern medicine

The notion of an organic, living, and spiritual universe was replaced by that of the world as a machine, and the world-machine became the dominant metaphor of the modern world (2).

Modern medical science tends to be equated with the philosophy of reductionism. Reductionism is the belief that complex data can be reduced to seemingly equivalent simple ones. Only phenomena that can be measured and quantified are of any importance. Galileo, Descartes and Newton come to mind. "Galileo's programme offers us a dead world: Out go sight, sound, taste, touch and smell, and along with them have since gone aesthetic and ethical sensibility, values, quality, soul, consciousness, spirit. Experience as such is cast out of the realm of scientific discourse. Hardly anything has changed our world more during the past four hundred years than Galileo's audacious programme," said RD Laing (3).

What the programmes of these men offered was a way of reducing the complexity of biological systems and life into easy, byte-size pieces that could be handled and measured. This simplistic scientific model, which was able to send astronauts to the moon, was applied increasingly to biology, reducing the laws of biology to those of physics and chemistry.

This was the phase of the domination of Order (logic, thought, math, science, measurement) over Change (art, creativity, right brain) and the French physicist Pierre Laplace would state that scientists would one day derive a mathematical equation so powerful that it would explain everything, a universal field theory of everything.

Clearly this approach has led to astonishing advances in physiology, biochemistry, pharmacology and surgery, and yet chronic disease has continued to increase, and the complex nature of biological organisms remains an enigma.

Nevertheless the development of cell theory, modern embryology, the increasing sophistication of microbiology and the development of the microscope continue to fuel the idea that this direction is where the future of medicine still lies.

The confounding truth is that this seems only partially true, and with each new discovery more questions than answers become obvious. Jan Smuts, the Prime Minister of South Africa from 1919 to 1924, with astonishing insightfulness in his book on Holism, pointed out that "In its analytic pursuit of parts, science has missed the whole, and thus tended to reduce the world to dead aggregations rather than to the real wholes which make up nature" (4). William Blake, a passionate critic of Isaac Newton proclaimed: "May God us keep us from single vision and Newton's sleep" (5).

Reductionism is based on the assumption that all apparently chaotic systems have an underlying order which just requires time to uncover, and that is the role of science. What the new science of quantum mechanics has shown is that this will never be possible, that living systems are non-linear and function far from equilibrium, and this makes possible the enormous breadth of creativity and change that is obvious all around us. Both Order and Change are the two dynamics of living systems allowing for homeostasis and creativity.

PARADIGMS

One aim of the physical sciences has been to give an exact picture of the material world. One achievement of physics in the twentieth century has been to prove that that aim is unattainable.

What is a paradigm? Thomas Kuhn in 1962 (6) defined a paradigm as "a constellation of achievements, concepts, values, techniques etc – shared by scientific communities and used by that community to define legitimate problems and solutions."

The conventional paradigm as it has developed over the last 200 years has defined itself more and more by a rigid scientific approach. This is especially true in the medical and biological sciences. There are a number of characteristics which define this approach in medicine:

- Emphasis on scientific investigation
- Focus on control of symptoms
- Treating end points, which are defined as "the disease"
- Belief in biochemical sameness. Normal individuals are all normal and therefore similar. Parkinson's patients, for example, have the same problem and disease development.
- Linear causation. A relatively straight arrow from the cause to its end point.
- Human beings are basically anatomy and biochemistry. All the rest, such as energy, emotions, mind and consciousness, are epiphenomena.
- Use of toxic drugs, anatomy, radiotherapy and other invasive approaches to treat the disease.

This approach is best exemplified by the evidence based medicine model (EBM) which now dominates conventional medical thinking. There is even the idea that EBM is the new paradigm and that modern medicine has been moving slowly towards this ideal. The goal of this approach is to have all diseases easily identifiable according to rigid criteria and management approaches narrowed down to practical and workable solutions, which would make it easy for medical aids, governments and national health schemes to manage according to various schemes worked out by these bodies.

According to Kuhn (6), paradigms are "universally acknowledged scientific achievements which, for some period of time, provide model problems and solutions for a community of practitioners of a given science". During this period of scientific development, which he called "normal science", scientists are occupied with solving problems based on what is understood within that paradigm, and tend to ignore exceptions and incongruities that may come up in their investigations as aberrations and chance only.

Kuhn (6) understood that paradigms were not eternal and that slowly more and more exceptions and anomalies would became so obvious that they could no longer be ignored.

Normal science soon becomes disorientated, and when this occurs, that is, when members of a profession can no longer avoid the anomalies that subvert existing tradition in scientific practice, extraordinary investigations begin that finally leads the profession to a new set of commitments, a new basis for the practice of science (6).

According to Ken Wilber (7) most scientists misunderstand Kuhn's description of paradigms, because he described any novel experiment that actually produced new data as a revolution or "new paradigm". I don't wish to argue with his definition but suggest that the way I understand a "new paradigm" is something much deeper and more complex. The shift is not just new ideas which expand the known, or new inventions or experiments which enlarge what one already knows, but a more fundamental change in the way we understand the world. Something much more akin to the "Big Bang", or what happens when a mixture suddenly turns into a compound, or that eureka moment when there is a sudden intuitive breakthrough, and the problem is seen in a completely different light.

In a mixture each ingredient still has its own fundamental properties and is moving towards its own unique activity and goals. In a compound each ingredient gives up its own identity and combines with the other ingredients to create a novel compound with new properties and goals.

In a similar way the eureka moment re-defines the way one understands something and frees the person to pursue his goals in a new and creative direction.

A paradigm shift is a fundamental change in the way one models reality and occurs because of a shift in consciousness.

SIGNPOSTS OF THE NEW PARADIGM

The "old" paradigm can be labelled as mechanistic, reductionistic, linear and logical. These are all left-brain ideas and concepts and exclude imagination, intuition, art.

What has happened, using our old model, is that logic and the intellectual application of left-brain thinking has become dominant and moved towards greater and greater rigidity and a more narrow view of disease. In the changing and emerging paradigm there is the recognition of the limits of this viewpoint, and the emerging of a more right brain, intuitive and creative approach to health and ill-health. This is manifesting in the following way: a human rights discourse; patient dissatisfaction with the mechanistic approach to disease; the idea that humans are more than body; patient-centred medicine, a multi-causal, multi-layered approach to underlying causes, complexity and unpredictability.

The language of the new paradigm is interesting and gives some insight regarding the shifting ways of thinking about health and disease:

Table 1. Language of the new paradigm regarding the shifting ways of thinking about health and disease

New Paradigm	Old Paradigm
Systems	Parts
Webs	Isolated functions
Non-linear dynamics	Linear dynamics
Energy	Matter
Fields	Points
Information transfer	Chemical processes
Patterns	Units
Probability dynamics	End Points
Sacred geometry	Classical Geometry
Complexity	Simplicity
Meaning and purpose	No meaning or purpose
Self organization	Genetic immutability
Turbulence order and chaos	Disease
Art of medicine	Science of medicine
Intuition	Logic
Experience	Experiment
Potential within the system	Genetic immutability
Holism	Reductionism
Integrative model	Conventional model
Epigenetics and Nutrogenomics	Genetic immutability
Quality	Quantity
New metaphors	Conventional metaphors
Subtle information	Chemical processes
Listening and feeling	Impersonal
Physician know thyself	Physician separate from process
Multi-causal	Single cause

It is clear from a perusal of the above table that the left column represents a much more creative, open-ended, personal and holistic kind of medicine, a medicine that seeks for meaning and patterns and recognises that there is a bigger picture and other dynamics at play; that there are known and unknown processes and the physician is important in the process, linking the hidden potential within the whole (known and unknown) to the present condition of the patient. The meaning and purpose of the illness are important to the client.

The conventional model expects the doctor to be impersonal, to deal with the parts that are broken and mend them in the best scientific way possible. Everything is out there to be measured, and what can't be measured is unimportant when a person is ill and wants symptomatic improvement. Meaning and purpose are of no special interest to the doctor who regards it as a waste of valuable time within the consultation process.

THE INTEGRATIVE MODEL

The scientific/EBM model continues to insist that human beings are physical objects that can be measured. If measuring of any part of the system is not possible (consciousness, soul, spirit etc), then generally this fact is ignored as having any influence on the way the system functions and becomes dysfunctional. It is possible, however that what can't be measured is intrinsic to the health of the system and that there may always be limits to what can be known (8). Quantum science has already explored the limitations to measuring the quantum potential, the fact that it is not possible to measure both the wave and particle properties of light at the same time, and that in any chaotic process it is not possible to know in which direction it will move or when order may suddenly emerge. Spontaneous remissions of cancer are an example of a shift from disorder or chaos back to a new order or health.

It is for this reason that prediction in living systems becomes impossible. Human beings are complex systems which are living and dying at the same time. Complex systems cannot be broken down into more simple "orderly" bits and pieces without losing something very intrinsic to the function of the whole. It is by excluding these confounding aspects that the conventional model of medicine slowly becomes more restrictive and limited in its ability to heal, and ends up treating disease.

Exceptions, anomalies and unique presentations to the conventional model are excluded and the integrative process discouraged. Mavericks, dissidents and independent thinkers are excluded from the conversation and their articles and viewpoints limited to their own independent journals. Spontaneous remission of disease, the placebo effect and independent and original healing techniques are not further investigated in a creative and open-minded way.

At the same time most medical scientists are aware that very little is known about the nature of consciousness, about the way that the electromagnetic recordings easily measured over the body can affect physiological functions, how thought can influence the body, and if people are believers in a higher being such as a God, how this could also influence the direction of matter, energy and information transfer. All this is excluded from the conventional model, which limits itself to what can be measured, and this despite the enormous limitations in this approach. While experience may be acknowledged as a valid way of learning, very little insight into what this is, how it functions and how the traditional healers, for example, acquire their knowledge and experience is pursued. Medical journals confine themselves to the scientific investigation of matter and assume that there is logic in this process, when the placebo effect, which is always lurking in the background, is itself an enigma. Comparing a drug to an enigma is not scientific and will always confuse results.

BIOCHEMICAL INDIVIDUALITY

No two individuals are alike. Even identical twins will have some characteristics that are different, and this may be most obvious at the level of chemistry, where blood characteristics such as individual chemicals (sodium, potassium, vitamin D levels, uric acid etc) will not match. They may be within "normal" limits but not the same. Not surprisingly, therefore, each person will respond or react in a unique way, and when they become ill will again respond to management and drugs in their unique way again. For this reason there are many drugs on the market to cater for these individual biochemical responses. This means that each person requires an individual management profile, and uniform approaches will not work for everyone.

Systems, not parts

Human beings are functioning systems, not parts strung together. There is a continual and dynamic flux of information through living organisms resulting in matter appearing and dissolving. There is growth, development and evolution in a continuous cycle or spiral of change. This is very unlike a machine made of parts, where each part is separate and functions in its own contained way. Living systems are self-organising webs or networks of activity interacting with the surrounding space. Fritjof Capra calls this "new synthesis" of understanding living systems as their "pattern of organisation". Identifying these "patterns" may help co-ordinate treatment approaches better than diagnostic labels (9).

Holons, holograms, wholes

The idea of parts strung together also tends to create the idea that causes lead to effects in some linear sequential way, and in theory therefore one should be able to trace backwards the end point, or disease, to its origins. This has not happened and tracing disease backwards within the complexity of the system is not possible. It is also not possible to even trace the cause of a crack in a wall to its origins. There are too many variables and interactions in biological systems, preventing any accurate assessment of causes.

While each of the above expressions (holons, holograms, wholes) may have slightly different meanings, they do refer to the idea that nothing in nature can really be seen in isolation. All natural systems are open systems connecting and interacting with other systems in a meaningful way. Each whole system is really a part within a greater whole defined by Arthur Koestler as a holon (whole/part). What becomes obvious is that trying to define a linear causation to any condition within living systems is impossible. There are so many points of activity weaving themselves through such systems within systems, on so many levels of activity and dimensions, that trying to identify the cause or causes of the specific illness in each person is not possible. It also could mean that in any specific disease such as cancer or Parkinson's disease the underlying causes are not the same in each group of diseases despite the similar end point. End points, or diseases, are merely the final destination as it were of a chain of events in a dynamic holon which is trying to maintain its integrity.

Ken Wilber suggested that there is a "profound tension" within that holon in order for it to exist and have its own identity, while at the same time participating in and being part of the surrounding space (10).

Upward and downward causation

The idea of upward and downward causation brings in the concepts of levels, or hierarchies.

> "It is often said that physicists invented the mechanistic-reductionistic philosophy, taught it to the biologists, and then abandoned it themselves. It cannot be denied that modern physics has a strongly holistic, even teleological flavour, and that this is due in part to the influence of quantum theory"
>
> Physicist Paul Davies (11).

Much of medical research is driven by funding by pharmaceutical companies with the main concern being the biochemistry of the body. Anything other than biochemistry is regarded as an epiphenomenon, despite the lack of evidence for this. Electrical recordings such as the ECG and EEG are of interest only as diagnostic or research tools. The complex electromagnetic wave of the heart passes through every cell of the body, yet possible effects of this electromagnetic activity on the body's biochemistry seems to be of little interest.

Conventional medical science tends to confine its research to the body as a physical structure which can be separated into parts, and chemistry which can be manipulated to relieve symptoms. There is little research into the electromagnetic fields which are everywhere within the body, and even extending out of the body and other electromagnetic fields into the surrounding space.

Electromagnetic fields carry information and physicists understand something of the relationship between matter, energy and information.

Ken Wilber refers to this idea as the "The great chain of being" (12) recognised by all the great wisdom traditions. "Reality is a rich tapestry of interwoven levels, reaching from matter to body to mind to soul to spirit. Each senior level 'envelops' or 'enfolds' its junior dimensions – a series of nests within nests within nests of Being, so that everything and event in the world is interwoven with every other, and all are ultimately enveloped and enfolded by Spirit, by God, by Goddess, by Tao, by Brahman, by the Absolute itself."

Body-emotions-mind-spirit or matter-energy-information-consciousness can be seen as finer or deeper levels or hierarchies, connecting and enfolding lower levels. Searching for electricity with chemical tools will not work, and looking for information with electrical tools won't work either. It is for this reason that trying to identify the nature of experience with tools that do not belong to that dimension will not ultimately resolve the problem of the nature of experience. The only tools that will work will be tools which belong to that dimension, which are the mechanisms within the human mind and consciousness where the experience is recorded.

EXPERIENCE, AWARENESS AND CONSCIOUSNESS

These are all very broad categories and this is not the place to define and tease them out. Nevertheless experience, awareness and consciousness are qualities which are identifiable even if they are not scientifically measurable in the same way that the objective world can be measured. The Integrative model acknowledges these qualities, encourages the development and refinement of experience, the enlargement of awareness beyond a self-centred view of the world and a greater understanding of consciousness.

> "Some scientists have been inclined to think that the psychological phenomena could ultimately be explained on the basis of physics and chemistry of the brain. From the quantum-theoretical point of view, there is no reason for such an assumption"
>
> Heisenberg (13)

Awareness, experience and the application of consciousness have been the way all traditional people have acquired their skills, and the way even babies and young children learn. Scientists, and in fact most medical professionals, use mind, intuition, feeling in their investigations and contact with patients, yet never mention this in their articles or discussion with peers.

BRINGING IT ALL TOGETHER

For the new integrative medicine to evolve and emerge the following ideas should be kept in mind:

- There are clear limits to what science can measure, and what is already known is a very small part of the whole.
- Experience and experiment should be given equal status and not kept separate. Medical journals should allow medical scientists to give their viewpoints and experiences, provided these are clearly explained and differentiated from the reductionistic measuring process. Experience, reflection, intuition and awareness are valid forms of investigation and need to be shared with other scientists from many fields of science.
- Each person is unique in every way; physically, chemically, energetically and spiritually.
- Human beings are conscious beings and Mind can clearly influence body, either directly or by calling up emotions.
- Integrative medicine as it is emerging at the moment has the following important criteria which define its philosophy:
- The human being is a multidimensional system. Parts and Wholes are two equally valid views of the system, depending on what is required. Nevertheless, it is as advantageous for the surgeon to recognise that he is dealing with a complex human being as it is essential that he knows his anatomy and surgical techniques.

- The multidimensional aspects must be investigated at the same level at which they are operating. The study of biochemistry is inadequate to understand emotions, mind and consciousness! Nevertheless it should be understood that the lower levels also do reflect what is happening at the higher levels. Body language is one way we gain information about the person's emotional state, but deeper insight requires physicists and engineers to become involved in measuring the dimensions of electromagnetism and information.
- There are no single causes for ill health. The human body/mind/spirit/ consciousness system and matter/electromagnetic/informational system have many points of stress which impact on the system as a whole. How the system deals with the stress will affect the outcome and the nature of the physical symptoms and the eventual disease. This means that while the end point may be diagnosed as Parkinson's disease, the underlying causes could be different in each person, and do not follow a linear progression, which also means that outcomes are not predictable.
- The system functions as a whole so that any change in one part is immediately recorded and recognised by the whole system.
- "Thus the whole system moves together and what is done to one particle is instantaneously registered by a change in the whole system, thus affecting the other particle" (14). This quantum understanding is referred to as Bell's Theorem. Systems theorist Peter Senge describes systems thinking as "a discipline for seeing wholes. It is a framework for seeing interrelationships rather than things, for seeing patterns of change rather than static snapshots" (15)
- The system is intelligent at the level of its control systems. Exactly where these control systems are has not been elucidated. Nevertheless it can be predicted that the higher dimensions or levels have a controlling influence over lower levels. Anatomy is controlled by biochemistry which is controlled by electromagnetic fields which are controlled by the informational circuits which are controlled by consciousness. Each level is more refined and more subtle and less easily subjected to reductionistic research approaches.
- Ill-health in the system has its origins in all levels. Chemical pollution has powerful toxic effects on the chemical level, cellphones disturb the electromagnetic level, ideas both positive and negative may influence the informational level. Thus ill-health is multi-causal and multi-level.
- The intelligence for healing is vested in the system as a whole. Health is an innate intelligence within the system. The systems move into illness only when equilibrium of all systems can no longer be maintained without producing symptoms and signs. Symptoms and signs are not the disease, but evidence of a system malfunctioning. Giving names of diseases to symptoms and signs misses the point and deflects management away from the dysfunctional system towards the symptoms and signs which have been designated the name of a disease.
- Science is an attempt to free the practitioner from uncertainty by reducing the whole to byte-size pieces. The limits of this approach now and in the future should be clearly recognised by medical scientists, as it is by physicists and other scientists. The real world is full of uncertainties, interrelationships and mutual dependencies that pervade all of nature. It is dynamic and constantly slips past any scientific

investigation. As Bertrand Russell said: "Physics is mathematical not because we know much about the physical world, but because we know so little: it is only its mathematical properties that we can discover" (16). Mathematics cannot represent the fullness and beauty of a rose or the expression of joy in a mother on seeing her baby for the first time.

CONCLUSION

Any theory is a limited understanding. It is now clear that science cannot know absolute truth and therefore what is known is not true, only a theory about possibilities. It is really useful to know this because it will allow a constantly creative approach to the problem that each person presents with. Any description of reality is not strictly about reality, but only a description which may work or not work depending on the circumstances which themselves are in a process of change. Reductionism in medicine is about attempting to reduce complexity to simple bytes which can be measured, and attempts made to control parts of the system with drugs or surgery. Reductionism is only one way of seeing the world, and gives a particular viewpoint.

Holism is another way of dealing with ill-health. Life itself is too big for the human mind to encompass and comprehend in its entirety. Integrative medicine is an attempt to combine both the reductionistic and holistic approach so that a better working relationship can exist between the doctor and the patient. It means being open-minded to outcomes, to the needs of the patient and to the dictum "do no harm". The incidence of iatrogenic disease (doctor induced disease) needs to be addressed and can no longer be ignored. Practitioners need to know the parts and how they function together, creating a unique body-mind profile; they need to know the techniques available for supporting health and how to respond in a creative way to these possibilities. Only then can the art and science of medicine, the Yin and the Yang which were never separate, participate in a creative dance and allow the new paradigm of medicine to emerge.

REFERENCES

[1]   Jones D, Bland J. Textbook of functional medicine. Introduction to functional medicine. Gig Harbor, WA: Inst Funct Med, 2006.

[2]   Capra F, ed. The web of life. A new synthesis of mind and matter. London: Harper Collins, 1996:19.

[3]   Laing RD. Uncommon wisdom. In: Capra F, ed. The web of life. A new synthesis of mind and matter. London: Harper Collins, 1996:139.

[4]   Smuts JC. Holism and evolution. Cape Town: NandS Press, 1987.

[5]   Blake W. Letter to Thomas Butts, 22 November 1802. In: Ostriker A, ed. William Blake: The complete poems. New York: Penguin, 1977.

[6]   Kuhn T. The structure of scientific revolutions. Chicago, IL: University Chicago Press, 1962.

[7]   Wilber K. The marriage of sense and soul. Integrating science and religion. New York: Random House, 1998.

[8]   Brom B. The limits of medical science. S Afr Med J 2005;95(1):35-8.

[9]   Capra F, ed. The web of life. A new synthesis of mind and matter. London: Harper Collins, 1996:153.

[10] Wilber K. The marriage of sense and soul. Integrating science and religion. New York: Random House, 1998:68.
[11] Davies P. The cosmic blueprint: New discoveries in nature's creative ability to order the universe. New York: Simon Schuster, 1988:165.
[12] Wilber K. The marriage of sense and soul. Integrating science and religion. New York: Random House, 1998:6-7.
[13] Heisenberg W. Physics and philosophy: The evolution in modern science. New York: Harper Row, 1958:106.
[14] Briggs J, Peat FD. Turbulent mirror. New York: Harper Row, 1990:184.
[15] Senge P. The fifth discipline. New York: Currency/Doubleday, 1990.
[16] Barrow J. The world within the world. New York: Oxford University Press, 1998:279.

Submitted: May 01, 2011.
Revised: June 15, 2011.
Accepted: June 24, 2011.

In: Alternative Medicine Research Yearbook 2012
Editors: Søren Ventegodt and Joav Merrick

ISBN: 978-1-62808-080-3
© 2013 Nova Science Publishers, Inc.

Chapter 4

DIMENSIONS OF HEALTH CARE AND THE BIOMATRIX

György Járos, MSc, PhD[*]

Independent Professional Training and Coaching and Faculty of Health Sciences and
Medicine, Bond University, Queensland, Australia

ABSTRACT

Health is much more complex than simply the absence of physical dysfunction. Caring
for it means much more than prescribing drugs or cutting out malfunctioning body parts.
Humans are sophisticated bio-psycho-social beings, whose bodies cannot be separated
from their inner feelings and outer connections to their total environment. Health Care
must start with caring and only end with curing. Unfortunately, the latter seems to be the
major, if not the only, preoccupation of the health care profession today. Health
promotion should take centre stage and should make use of the fantastic healing potential
in the human organism that ensured that we are still here in a dominant position after the
tribulations of the millions of years of our existence on this planet. The biomatrix
approach was developed at the University of Cape Town in South Africa during the
1980s for the study of complex living systems. It looks at life on earth as composed of
many levels that stretch from the atomic to the universal. It studies the processes that
connect these levels as well as those that take place within the levels. It also looks at the
contributors to the processes, as well as the way the various factors, such as technology,
economics, politics and culture affect the processes. The biomatrix approach is eminently
suitable to provide a framework within which the complex questions of health care could
be studied.

Keywords: Health care, biomatrix

---

[*] Correspondence: György Járos, PhD, Faculty of Health Sciences and Medicine, Bond University QLD 4229,
Australia. E-mail: gjaros@bigpond.com and gjaros@bond.edu.au.

INTRODUCTION

> We are one with Nature: her genetic fibres run through all our being; our physical organs connect us with millions of years of her history; our minds are full of immemorial paths of pre-human existence
>
> Jan Smuts (1)

In 2010 it was my privilege to attend a small group of practitioners from the mainstream and alternative health care professions in Stanford, South Africa. Our brief was to think creatively and to talk about a new paradigm in medicine that would integrate the different facets of health care into a cohesive whole. In an atmosphere of uninhibited and caring openness, each of the participants expressed his or her vision of such new health care. The purpose of the series of papers in this specil issue was to formalise each participant's original vision in light of the conversations that took place in the Stanford meeting.

My personal vision was the creation of an integrated model of health care that would bring together all dimensions of health care into a unifying framework, which could easily be understood by all concerned and which could act as a cohesive force for future developments in health care. The framework I had in mind was the biomatrix approach to complex multilevel problems in living systems (2) that a group of researchers under my leadership developed at the University of Cape Town about 25 years ago. The aim of this article is to introduce the principles of the biomatrix approach and to apply them to questions of health and disease with a special focus on integration.

Before proceeding with our task, it is necessary to define what health care and its dimensions mean. In the minds of many people "health care" is synonymous with "medicine" and when politicians allocate funds to health care, they mean building of hospitals and educating doctors and nurses. Obviously, health care is much more than the above perception would suggest: it has many dimensions that are concerned with levels of life where health care takes place, processes that are performed in the pursuit of health, contributors to the processes of health care, evidence that underlies our understanding of health and disease, treatment and technology that are applied within its processes, politics and economics that influence health care decisions and culture that determines how people think about health. There are possibly other dimensions, which we shall not be addressing in this paper. In a truly integrated health care model, all these dimensions, as well as the factors that contribute to them, should be considered.

In this paper, we shall discuss briefly the first three of the above dimensions, namely, levels, processes and contributors. This will be followed by a short summary of the relevant principles of the biomatrix approach with a few examples about the way it may be used for the integration of the various dimensions into a greater whole.

THREE DIMENSIONS OF HEALTH CARE

By dimensions we mean those considerations that can be subdivided into a whole spectrum of inter-related aspects. Thus, the dimension of levels refers to the existence of several interacting levels as part of the totality of life on earth, and tells us where we focus our efforts. The dimension of processes acknowledges the existence of the multitude of processes that interconnect these levels and defines what we do and should do. The dimension of contributors takes into consideration the different people, groups of people and organisations that contribute or have the potential to contribute to health care. Apart from these dimensions, there are others, some of which we have identified, but will not elaborate upon.

The dimension of levels

In 1948, as the world was recovering from the ravages of the Second World War with all the problems of injury, disease, disability, personal psychological trauma and social harm that accompany such a calamity, it became clear that health is much wider concept than just a lack of physical disturbance to the molecules and structures that make up the human body.

The United Nations (UN) was set up to prevent disasters like world wars in the future, and one of its constituent bodies, the World Health Organisation (WHO) was given the mandate to improve the state of health of the world. The WHO started off by redefining health "as a state of complete physical, mental and social well-being, and not merely the absence of disease or infirmity" (3).

It was to ensure that such complete health is achieved for every human being in the world within the foreseeable future. Both the UN and the WHO have failed in their mandate. Although there have been no world wars since 1945, one cannot describe the world as being peaceful either. Clearly, the UN has failed to secure a peaceful world, just as the WHO failed in creating a healthy one.

The above-named physical, mental and social aspects of health refer to the various levels of life of relevance to human beings. The physical level (also called the biological level) refers to the things that constitute our bodies and the processes that take place in them. The mental (also called the psychological level) level refers to the human being as an individual as it functions in the world. The social level looks at relationships between individuals as they form groups, communities, nations and eventually the world community. We all live in all three of these levels simultaneously: we are multi-leveled, bio-psycho-social beings. The physical, mental and social aspects of our being cannot be separated from one another. Indeed, they greatly influence one another, and as a consequence they cannot be treated separately from one another.

It is, therefore, unfortunate that the main players in health care, the medical and allied professions, still overwhelmingly concentrate on physical disease, on damage done to the structures of the body, i.e. organs, tissues, cells and molecules.

Although some lip service is being paid to the psychological and social aspects of disease, these are considered as being additional to, rather than integral within health care. Medical students, mostly very reluctantly, learn a minimum amount about psychology and sociology, and patients are often referred to psychologists and social workers. Although it is increasingly acknowledged that psychological and social stress play a role in the development of many physical diseases, they are only considered as aggravating factors rather than one of the many causative factors that can lead to disease.

In my opinion, this problem will not be solved until we realise that the bio-psycho-social aspects are simply levels of an inseparable whole.

The interaction between them may be much more important than presently realised. Whether these aspects should be included in any health care action or not is not disputed.

36 *György Járos*

What needs further investigation are the interactions between these aspects, and the way these interactions can contribute to the maintenance of health as well as to the prevention and treatment of disease.

To enable such investigation, we need a framework in which the inter-relationship between the biological, psychological and social levels can be examined.

The dimension of processes

Health care processes relate to the things we do to care for health. According to its name, the very first thing we should be doing is caring for, viz, cherishing, enhancing and promoting health. Surely, this must be the primary function of healthcare professionals, if they are to deserve that name. Only if they fail in their caring function and disease still threatens, must they prevent it from causing havoc. If they fail in this as well and people get ill, then they should remedy this failure by curing the resulting disease. And, if they fail in that too, they should at least alleviate pain and manage its symptoms in a humane way. If they succeed in curing a biological disease, their job is still not finished, as they should still psychologically rehabilitate and socially reintegrate the person into mainstream life before they can claim to be involved in a health-related activity. Thus the main processes of broader health care are:

1. Health Promotion
2. Disease Prevention
3. Disease Cure
4. Disease Management
5. Psychological Rehabilitation and
6. Social Reintegration

Caring for health should be a proactive process that enhances the health status of individuals. Of the processes mentioned above, only one, viz, health promotion, is proactive. All the other processes are reactive: they are responses to something that has already gone wrong, namely, disease. The present "health care" professions respond to disease, and even in that in the wrong order and incompletely. They start by managing disease by removing its symptoms and alleviating pain and discomfort. It can be said that they provide processes that take the patient towards health. However, most of the time even in this reactive manner they only go part of the way. Total rehabilitation and even a semblance of reintegration are often given less than what would be desirable.

Caring for health is often regarded as a commodity, not as a process, something that can be provided or dispensed to the patients. And health care is often referred to as an industry that dispenses its products. This is reinforced by the belief that people have the right to health care. They expect to be given something: a drug, a new kidney or at least a walking stick. But real health care is not what we are given, but what we do to preserve or improve our health: it is a process or series of actions that fit in with the natural bio-psycho-social processes that take place inside and around us: processes that connect us with our internal and external worlds. These processes have served us for millions of years, as manifested by the fact that we survived all the hardships during that time. The function of these processes is to keep us whole and functioning optimally and all our efforts to maintain and enhance our health should be in harmony with them. We need a framework in which our health care efforts can be linked to the processes that naturally run through our being and all that surrounds us.

The dimension of contributors

The dimension of contributors to health care can be divided into five groups: Official medicine, alternative or complementary medicine, personal wellness, organisational health and hygiene, public or societal health.

Official medicine (disease management and cure) During the last one hundred years health care has been dominated by the medical profession ably helped by the so-called allied professions that include pharmacy, physiotherapy, occupational therapy, radiography and logopaedics, among others. The great scientific progress of the 18th and 19th centuries brought about a tremendous confidence in our abilities. We assumed that if we could conquer the physical world we could do the same with the living world as well. Indeed, the dominant medical paradigm that was based on scientific foundations achieved great successes and clinical medicine reigned supreme. Unfortunately, the medical profession also became over confident and assumed that all disease would be conquered before the end of the 20th century, or soon thereafter. Obviously, this did not happen, and in spite of all the successes the overall health level of the world's population is not getting better.

Our scientific medicine is failing us in both developed and developing countries, albeit for different reasons. Disease is on the increase in the former because of want, while in the latter it happens as a result of excess. The cost of health care is increasing everywhere and medical activities consume an increasing share of national budgets and personal income. People are demanding better health care and governments are throwing more money at it without any real success. There is a great disappointment with the current situation, even though medicine is coming up with fantastic new technologies to "combat disease" on a daily basis. In spite of these disease-oriented successes, many (who can afford it) are looking for alternative methods for maintaining and enhancing their health.

Why would people leave mainstream health care, which has served them so well in the past with its many dedicated doctors, excellent techniques, medications and equipment? The answer probably lies in what we have already mentioned in previous sections. Modern medicine has been concentrating on biological aspects of disease, omitting the psychosocial. It has also limited itself mainly to disease management and cure, with minimum effort on disease prevention and rehabilitation and leaving health promotion and social reintegration to others.

ALTERNATIVE AND COMPLEMENTARY MEDICINE

Modern "scientific" medicine came into prominence at the beginning of the 20th century to replace the myriad of so-called "non-scientific" methods that were practised previously, some of which have been around for thousands of years. What also helped this development was that scientific feats were transformed into technologies, which in turn provided economic incentives, especially for the pharmacological industry, which in turn fuelled a drug and technology-driven medical activity. The "non-scientific" methods were labelled as backward or as based on superstition or "old wives tales". But, obviously, some of them must have had some merit as they were in use for such a long time.

Some of these methods, such as acupuncture, Ayurveda and traditional medical practices were preserved in certain countries. Many of them have been rediscovered in other countries and are now practised as part of alternative and complementary medicine. There are also new therapeutic modalities that have been developed more recently and are practised widely.

Alternative and complementary medicine can be divided into the several groups, listed below. Some examples of each group are given. However, these examples are only meant to illustrate the fact that there are many of them in each group. Some disciplines can be classified in several groups:

1. Whole medical systems: such as Ayurveda, Yoga, Homeopathy, Anthroposophical Medicine, Alexander Technique, Naturopathy, Osteopathy, Chiropathy, Life Extension, etc.
2. Biologically-based therapies: such as diet-based therapies, Bach Flower therapy, Buteyko method for asthma, Rebirthing, herbal therapy, etc
3. Energy medicine: such as Therapeutic Touch, Shiatsu, Magnet Therapy, Reiki, Medical Qigong, Jin Shin Jyutsu, Wise Method, Eden energy medicine, etc
4. Manipulative therapy: such as Bodywork, Rolfing, Bowen technique, Myofascial release, Metamorphic technique, Massage therapy, Reflexology, Feldenkrais, Pilates, etc
5. Mind-body interventions: Autogenic training, Vivation, Progressive Relaxation, Transcendental Meditation, Hatha Yoga, Hypnotherapy, etc
6. Traditional medicine: Chinese, African, America Indian, Australian aboriginal traditional therapies among many others. In almost every country, some kind of traditional therapy has survived to a greater or lesser extent.

There is definitely a need for an overarching framework within which these therapies can be placed and evaluated. One needs to know which natural processes are influenced by these methods at what level of the complex life on earth.

PERSONAL WELLNESS MANAGEMENT

There are many things that one can do for one's own health. Unfortunately, it is not easy as we all carry the burden of our bad habits, which means a solidly-wired brain circuitry that is very hard to change. We are also exposed to signals from our environment that reinforce this circuitry. These include the bad habits of our parents, the pressure from our peers and the constant barrage of advertisements from industry through the media, among other things. But we know today that brains are plastic, ie, they can change themselves. This plasticity has led to our behaviours today, and fortunately it can be also be used to change that behaviour for something better suited to maintain and enhance our health.

The things we can do for our health include brain fitness, active hobbies, recreation, pastimes, gym and water exercises, brain fitness activities, diet management, stress management, body care, dyadic activities (those we do with one partner or friend), social activities (those we do in groups). Each of these includes many possible activities, which will not be mentioned here. If we could locate our activities in a larger framework, we could see where they are focused and where they make an impact. In such a framework we could see whether our action deals with the inputs into our body, or with the way the body maintains the environment of our cells, or with the way it musters cellular activity for a common cause, or with the way it interacts with and contributes to the environment. In fact, we should be contributing to all these modalities. Knowing what they are could help us direct our efforts to all in a balanced way.

ORGANISATIONAL HEALTH CARE

In most large corporations, such as those of mining, there are divisions of Health and Hygiene, charged with the task of looking after the health of their workers by preventing accidents and rehabilitating workers returning from an absence due to disease and disability. Most people spend a large proportion of their lives at work, and work providers have a great influence on their lives. This influence could be used to promote health through correct diet, recreation, stress release and exercise.

SOCIETAL HEALTH CARE

An aspect of health care that gets some political support is Public Health which mainly deals with the prevention of diseases that might affect large populations. It is largely a reactive activity in response to the threat of disease. Societal health care could be much more proactive in advocating health promotion independently of disease. It could spend more effort on educating people on the advantages of healthy living.

OTHER DIMENSIONS

Apart from the above three dimensions, namely, those of levels, processes and contributors, there are many others that need to be taken into consideration. Examples of these are dimensions of evidence, treatment, technology, economics, politics and culture as they relate to health care. Because of limited space, we shall not elaborate on these.

THE BIOMATRIX

As has been mentioned in the introduction, the biomatrix approach was developed during the 1980s with the aim of creating a framework within which complex living systems could be studied. It was based on cybernetic principles and first used to analyse physiological systems. It was later realised that the method could be extended to many different kinds of systems right across all levels of life that exist on earth. Many articles, as well as a book, have been published on the subject during the last 25 years (4).

Life on earth is a complex indivisible web of natural and man-made actions that stretches from atomic proportions to those of the universe. It is a single web that encompasses biological, psychological, societal, ecological, technological and economic aspects of our lives, being responsible for all life's beauty, and alas, also for all its ugliness that manifests in overpopulation, famine, violence, wars and disease. For the ancient Greeks the word *bios* used to cover all life on earth, not just the activities that go on within living cells. They considered all activities that contained living beings as being alive. Indeed anything we use as human beings is part of the complex living web that we decided to call the Biomatrix.

As time goes on, the complexity of the biomatrix increases, with man's actions being responsible for an increasingly greater proportion of activity within the living web. As our actions are not always well considered with respects to the natural laws that underlie the web, the problems they cause are starting to reach seemingly unmanageable proportions. We often feel as though we are in a maze from which there is no way out.

Luckily, the web is not like an entangled heap of knitting wool, but more like a woven spider's web, viz, its actions are arranged in a definite pattern (mould, matrix). The pattern of a well functioning web (biomatrix) is different from that of a malfunctioning one. Thus knowing the healthy pattern can help us identify actions that might cause the problems. The most important characteristic pattern in the web of life is that the main actions, like the thicker radial threads of the spider's web, aggregate (cluster) and cross many levels. As the radial threads impart strength to the spider's web, these clusters are also dedicated to achieve specific outcomes within the Biomatrix. For this reason they have been named teleons (*teleos* in Greek means outcome, end-point, object, goal, reason, aim, purpose). The substance of the universe, viz, matter-energy-information (MEI) flows in teleons driven by the common teleos that drives them. Teleonics is the study of teleons, their internal organisation and their interactions within the biomatrix.

If we realise that life on earth is a system of actions, what we do or don't do becomes of vital importance. We do not have to change things, only what we do with them. It is much easier to change actions than to change things: to put on a smile rather than to change a face through plastic surgery! This may be both good and bad at the same time. It is good as it makes the web flexible and changeable to meet new challenges, but can be bad as ill-considered actions cause serious problems. If teleons become less efficient in achieving their intended outcomes, we have a "disorder relating to the success of outcome" (*telentropy*). Consider cutting one of the threads of a spider's web. That thread will be unable to fulfil its role in the web, viz, its telentropy will be infinitely high. However, other surrounding (weak) cross links will readjust their tensions to try bringing about a new balance in the web, and thus eliminating the telentropy created by cutting the thread in the first place. Whether their efforts will be successful or otherwise depends on the internal functioning of the involved threads as well as their contributions to the overall balance of the living web.

The biomatrix approach (teleonics) describes actions or processes, viz, what is being done on all levels within the web of life, from the atomic to the universal. It is like language that describes actions by use of verbs. In fact, the action word (verb) is an essential component of a sentence. While an expression, such as "I am walking" simply describes general action, it becomes much more meaningful if we specify its teleos, as in "I walk everyday to improve my fitness" or "I am walking to work". In these cases, my "walking" becomes part of the teleon of "my quest for fitness" or the teleon of "my earning a living". I can use my walking in the morning and afternoon for both reasons: for fitness and getting to work if I am close enough to my office. This is like killing two birds with one stone, which is wonderful. But let us assume that this is all I do for fitness, which can be sufficient under certain circumstances. Now, consider the scenario that I am transferred to another office, which is too far to walk to. I remove the "walking to work" from the "earning my living" teleon and replace it by "driving to work". This will throw a hammer (telentropy) into my "fitness teleon", viz, the chances that I can maintain my level of fitness diminishes, unless I replace the early morning and afternoon walks with some other activity, or do these before going to work or after arriving at home, or going to the gym or swimming pool. This example illustrates the transfer of telentropy from one teleon, caused by moving of a workplace, to another teleon that can seriously influence our health. While this might sound a trivial example, it is not. The uncontrolled transfer of telentropy can occur between many levels. The effects of lack of physical exercise, coupled with unhealthy eating habits has been shown to result in obesity, diabetes, arteriosclerosis and heart disease, with very serious consequences right down to the atomic and right up to the universal levels.

The stretching of teleons between the atomic to the universal level has important implications. Let us take nutrition as an example. Its aim is to provide the molecules of our bodies with the energy needed to perform all our bodily functions. However, for proper nutrition, we need the support of our family to buy and prepare the food we eat, the community to provide places where we can buy it, society that allows growing and processing it, the whole world that provides places from where we can import it and knowledge that allows our agriculture that can grow it. We also need sunshine and rain to make our crops grow. If our molecules are well provided for, we can act as whole people and can contribute to the functioning of our families, communities, society and, indirectly, to the entire world. One can visualise a complex web of actions that stretch up and down in the multilevel hierarchy. A disease like kwashiorkor is not simply a medical disease, but a complex combination of actions that have gone wrong on many levels. The lack of provision of rain, grain, money and knowledge, combined with fighting, maiming the able and destruction of the sick, reduced abilities to work and play have as much to do with the disease as protein deficiency on a cellular level. Only by re-establishing the balanced web of actions can a problem like this ever be solved. This also applies to obesity, HIV-Aids, heart disease, arteriosclerosis, Mad Cow Disease, smoking, overpopulation, urban sprawl and violence, among many others.

Until the structure of the complex problems we face is clear to us all, our effort to solve them will undoubtedly fail. The Biomatrix approach allows us to rise up to a level above our problems and to look at them from a comfortable distance with a clear mind, without local personal and political bias.

The examples given in this short introduction were meant to whet the appetite. There is no problem in this world in which actions can be restricted to a single level and no systems that generate no telentropy and do not pass it on to others. Health is not simply a matter for the medical profession; it has implications from the atomic to the universal. Although the problems can be very complex, we are given a saving grace by the existence of manageable action patterns that can be described in the biomatrix approach.

CONCLUSION

Health is a very complex issue that has many dimensions that intertwine with one another, and fully caring for it requires many processes by many contributors. The new paradigm in health care is the creation of a truly holistic approach, in which all dimensions are integrated. In order to deal with such complexity we need a framework, which can position all the dimensions and reveal the interactions between them. The biomatrix approach is such a framework.

REFERENCES

[1]   Smuts J. Holism and evolution. New York: MacMillan, 1926:336-7.
[2]   Járos GG, Cloete A. Biomatrix: The web of life. World Futures 1987;23:215-36.
[3]   Preamble to the Constitution of the World Health Organisation as adopted by the International Health Conference, New York, 19-22 June 1946; signed on 22 July 1946 by the representatives of 61 States (Official Records of the World Health Organization, no 2, p. 100) and entered into force on 7 April 1948. The Definition has not been amended since 1948.
[4]   Dostal E, Cloete A, Járos GG. Biomatrix. Stellenbosch: Sun Press, 2004. Available though the website http://www.biomatrixweb.com/history1.htm

Submitted: May 01, 2011.
Revised: June 15, 2011.
Accepted: June 24, 2011.

In: Alternative Medicine Research Yearbook 2012
Editors: Søren Ventegodt and Joav Merrick

ISBN: 978-1-62808-080-3
© 2013 Nova Science Publishers, Inc.

Chapter 5

A-CAUSALITY, CONSCIOUSNESS AND ORGANISATIONS

Walter Baets, BSc, MSC, PhD [*]

Graduate School of Business, University of Cape Town, Cape Town, South Africa

ABSTRACT

A tendency is emerging in management theory and practice today to accept that our linear and deterministic ways of thinking about managerial problems create more problems than they solve. In the field of strategy studies, for instance, one can observe a growing interest in learning and organisational flexibility. It gives importance to distributed cognition and adaptive systems. Management theorists are keenly observing developments surrounding the complexity and chaos theory in science, and management researchers are attempting to apply emerging theories to managerial problems. The current economic reality is harsh and tough in showing the consequences of choices we have made over the last decade. This contribution is an attempt to explore the essence of such a quantum ontology and its consequences for a more consciousness-oriented approach to management and organisations.

Keywords: Mind, body, consciousness, integrative medicine

INTRODUCTION

Wanderer, your footprints are the path, and nothing more; Wanderer, there is no path, it is created as you walk By walking, you make the path before you, and when you look behind you see the path which after you will not be trod again. Wanderer, there is no path, but the ripples on the waters.
Antonio Machado

A tendency is emerging in management theory and practice today to accept that our linear and deterministic ways of thinking about managerial problems create more problems than they

---

[*] Correspondence: Professor Walter Baets, Director, Graduate School of Business, University of Cape Town, Private Bag X3 Robndebosch 7700, Cape Town, South Africa. E-mail: walter.baets@gsb.uct.ac.za.

solve. In the field of strategy studies, for instance, one can observe a growing interest in learning and organizational flexibility. It gives importance to distributed cognition and adaptive systems. Management theorists are keenly observing developments surrounding the complexity and chaos theory in science, and management researchers are attempting to apply emerging theories to managerial problems. The current economic reality is harsh and tough in showing the consequences of choices we have made over the last decade.

The ideas that many simple, non-linear deterministic systems can behave in an apparently unpredictable and chaotic manner is not new. It was first introduced by the great French mathematician Henri Poincaré. Other early pioneering work in the field of chaotic dynamics is found in mathematical literature by scientists such as, amongst others, Birkhoff, Levenson and Kolmogorov. More recently, several Nobel prizes have been awarded in this field of research, for instance to Prigogine and Kauffman.

Complexity as an emergent organizational paradigm in the knowledge-based economy primarily questions the concept of causality. Despite relativity and quantum mechanics, most physics (and certainly all managerial thinking) is still Newtonian, based on a fixed space-time frame. In the meantime, further developments have taken place in the area of biology (such as the concept of Sheldrake's morphogenetic fields) (1) and mind/body medicine seems to point to a federating idea of a quantum interpretation of social phenomena (non-locality, synchronicity and entanglement). Isn't a-causality the basis for a quantum ontology of complex systems?

Once we have accepted such a quantum ontology, the concept of "mind over matter", or the prevailing role of consciousness, becomes more obvious.

This contribution is an attempt to explore the essence of such a quantum ontology and its consequences for a more consciousness-oriented approach to management and organizations.

THE PHILOSOPHY OF QUANTUM MECHANICS

The foundational concepts in the complexity realm emerge from such fields as neurobiology, cognitive sciences, physics, and organizational theory. New developments in knowledge management such as connectionist approaches (complex adaptive systems) for the visualization of emergence give promising results (2). In fact, instead of causality, it appears that the networked economy is rather ruled by synchronicity (appearing at the same time) as many quantum researchers suggest. Is economy and management, and in particular the more dynamic aspects of it like innovation or leadership development, indeed based on a quantum ontology?

Given the insight into complexity that we have developed over the last decade and its consequences for management the way we have discussed it in earlier work (3,4), we are now ready to explore the ontological basis of complex systems, and possibly draw some far-reaching conclusions for the way ahead. In the current economic turmoil, the necessary shift towards transformational leadership will have to be based on a different set of assumptions about reality.

What Prigogine and complexity theory in general discussed fundamentally was the existence of any causal relationship. In fact he was surprised that despite the two fundamental revolutions in physics in the last century, relativity theory and quantum mechanics, physics is still mainly Newtonian. It presumes a fixed time and space concept, in which the future is causally related to the past. Complexity theory shows the impossibility of this assumption, and so does quantum mechanics.

The discontinuity versus continuity dichotomy can be seen as contingently rooted in philosophical commitments and in the physical phenomena studied. By the late 19th century, there were already significant, even if not overwhelming, philosophical precedents for the concept of indeterminism (including the possibility of inherent chance) in nature, as opposed to the straightforward determinism often associated with classical physics. Soren Kierkegaard believed that objective uncertainty can force one to make a leap into the unknown so that decisions cannot always "even in principle" be based on a continuous chain of logic. For example one of Hoffding's tenets was that in life, decisive events proceed through sudden "jerks" of discontinuities, an idea incorporated into Bohr's view of atomic phenomena (5).

There was a split in philosophical outlook along generational lines: the "older" essentially classical world view of people like Einstein, Schrödinger and de Broglie versus a radically different, eventually indeterministic conception of physical processes engendered by a generally younger generation (Bohr and Born being the exceptions here) including Heisenberg, Pauli, Jordan and Dirac (6).

On the standard or so-called Copenhagen interpretation of quantum mechanics, in particular the Schrödinger equation, we no longer have event-by-event causality, and particles do not follow well-defined trajectories in a space-time background. The theory predicts, in general, probabilities and not specific events.

We now come to one of the most profound issues in the interpretation of quantum mechanics – that of causality (in the sense of a specific, identifiable cause for each individual effect). Dirac (7) observes: Causality applies only to a system which is left undisturbed. If a system is small, we cannot observe it without producing a serious disturbance and hence we cannot expect to find any causal connection between the results of our observations.

In this same spirit Heisenberg, too, felt that since the mathematical structure of quantum mechanics is so different from that of classical mechanics, it is not possible to interpret quantum mechanics in terms of our commonly understood notions of space and time with classical causality (8).

We characterized the standard, or Copenhagen view of quantum mechanics as requiring complementarity (such as wave-particle duality), inherent indeterminism at the most fundamental level of quantum phenomena and the impossibility of an event-by-event causal representation in a continuous space-time background. So, on the Copenhagen interpretation of quantum mechanics, physical processes are at the most fundamental level both inherently indeterministic and non-local. The ontology of classical physics is dead. The heart of the problem is the entanglement (or non-separability) of quantum states that gives rise to the measurement problem. This entanglement makes it impossible to assign independent properties to an arbitrary isolated physical system once it has interacted with another system in the past – even though these two systems are no longer interacting. The non-separability characteristic of quantum systems can be seen as an indication of the "holistic" character of such systems.

A bell-type theorem is proven and taken as convincing evidence that non-locality is present in quantum phenomena. Quantum mechanics has undeniably introduced us to non-locality, entanglement and synchronicity; concepts that thus far have not yet been applied to business, economics or social sciences at large.

THE SOCIAL SCIENCE IMPLICATIONS

In earlier work (3) I already suggested that the solution might be, in effect, to go as low as possible on the aggregation level (human emotions, team members) to allow innovation to produce itself through the emergence processes. In fact we want to explore the quantum reality of management or any other social phenomenon. The remaining question is a double question: can, and how can, you make the concept of innovation holistic, and so encapsulate the personal emotional side; but on a deeper level we can ask ourselves this question with reference to conscience and causality, and the "seat" of consciousness.

The more on-the-ground question is: on what level can we find consciousness; is there something like a collective consciousness (for example in a company; on the subject of innovation): does everyone have a sort of essential element of incorporated consciousness with a possibility of connection with others (at the level of consciousness)? Translated to companies: do consciousness, engagement and emotions make a difference for a company; does a company have a "soul", a consciousness; is there a link between this "consciousness" and the success of a company; are vision, emotions and consciousness linked? More concretely, who determines the choice of a client who has a preference for one company rather than another? What lets potential clients make a distinction between two companies which offer the same services (for example, two big banks such as BNP and ING, or two consultancy companies such as PWC and Accenture)? And finally, can we arrive at an approach, accepted as scientific, that gives at least the beginning of a response to these questions? Although these questions are, of course, a little metaphysical, this does not prevent them from remaining important questions. Is the current crisis a quest for a more conscious approach to management and responsibility, and are we able to think on a level of consciousness if we talk business? Indeed, our managerial thinking is still Marshallian, the economic thinking of the 19th Century (9).

At the end of his scientific career, Wolfgang Pauli (10) asked himself how we can know if human cultures can live with a clear distinction between knowledge and belief (an idea, moreover, of Max Planck). For this reason, according to him, societies are in difficulty if new knowledge arrives and puts the classical spiritual values in question. The complete separation between the two can only be a solution in the short term, and one of facility. Pauli predicted (and we see how much reality seems to support him today) that there will be a moment in the near future when all the images and metaphors of classic religions will lose their strength of conviction for the average citizen. We will be in a situation where classic ethical values explode and we have a period of hitherto unknown barbarism. He was touched and very interested by what he himself called "background physics": the spontaneous appearance of quantitative concepts and images concerning the physical in fantasies and dreams. He admitted he also had them himself. Their character was very dependent on the dreamer himself. Background physics has an archetypal origin and that leads (always, according to him) to a natural science which will work just as well with matter as with consciousness. He was also sufficiently realist to say that if a researcher in physics has observed a sub-system, the observations are as much dependent on the observer as on the instruments.

According to Pauli, the physical concept of "complementarity" physics (10) illustrated a profound analogy with concepts such as conscience and the unconscious. Two extreme cases which can never be attained in practice are "someone with a perfect conscience" (Eastern philosophy suggests that this can be attained uniquely in death, also called Nirvana) and something like a "bigger spirit" which will never be influenced by a subjective consciousness. This "bigger spirit" is what Eastern philosophy calls the "consciousness", and western psychology calls "collective unconsciousness". Pauli accepted that physical values, as much as archetypes, change in the eyes of the observer. Observation is the result of human consciousness.

Pauli wrote a book with Jung on this issue (11). Where Jung talked about defined archetypes as primordial structural elements of the human psyche, Pauli introduced the notion of the "collective unconsciousness". They both believe that we are moving towards a joining of the psyche and the physical.

The introduction of the notion of "synchronicity" in this co-authored work is not only interesting but we also find it with some other authors in other disciplines.

Synchronicity (being united-in-time) (according to Pauli) appears in all the sciences and the techniques in which simultaneity plays a role. We must take into account that we are not speaking about a causal coherence (from cause to effect) but about a coincidence (=being together in time) which must be considered as useful even if we cannot explain the deep cause of this simultaneity. We must remember that we always speak about synchronicity if the events concerned occur in the same time period. The concepts of statistics or the theory of probability are of another order. Probability can be calculated with mathematical methods, which is impossible when speaking about synchronicity.

Synchronicity (10) is considered as the basis of a lot of phenomena which are difficult to explain and which are often called non-scientific. In the context of this paper, we do not go into these aspects. The way to understand this better is that the widening of consciousness and the dissolving of borders is only possible when we keep, besides our energetic causal thinking (classical), a space for synchronicity and information. It is to Pauli's great credit that he indicated the necessity to create space for the concept of synchronicity in scientific thinking. Jung speaks about this as the "a-causal" link. Sheldrake later confirmed these ideas with his theory of morph(ogenet)ic fields.

Pauli and Jung (11) proposed that the classic triad of physics (space, time and causality) be extended with synchronicity to then form a tetrad. This fourth element works in an a-causal manner, and it is in effect, the polar opposite of causality. Pauli and Jung believed that these oppositions were orthogonal in time and space. The idea of an a-causal link, or non-locality, are new concepts which should contribute effectively to the science of management.

CONSCIOUSNESS IN COMPLEX SOCIAL SYSTEMS

One of the illustrations of this quantum concept, and with the goal of doing a thought experiment, is developed in Mitchell's "dyadic model" as he describes it in his book (12). Stated simply, the concept of non-locality is derived from quantum physics (as explained before). In fact, in the experiments he demonstrated that particles (photons) stay attached in a "mysterious" manner, even if they displace in directions contrary to the speed of light.

The dyadic model is built on the idea that everything is energy. This basic energy is linked to information, what Mitchell calls structures of energy. The energy and the information form a dyad. The information, in this context, is the basis of the capacity of matter to "know" (and so has nothing to do with information as treated in information systems).

All matter contains a sort of "awareness" or, in other terms, a capacity to "know". If not, how can molecules "know" that they must join up with others to form cells? In a subsequent state (a more complex state), it could be that in the human body/brain matter evolves such that it knows what it knows. It is therefore capable of self reflection.

Another dyad in his model is "awareness" and intention which equally make up part of the evolutionary process which leads to consciousness. Consciousness and innovation, accepted elements of the energy-information scheme, are the basis of self-reflective consciousness.

The non-locality is illustrated by the famous connection, proven and explained, ("entanglement") between partner photons which are sent in opposite directions. They still stay in a position to ("instantaneously") communicate between themselves over large distances. This is a relationship with the "knowledge" of these particles. Man is equally made up of these sorts of particles.

So how does such communication function according to Mitchell (12)? The groups of particles seem to have special characteristics of resonance and coherence which are evoked by the groups themselves. This resonance includes historical knowledge about universal matter. This idea strongly corresponds with Rupert Sheldrake's observations. The body/brain can receive holographic information in the form of virtual long wave signals. Mitchell's dyad suggests that the particles "know" by their inherent qualities of conscience and intention. The groups of particles communicate between themselves on the basis of quantum holograms (what Sheldrake calls the morphogenetic fields) which includes information about the universe. As our body/brain also works in a holographic way, it can recuperate this information. Apparently, Nature does not lose its memory concerning its own evolution. Mitchell believes that it is our intention or directional attention which links us holographically with the signals or non-local long waves.

The greater the experience of satisfaction, the more the consciousness of each cell in the body will resonate with the holographic information engraved in the "quantum zero point" (the lowest possible state of energy, in an almost resting, but not quite, state)(6) of the energy field. This phenomenon refers to what we know as to be "carried along". If a person lives in harmony with his biological rhythms (all sorts of rhythms) the body is in balance and the person will fall ill less quickly. In the material world we can witness a phenomenon of "being carried along" if we put two pendulums beside one another. Although the movement of the pendulums in the two clocks seems at first to be totally arbitrary, after a certain time, the movements adapt to each other and move in harmony. The two clocks are "carried along". In the world of medicine a lot of these ideas are found in Ayurvedic (holistic) medicine.

This quantum approach of energy, information and communication, allows us to suggest causality at a much lower level of aggregation; that is to say, at a quantum level. In effect, we should really speak about synchronicity or coincidence rather than causality. It is important that it is this structure which allows people to realize what they want to realize; that could be, for example, to protect themselves against viruses, to simply survive or to innovate in companies. It is therefore a question of elementary particles (let us say the characteristics of people if we translate them into economic behaviour), which are linked in solid networks with all sorts of matter (the context) which in turn interact with this matter, and in doing that, become part of the wider energetic field (morphogenetics) which contains knowledge and information. When more members of a team (or a company) are "carried along", their actions will be more successful. This can be seen in teams working on product innovation.

Once we relax the five basic assumptions that physics gave us on the fabric of reality: reality, locality, causality, continuity and determinism (13), we are able to see and develop consciousness.

SUSTAINABILITY

A transformational view in management or organizational theory today has to be based on the concept of sustainability. The currently prevailing definition of sustainability emphasizes cross-generational equity, clearly an all-important concept for any society that wishes to endure, but one that is operationally insufficient. Anchoring an alternative definition directly to the relationship between a population and the carrying capacity of its environment (a here and now concept) offers some advantages. Ben-Eli suggests the following definition:

Sustainability: A dynamic equilibrium in the processes of interaction between a population and the carrying capacity of an environment such that the population develops to express its full potential without adversely and irreversibly affecting the carrying capacity of the environment upon which it depends.

This definition points to the dynamic nature of sustainability as a state. This state has to be calibrated with time, again and again, as changes occur in population numbers, or in the resources available for supporting all humans at a desired level of wellbeing. It does not seek to define specifically what such a level is, nor to limit yet unimaginable possibilities for social evolution. It recognizes, however, boundaries and limits that must be maintained by stone-age tribes and industrial societies alike. As long as the underlying conditions for equilibrium are maintained, the well being of future generations is assured.

The set of sustainability principles which follows is grounded in Ben-Eli's definition. The principles are articulated in broad terms but can receive a specific operational meaning in relation to particular sectors of the economy, development issues, business strategies, investment guidelines, or initiatives taken by individuals. We express them in relation to the following five fundamental domains (all representing essential aspects in the interaction of human populations and the environment):

1. The Spiritual Domain: Which identifies the necessary attitudinal orientation and provides the basis for ethical conduct.
2. The Domain of Life: Which provides the basis for appropriate behaviour in the biosphere with respect to other species.
3. The Social Domain: Which provides the basis for social interactions.
4. The Economic Domain: Which provides a guiding framework for creating and managing wealth.
5. The Material Domain: Which constitutes the basis for regulating the flow of materials and energy that underlie existence.

The result is a set of five core principles, each with its own derived policy and operational implications. The set is fundamentally systemic in nature, meaning, that each domain affects all the others, and is affected by each in return. Rather than a list, the set should be approached and understood as a coherent whole. The framework of these principles enables a nurturing context for talking about values.

In respect to the role and necessity for consciousness in organizations, I would like to highlight only the first principle. It relates to the spiritual domain, to the basic assumptions we hold about the very nature of reality and the values we hold. It calls for recognizing the fundamental mystery that underlies all existence, and the seamless continuum that links humans and our technology with the rest of the biosphere, and with the outermost reaches of the cosmos. This principle means honoring the earth with its intricate ecology; fostering compassion and an ethical perspective in all human affairs; reintroducing a sense of sacredness and reverence to all interactions; linking inner transformation of individuals to transformations in the social collective; and fostering the emergence of a genuine, wise, planetary civilization. With some creativity we can see in this list a first draft of attributes to consciousness in management.

CONSCIOUS BUSINESS

Would it help to start even a little more a-centric? Would the culture shock be made bigger by limiting the values to consciousness-related values in line with Kofman's (14) view that conscious business means finding your passion and expressing your essential values through your work? A conscious business seeks to promote the intelligent pursuit of happiness in all its stakeholders. It aims to produce sustainable, exceptional performance through the solidarity of its community and the dignity of each member.

Ken Wilber (14) talking about Kofman's book "Conscious Business: How to Build Value through Values" says that integral mastery begins with mastery of self, at an emotional level, a mental-ethical level, and a spiritual level. Anything more than that is not needed; anything less than that is disastrous, according to him. Peter Senge, in the same book (14) highlights yet another important issue; the key to organisational excellence lies in transforming our practices of unilateral control into cultures of mutual learning. When people continually challenge and improve the data and assumptions upon which their map of reality is grounded, as opposed to treating their perspectives as the truth, tremendous productive energy is released.

Collins (15) studies what drives average companies to take a quantum leap and become extraordinary. He concludes that a crucial component of greatness is a group of leaders with a paradoxical blend of personal humility and professional will. These leaders, whom Collins calls "level five", channel their ego ambition away from themselves into the larger goal of building a great company. Conscious employees are an organization's most important asset; unconscious employees are its most dangerous liability. So what are conscious employees?

Kofman (14) used seven qualities to distinguish conscious from unconscious employees. The first three are character attributes: unconditional responsibility, essential integrity and ontological humility. The next three are interpersonal skills: authentic communication, constructive negotiation and impeccable coordination. The seventh quality is an enabling condition for the previous six: emotional mastery. Conscious employees take responsibility for their lives. They don't compromise human values for material success. They speak their truth and listen to others' truths with honesty and respect. They look for creative solutions to disagreements and honor their commitments impeccably. They are in touch with their emotions and express them productively.

Buckingham and Coffman (14) reported on a 22 year study on organizational effectiveness. According to them, exceptional managers create a workplace in which employees emphatically answered "yes" when asked the following questions:

- Do I know what is expected of me at work?
- Do I have the materials and equipment I need to do my work right?
- At work, do I have the opportunity to do what I do best every day?
- In the last seven days, have I received recognition or praise for doing good work?
- Does my supervisor, or someone at work, seem to care about me as a person?
- Is there someone at work who encourages my development?
- At work, do my opinions seem to count?
- Does the mission/purpose of my company make me feel my job is important?
- Are my co-workers committed to doing high-quality work?
- Do I have a best friend at work?
- In the last six months, has someone at work talked to me about my progress?
- This last year, have I had opportunities at work to learn and grow?

Kofman proposed a systemic organizational map that comes very close to our own development that is laid out in our recent book (16). In this book we give very practical tools for managers that are interested to make the shift into transformational leadership for a more sustainable performance of the company. Finally, Kofman illustrated (14) the difference between unconscious and conscious attitudes in the following:

A big, tough samurai once went to see a little monk. "Monk", he barked, in a voice accustomed to instant obedience, "teach me about heaven and hell!"

The monk looked up at the mighty warrior and replied with utter disdain, "Teach you about heaven and hell? I couldn't teach you about anything. You're dumb. You're dirty. You're a disgrace, an embarrassment to the samurai class. Get out of my sight. I can't stand you."

The samurai got furious. He shook, red in the face, speechless with rage. He pulled out his sword, and prepared to slay the monk.

Looking straight into the samurai's eyes, the monk said softly, "That's hell."

The samurai froze, realizing the compassion of the monk who had risked his life to show him hell! He put down his sword and fell to his knees, filled with gratitude.

The monk said softly, "And that's heaven."

Zen parable

CONSCIOUSNESS AND MIND

This only presents an outline of my understanding of consciousness and organisations, and in some way the mind over matter orientation this might take. Of course, some of this is still a working hypothesis, but at the same time there is growing evidence for these theories and their appearance in real life. Essential to me is a new paradigm, a paradigm shift, in order to be or to become the transformational leaders we need, putting consciousness in the forefront of their managerial practice. This paradigm shift is based on what I call a quantum ontology, as I have tried to briefly develop in this contribution.

This ontology shifts our assumptions and beliefs into a set of other assumptions that not only allows definition of the role of consciousness, but also illustrates its great necessity for a different economy and society. The current crisis, unfortunately, is hard proof of this. The point is no longer to re-invent capitalism, with or without a human face, but rather to reinvent a social fabric that is based on interconnectedness and the realization of values, including economic added value. Some might want to call this a stakeholder economy, but yet again, this fabric needs another soul.

This new paradigm and its related managerial approach manifestly contain different aspects. Some of those aspects we could label as more spiritual (dealing with connectedness and the inner self), as value driven, as related to awareness in action, as giving meaning to actions.

The consequence of those choices will cause companies and organizations to develop an orientation towards sustainable performance that would be able to define a coherent answer to the crisis we observe today. Other than being based on another paradigm or another ontology, it is characterized by another performance orientation. The contemporary economy has developed a strict orientation on short term shareholder return, and by doing so it has put itself artificially outside the necessary interconnectedness that we have referred to in this contribution. Hence there is little role for consciousness and conscious action in today's managerial paradigm.

For managers or people with responsibility that would like to make the shift themselves into conscious leaders, concepts and tools are available. I gladly refer to the new book (16), that exclusively deals with this and that gives a workbook in the annex.

We are all linked by a fabric of unseen connections. This fabric is constantly changing and evolving. This field is directly structured and influenced by our behaviour and by our understanding. Hence, the shift is ours to make.

REFERENCES

[1]   Sheldrake R. The presence of the past: Morphic resonance and the habits of nature. London: Fontana, HarperCollins, 1988.

[2]   Baets W. Knowledge management and management learning: Extending the horizons of knowledge-based management. Berlin: Springer, 2005.

[3]   Baets W. Complexity, learning and organisations: A quantum interpretation of business. London: Routledge, 2006.

[4]   Baets W. Complexity theory: dynamics and non-linearity are the only reason for knowledge management to exist. In: Boughzala I, Ermine J-L, eds. Trends in applied knowledge management. London: Hermes Penton Science, 2006.

[5]	Cushing J. Philosophical concepts in physics. Cambridge: Cambridge University Press, 1998.
[6]	Polkinghorne J. The quantum world. New York: Penguin, 1990.
[7]	Dirac P. The principles of quantum mechanics, 4th ed. Oxford: Oxford University Press, 1958.
[8]	Heisenberg W. [Uber den anschaulichen Inhalt der quantentheoretischen Kinematik und Mechanik]. Zeitschrift für Physik 1927;43:172-98.
[9]	Arthur B. The end of certainty in economics. In: Aerts D, Broekaert J, Mathijs E, eds. Einstein meets Margritte. Dordrecht: Kluwer Academic, 1998.
[10]	van Meijgaard H. Wolfgang Pauli: A man of this age. Enschede, Holland: Twente University Technology Press. 1998.
[11]	Pauli G, Jung H. The interpretation of nature and psyche. London: Routledge K Paul, 1955.
[12]	Mitchell E, Williams D. The way of the explorer: An Apollo astronaut's journey through the material and mystical world. New York: Putman's Sons, 1996.
[13]	Radin D. Entangled minds. New York: Paraview Pocket Books, 2006.
[14]	Kofman F. Conscious business: How to build value through values. Guatemala: Sounds True, 2006.
[15]	Collins J. Good to great: Why some companies make the leap and others don't. New York: HarperBusiness, 2001.
[16]	Baets W, Oldenboom E. Rethinking growth: Social intrapreneurship for sustainable performance. Basinstoke, UK: MacMillan Palgrave, 2009.

Submitted: May 03, 2011.
Revised: June 18, 2011.
Accepted: June 24, 2011.

In: Alternative Medicine Research Yearbook 2012
Editors: Søren Ventegodt and Joav Merrick
ISBN: 978-1-62808-080-3
© 2013 Nova Science Publishers, Inc.

Chapter 6

SUSTAINABILITY AND HEALTH:
BACK TO THE ROOTS AND FEEDING THE SOIL

*Jeanne Viall, BA**
Freelance journalist, Dennesig, Stellenbosch, South Africa

ABSTRACT

It has become apparent that a new vocabulary has emerged, which has applications in the many fields where paradigms are shifting. The challenges of agriculture and the importance of soil health is dovetailed closely with the challenges of medicine and supporting the body's health rather than treating disease. Concepts such as "restoration", a focus on soil biology rather than just chemistry, and changing the way we measure wellbeing is underpinned by the stark facts that one billion people are underfed and 1,6 billion overfed – and obesity, diabetes and heart disease are a growing problem worldwide.

Keywords: Health, medicine, integrative medicine, future

INTRODUCTION

The conversation around sustainability in relationship to health has just begun. This article is based on a discussion around the principles of sustainability applied to health care with Professor Mark Swilling, Dr Bernard Brom and Professor Milla McLachlan.

Sustainability is not an area that has been much debated, and a search on the internet indicated that sustainability in medicine or health care is seen largely in terms of spending, whether it be the financial sustainability of medical aids, or public health spending. It is framed in terms of rising costs and the merits of privatisation (or not). Another use of the word sustainability is in terms of the bio-waste produced from the manufacture and use of

---

* Correspondence: Jeanne Viall, BA, POBox 2229, Dennesig, Stellenbosch, 7601 South Africa. E-mail: jeanne@creatinghealth.co.za.

medications, and the packaging used. On a business level, sustainability is seen as creating the least invasive carbon footprint.

None of these question the basic paradigm underpinning the western allopathic medical model. Sustainability in health care seems to me to require us to go much further and ask more fundamental questions about health, and all the factors which contribute to health and disease. Sustainability is a word used with increasing frequency, but often with different meanings and underlying assumptions. A 1987 United Nations conference defined sustainable developments as those that "meet present needs without compromising the ability of future generations to meet their needs". Sustainability, then, brings to mind ecosystems in distress, dwindling natural resources (including oil), carbon emissions, soil degradation, water and air pollution, among others. Much of the way sustainability is viewed today is not about sustainability at all, but about "retarded collapse". According to Professor Swilling:

> "Minimising damage is not the way to get to sustainability. The new discourse emerging to replace minimisation of damage is restoration of life. Less bad is not good enough. We need to fundamentally question what we mean by development. Restoration becomes the key objective, and it does mean fundamentally questioning development and redefining it in terms of restoration" (1)

One aspect of this is rethinking "growth" and GDP as an economic measure of progress. "The problem with this index is that beyond a certain economic point, people don't get happier. What is the point of growth if people don't get happier?" (1). The debate now is that GDP alone doesn't have a future, and the suggestion is to expand it with a 'happiness index'. Which then asks us to reflect on happiness/unhappiness, and what it is. This has major implications for how we use resources and our understanding of identity and quality of life.

In medicine there is also some movement towards evaluating healthcare using the concept of "quality of life" as a better way to measure outcomes than morbidity and mortality rates only. The question with which we started our group conversation was "what is unsustainable about medicine?"

One concern is the disconnection between health and medicine. In general the health of the world's population is declining. Diseases of lifestyle, such as diabetes and heart disease, are becoming endemic. Denmark has had free health care for 30 years, but it has not made for a healthy nation – half the population is now on chronic medication.

Robert Verkerk, in his article "Can the failing western medical paradigm be shifted using the principle of sustainability?" (2) suggested that existing models of western, evidence-based medicine have resulted in a medical paradigm that is "relatively ineffective, untenable and almost certainly unsustainable".

Inadequate attention to chronic disease prevention and overuse of drugs (with their high cost and relatively low and unpredictable efficacy) contribute to the unsustainability of this model of medicine, he contends. He points out that while rates of infectious diseases have declined (thanks to improvements in public health, nutrition and the use of antibiotics), chronic disease rates have risen significantly, partly because of the extension to lifespan. Chronic diseases are expected to account for almost 75% of deaths worldwide by 2020.

While chronic diseases are largely dependant on lifestyle and nutrition, nutrition education in medical schools is considered inadequate by public health researchers, he writes.

Doctors, nurses and pharmacists have very limited formal training in nutritional or lifestyle strategies.

Healthcare's primary focus on the symptomatic treatment of chronic disease, rather than prevention, is relatively ineffective and uneconomic compared with preventative strategies in the early years of life.

Some of what he calls the "constraints" of the present-day medical paradigm are the mechanistic nature of medicine; its intrinsic reductionism; its limited and linear view on causality; the avoidance of considerations of the whole organism and interactions with humans and environment and the overuse of "new-to-nature" molecules as therapy.

The medical system's emphasis on drug treatment is problematic: One aspect of this is that the vast majority of drugs – more than 90%, only work in 30 to 50% of people, he writes. Another is that adverse drug reactions, which increase exponentially in people taking four or more medications, is the fourth leading cause of death in the USA, ahead of pulmonary disease, diabetes, AIDS, pneumonia, accidents and MVA. If you add surgical deaths, investigation deaths, and hospital acquired infections, then orthodox medicine is the third leading cause of death. The situation is similar in other western countries.

Medicine also has limited success in dealing with the major disease burden, chronic diseases. Because there's little emphasis on the psychological and emotional health of individuals, quality of life considerations are to a large extent ignored. Most clinical decisions are made on limited consultations of 5 to 10 minutes, and in the majority of cases lead to prescription of pharmaceutical drugs.

In terms of environmental sustainability, Verkerk highlights that "natural" is not neccessarily sustainable; for example the use of a rare herbs which ravage a rainforest; and closer to home the over-exploitation of some indigenous medicinal plants. Other environmental issues are the pollution of waterways by pharmaceuticals and the pillaging of indigenous knowledge and products.

In addition, Western medical care is expensive, and not accessible to many people, except at a very basic level. It would seem then that the present, largely drug-based, approach to treatment of disease is not contributing to better health, and new ways need to be explored.

Sustainability in health care, as in the environment, needs a broader vision. Harm reduction is not enough. We need to look deeper into the underlying causes of ill health, and "treat" them, not just the symptoms. One place to start would be at the root of much of ill health, the food we eat. Nutrition is not the only contributor to ill-health, but it is a major one. A malnourished or under-nourished body is less able to fight disease and deal with environmental toxins.

SOIL HEALTH

"I'm interested in the big macro questions," says Professor Swilling. "The challenge is that 1,6 billion people are obese and 1 billion people in the world are hungry" (1). These figures come from the International Assessment of Agricultural Science Technology and Development (IAASTD) report (3), which stated that "over 800 million people are underweight and malnourished, while changes in diet, the environment and lifestyle worldwide have resulted in 1,6 billion overweight adults; this trend is associated with increasing rates of diet-related diseases such as diabetes and heart disease".

"Obesity is no longer a problem of the overfed, but also the underfed," states Professor Swilling. "You can be rich and malnourished, you can be poor and malnourished. It's got a lot to do with the difficult problem of a globalised food-production system, which maximizes profit through the continuous integration of the value chain, through homogenous foods on the one hand, and the degradation of the key resource we need to produce food, that is, soil (1)."

"In my view supermarketisation is one of big culprits holding the system in place, it's very new, taking place over the last 10 to 15 years. South Africa has the highest amount of food sold in supermarkets in the world, bought through powerful intermediaries who start buying up the value chain, and horizontally integrate through the value chain. They can then dictate to farmers" (1).

There is enough food in the world to supply every person on the planet with 2,720 Kilocalories (kcal) per day which is what the average person needs to live well (4). The question is not whether there is enough food for everyone, but who gets it, who produces it for whom, and the nutritional quality of the food. The key to the issue, believes Professor Swilling, is soil health, and the degradation of soils, which is seldom mentioned in discussions on sustainable agriculture (1)

> "For me, as a non health person, we must ask what is the relationship between soil degradation and the decline in the mineral content of food, the problem of the 'stuffed and starved' (3) and the global food industry? There must be a link, and if the medical profession is only treating symptoms, in a system that is resulting in an increasingly expensive set of diseases, is that really health care? I see the health care system as reactive, reacting within its own paradigm to the symptoms, which are getting worse, not to the deeper underlying set of conditions" (1)

In our discussions we realized there are many parallels between the western medical paradigm and the dominant agricultural paradigm. Agriculture has favored soil chemistry over soil biology. So, too, in Western medicine, where biochemistry favors treating disease rather than improving health. It's interesting to note that whereas the so-called "green revolution" (using chemical fertilizers, irrigation, hybrid seeds and micro-credit to transform agricultural practices) initially boosted crop yields, by the end of the 1990s every major report and researcher expressed concerns about declining rates of growth of agricultural yields (2).

Similarly in medicine, where the era of antibiotics was heralded as the "end of disease" in the mid-1900s, that promise has failed to materialize. In many hospitals there are antibiotic resistant organisms, and infection control is a serious concern. Drugs are no longer seen as a "quick fix" to chronic diseases, and their side-effects are often seen as intolerable.

Declining crop yield is directly related to soil degradation. "Soils however are not seen as a limited ecological resource because soil science has privileged soil chemistry over soil biology, thus making possible a reductionistic focus on NPK (Nitrogen, Phosphorus, Potassium) as the only variable worth worrying about (1).

So too in medicine, where a similar reductionistic approach to disease management leads to using synthetic isolates to manage disease, rather than improving the health of the organism through better food choices and other lifestyle shifts as a management profile for treating ill health.

During the green revolution, as crop yields increased, soil fertility has decreased and as soils become exhausted, crop yields are more and more dependent on fertilisers. Over the past 40 years soil nutrition – the amount of nutrition food takes from the soil – declined from 45% to 20%, according to Professor Swilling, which means we are now eating more food grown using chemically based nutrients (NPK). "Soil fertility decline includes the deterioration in the chemical, physical, and biological properties of the soil that affect plant nutrition, and is a result of specific processes such as reduction of SOM [soil organic matter] and soil biological activity, adverse changes in soil nutrient resources and development of nutrient imbalances, and build-up of toxicities and acidification through incorrect fertilizer use, etc" (4). "This is a remarkable indictment of a chemistry-centred soil science paradigm that has been dominant since at least the 1960s," writes Professor Swilling (4).

The techno-fix of the global food industry proposed to address declining food production is genetically modified crops, the "gene revolution". However, already there are signs that this will not be the success story it's touted to be, with increasing pest-resistance and crop failures.

NUTRITION AND FOOD PRODUCTION

Our health is also affected by the kind of foods being produced. One problem with the global food industry is that it produces energy and resource intensive food (that contains too much fat and sugar) to supply the world's billion over-consumers via the supermarket chains (4). The large majority of poor urban households can only afford nutritionally poor mass-produced cheap foods, and hence the new correlations between obesity/diabetes and malnutrition.

The same reductionistic scientific paradigm informing agriculture informs medicine. Adding fertilizer and chemicals in agriculture, treating with drugs in medicine, are seen as the answer. However, as we have mentioned before, these approaches are proving to be problematic. If not sustainable in agriculture, when we thought it was, is it not the same thing in medicine? Few doctors know about diet, nutritional deficiencies (for example vitamin D deficiency) or heavy metal toxicities. The body, depleted of nutrients, is the 'soil' into which we're putting drugs. It has been pointed out that much of what we discussed around soil health could apply to human health: just as a fertile soil can deliver nutritious food better than one which is fed fertilizers, the body fed the right nutrients will be able to function better at all levels and be able to resist diseases and be healthier. Treating disease using drugs without correcting the malfunction at the level of the system, and without optimizing nutrient deficiencies, makes no more sense that trying to grow good quality food on soil which is mineral rich through fertilizers, but of poor quality. There are many problems related to soil degradation, according to Professor Swilling: "If we want food security, we must grow more food by restoring the soils. That's a completely different phrase from 'food production which minimizes environmental damage'. You don't restore soils by slowing down destruction. Less bad is just as bad. You need good. And so we asked, is there a science that allows you to conceive of soils so you can use them in such a way that it restores them? And there is a body of science emerging, called agro-ecology (1)."

Similarly, in medicine there is a more integrative way: instead of using drugs to block functions and treat symptoms, we improve health through various means and take a systems approach to dysfunction. "Agro-ecology returns to science and the information needed for advancement; but we need more than reductionistic science; we need systems thinking – for example moisture sensors to tell us when to irrigate. We need the added intelligence of information technology on how to use natural resources."

RESTORATION

The agro-ecological revolution is a paradigmatic shift, and it boils down to moving soil biology into soil science and displacing soil chemistry. "You start taking into account the full life of the soil, not just the NPK (Nitrogen, Phosphorus, Potassium), but soil organic matter, microbes, humus content, filtration, all the dynamics of soil, treating it as a living organism with its own life. Once you've made that paradigm shift, you can start to understand why adding more NPK actually makes things worse," states Professor Swilling. "Once you realize you have to treat the whole soil in an holistic way, you bring animals and bees in, plant the right trees around to capture nitrogen out of the air, then you have a way of thinking about restoration of soils as a means for producing healthier foods."

In our discussions it was agreed there was a parallel in the way integrative medicine thought about health and healing and the emphasis needs to shift away from the end point/disease model towards improving the 'soil' in an holistic way. Making the shift, however, is a process. While agro-ecology is becoming more mainstream intellectually, in practice it's not how agriculture works. It is a completely schizophrenic environment; the world of what should happen is different to the world of real power, who owns the land and who plants the seed and who buys the product.

In health care there is talk about lifestyle change and doctors know about lifestyle change, but few use it. It is still not part of medical training. The same thing is happening in the medical chain as in the food chain – pharmaceutical companies dictate what research is done and this tends to direct what treatment is followed, and medical doctors then follow the various protocols suggested by their peers.

In our discussions it was noted that, particularly in medicine, it is "both and". Professor McLachlan stated:

> "You cannot throw out everything, but the question is how do you bring them together? A real understanding of how biology works, how everything is interrelated, is where the next leap is going to be". "What we are seeing now is an intellectual understanding, but the real deep mindset change - what it says about our relationship to the earth, how humans are on the earth - has not happened yet. It's like we are seeing practices, scientists understand it, but our psychology is out of whack: we still have the mindset, we still want instant, still want quick. We don't know where our food comes from. If we think about the chemicals we use, we are mining the only earth we have."

While many have heard of "peak oil", few know about peak phosphorus, which has serious implications for agriculture and food. Unlike nitrogen, phosphorus does not exist in the atmosphere or disperse after use. It gets mined, transformed for use in agriculture, embodied in food and ends up in toxic concentrations in our rivers, lakes and oceans after leaching out from the soils or being processed through our bodies and the sewage treatment systems of the world's cities and towns. The problem is that phosphorus – like oil – is a finite resource.

> "We're using all this stuff, but we don't think: what does it mean to be humans on the earth? There are pockets where discussions are happening – the challenge is to develop that kind of consciousness. We haven't challenged fundamental beliefs in a linear, cause-and-effect world, in which you as an atom are more important than the molecule of which you are a part of. As long as that paradigm isn't challenged, all the rest is something we put on top, and we haven't fundamentally changed the way we engage with the world (1)."

INDIVIDUAL AND CONTEXT

An important element in a paradigm shift is the idea that in medicine doctors are dealing with individuals, and no two individuals are bio-identical. The notion of biological individuality is upsetting for researchers, as it makes nonsense of much research, which looks at groups, not individuals. Dr. Brom observed:

> "There is not one diet for everyone; statins work for one, not the next. I don't treat sinusitis, I treat the person and may not treat the sinus, but rather the GI tract. You have to see the whole problem. But medicine has stepped away from that and tends to stick to a narrow focus by its concentration on disease diagnosis."

> "Yes, you take the results of something, and say it's 'the truth', rather than it's the best evidence we have. We live in a world which believes there is one way of knowing, that is the current scientific paradigm, and it's the only way. It's not wrong, it's just not complete." (1)

A key element of the paradigm shift in agro-ecology is that 'context matters'. High external input (HEI) agriculture tried to eliminate context: that is, that no matter where you farm, micro-ecology is irrelevant, local varieties are irrelevant, everyone must use the same seed; the soil may have slight variations, but you adjust that with chemicals. In agro-ecology, each specific locality, each hectare is different. The reason why agric-ecology is more favourable to small farmers is this focus on context: small farmers have greater micro-knowledge of their small patch; they have to maximize output. Agro-ecology is dependent on local knowledge for context to figure out what applications or systems you need to maximise production.

Across all paradigms there is a shift from generality to context; but we cannot do anything without maps and models to establish general trends, and to train professionals to relate to the general trend by being able to read them.

TRANSITIONS

Having established the need for change, we used the idea of "transitions" (1) to find out how transitions can happen. It was realized that you have to get into the interactions between epochs: there's a broad historical macro-trajectory, referred to as 'landscape'. The next level down is 'regime': a configuration of norms, regulations, ways of doing things, technologies - what you would call the existing health paradigm. The paradigm sits inside a broad landscape, the larger epochal historical framework. The important thing is the 'niche': regimes are not going to change, change comes from niches, when nodes start to coalesce to explore alternatives as the landscape puts pressure on the regime. Niches are the places where it is possible to create Otto Scharmer's "landing strips for the future" (6).

Nodes are small groups of people looking at different ways of doing things. This could be NGOs, eco-villages, alternative energy, alternative ways of growing food. Alternative ways of thinking are protected from the market, and some start bursting out, such as solar energy which is now becoming big business. However, this still fits into the techno-fix mentality.

> "The real shift needs to be in our consumerist lifestyle and to change the drive for high consumption requires us to reprogramme satisfactions. We need to ask, how do we live on the earth (1)?"

This takes us back to the need for new measures of "growth". Measures of contentment, quality of life and how to assess that come to the fore. The idea of a "happiness index" or "Genuine Progress Indicator" rather than GDP/capita is now entering mainstream discussions.

Cultural transitions include a redefinition of what everyday life means: contentment, generosity; living life in a way that restores, in community; re-establishing ecologies – restoring systems. In all fields of life, whether it be agriculture or health or whatever, new ways of doing things are required.

> "To farm sustainably means working with rather than against nature, and this can only happen if agro-ecological systems are understood as complex systems"

In a similar vein, healing the body sustainably means working with rather than against nature, and this can only happen if human body systems are understood as complex systems.

We also discussed our relationship with nature. We are a community of subjects, not a community of objects. You need to see yourself as embedded in the unique local ecology.

> "If we see ourselves extended, as the other, and we don't see my skin as the end of my body, and we don't see the mind as being in one place, there is little room for self-importance. Our story is the world's story. This allows for exploring the unknown through daily practices, activism, changing things and moving to radically pragmatic alternatives, and being authentically with self. In our world today 85% of resources are consumed by 20% of the population. The hunger for more 'stuff' is problematic. It's not fashionable to scale down. It's not the poor screwing things up, it's not animals, it's really us as people who consume too much" (8) this should be 7

We were left with the question: Who is responsible for change? And a thought: There is no single leader, no single text, no single modus operandi driving change. When Paul

Hawken wrote a book to analyze this question (5) this should be 8,not 5 he entitled it ÏBlessed UnrestÒ. We can choose to be part of the transition by being part of this global grassroots movement of change to work with, rather than against, nature.

REFERENCES

[1] Discussion held with Professor Mark Swilling, Dr Bernard Brom, Professor Milla McLachlan and Jeanne Viall in October 2010 in Stellenbosch to examine questions around sustainability and medicine.

[2] Verkerk R. Can the failing western medical paradigm be shifted using the principle of sustainability? Aust Coll Nutr Environ Med 2009;28(3):4-10.

[3] International Assessment of Agricultural Knowledge, Science and Technology for Development. Agriculture at a crossroads: The global report. Johannesburg, SA: IAASTD, 2009.

[4] Swilling M, Annecke E. Just transitions. Explorations of sustainability in an unfair world. Cape Town: Juta, 2011.

[5] Patel R. Stuffed and starved: Markets, power and the hidden battle for the world's food system. London: Portobello, 2009.

[6] Scharmer O. Theory U. Learning from the future as it emerges. Cambridge, MA: Society Organisational Learning, 2007:18.

[7] Anneke, E. Presentation on sustainability. Forum for a Changing Health Paradigm, Stanford, South Africa, 2010.

[8] Hawken P. Blessed unrest. How the largest movement in the world came into being and why no one saw it coming. New York: Viking Press, 2007.

Submitted: May 01, 2011.
Revised: June 01, 2011.
Accepted: June 10, 2011.

In: Alternative Medicine Research Yearbook 2012
Editors: Søren Ventegodt and Joav Merrick

ISBN: 978-1-62808-080-3
© 2013 Nova Science Publishers, Inc.

Chapter 7

THE SCIENCE OF THE ART OF MEDICINE

Bernard Brom, MB ChB (UCT), CEDH (France) and Dip Acup[*]
Private practice, Dennesig, Stellenbosch, South Africa

ABSTRACT

Health and disease remain an enigma. We seem no closer to understanding the cause of most ill health and disease. Medical interventions in the form of drugs, surgery, and investigations now contribute to an enormous amount of ill-health, and even death. This even has a name, iatrogenic disease. Science it seems has a downside, or perhaps there are just limits to what can be known.

Keywords: Medicine, integrative medicine, alternative medicine

INTRODUCTION

The rapidity with which science has advanced has created the idea that we know so much that there is not much more that needs to be known, and that the basic laws of the universe are already sufficient for scientists to move rapidly ahead to ever more complex tools, equipment and machines.

The same approach is expected of medical scientists, who are expected to create more effective drugs, better diagnostic equipment and tests and better surgical techniques which are less invasive. Medical scientists have mapped the genome, discovered more of the biochemical pathways within the body, the complex nature of the interactions of hormones and the almost miraculous nature of brain function.

Yet despite all these advances in medical science, health and disease remain an enigma. We seem no closer to understanding the cause of most ill health and disease. Medical interventions in the form of drugs, surgery, and investigations now contribute to an enormous

---

[*] Correspondence: Bernard Brom, MB ChB (UCT), CEDH (France), Dip Acup, POBox 2229, Dennesig, Stellenbosch, 7601 South Africa. E-mail: bernard@creatinghealth.co.za.

amount of ill-health, and even death. This even has a name, iatrogenic disease. Science it seems has a downside, or perhaps there are just limits to what can be known.

LIMITS OF SCIENCE

Newtonian science made reality seem quite simple. Like billiard balls moving around a table, knowing a few easily measurable numbers such as weight, direction, speed etc, it was possible to predict what could happen to the ball. Human beings are however much more complex than billiard balls and the deeper science went, the more complex things became, not only for living systems, but even for the simple billiard ball. The fact is that turbulence, irregularity and unpredictability are now recognised to be everywhere and will constantly confound all our efforts to make absolute sense of the world. Weather prediction still remains a prediction despite all the satellites in the sky. This suggests that in the end it is just a good guess, based on some very complex measurements. The observer in the form of the meteorologist is still required to use his/her experience in order to read the signs and numbers. This is due to the fact that complex systems are so complex and so many factors are involved at any one time that no one can predict how a small shift in the weather will eventually manifest as a storm or just peter out and disappear. Edward Lorenz, a meteorologist, introduced the world of scientists to "chaos theory" and the "butterfly effect", showing that long-range weather forecasting could never be perfect, but just a good guess.

Chaos theory is not suggesting that the world is chaotic but that so many things are happening in every moment that it is impossible to measure or know all the factors involved in weather control. The science of weather prediction is thus limited to an increasingly sophisticated measuring technology but also an increasingly limited prediction ability, where experience and gut feeling become just as important. The more information and experience we have, the better our guess is likely to be.

EVIDENCE-BASED MEDICINE

The conventional medical model is sometimes referred to as the biomedical model, and still insists on following the deterministic laws postulated by Descartes in the 17th century. The four essentials of the scientific method as postulated by Descartes are the following:

- Accepting only that which is clear in the mind
- Breaking down large problems into smaller ones
- Arguing from the simple to the complex
- Repeatability

These essentials of Descartes were the early stirrings of the scientific method, which led to the following approaches over the subsequent centuries:

- Reason and logic - mathematics and statistics.
- Reductionism - breaking wholes into their constituent parts.

The science of the art of medicine

- Examining the parts - using this information to understand the whole.
- Reproducibility

Reason and logic dealing with reality confines itself to the objective world. It is here that Newtonian physics is admirably useful and had laid the basis for the rapid advances seen in the early part of the last century. The objectification of medicine had established the diagnosis of disease as a priority. The earlier idea of "humors", with its vague edges and subjective approaches, was replaced by an objective concept of "disease" which could be clearly defined and measured. The sickness became more important than the sick.

> "The concept of disease is now so pervasively woven into the fabric of medicine that it is almost impossible to imagine the practice of medicine without considering the disease..." wrote Tavassoli in 1987. Before the 19th century, physicians dealt with the sick, and not the sickness. This is in contrast to our time when we delve so deeply into the disease that the patient frequently remains out of focus. The 'disease' as an entity with an identity independent of the patient did not exist" (1).

The focus on disease resulted in doctors spending most of their clinical time trying to find this disease, and writing out a script to treat the disease. The cause of disease became lost in the process, and so did the mechanism leading up to the disease. The patient became much less important.

The idea of a patient-centred medicine has become necessary to combat the scientific rationale that the disease is what counts, rather than the patient.

In seeking to find the disease the machine metaphor was applied: The human being was like a machine which could be taken apart and the various parts examined in order to establish how the human machine body worked. This idea has indeed been most helpful and established the field of physiology, anatomy and biochemistry. The idea was that by understanding the parts, the whole would be better understood. While this idea has been extremely helpful, it has major limitations with regard to living systems. The focus on parts misses out the way the system operates as a whole. There is a major difference between a mixture and a compound. In a mixture each different substance functions in its own way according to its own particular nature. In a compound each individual item gives up, as it were, its own individual property to the whole, and new properties develop which were not there before. Examining oxygen and hydrogen, for example, will not give much indication about the properties of water, which now has new emergent properties that could not have been deduced from examining oxygen and hydrogen. So while every "normal" human being may have certain biochemical features in common, the way all the different features come together and respond will always be unique, in each and every case. Human individuality is remarkable for its uniqueness and no two individuals will be the same.

Keeping the above in mind, one can then understand that reproducibility of living systems is a scientist's dream only. In the real world no such thing is possible. An individual, for example, that responds to a placebo may not respond again when the test is repeated. Even experiments in laboratories may show a high degree of difference when repeated. By using large numbers and various statistical manipulations the difficulties inherent in living systems and especially human beings is ironed out, and reproducibility suddenly appears, But at the individual level and in small numbers, the true variation, complexity and chaotic appearances become more obvious.

GOING DEEPER

Going deeper means recognising the unique nature of each person, both physically, emotionally and mentally. At the physical level, despite being classified as "normal" each person exhibits a unique fingerprint, unique biochemical profile, unique anatomical features and unique genetic profile. This shows itself also in the way each person's system functions and responds to environment, food, micro-organisms and a range of different stressors. At the emotional level, each person is unique and will respond in a particular, characteristic way. At the mental and spiritual level, again, there are a range of specific and non-specific responses.

QUANTUM SCIENCE

On another level, quantum science has also discovered the very strange nature of matter, and even here reproducibility is a strange affair. The very act of observation has an influence on the outcomes (the observer and what is observed) and particles are affected by the movement of other particles at a distance (Bell's Theorem). This effect is even immediate.

The science of medicine as indicated above has major limitations that need to be recognised. In a recent paper describing the enormous advances of technology as applied to medicine combining different streams in new and creative ways, the author concludes with the following statement:

" …but it will always be the clinician's skill and art that counts most" (2)

Most doctors, I think, would agree with this statement, yet few acknowledge it enough in peer-reviewed journals, where personal opinion is not encouraged. What does it actually mean to talk about the art of medicine as opposed to the science of medicine?

Science: "Systemized knowledge derived from observation, study and experimentation" (Collins Dictionary): Words which characterize science: objectivity, energy, fields, chemistry, anatomy, impersonal, nature is mechanical, reductionistic, basic building blocks, human beings are bodies and chemistry, parts, experiment, research, logic.

Art: "Human creative skill or its application" (Collins Dictionary): Words which characterize art: sacred, meaning, spirit, experience, inspiration, knowing, relationship, the journey, dance, passion, mystical, insight, holistic.

Using language and logic there is a way of separating these two ways of doing things, but in the real world this becomes very difficult. In the effort to make medicine a pure scientific endeavour, scientists must leave out all that one may call "art" for the sake of the science. But in doing this the scientist is no longer dealing with the real world, unless the scientist believes that the real world is made of objects only that can be subjected to scientific research. Human beings, however, are not machines, but open systems with connections to the outer world, and an inner world full of mystery where consciousness reigns supreme.

MEDICAL SCIENCE

Is there a way of using scientific principles to enter the unknown? Clearly all scientific discoveries have happened because the most creative scientists have explored areas which other scientists have not dreamed of exploring.

In order to do this they have used human faculties which are well known but not acknowledged in scientific papers. Imagination, intuition and even mind-altering substances have been ways to get around the logical mind and access the unknown, The logical mind uses thought strung out in linear patterns to make sense of the world, but that is only one way of knowing. Weather forecasting as indicated above reminds us of the chaotic potential always present. In the end it is a good guess, based on experience and the numbers generated by computers. Logic always has its own limitations.

The thinking mind will always be limited. Entering the unknown is about slipping through the threads of logic and using faculties that are not uncommon to all of life, and may even have preceded logical thinking.

The way animals for example find food, migrate, fly, escape from danger may all be examples of using non-linear ways of operating. The right brain works differently to the left brain. The human "mind" probably works as a whole in which right and left brain complement each other. The problem comes about when the left brain using logic denies the inspiration and intuitive thrust it receives from the right brain. Scientists do this every day when they write articles and exclude from the article any indication of inspiration and intuition, and use large numbers and statistics to create a sense of uniformity and repeatability of results.

The science of the art of medicine is all about honouring these strange and immeasurable qualities that lie behind creative science, and using these qualities to approach the unknown.

THE UNKNOWN

The unknown is clearly unknown. One can say that the unknown is in the process of becoming known, and there still may be a great deal that will remain unknowable. The science of complexity suggests that the real world is in fact so complex and chaotic that it will always remain unknowable. By definition "infinity" cannot be finite and therefore will remain unknown, except as a mathematical formula. Any suggestion that the infinite or unknowable has no influence on what can be measured and known by science seems highly unlikely.

The quantum potential is another name for the unknowable. Giving it a name (like infinity) does not mean that we know exactly what we are talking about. What it does mean is that we have enlarged our world view and can find ways of relating to this potential. Intuition, imagination, inspiration may all be ways of accessing information and finding ways to relate to our own hidden potential. This is also the science of the art of medicine. It is the way shamans, traditional healers, spiritual seekers and healers have researched life to discover its hidden depths.

Modern medical science, by denying these human attributes, leaves out our most treasured gifts and reduces humans to physical machines.

THE MAP IS NOT THE TERRITORY

Maps are essential and help create order of the chaotic view of life. Without maps we would soon get lost, or take a whole lifetime to get to where we want to get, but the map is not the territory. Words are not the experience. Logic and mathematics is all about map making. The work of the left brain is to make maps of reality, but the maps are not the reality. One needs to learn driving from a book, and use the logical mind, but somewhere along the way it becomes necessary to drop the logical mind and start driving with right and left brain working together. In fact left brain in the best drivers probably takes a back seat. To be present in the NOW requires the thinking mind to be out of the way in order to allow the creative, non linear mind to operate. The territory can only be entered without the mapping, thinking mind.

INTEGRATIVE WAY

Integrative medicine acknowledges the complex nature of the human being. It recognises the unique nature of each individual. At the individual level one is always dealing with the unknown. The cause of ill health involves a whole range of factors, and in each individual the background causes will be unique. Searching for a single cause for each disease will only reveal the complexity of that person. Food choices, exercise, weight, smoking, toxin exposure, climate, genetics, nutritional status, sun exposure, pollution, electromagnetic influence, emotions, world view, childhood, birth trauma etc will all be responsible for that person's ill health, and it will be a unique combination of these, together with the body's fundamental response that will dictate the direction and end point of the disorder. Medical scientists will never find a single cause for each person's ill health, or even for a particular disease. There will always be a whole range of confounding factors.

In the doctor-client interaction there is the acknowledgement of the full potential hidden in each person and that the disease is only a part of the whole drama. Integrative doctors do have maps (practice guidelines, holistic diagnosis approaches, lifestyle management procedures, various techniques etc) but they also understand that so much is unknown that they remain open-minded and open-hearted (left and right brain functioning) to the process of listening and responding to the client's particular story, and the direction in which it needs to go.

In this approach science has two arms. The first is the conventional approach using measurements and the understanding gained from conventional scientific investigation using large numbers and statistics. The second arm is what is gained by experience over many years, and applying wisdom and compassion to the needs of the client.

REFERENCES

[1]   Tavassoli M. The concept of disease and the birth of modern medicine. Adler Museum Bull 1987;13(2):48.
[2]   Freiherr G.3-D ultrasound: will it become a clinical tool? Diagn Imaging (San Franc) 1998;20(7):52-7.

Submitted: May 01, 2011.

Revised: June 15, 2011.
Accepted: June 24, 2011.

In: Alternative Medicine Research Yearbook 2012
Editors: Søren Ventegodt and Joav Merrick

ISBN: 978-1-62808-080-3
© 2013 Nova Science Publishers, Inc.

Chapter 8

ON THE PARADIGM OF CONSCIOUSNESS-BASED MEDICINE AND QUALITY OF LIFE AS MEDICINE

Søren Ventegodt, MD, MMedSci, EU-MSc-CAM[1,2,3,4,5]*

[1]Quality of Life Research Center, Copenhagen, Denmark
[2]Research Clinic for Holistic Medicine
[3]Nordic School of Holistic Medicine, Copenhagen, Denmark
[4]Scandinavian Foundation for Holistic Medicine, Sandvika, Norway and
[5]Interuniversity College, Graz, Austria

ABSTRACT

Quality of life as medicine is a classical strategy of improving health by improving life in general. It has been used by physicians in Europe since Hippocrates and by medicine men, shamans, African Traditional Healers, druids and healers in all known pre-modern cultures. The physician can intervene in the philosophy of life of his patient, state of consciousness, state of existence, or in the quality of life, subjective mental and physical health, and subjective ability of social, sexual, work-related and study-related functioning. Any interventions that will improve one or more of these factors are likely to also improve objective health and survival. The physician using quality of life as medicine is basically intervening at the level of consciousness and lifestyle, encouraging the patient's exploration of self, leading to increased self-awareness and self-insight. A better understanding of a person's own talents and physical, mental, spiritual and sexual character leads to a more loving and generous attitude, better use of character and talents in all relationships. The improved creation of value to self and others leads to an improved quality of life, which leads to better physical and mental health. Interventions help the patients address one of the following dimensions: Philosophy of life: a) conception of life; b) conceptions of self; c) conception of the surrounding world; State of consciousness: positive doing, positive being and existential healing (salutogenesis); State of being: subjective mental health, subjective physical health, quality of life, and subjective ability of functioning (social, sexual, work-related, study-related etc.)

---

* Correspondence: Søren Ventegodt, MD, MMedSci, EU-MSc-CAM, Director, Quality of Life Research Center, Frederiksberg Alle 13A, 2tv, DK-1661 Copenhagen V, Denmark. E-mail: ventegodt@livskvalitet.org.

74 Søren Ventegodt

Keywords: Medicine, integrative medicine, alternative medicine, quality of life

INTRODUCTION

"Health comes from happiness; happiness comes from stepping into character, knowing all one's talents, and using these talents to create value for other people and oneself," was already said by Hippocrates in 400 BCE in the teaching of the Corpus Hippocraticum (1). Wellbeing, whether you call it happiness, satisfaction, or the meaning of life, has for a very long time been the sign of the good human life. Today we often call this dimension "quality of life". We call it quality of life because we acknowledge that it is a complex term (2). It is happiness, but sometimes even the most difficult and unhappy times carry meaning and value for us, because we learn more about life when difficulties force us to stop and reflect. This understanding of our self, other human beings and the world at large, gained from overcoming our challenges, will often lead to future happiness (3,4).

A philosophical difficulty with the concept "quality of life" is that we are human beings in space and time; we are travelers on the journey of our souls. According to the existential philosophers, even personal crises, disease and great loss can contribute to our personal development of wisdom and intimate contact with life (5,6).

Evolution is ongoing and we are all part of the creation of the future human being; therefore our personal struggles can even be seen as part of the bigger struggle of human beings to evolve to a species that can inhabit this planet in harmony with all the other species that inhabit it. Spiritual and religious people, believing in concepts like karma and divine order, would believe that the universe contains more subtle energies than just matter, and elements from the development of our consciousness are considered in the grand equation of the development of the universe (7).

In this immensely complex universe, of which contemporary science only covers a small part, we strive for order. We strive to organise our knowledge for the benefit of humanity, to facilitate growth and healing of the unhappy and the ill. A holistic medical science must therefore include as many possible layers, structures and aspects of the world, without losing simplicity, efficacy and direction (8-12).

We cannot be naïve and deny the complexity of the world or of human life. On the other hand we cannot afford to be mystics if we are to create a medical science that in a simple, rational and efficient way can guide our daily actions. So we need to simplify the world in our description to make it a science, but we also need to keep our model in accordance with truth, knowing that we always will lose some depth and truths in the process of simplification.

CASCADE OF LIFE

Seen through time, life is like a cascade. A fertilised egg becomes a conscious human being that interprets, makes choices and acts in a complex world. Actions lead to experiences, which lead to re-interpretation of the world, new choices, new actions and so forth. Sometimes we get sick, and sometimes we get better again fast. Other times we lose our health on a continuous basis though time, until we die. Other times again we are close to dying from cancer or a heart condition, but on our way down we learn something of extreme importance that allows us to turn around the sad development and regain health and happiness. Sometimes we have a bad start, with parents who are sick or dysfunctional. In spite of this we break the patterns of the family and lead great lives. Sometimes we come from the most privileged of families, with incredible wealth and unlimited possibilities for doing good, but for some inner reasons we do not appreciate what we have, and end up losing it all by for example abusing alcohol, sex and drugs.

Life is highly dynamic, and it seems that we create our own life, future and destiny though our philosophy of life, state of consciousness, strategy of self-realisation and the way we use our character and talents to be fit and able and create value in this world (13). Can the way we create or destroy our own health, happiness and ability be understood in scientific terms? Can we make the dynamic of life a science? Yes, we believe we can. During the last four or five decades about 1 million scientific papers have explored different aspects of the dynamic of human life, and quality of life is a central concept in close to 125,000 papers in biomedicine alone if you search for "quality of life" in Medline/PubMed. So we know a great deal about these dynamics now. Many research centres all over the world have started to use this knowledge to cure even the most severe diseases, like poor quality of life (14-16), chronic pain, metastatic breast cancer (17) and coronary heart disease (18,19).

Recent reviews have shown that holistic non-drug medicine can be as safe and efficient as medicine (20-27), which might be the main reason for the inclusion of mind-body medicine in the curriculum of most American medical schools (28).

The therapeutic value of medical systems based on the idea of quality of life as medicine should not surprise us too much, as all medical systems in the pre-modern cultures have used such strategies of medicine for as long as man has existed.

Modern European medicine started in Greece and was highly developed about 400 BCE, when Hippocrates and his students wrote about 70 books on the science of medicine. This well-preserved source of medicine is called the Corpus Hippocraticum and was in its time translated to all European languages, becoming the basis for European medicine for the next two millennia (1). The essence of the Greek character of medicine was that the patient was ill because he or she did not know him or herself well enough to acknowledge his/her own talents and step into character to contribute and create value in all relationships. The key to health was surprisingly simple: The physician helped the patient to gain self-insight and coached the patient to better use his or her talents on all levels of existence – physical, mental or spiritual – in all relationships, to family, friends and the world at large. Sexuality was ascribed a lot of importance, and a normal cure for female conditions of all kinds, from physical to mental illnesses, was rehabilitation of female sexuality and normal sexual function. It is clear from the writings that the concept of character included the patient's sexual character as man or woman. In today's holistic cures, ie the cure for coronary heart disease developed by Dean Ornish (18,19), the rehabilitation of a patient's ability for close emotional contact and intimacy is still a cornerstone, indicating that even the most modern of today's "quality of life as medicine" cures are paying tribute to the character medicine of Hippocrates (1).

KEY CONCEPTS

Table 1 lists the key concepts that most often have been the focus of research in human life. The table uses the somewhat artificial compartmentalisation of human existence into an inner part (life), an outer part (surrounding world), and a middle part (self). There is a strong mirroring of the inner world into the outer world, and vice versa, making such a description of a person somewhat rigid; the Asian spiritual understanding has always believed that the outer life is a materialisation of the inner life (the person's consciousness) (7). Material western cultures have often stressed the positive or negative impact of the surrounding world on the person.

**Table 1. The most important dimensions of quality
of life as medicine**

Self-rated quality of life
Philosophy of life and state of consiousness
Self-rated physican health
Self-rated mental health
Self-rated quality of human relations
Self-rated qualtiy of one-to-one relationship
Self-rated self-esteem
Self-rated sexual functioning
Self-rated social functioning
Self-rated working ability
Survival

**Table 2. Hierarchy of Outcomes – most valuable
to least valuable as documentation for *cure***

Excellent
Self-assessed global QOL
Survival
QALY (survival time x global OQL)
Good
Self-assessed sense of coherence
Self-assessed physical and mental health
Self-assessed ability of functioning (social, sexual, working/studying)
Self-reported cure from experienced severe, chronic physical or mental disease.
Fair
Objectively measured physical and mental health
Objectively measured ability of functioning (social, sexual, working/studying)
Poor
Objectively measured local aspects of health (i.e. coughing, motility etc.)
Health related QOL
Patient satisfaction

Life can be seen as a cascade in time and space that is determined by a series of factors that determines the next level, that again determines the next level etc. At each level there is inner, outer and intermediate factors called "life", "self" and "surrounding world". The subject is further complicated by interactions on all levels at all times. The physician can thus interact with a patient's philosophy of life, state of consciousness, ability to live, or his objective health and survival (see table 1). This is closely related to the hierachy of outcomes (see table 2).

The cultures of the East have always stressed the causal importance of the content of a person's consciousness, like divine potentials, the potential Buddha-hood, and karma, i.e. inherited impurities to be processed during one's lifetime. Modern western cultures stress material factors like the impact of DNA and genes on health and happiness. Most pre-modern cultures seem to agree with the eastern traditions on the importance of consciousness in the creation of a person's life and destiny.

In this article we look for a balanced view that can be accepted by people of all cultures and all over the world. We believe that the work of Aaron Antonovsky (1923-1994) (29,30) might be especially valuable as a basis for such an endeavour.

1. Early factors

Most researchers in the dynamics of life use a timeline to organise the events of life and usually start with conception (13). Materialistic researchers insist that at this point in time the only information in the zygote is carried by the DNA and the biological structures of the cell and its cytoplasm. Spiritual researchers suggest that this first cell already has a consciousness and makes conscious choices. It has been difficult for science to establish the truth regarding these matters as our science of consciousness is still insufficient for the final documentation of early consciousness. Evolutionary theory has not been able to establish the evolutionary value of consciousness, but many appealing theories have been presented that could potentially expand our understanding of the role of consciousness in evolution and individual ontogenesis.

2. Philosophy of life

As soon as the individual is established with his or her own consciousness, whether this happens at the minute of conception, in the middle of embryonic life when the brain and nerve system gets active, or early in childhood when the brain is mature, the individual starts interpreting the world and making choices that guide behaviour. To understand what is going on, the individual needs to discriminate between self and other, between me and you, internal life and external life. This need gives birth to the perception of internal life, world and self. These three fundamental dimensions of the interpretation of reality become fixed and stable in time and constitute the person's philosophy of life. This collection of ideas, conclusions and descriptions of reality is used for perception, interpretation and choice. Philosophy of life can be seen as the axioms of consciousness; the invisible structures holding the content of consciousness, very much the same way as a mathematical universe is determined by its axioms. As soon as the axioms are in place, the mathematical universe can have its content. In a similar way, the content of human consciousness is sourced by the philosophy of life.

3. The six central states of consciousness

We know our consciousness from its content; we know that we can be in different states of consciousness, and many scientists have explored altered states of consciousness, with the aim of understanding the nature of human consciousness.

Unfortunately we do not yet have a satisfactory theory of consciousness, or a science of consciousness. The deeper structures of consciousness have been subtle, elusive and hard to identify; many scientists that have pursued this endeavour have ended up using religious terms. In Table 1, three states of consciousness are listed: the salutogenetic state (5-7,31), the state of sense of coherence and the dynamic state of self-realisation using talents and character to create value for self and others.

The state of salutogenesis means the state of existential healing; it is a kind of existential crisis where you heal the damage to your existence caused by emotionally painful life-events and destructive decisions earlier in life.

The state of "sense of coherence" is a state of being where you acknowledge that you are coherent with everything else in the world; that you are an integrated part of the world and inseparable from it. The classical experience is sat-sit-ananda (to use a Hindu term), meaning "being-knowing-happiness". In many religions and pre-modern cultures this state of being is seen as "home", the natural, true state of being.

The state of self-realisation has been seen by sages, philosophers and scientists (like Buddha, Frankl, Gurdjieff, and Maslow to mention a few) as the highest obtainable state of action in the human being (5-7). In this state of consciousness you step into character and use all your talents on all levels of existence to create value for self and others. You can play music, you can be a skilful carpenter, you can dance, talk, think, write poems… it does not matter what you do, as long as you fulfill your existential determination.

To help the patient achieve these states of consciousness seems to have been crucial in non-drug medicine at all times. The physician often used a threefold strategy of helping the patient to heal, helping the patient to be and helping the patient to do. When the patient healed, being and doing improved; with improved doing and being, more resources were available for the process of healing.

If you want health and happiness, you need to shift among three positive states of consciousness: positive doing, positive being and positive re-organisation of your internal realm: existential healing or salutogenesis.

If you live in states of negative doing, negative being and negative crisis, where you continuously stretch your own existence to survive and fit to the environment, while compromising your contact to your true self, you will eventually end up with unhappiness and ill-health.

Thus good consciousness-based medicine will build you up by leading you into states of good doing, good being, and the crisis of healing; while a hard, exhausting life will take you down by leading you into the destructive states of negative doing, negative being and degenerative crises.

4. State of existence

The good life or human existence has three key dimensions: quality of life, health and ability. Poor health is often what brings the patient to the physician, but almost as often are unhappiness or problems of sexual or social functioning, or problems at work or study. You could say that the skilful physician knows how to bring health, quality of life and ability to the patient. To do this is the core of good medicine.

The same way as philosophy of life is the hidden basis of the states and contents of consciousness, the states and contents of consciousness are the hidden basis of the state of existence: the person's subjective physical and mental health, quality of life, and general ability to function.

5. Disease

If a patient is ill the patient will often also be unhappy and poorly functioning. Vice versa: it is also correct that a poorly functioning person often will be unhappy, and an unhappy patient often will be ill. We know of countless examples of this from medical science. If you are depressed you are likely to have chronic pains; if you are unhappy you are much more likely to develop cancer or a bad heart. If you have a crisis in your marriage and repress your sexuality you will become unhappy, emotionally unstable and often also depressed. We all know from personal experience that our allergy, flu or common cold comes in periods of bad thriving. It is not a new idea. It is an old truth, old as medicine itself.

Mental and physical disorders have for millennia been cured by interventions that improved quality of life and related dimensions. Often the strategy for improving health, happiness and ability has been to improve the patient's state of consciousness. This has been the basic tool of shamanistic healers, but so too have many physicians and healers worked directly with the patient's philosophy of life.

Fundamental beliefs about self, life and the world have often been found to be very negative by classical physicians, and debugging the patient's negative beliefs has been their art of medicine. If we go back to Hippocrates and his students, most of the interventions seem to address philosophy of life, while other interventions address the patient's state of consciousness and subjective feeling of health, happiness and ability.

It seems that most of the modern strategies of non-drug medicine also address all layers of human existence, both philosophy of life, state of consciousness, and the dimensions we call ability to live, or the "art of living" – subjective health, quality of life and ability in general.

6. Death

The final outcome of life, with or without disease, is death. Spiritual cultures, like the Japanese Zen tradition, describe the good death as the chosen death; often the Zen master invites his students to a special ceremony, under which he reads a Zen poem written for the occasion. After reading the poem, the Zen master simply sits down to die.

In materialistic cultures death is often seen as something bad or negative, something that should be avoided at any cost, something that only comes from disease and disaster.

We know from many studies now that the strongest predictor of survival is good self-assessed health and good quality of life (32-34). We know that people with little meaning in life often die: for example we often see disease and sudden death occurring after we have retired from work. We thus know that feeling good, healthy and actively participating in reality are important for survival. Preventive medicine is therefore about helping people to experience good health, high quality of life and a valuable presence in their world. Good and efficient non-drug medicine is about helping people to a positive philosophy of life and happy, healthy, healing states of being. Good medicine is about helping the patient to know him or herself, to self-realisation, where all talents, physical, mental and spiritual are taken into use.

The good physician helps the patient gain self-awareness and self-insight by the examination of both body, mind, spirit and whole life, together with the patient, in order for the patient to explore negative philosophy of life, destructive states of consciousness, compromised quality of life and abilities, a poor physical, mental and sexual health.

The classical tools for doing this are talk and touch. Everything can in principle be used as medicine as long as it has a positive impact on the patient's philosophy of life, state of consciousness and ability to live. A positive impact on any level will have a positive impact on subjective health, objective health and survival.

Table 3. Estimated NNT-numbers (Number Needed to Treat) of CAM treatments of physical, mental, existential and sexual health issues and working disability (mostly based on observational research, clinical studies using chronic patients as their own control, see text)

	NNT
Quality of life (QOL)	2
Physical health	2
Mental health	2
All patients	2
Self esteem	1
Working/studying ability	2
Sexual functioning	1
Specific sexual problems	
Anorgasmia	1
Sexual dysfunction	2
All sexological patients	1

EFFICACY AND SAFETY

While there is broad agreement in the literature that consciousness-based medicine (non-drug medicine) is completely harmless (35) there has been discussion about the efficiacy of this kind of medicine, and the variety of clinical conditions that can be improved by this kind of intervention. In a recent review we have analysed this and found QOL as medicine to be efficient with most clinical conditions (see table 3) (36,37).

Most of the sources are from observational research, done in rigorous research designs, making us believe in the validity of the results. If you accept this data, you will also acknowledge the fact that consciousness-based medicine is both safe, efficient and applicable in most clinical conditions. All this together might be an important reason to choose the paradigm of consciousness-based medicine and to start learning and practising quality of life as medicine.

CONCLUSION

Classical medicine has for millennia, independent of the culture you investigate, been about helping the patient back into happiness, good health and a constructive role in society by helping the patient to increased self-awareness and self-insight. The fruits of realising your own talents and character is the experience of being of value to oneself and other people – being of value in all relationships, private or professional. From the experience of this happy and constructive state of being comes all good things, a positive understanding of life, a positive state of consciousness, a positive state of existence and finally good physical and mental health, high quality of life, and excellent ability to function in all areas of life.

Whether we call this classical medicine, quality of life as medicine, consciousness-based medicine, character medicine, placebo medicine, holistic medicine or any other equivalent label, it is basically about helping the patient to know him or herself and to live in accordance with this knowledge.

Life is simple for the wise and complex for the fool. It is difficult for the person who does not understand it, and easy for the person who understands this much: that the good life comes from sharing, giving and contributing.

You could say that the good life is about loving. This might be the simplest way to express the wisdom of Hippocrates and his students, of the Native American shamans, of the African Traditional Healers, the Australian Aboriginal medicine men, the Celtic druids or the Same healers. This is also the simple message of all sages at all times and it is the core of all religions. The good healer loves his patient and this love brings back the patient's ability to love life, self and other living beings. In principle it is really that simple.

How powerful is quality of life as medicine then? If we go to religion we will hear that everything can be healed if your faith is strong enough. If we go to the most skeptical of the skeptics, you will learn that placebo has no healing power at all - at least in the form it is used in the pharmaceutical randomised clinical tests (38). We need to come to a balanced answer to this question, based on four or five decades of establishhed science in the dynamics of life.

REFERENCES

[1]   Jones WHS. Hippocrates. Vol. I–IV. London: William Heinemann, 1923-1931.
[2]   Ventegodt S. Measuring the quality of life. From theory to practice. Copenhagen: Forskningscentrets Forlag, 1996.
[3]   Kierkegaard SA. The sickness unto death. Princeton, NJ: Princeton Univ Press, 1983.

[4]   Buber M. I and thou. New York: Charles Scribner, 1970.
[5]   Maslow AH. Toward a psychology of being, New York: Van Nostrand, 1962.
[6]   Frankl V. Man´s search for meaning. New York: Pocket Books, 1985.
[7]   Goleman D. Healing emotions: Conversations with the Dalai Lama on mindfulness, emotions, and health. Boston, MA: Mind Life Inst, 1997.
[8]   Ventegodt S Kandel I Merrick J. Principles of holistic medicine. Philosophy behind quality of life. Victoria, BC: Trafford, 2005.
[9]   Ventegodt S Kandel I Merrick J. Principles of holistic medicine. Quality of life and health. New York: Hippocrates Sci Publ, 2005.
[10]   Ventegodt S Kandel I Merrick J. Principles of holistic medicine. Global quality of life. Theory, research and methodology. New York: Hippocrates Sci Publ, 2006.
[11]   Ventegodt S Merrick J. Principles of holistic psychiatry. A textbook on holistic medicine for mental disorders. New York: Nova Science, 2011.
[12]   Ventegodt S Merrick J. Sexology from a holistic point of view. A textbook of classic and modern sexology. New York: Nova Science, 2011.
[13]   Ventegodt S Flensborg-Madsen T Andersen NJ Nielsen Morad M Merrick J. Global quality of life (QOL), health and ability are primarily determined by our consciousness. Research findings from Denmark 1991-2004. Soc Indicator Res 2005;71;87-122.
[14]   Fernros L,Furhoff AK Wändell PE. Quality of life of participants in a mind-body-based self-development course: a descriptive study. Qual Life Res 2005;14(2):521-8.
[15]   Fernros L Furhoff AK Wändell PE Improving quality of life using compound mind-body therapies: evaluation of a course intervention with body movement and breath therapy, guided imagery, chakra experiencing and mindfulness meditation. Qual Life Res 2008;17(3):367-76.
[16]   Fernros L. Improving quality of life with body-mind therapies. The evaluation of a course intervention for personal self-awareness and development. Dissertation. Stockholm: Karolinska Institutet, 2009. Accessed 01 May 2011. URL: http://diss.kib.ki.se/2009/978-91-7409-356-8/
[17]   Spiegel D Bloom JR Kraemer H Gottheil E Effect of psychosocial treatment on survival of patients with metastatic breast cancer. Lancet 1989;2(8668):888–91.
[18]   Ornish D Brown SE Scherwitz LW Billings JH Armstrong WT Ports TA et al. Can lifestyle changes reverse coronary heart disease? Lancet 1990;336(8708):129–33.
[19]   Ornish D. Love and survival. The scientific basis for the healing power of intimacy. Perennial, NY: HarperCollins 1999
[20]   Harrington A. The cure within: a history of mind-body medicine. New York: WW Norton, 2008.
[21]   Goleman D Gurin J Connellan H. Mind, body medicine: How to use your mind for better health. New York: Consumer Reports Books, 1993.
[22]   Sobel DS. Mind matters, money matters: The cost-effectiveness of mind/body medicine. JAMA 2000;284(13):1704.
[23]   Astin JA Shapiro SL Eisenberg DM Forys KL. Mind-body medicine: State of the science, implications for practice. J Am Board Fam Pract 2003;16:131-47.
[24]   Bø K, Berghmans B Mørkved S Van Kampen M. Evidence-based physical therapy for the pelvic floor. Bridging science and clinical practice. New York: Butterworth Heinemann Elsevier, 2007.
[25]   Vickers A Zollman C. ABC of complementary medicine. Massage therapies. BMJ 1999;319(7219):1254-7.
[26]   Ventegodt S Omar HA Merrick J. Quality of life as medicine: Interventions that induce salutogenesis. A review of the literature. Soc Indicator Res, in press.
[27]   Ventegodt S Merrick J. A Review of side effects and adverse events of non-drug medicine (non-pharmaceutical complementary and alternative medicine): Psychotherapy, mind-body medicine and clinical holistic medicine. J Complement Integr Med 2009;6(1):16.
[28]   Wetzel MS Eisenberg DM Kaptchuk TJ. Courses involving complementary and alternative medicine at US medical schools. JAMA 1998;280(9):784-7.
[29]   Antonovsky A. Health, stress and coping. London: Jossey-Bass, 1985.
[30]   Antonovsky A. Unravelling the mystery of health. How people manage stress and stay well. San Francisco: Jossey-Bass, 1987.

On the paradigm of consciousness-based medicine

[31] Long MJ, McQueen DA, Banga-lore VG, Schurman JR2nd. Using self-assessed health to predict patient outcomes after total knee replacement. Clin Orthop Relat Res 2005;434:189-92.

[32] Idler EL Russell LB Davis D. Survival, functional limitations, and self-rated health in the NHANES I epidemiologic follow-up study, 1992. First national health and nutrition examination survey. Am J Epidemiol 2000;152 (9):874-83.

[33] Idler EL Kasl S. Health perceptions and survival: do global evaluations of health status really predict mortality? J Gerontol 1991;46(2):S55-65.

[34] Burström B Fredlund P. Self-rated health: Is it as good a predictor of subsequent mortality among adults in lower as well as in higher social classes. J Epidemiol Community Health 2001;55(11):836-40.

[35] Ventegodt S Merrick J. A Review of side effects and adverse events of non-drug medicine (nonpharmaceutical complementary and alternative medicine): Psychotherapy, mind-body medicine and clinical holistic medicine. J Complement Integr Med 2009;6(1):16.

[36] Ventegodt S Omar H Merrick J. Quality of life as medicine. Soc Indicator Res 2011;100:415-33.

[37] Ventegodt S Andersen NJ Kandel I Merrick J. Effects, side effects and adverse events of non-pharmaceutical medicine. A review. Int J Disabil Hum Dev 2009;8(3):227-35.

[38] Hròbjartsson A Gøtzsche PC. Placebo interventions for all clinical conditions. Cochrane Database Syst Rev 2004;(3):CD003974.

Submitted: May 05, 2011.
Revised: June 20, 2011.
Accepted: June 28, 2011.

In: Alternative Medicine Research Yearbook 2012
Editors: Søren Ventegodt and Joav Merrick

ISBN: 978-1-62808-080-3
© 2013 Nova Science Publishers, Inc.

Chapter 9

THE MATTER-ENERGY-INFORMATION (MEI) BODY OF THE HUMAN BEING

Bernard Brom, MB ChB (UCT), CEDH (France) and Dip Acup[*]
Private practice, Dennesig, Stellenbosch, South Africa

ABSTRACT

Despite the enormous advances made in medicine during the last century, chronic ill health remains a major challenge, consuming an increasing amount of the national budgets in most countries of the world. The main emphasis of healthcare is on the management, treatment and (some) prevention of disease rather than on the promotion or enhancement of health. Medicine today has become so specialised that most doctors do not realise how narrow their field of interest has become, and that pharmaceutical companies, by financing most research, have tended to monopolise the education of medical students. This needs to change if medical scientists are hoping to find answers to cancer and many of the other diseases which contribute to the increasing burden of chronic disease today. One cannot expect biochemists to have all the answers when dealing with the complex human being. Biochemistry is not all there is and moves much too slowly throughout the body to be able to maintain homeostasis in a system that requires instant communication throughout its domain. Electricity, magnetism and light offer not only a powerful way of understanding the complex dynamics of the human organism, but also new possibilities of integrating the present approaches to management with complementary electromagnetic tools and low energy lasers. It is probably only in the domain of energy-information medicine that we will find a way of incorporating consciousness.

Keywords: Medicine, integrative medicine, alternative medicine, energy medicine

---

[*] Correspondence: Bernard Brom, MB ChB (UCT), CEDH (France), Dip Acup, POBox 2229, Dennesig, Stellenbosch, 7601 South Africa. E-mail: bernard@creatinghealth.co.za.

INTRODUCTION

The biomedical model (or biomedicine) that dominated medical thinking during most of the twentieth century has been the basis of medical education, and initiated enormous advances in technology, surgery, pharmacology and genetics, which have been life-saving and contributed considerably to the extension of human life span. The problem with biomedicine is that it is based on a reductionistic Newtonian paradigm, which places too much emphasis on easily identifiable diseases of the body, leading to the de-personalisation of the patient.

During the latter part of the twentieth century the bio-psycho-social approach came to the fore. It shifted the focus towards the patient and to the recognition that the environment also contributed to health and ill health. Today this approach forms the basis of curricula at many medical schools all over the world. While the bio-psycho-social approach is more holistic, and medical students get a more rounded and inclusive education, health in general is not improving. More and more money is spent on medicine, while diseases, such as heart disease, diabetes and cancer are on the increase. The economic nature of medical practice continues to reduce the amount of time a doctor spends with the patient. A ten to fifteen minute consultation unavoidably means that "disease" is still a priority, for which the easiest answer is a pharmacological product. The emphasis of medicine is still on measurable "materialistic" aspects, such as matter embodied in molecules, cells, body parts and pharmacological products, and energy variations, such as electromagnetic (heat, light, etc), electrical (stimulation and diagnosis), or mechanical (motion, sound, etc) energy. In general these energy variations are often high-powered and invasive, such as electroconvulsive therapy and high powered lasers used in surgery, while the "softer" varieties are used by integrative doctors, physiotherapists and other health practitioners to stimulate healing, for example ultrasound therapy, low energy lasers and low energy electrical devices.

Many people are beginning to realise that matter and energy are much more complex than we thought, and should not simply be used in isolation. Niels Bohr, the Nobel Prize winner of physics said: "There is no such thing as matter ...all is energy". Ervin Laszlo, of the Club of Rome, in his book "Quantum Shift in the Global Brain" (1) pointed out that "matter is vanishing as a fundamental feature of reality, retreating before energy, and continuous fields are replacing discrete particles as the basic elements of an energy-bathed and information-filled universe". A group of authors from the universities of Cape Town and Sydney with their biomatrix theory (2) has suggested that the substance of life in the universe is actually an inseparable amalgam of matter-energy-information, which they called "MEI" (3). Life is a pattern of MEI. The biomatrix theory incorporated the idea of MEI and systems theory with ideas of webs, flowing systems, networks and patterns of organisation. When living systems die, the pattern is destroyed and we are left only with components. Fritjof Capra in his bestseller "The web of life" (4) argued that there needs to be a synthesis of two very different approaches, the study of substance (or structure) and the study of form (or pattern). Patterns, he points out, cannot be measured or weighed; they must be mapped.

A new modality of medicine that many doctors are already using successfully in their practices is so-called "bioenergy medicine". Although its name indicates a focus on energy, the author believes that it is based on a paradigm that takes the unity of MEI into consideration. The interchangeability between the components of MEI allows very small amounts of energy to be used for considerable information transfer that can be useful in the healing process. Perhaps a better name for this modality would be "matter-energy-information medicine" or simply "MEI medicine". The aim of this paper is to discuss some examples of this exciting new modality, through which one might explain the way stress and personal loss can lead to disease, and even throw light on some hitherto mystical methods such as healing through prayer, love, positive thinking, placebo and willpower.

Bioenergy medicine shifts the focus from an emphasis on matter as being the cause of "the disease" to the possible role of MEI as the underlying problem in ill health. Practitioners using these approaches have found that low-level energy variations carrying information can cause measurable physiological changes over time, and are acceptable to the body because of their non-invasive properties.

In this article I will discuss some of the "MEI" modalities in use by practitioners with special reference to studies that have been done.

ENERGY INFORMATIONAL MEDICINE

The biomedical model is about matter and energy, nevertheless medical doctors as taught in medical school still follow a model of medicine which studies human beings as matter, searching for the "disease" which can be controlled with drugs, destroyed with radiation or removed with surgery. The early Newtonian science model still pervades the corridors of medical schools and the central premise of this approach, as referred to by the celebrated physicist Richard Feynman (5) - that things exist independently of each other - still dominates a great deal of modern medicine. Students coming out of medical school are still tremendously influenced by the mechanistic and reductionistic view that underlies classical physics, reducing complex phenomena to basic building blocks and looking for mechanisms through which these interact. These building blocks and mechanisms are generally seen as matter working on matter.

Modern science on the other hand is no longer stuck in the machine model and this is largely due to an understanding of energy-information and systems theory, flowing systems that are connected and interdependent. Medical scientists do study chemical energy (ATP and related compounds), mechanical energy (heart and muscle movement), concentration energy (diffusion, osmosis, active transport etc), electrical energy (osmosis, nerve conduction), electromagnetic energy (heat, UV activation of vitamin D etc). Nevertheless the basic premise of medical school education does not include an understanding of how matter, energy and information flows, controls and influences the nature of health and ill health.

While scientists have worked out ways to use energy, energy itself is an enigma. Richard Feynman (5,6) the physicist said: "It is important to realize that in physics today we have no knowledge of what energy is. We do not have a picture that energy comes in little blobs of a definitive amount." David Ross, MIT engineering professor, added (6): "Energy is an abstract concept invented by physical scientists in the 19th century to describe quantitatively a wide variety of natural phenomenon." So scientists know what energy can do, but very little about what it is. This makes the study of "bioenergy" difficult, and is why it is possible for everyone to use "energy" terminology but often mean different things which may not make sense to most scientists.

There is a recognised relationship between matter and energy as defined by Einstein, and matter can be transformed into energy and vice versa. At the same time we know that energy carries information. Matter-energy-information is thus inseparable, the substance of life. Some substances are more matter dense and low in information (rocks) while other phenomena are low in matter-energy but high in information (psychic phenomenon, homeopathic medicines, e-mails). Still in other situations we can see high energy-information, but low levels of matter (laser). The relationship between energy and information may vary. For example, the information in low energy lasers is used to stimulate healing, while the ratio between energy and information is very different to high energy lasers, which are used as surgical knives with the aim of coagulating and thus destroying tissue.

These new insights gained about matter, energy and information and their intrinsic relationship could help to shift and enlarge our understanding of the human being. Human life is a manifestation of the flow of MEI. Sometimes it reveals itself as matter through its physical, observable, touchable form. Other times it masquerades as energy, revealed by heat, movement or in measurements such as the electrocardiogram and electroencephalogram: at still other times as pure information, such as consciousness and the workings of the mind.

This deeper understanding of matter, energy and information and its relationship to health and disease appears to be missing in the conventional models of medicine (biomedicine and even in bio-psycho-social medicine).

The adoption of the Newtonian scientific model in medicine and the influence of pharmaceutical companies which drive a great deal of scientific research has meant that most research sticks to the investigation of matter, and a small window of energy that comes into focus during physiological research. Physiology is all about the science of the functions of the living organism and its components, and the chemical and physical processes involved. While physiologists understand that energy drives chemical processes, the subtle nature of the energy involved in biological living systems and its interaction with informational systems within and outside the body generally means that the focus of health and disease is more on the chemical processes and finding drugs to control these chemical processes.

Tavassoli (7) in 1987 said: "The prevailing paradigm that has shaped medical education, medical practices and medical research for most of the 20th century envisages disease as the end result of disordered molecular and biochemical processes. Such processes lead to cellular, tissue, organ, and system disturbances or destruction, resulting in disease, a characteristic constellation of specific biochemical, physiological and pathological anomalies. These anomalies are responsible for the specific loss of physical and other functions experienced by the patient and observed by the physician" (7).

The concepts of matter-energy-information as a functional integrated understanding are not really part of the older biomedical paradigm as described by Tavassoli quoted above, where the focus is on chemistry and pathology. As indicated, chemistry and pathology have to a large extent shaped the training of medical doctors.

As physicist Paul Davies (8) said: "It is often said that physicists invented the mechanistic-reductionistic philosophy, taught it to the biologists, and then abandoned it themselves. It cannot be denied that modern physics has a strongly holistic, even teleological (design or purpose) flavour, and this is due in large part to the influence of quantum theory."

Biomedicine confines itself to a particular viewpoint which is largely anatomical and physiological, with little emphasis on energy and information. Its journals support this more narrow perspective and the training of doctors keeps students very focused on the human being as a body-chemistry being. The increasing evidence of the role of energy-information tends to be downplayed and underrated. There is an assumption, for example, that the electrical conduction from the heart passing through every cell of the body is just a recording, without any physiological effects and without the possibility that it also carries information. The Institute of Heart Math (9) has found that "the heart generates a continuous series of electromagnetic pulses in which the time interval between each beat varies in a dynamic and complex manner. We have demonstrated, for example, that brain rhythms naturally synchronize to the heart's rhythmic activity, and also that during sustained feelings of love or appreciation the blood pressure and respiratory rhythms, among other oscillatory systems, entrain to the heart rhythm."

Bruce Lipton (10) in his book "The biology of belief" sums up much of the work which has revealed the extent to which energy and information influences matter. "Hundreds upon hundreds of other studies over the last fifty years have consistently revealed that 'invisible forces' of the electromagnetic spectrum profoundly impact every facet of biological regulation...Specific frequencies and patterns of electromagnetic radiation regulate DNA, RNA and protein syntheses, alter protein shape and function, and control gene regulation, cell division, cell differentiation, morphogenesis, hormone secretion, nerve growth and function. Each one of these cellular activities is a fundamental behaviour that contributes to the unfolding of life." He further states that energetic signalling mechanisms are many times more efficient at relaying environmental information than physical signals such as hormones, neurotransmitters and other biochemical messengers (11).

Professor Fritz Popp (12) has consistently demonstrated that biological systems can emit electromagnetic waves and also show sensitive responses throughout the whole spectral range. It seems, he says, that "nature utilises such waves for regulatory processes, or more generally for communication within living systems".

The Institute of Heart Math, where much work has been done on the electromagnetics of the heart and brain, suggests that "the heart's field acts as a carrier wave for information that provides a global synchronizing signal for the entire body". "Specifically, we suggest that as pulsing waves of energy radiate out from the heart, they interact with organs and other structures. The waves encode or record the features and dynamic activity of these structures in patterns of energy waveforms that are distributed throughout the body. In this way, the encoded information acts to in-form (literally give shape to) the activity of all bodily functions – to coordinate and synchronize processes in the body as a whole" (9).

Beverly Rubik (13) has performed extensive research in the field of bio-electromagnetics and cellular biophysics and has written extensively on the concept of "the biofield". She described the biofield as an "endogenous, complex dynamic field resulting from the superposition of component fields of the organism: the oscillations of the homeodynamic life processes and of the EMF contributed by each electrically charged, moving constituent of the organism (ion, molecule, cell, tissue etc). The resulting biofield may be conceived of as a complex dynamic standing wave both inside and enveloping the organism. This field is hypothesized to regulate homeodynamic life processes. It orchestrates the activity of the components of the organism...life is a self-organizing system. The body constituents and their interactions give rise to the biofield; and the biofield in turn directs the functions of the body constituents" (13).

There is thus increasing consensus amongst many scientists involved in this kind of research that information may be moved around the body by electromagnetic waves, photons or even by quantum means in which this transfer is instantaneous (non linear) and does not follow the more conventional electromagnetic process. It is possible that every cell is a coherent pattern of information in constant contact with every part, as suggested by Rubik (13), and that this is not a linear process. A holistic coherent system, a web of activity in which energy information drives matter and not the other way around. This is exciting work and could help to explain the way mind-body communicates so rapidly and how the whole body is able to respond so dynamically to the changing patterns of the external environment and shifting processes within the body, maintaining homeostasis despite all these forces and the play of emotions.

The human body is a complex of different energies; mechanical (breathing), sound (heartbeat), electricity, magnetism and light (photons). Anatomy and biochemistry have been extremely valuable ways of investigating the complex nature of the human body, but is clearly only one facet of this investigation. There is enough evidence now that more attention, money and research should also be directed to energy in all its many expressions, and the way the informational content of the transmission signals may have an effect on the physiological processes and controls in the body. Chronic disease continues to be a serious problem and the millions of people having to take drugs for life does not suggest that the present model is really curing people of their disease. This approach does not appear to be sustainable over time. The use of "energy tools" described below suggests another way to heal and the fact that they work is a powerful indication that this approach should be taken more seriously.

ENERGY INFORMATION RESEARCH: LOW ENERGY LASER TECHNOLOGY (LLL)

It would probably surprise most doctors to know that there are literally thousands of scientific articles and studies on LLL (low-level laser) technology and treatment, a number of peer reviewed journals, major textbooks and world congresses. There is an idea that if something works, then doctors would be told about it. The conventional model is focused on biochemistry and the treatment of disease using drugs. Energy medicine does not fit into the model and is not taught to medical students despite its efficacy and use by other health practitioners. LLL is a case in point. This writer has had more than 20 years experience in this therapy and finds it indispensable to the practice of medicine. It is especially useful in sports injuries and any inflammatory condition of soft tissue, arthritis, sinus infections, mastalgia and many other pain conditions. In Russia it has even been used to treat internal organ problems such as angina and some abdominal conditions. The LLL improves the local microcirculation, improving oxygen supply, decreases muscle tension and reduces swelling and inflammation. The results can be quite dramatic with observable effects even after the first treatment.

A laser produces coherent light, and in high power can be used as a surgical knife, while in low power it appears to stimulate physiological processes towards homeostasis. Normal living systems, such as human beings, are able to spontaneously produce active biological light. This photon emission can be measured with sensitive photon counting devices. Under certain circumstances, biological tissue emits ultraviolet light, which is able to stimulate mitosis in other cells and there is some evidence that mitochondria may be a source of photon emission from cells (14).

In the animal model, laser irradiation reduced the healing time for severed Achilles tendons significantly. Of particular interest was the frequent presence of new tendon cells in the laser treated group after 4 weeks, a condition that is not usually seen. Treatment was six minutes daily (15). Hundreds of other studies in human have also shown the efficacy of LLL (16-20). In the study by Gur and colleagues (20), LLL significantly improved pain intensity, morning stiffness and depression, as did the drug, but without any side effects.

MAGNETIC FIELD TECHNOLOGY

The studies on the effects of magnetic fields on biological systems continues to increase, but again do not appear in journals specialising in drug approaches to health and disease. Magnetic effects should not be doubted, as biological systems have developed within the earth's magnetic field and it should not be surprising that this magnetic field in some way contributes to the health of the organism. Of special interest is the use of Pulsating Magnetic fields (PMF) in the extremely low frequency range for its effects in human physiology. The pulsing brings in a dynamic component such that a pushing and pulling effect takes place across the cell membranes.

The human body is penetrated completely by the magnetic field. Human and animal organisms consist of a large number of cells which function electrically. The flow of ions (sodium flowing outwards and potassium flowing into the cells) constitutes a small electric current, producing a miniscule but virtually undetectable magnetic field. If cells are damaged by accident or disease, then this flow inwards and outwards of the ions is disturbed with leaking of ions into the tissues and swelling of the area. If there is no electrical potential left in a cell, it is no longer viable. If the ions (electrical charged particles surrounding the cells) move into an area of pulsating magnetic fields, they will be influenced by the rhythm of the pulsation and a restoration of the ion balance could occur. The ion exchange is responsible for the oxygen utilisation of the cell. PMF can dramatically influence the ion exchange at the cellular level and thereby greatly improve the oxygen utilisation of diseased or damaged tissues. PMF has now developed a wide range of uses and is increasingly used by professionals and the public (21-24).

In the following study the authors showed that a combination of weak pulsed electromagnetic fields with antioxidants supplementation is beneficial in the treatment of patients suffering from tongue cancer, improving speech, pain control, and tolerance to chemotherapy (25). This double-blind placebo-controlled study found that low frequency, low intensity electrostatic fields administered for 12-14 minutes per day helped normalise blood pressure in patients suffering from hypertension (26). This study examined the effects of alternating magnetic fields in patients suffering from chronic venous insufficiency, varicose veins and trophic shin ulcers. Good effects were obtained in 236 of the 271 patients; 34 had satisfactory results and only one patient experienced no improvement (27). The above examples are just a small indication of work done with magnetic fields.

Much of the research on energy medicine has been performed in Europe and Eastern Europe in particular, and this work has not been recognised or widely disseminated in the

West. On a visit to Russia I discovered that many medical schools are doing research on a variety of energy medical approaches using sophisticated equipment.

ELECTROMAGNETIC TECHNOLOGY

This is not a complete treatise on the subject, as there is extensive scientific research on the subject of electromagnetism in biological systems. Both Robert Becker, a surgeon, and Bjorn Nordenstrom, a radiologist, have done extensive work on electromagnetic devices in the treatment of disease. Both recognised that there is a current of injury in which the polarity at the site of an injury in the body turns positive almost immediately, then gradually back to negative as healing begins and continues. Robert Becker believed that it was the current of injury that was driving the healing process rather than just an epiphenomenon of chemical reactions (28,29).

I wish however to review one therapy called cranial electrotherapy stimulation (CES). This is the application of extremely low levels of electricity to the brain for the treatment of a wide range of psychiatric and medical disorders. All doctors are familiar with the use of the much more powerful electrical devices used in hospitals such as the electrical defibrillators, shock therapy for treating severe depression, and many other uses of electricity, but of a different kind. Like low energy laser, CES is much "softer" and less invasive. It seems to operate at physiological doses so that the body is not stressed to react but rather responds in a healing way. The early work by the Russians who developed electrical devices to induce electrosleep "sleep states" stimulated some researchers to go further. The FDA approved these devices in 1978 already, and the name CES was registered at the time. Their use was extended to pain management when electrodes were place on the body.

CES seems to prod the various neuro-hormonal systems in the brain back into their pre-stress homeostatic relationship so that the person is able to stop treatment after completing the course of treatment. CES has been shown to be both cost effective as well as being therapeutically effective (30). Kulkarni and colleagues (31) studied microcurrent electrical therapy (MET) and CES study in pain patients. The study reported that Fibromyalgia patients in the group responded "extremely well" with an 80-90% relief (31).

Lichtbroun and colleagues (32) have also shown that CES technology significantly eases the pain of fibromyalgia and was as effective as prescription drugs in relieving pain without major side effects. Patients treated with CES had a significant improvement in tender point scores, quality of sleep improved and there were significant gains in the feeling of wellbeing.

Rat studies demonstrated as much as a three-fold increase in b-endorphines concentrations after just one CES treatment. Other animal studies have shown similar results with an overall physiological effect to be anticholinergic and catecholamine-like in action. A recent review by Kirsch (33) listed an aggregate of more than 126 scientific studies of CES involving human subjects and 29 animal studies.

A review of CES in anxiety disorders suggested that it is capable of producing significant benefit in the short term both in anxiety and other stress-related disorders (34). Other studies indicate its usefulness and efficacy in anxiety, depression and insomnia (35).

SUBTLE ENERGY

In this paper I have confined myself to energy systems which are familiar and relatively easily measured. There are indications however that the understanding of energy could be much more complex than indicated above. The nature of consciousness, remote viewing (36,37), healing through the laying on of hands, the power of prayer (38,39), meditation and many other approaches have not been discussed in this paper although this work has been extensively researched and reviewed, and there appears to be sufficient positive results to convince many scientists of the efficacy of these approaches.

Quantum mechanics predicted many of these possibilities and the strangeness of quantum truths should at the very least open our minds to the fact that the biomedical model as practised today is not sufficient to incorporate an understanding of complexity, chaos, turbulence and entanglement. While many of these quantum truths seem of only abstract interest to medicine as they deal with the microscopic world of elementary particles, that view may need to be revised. Scientists are now finding that there are ways in which the effects of microscopic entanglement for example "scale up" into the macroscopic world. The whole concept of entanglement, which can explain the way all systems in the body function as one whole, how human beings connect to each other, how prayer works and how birds fly together, has been repeatedly demonstrated as fact in physics laboratories around the world since 1972. Entangled connections are proving to be more pervasive and robust than anyone had previously imagined (40).

A review of developments on entanglement research in March 2004 by New Scientist writer Michael Brooks concluded that "physicists now believe that entanglement between particles exists everywhere, all the time, and have recently found shocking evidence that it affects the wider, 'macroscopic' world that we inhabit" (41).

Read more about entanglement and what it means to medical scientists in "Entangled mind" by Dean Radin (42). Radin has performed a great deal of scientific research with "sensitives" in the field of telepathy, remote viewing and prayer (42).

While scepticism is healthy, one does need to keep in mind firstly one's own experience of "feeling connected" to another human being, an animal, a space in one's house etc, and secondly how little we know of cancer and yet have no problem accepting the various treatments offered despite our ignorance. We have not even approached the question of consciousness. This remains an enigma and yet cannot be dismissed as just an epiphenomenon and of no consequence to medical scientists.

The sad truth is that this most amazing of human traits gets banished to the periphery despite the fact that consciousness itself is the author of every possible experiment in science. Doctors then get blamed for not dealing with human beings, but being only interested in bodies, the physical part of human beings. Science may attempt to measure the physical magnitude and regularity of the wind's velocity, to determine its direction, or to ascertain its implication for tomorrow's weather, but usually fails to hear its sublime harmony or grasp its profound message. On rare occasions, when the analytic mind is still, the heart of the scientist may vaguely sense the wind's mystery, but the challenge of its translation and response seems insurmountable, and so the mind typically dismisses it as unworthy of scholarly attention. Yet, throughout human history, it is this whisper of the spirit that has moved many who have heard it to deep contemplation of their role in the creation of reality (43).

CONCLUSION

Despite the enormous advances made in medicine during the last century, chronic ill health remains a major challenge, consuming an increasing amount of the national budgets in most countries of the world. The main emphasis of healthcare is on the management, treatment and (some) prevention of disease rather than on the promotion or enhancement of health.

However, there must be an intermediary functional region between health and disease. This means that long before a disease becomes apparent there must already be a change in the functional integrity of the organism. During this phase homeostatic mechanisms come into play to maintain balance. Only when these fail to halt the development of structural and functional changes does the classical symptomatic picture of the disease emerges.

According to the "bioenergy model" the MEI (matter-energy-information) systems of the body are sensitive to stress that could be caused by physical (due to toxins, radiation, physical abuse etc) or psychological (emotional or cognitive) disturbances. This stress can cause physiological changes that either succeed in returning the organism to normal function or fail, leading to disease in the organism.

Treating a disease without changing the underlying MEI dynamics does not remove the underlying problem, and results in symptomatic treatment only. It has been shown in this paper that low intensity MEI tools may help to maintain coherence in the system, which over time strengthens the normal homeostatic mechanisms and shifts the organism towards normal function and better health.

Bio-energy has more than come of age. Very clearly studies and papers related to energy in medicine do not appear in journals which specialise in biochemistry; they appear in journals which specialise in energy/consciousness research. Medicine today has become so specialised that most doctors do not realise how narrow their field of interest has become, and that pharmaceutical companies, by financing most research, have tended to monopolise the education of medical students.

This needs to change if medical scientists are hoping to find answers to cancer and many of the other diseases which contribute to the increasing burden of chronic disease today. One cannot expect biochemists to have all the answers when dealing with the complex human being. Biochemistry is not all there is and moves much too slowly throughout the body to be able to maintain homeostasis in a system that requires instant communication throughout its domain.

Electricity, magnetism and light offer not only a powerful way of understanding the complex dynamics of the human organism, but also new possibilities of integrating the present approaches to management with complementary electromagnetic tools and low energy lasers. It is probably only in the domain of energy-information medicine that we will find a way of incorporating consciousness.

ACKNOWLEDGMENT

I would like to thank Professor Jaros for his interest and input in helping me gain new insights into the nature of energy during the writing of this paper.

REFERENCES

[1] Laszlo E. Quantum shift in the global brain. Rochester, VT: Inner Traditions, 2009:5.

[2] Jaros GG, Cloete A. Biomatrix: The web of life. World Futures 1987; 23:203-24.

[3] Dostal E, Jaros GG, Baker B. Some fundamental questions concerning healthcare from a process-based systems perspective. J Soc Evolutionary Systems 2000;21(2):193-211.

[4] Capra F. The web of life. A new synthesis of mind and matter. New York: Harper Collins, 1996:81.

[5] Feynman RP. Six easy pieces. The fundamentals of physics explained. New York. Penguin, 1995:24.

[6] FT Exploring. Accessed Jun 30. URL: http://www.ftexploring.com/energy/definition.html

[7] Tavassoli M. The concept of disease and the birth of modern medicine. Adler Museum Bull 1987;13(2):48.

[8] Davies P. God and the new physics. New York: Simon Schuster, 1983.

[9] McCraty R. Enhancing emotional, social, and academic learning with heart rhythm coherence feedback. Biofeedback 2005;33(4):130-4.

[10] Lipton BH. Biology of belief, Unleashing the power of consciousness, matter and miracles. Santa Rosa, CA: Mountain of Love/Elite Books, 2005:111.

[11] McClare CW. Resonance in bioenergetics. Ann NY Acad Sci 1974;227:74-97.

[12] Popp FA. Electromagnetic bio-information. Munich: Urban Schwarzenberg, 1989.

[13] Rubik B. Sympathetic resonance technology: Scientific foundation and summary of biological and clinical studies. A white paper. Unpublished, November 2001.

[14] Ruth B. Experimental investigations on ultra-weak photon. emissions. In: Popp FA, Warnke U, Konig HL, Peschka W, eds. Electromagnetic bio-information, 2nd ed. Munich: Urban Schwarzenberg, 1989:128.

[15] Kokino M Tozun R Alatli M, et al. International Congress on Laser in Medicine and Surgery. Bologna, June 1985.

[16] Rochkindd S Barr-Nea L Vogler I. Spinal cord response to laser treatment of injured peripheral never. Spine 1990;6:435-8.

[17] Palmgren N, et al. Low powered laser therapy in rheumatoid arthritis. Laser Med Sci 1989;4:193.

[18] Pinheira AL Cavalcanti ET Pinheiro MJ, et al. Low level laser therapy is an important tool to treat disorders of the maxillofacial region. J Clin Laser Med Surg 1998;16(4):223-6.

[19] Simunovic Z. Low level laser therapy with trigger points technique: a clinical study on 243 patients. J Clin Laser Med Surg 1996;14(4): 163-7.

[20] Gur A Karakoc M Nas K, et al. Effect of low power laser and low dose amitriptyline therapy on clinical symptoms and quality of life in fibromyalgia: a single-blind, placebo-controlled trail. Rheumatol Int 2002;22(5):188-93.

[21] Nicolakis P, et al. Pulsed magnetic field therapy for osteoarthritis of the knee – a double-blind sham-controlled trial. Wien Klin Wochenschr 2002;114(21-22):95.

[22] Vavken P, et al. Effectiveness of pulsed electromagnetic field therapy in the management of osteoarthritis of the knee: a meta-analysis of randomized controlled trials. J Rehab Med 2009;41(6):406-11.

[23] Basset CA, et al. Treatment of therapeutically resistant non-unions with bone grafts and pulsing electromagnetic fields. J Bone Joint Surg 1982;64(8):1214-20.

[24] Basset CA. The development and application of pulsed electromagnetic fields for un-united fractures and arthrodeses. Clin Plast Surg 1985;12(2):259-77.

[25] Randoll U Pangan RM. The role of complex biophysical-chemical therapies for cancer. Bioelectronchem Bioenerg 1992;27(3):341-6.

[26] Kniazeva TA. The efficacy of low intensity exposures in hypertension. Vopr Kurortol Lech Fiz 1994;1:8-9.

[27] Pasynkov EI, et al. Therapeutic use of alternating magnetic field in the treatment of patients with chronic diseases of the veins of the lower limbs. Vopr Kurortol Fizioter Lech Fiz Kult 1976;5:16-9.

[28] Becker RO. The basic biological data transmission and control system influenced by electrical forces. Ann NY Acad Sci 1974;238:236-41.

[29] Nordenstrom BEW. Biologically closed electric circuits: Clinical, experimental and theoretical evidence for an additional circulatory system. Stockholm: Nordic Med Publ, 1983.

[30] Gilula MF Kirsch DL. Cranial electrotherapy stimulation review: a safer alternative to psychopharmaceuticals in the treatment of depression. J Neurotherapy 2005;9(2):7-26.

[31] Kulkarni AD Smith R. The use of microcurrent electrical therapy and cranial electrotherapy stimulation in pain control. Clin.Proct Alt Med 2001;2(2):99-102.

[32] Lichtbroun AS Raicer MC Smith R. The treatment of fibromyalgia with cranial electrotherapy stimulation. J Clin Rheumatol 2001;7(2): 72-8.

[33] Kirsch DL. The science behind cranial electrotherapy stimulation. Edmonto, Alberta: Meical Scope Publishing, 2002.

[34] DeFelice EA. Cranial electrotherapy stimulation (CES) in the treatment of anxiety and other stress disorders: a review of controlled clinical trials. Stress Medicine 1997;13:31-42.

[35] Smith RB. Cranial electrotherapy stimulation. In: Myklebust JB, Cusick JF, Sances A, Larson, SJ, eds. Neural stimulation. Boca Raton, FL: CRC Press, 1985:129-50.

[36] Targ R. Remote viewing replication evaluated by concept analysis. J Parapsychol 1994;58:271-84.

[37] Dunne BJ, Jahn RG. Information and uncertainty in remote perception research. J Sci Exploration 2003;17(2):207-41.

[38] Byrd RC. Positive therapeutic effects of intercessory prayer in a coronary care unit population. South Med J 1988;81(7):826-9.

[39] Harris W, et al. A randomised, controlled trial of the effects of remote, intercessory prayer on the outcomes in patients admitted to the coronary care unit. Arch Intern Med 1999;159(19):2273-8.

[40] Johnson G. Refining the cat's eye view of the cosmos. The spooky connection between tiny particles is appearing everywhere, and its consequences are even affecting the world that we experience. New York Times 2001 Jul 16.

[41] Brooks M. The weirdest link. New Scientist 2004 Mar 27.

[42] Radin D. Entangled mind. Extrasensory experience in a quantum reality. New York: Paraview Pocket Books, 2006.

[43] Dunne BJ, Jahn RG. Consciousness, information, and living systems. Cell Molecular Biol 2005;51:703-14.

Submitted: May 07, 2011.
Revised: June 25, 2011.
Accepted: June 30, 2011.

In: Alternative Medicine Research Yearbook 2012
Editors: Søren Ventegodt and Joav Merrick

ISBN: 978-1-62808-080-3
© 2013 Nova Science Publishers, Inc.

Chapter 10

REFLECTIONS ON A HEALTH PARADIGM

*Saadiq Kariem, MBChB, MPhil, FCPHM, OTF, EMBA**
General Specialist and Emergency Services,
Department of Health in the Western Cape,
Cape Town, South Africa

ABSTRACT

The biomedical model that governs mainstream western medicine has a number of examples of how allopathic medicine is only regarded as "medicine" when it can be reduced to a hard anatomical science. However for even the hardest and sharpest of critics, the demonstration of energy fields that surround the human body through the technique of Kirlian photography should be proof enough that these energy fields, if unbalanced, can cause severe illness and disease. The discipline of integrative medicine within the medical fraternity and hence within the Departments of Family Medicine at the Medical Schools. This will hopefully result in integrative medicine becoming a part of the medical curricula and will hopefully therefore result in health therapists, including medical practitioners, developing skills in integrative medicine practice.

Keywords: Medicine, alternative medicine, integrative medicine

INTRODUCTION

The invitation to participate in a workshop to discuss a "changing health paradigm" proved irresistible to me and I was excited by the prospect of sharing my thoughts and experiences with like-minded souls. Not being an integrative medicine practitioner, the invitation sparked my curiosity in the topic as I had not kept abreast of all of the latest developments in integrative medicine issues. I hail from the old school still, when the topic was referred to as "complementary medicine". This brief paper explores my thoughts and reflections around the topic.

---

* Correspondence: Saadiq Kariem, POBox 36061, Glosderry 7702, South Africa. E-mail: skariem@pgwc.gov.za.

CONTEXTUAL ENVIRONMENT

One of the aspects of a good qualitative reflective paper is to demonstrate how I locate myself within the context of the environment within which my reflections are taking place. This is important in that it provides the reader with a sense of my own worldview as an individual and how I approach these reflections. Whilst being medically qualified does allow me a particular insight into the issues discussed, it also perhaps places me at a disadvantage in that my worldview is generally steeped within the biomedical paradigm. Having been involved in strategic and management related issues for a lengthy period of time has also given me particular insights into the application of integrative care in the real world. My general approach to this topic therefore is from a systems-thinking point of view rather than as a practitioner of integrative medicine.

HEALING ENVIRONMENT

An important aspect that I believe contributed to the success of the workshop was the fact that it took place on a farm, far from the madding crowd and in a place that was conducive to the flow of energy between the participants. I believe that this allowed us to connect with each other and with the process, which in turn allowed the conversations to be conducted in a truthful and enlightened manner.

I found the use of storytelling and conversations a particularly interesting method of eliciting the very best that the Forum participants had to offer. This allowed for productive conversations to take place that were frank and honest without inhibiting the natural flow of ideas and emergent themes. The café conversational format where participants rotated through the different stations allowed for a saturation of ideas in the shortest possible time whilst also allowing for deeper reflection to take place.

A number of topics were presented and discussed that essentially focused upon integrative medicine as a hard science with its origins to be found in the works of Hippocrates. What I find interesting is exactly how far modern medicine appears to have digressed from the original methods and indeed concepts of healing. Ancient healers were far more perceptive to the inherent energy that we all possess, and how this contributes to disease. The demonstration of the method of healing used by these ancient healers and based upon ancient healing methods is an important aspect of healing the whole body in the mind-body-soul paradigm.

The biomedical model that governs mainstream western medicine has a number of examples of how allopathic medicine is only regarded as "medicine" when it can be reduced to a hard anatomical science. However for even the hardest and sharpest of critics, the demonstration of energy fields that surround the human body through the technique of Kirlian photography should be proof enough that these energy fields, if unbalanced, can cause severe illness and disease.

TRADITIONAL VERSUS WESTERN MEDICINE

There are many traditional African therapies that are available to people and are used quite frequently. However, whilst some research is being conducted upon some of the healing properties of the products used, African Traditional Medicine still struggles to integrate into the more traditional western concepts of healing.

Over time, western medicine had lost the consciousness-based approach to healing. This has resulted in a dissonance between the heart-mind-body connection that can result in illness. The discussions reflected upon the matter-energy-information triad and how these concepts are all inter-related with each other as well as with the universe. We learnt about the 'dyad' – the smallest social unit that can exist, even between humans and plants or humans and animals, and how these interactions form a relationship. Evidence of this exists in today's world of healing where people who develop relationships with animals or plants recover faster from their illnesses.

The café conversation explored the concepts of medicine as a "hard science" versus medicine as a "soft science". This is perhaps one of the themes that we should explore further.

Much of the perception within the biomedical world is that integrative medicine is seen as "soft science". Even traditional healing in South Africa is seen as part of this soft science approach. Thus if we are to ever succeed in developing a new paradigm for Integrative Medicine, this is one of the issues that must be addressed.

INTEGRATIVE MEDICINE

There are a number of challenges that face the integrative medicine practitioner in today's world where the focus is primarily on bio-medical quick-fix cures. One of these key challenges in my view is the fact that integrative medicine struggles to find a voice in this bio-medical western world. Whilst the practice of integrative medicine has for centuries found resonance amongst the Eastern cultures, it has not as yet penetrated the mainstream medical model of the western world. As I reflect upon the many different variations and forms of integrative medicine as a client of some of these therapies, I find that the myriad of options that exist to be quite confusing. It would make the "mainstreaming" of these practices far simpler if these therapies could be demystified by practitioners of the system. This will also therefore make these therapies more accessible to the general public. Other than the practice of African Traditional Medicine, which has deep cultural roots, the other practices are often limited to particular portions of the population who generally are already converts to such therapies.

It is important then to identify which of essentially four scientific paradigms would form a relevant scientific basis within which integrative medicine can function. These four paradigms are: positivism, post-positivism, critical theory and constructivism.

Positivism is where one believes in the hard science of inquiry whilst constructivism represents the other extreme in which one believes that knowledge is socially constructed, and hence, differs from person to person, so no objective reality exists. Post-positivism on the other hand is a straightforward affix to positivism, with the hope to correct its faults by incorporating qualitative techniques at the methodological level.

Critical realism, however, incorporates the lived experience by focusing on the real, actual and empirical levels of this lived experience. Critical Realism can be described as a socially sensitive philosophy, which has an underlying ontological claim that there exists an objective reality which is external whilst, at the same time, acknowledging the roles of perception and cognition (1,2).

Critical realism (CR) has elements of both positivism and constructivism and is also known as post-positivism or neo-positivism. Critical realism determines the reality of a social phenomenon through the triangulation of cognition processes.

Critical realism can also be described as a philosophy in need of a methodology grounded in ontology, as opposed to epistemology. These methods include: Iterative abstraction, grounded theory, triangulation, causality, emergent theory, qualitative methods, quantitative methods such as structural equation modeling, stratification of knowledge, dialectic engagement, as well as probing realities.

As a philosophy, CR informs our approach to our research, data analysis, process of conceptualisation and theory building. It can be argued (1) that CR interprets the world, that is, mechanisms, events and experiences, in three domains of reality.

- The real domain consists of the processes that produce events, in which generative mechanisms or causal powers exist independently with a tendency to produce patterns of observable events under contingent conditions.
- The actual domain is where events actually occur, whether they are observed or not.
- The empirical domain is where experience can be obtained by direct observation.
- Within this framework the discovery of observable and non-observable structures and mechanisms, independent of the events they generate, is the goal of realism research. In other words, realism researchers observe the empirical domain to discover by a "mixture of theoretical reasoning and experimentation" a knowledge of the real world, by naming and describing the generative mechanisms that operate in the actual world (1).
- The basic belief system of CR can be best understood by examining the ontological and epistemological elements:
- Ontological: reality is 'real' but only imperfectly and probabilistically apprehensible; thus triangulation from many sources is required to know it.
- Epistemological: the findings are probably true but the researcher needs to be aware of the values between them.

The realist research methodology of qualitative case studies is process- orientated and does not deal with cause and effect relations, but with underlying causal tendencies. Realism attempts to explain the world through research that is aimed at the discovery, identification, description and analysis of the variables in a complex situation.

Having at length described critical realism as a possible scientific paradigm within which integrative medicine could function, the discussion on the value of quantum mechanics makes me rethink this proposal. From my limited understanding of what was presented at the Forum, quantum mechanics can easily serve as the scientific basis for Integrative Medicine. This will allow for a more holistic scientific model that can accommodate both the 'hard' scientific aspects of integrative medicine as well as the 'soft' more artistic aspects of the discipline.

Having identified a possible scientific paradigm for the discipline of integrative medicine, the next crucial step is to find the appropriate "home" for integrative medicine. This issue was raised during one of the plenary sessions and we had some brief reflection on this issue.

Being healers and essentially artists practising our art of healing, our natural inclination would be to establish integrative medicine as a discipline on its own. This would essentially mean developing the practice of integrative medicine as a healing art in parallel with the more established biomedical model of care. However, I believe that we are still a long way away from this concept which remains elusive.

This therefore calls for a more pragmatic approach. Given that in South Africa as in the rest of the Western World, the various sub-disciplines of integrative care are not seen as major therapeutic disciplines, we need to find a home for integrative medicine within existing recognised structures.

There are therefore essentially two options that I believe are open to us: Firstly, we lobby for the placement of integrative medicine within the family medicine structures attached to the Medical Schools. The advantage of this approach is that we could begin integrating the discipline of integrative medicine with one of the more established and recognised disciplines within the biomedical model. The great disadvantage however is that it may limit the growth and practice of integrative medicine in that the biomedical model in itself has severe limitations.

The other option is that we seek to place the discipline of integrative medicine within, say, a Business School or some other Department within university structures that can accommodate a new paradigm of thinking.

This has the advantage of bringing innovation to the fore and finding new ways of healing. The disadvantage however is that it may further alienate integrative medicine from the mainstream medical disciplines and practices.

CONCLUSION

My recommendation is that we seek to lobby for developing the discipline of integrative medicine within the medical fraternity and hence within the Departments of Family Medicine at the Medical Schools. This will hopefully result in integrative medicine becoming a part of the medical curricula and will hopefully therefore result in health therapists, including medical practitioners, developing skills in integrative medicine practice.

I believe that as health activists we need to be striving towards this objective and working hard at including integrative medicine in the curricula of medical schools. This also needs to be done in conjunction with the formal established professional bodies in order that we could achieve a "ripple effect" and establish the practice of integrative medicine on a national scale.

Lastly, I believe that the energy that the Forum had ignited needs to be carried forward by ourselves with the same passion with which we had engaged these complex issues.

REFERENCES

[1] Plant M. Critical realism: a common sense philosophy for environmental education. ATEE Conference, Stockholm 2001.
[2] Yeung HW. Critical realism and realist research in human geography: a method or a philosophy in search of a method. Prog Hum Geogr February 1997;21(1):51-74.

Submitted: May 08, 2011. *Revised:* June 27, 2011.
Accepted: June 30, 2011.

In: Alternative Medicine Research Yearbook 2012
Editors: Søren Ventegodt and Joav Merrick

ISBN: 978-1-62808-080-3
© 2013 Nova Science Publishers, Inc.

Chapter 11

AN INTEGRATED APPROACH FOR HIV DISEASE

Gary Orr, MBBS, MSc, DIC, MRCPsych(UK) *

Consultant Psychiatrist, Hutt Valley District Health Board, Lower Hutt, New Zealand

ABSTRACT

A group of medical professionals and allied academics were brought together in South Africa to generate ideas to tackle the current issues with integrated healthcare in Southern Africa and elsewhere. I was invited to attend the meeting, which generated a series of conversations over wide ranging topics related to the problems that those interested in working in an integrated and holistic paradigm face. This paper outlines some perspectives on the issues of HIV disease and mental health. An initial outline of the current failures of a biomedical approach to the HIV epidemic in Southern Africa will be followed by a brief review of the poor mental health of those with HIV disease. It is also recognised that those with HIV disease have poor socio-economic outcomes in comparison to their healthy colleagues. The commercial sectors in South Africa have been at the forefront of delivering an integrated approach to caring for a workforce with benefits on productivity. I will briefly describe my personal experience of working in a specialist HIV Psychological Medicine Unit attached to one of the largest HIV Health Services in Europe at the Chelsea and Westminster Hospital in London, United Kingdom. Finally the paper will review some of the evidence for the role of traditional healing and a physical, psychological and spiritual perspective to a holistic approach. This paper is necessarily brief with an outline of the fundamental issues that could influence the evolution of an integrated healthcare system.

Keywords: Medicine, alternative medicine, integrative medicine, HIV

INTRODUCTION

The failure of the millennium development goals has been widely documented, and although remarkable progress has been achieved, the original targets of the "3 by 5 Initiative" have still

---

* Correspondence: Gary Orr, POBox 442, Wellington 6140, New Zealand. E-mail: drgorra@aol.com.

not been reached. The psychological and socio-economic impact of HIV disease has been well established and it is recognised that those living with HIV disease have poorer socio-economic outcomes, and are at greater risk of the effects of poverty including malnutrition that has a negative impact on the body's ability to contain the progressive decline of HIV disease to full blown AIDS. Additionally South Africa now faces another epidemic of tuberculosis (TB) and it is recognised that approximately 50% of those with TB are also co-infected with HIV, making treatment more difficult and the effects of malnutrition even more pronounced. HIV increases the risk of reactivating latent TB, and increases the progression of TB. TB is becoming one of the most common causes of morbidity in countries with high prevalence rates of HIV infection, and is the most common cause of death in HIV positive adults in such countries (1).

Sadly the South African Food Fortification programme has also failed to achieve desired benefits of enhanced micronutrient repleteness amongst the population. Vitamin A, particularly amongst children has increased since the previous survey of 1999. Iron levels were shown to be a problem with a third of women and children showing evidence of anaemia on the basis of Haemoglobin concentration. 45.3% of children were shown to have an inadequate Zinc status. The survey also noted the "persistence and possible worsening of the prevalence of hunger". The survey did make several helpful recommendations to overcome the issues of micronutrient depletion and acknowledged the limitations of the existing evidence base about the role of micronutrients. A significant recommendation was the issue of socio-economic uplift. This suggests recognition that in order to combat some of the major health issues in the country there needs to be a concerted effort to create an integrated approach (2).

SOCIO-ECONOMIC CONSEQUENCES

The socio-economic consequences of HIV disease have been well documented, but limited systems have evolved to tackle this concern. The private sector has long recognised the negative impact of HIV disease on the workforce and there are now well established HIV programmes in many large national and multinational organisations operating in South Africa, with many of the most effective examples being in the mining industry. Several mining multinational corporations have been pioneers in creating healthcare systems that aim to deliver anti-retrovirals to their workforce, with benefits on reduced absenteeism and productivity.

Integrated wellness approaches have now been set up in other commercial sectors that also include a nutritional component as well. This approach has shown benefits to the workforce with evidence of improved productivity, reduced absenteeism and a greater sense of health and wellbeing in the workplace. "andBeyond" (a high end eco-friendly safari and tourist operator throughout Africa and elsewhere) is a leader in the positive health market in the commercial sector and has promoted health and wellbeing amongst its work force for many years. Their "positive living" programme is actively promoted amongst its workforce at a grass roots level. This programme aims to deliver health and wellbeing messages across the workforce with support for access to nutrition by promoting the development of gardens to deliver fresh fruit and vegetables to its workforce. "andBeyond" have also invested in providing a bio-available micronutrient supplement that has shown improved health and wellbeing outcomes across its workforce. There is increasing evidence that the provision of a bioavailable micronutrient supplement provided to integrated health and wellness programmes in the commercial sector in South Africa has the capacity to improve health outcomes for those who are HIV positive (3).

NUTRITION

Neil Orr and David Patient have eloquently argued for an integration of biomedical and behavioural approaches to viral load reduction in primary HIV infection. They have been pioneers in the evolution of "positive living" programmes across Southern Africa, and are clear advocates of the role of bioavailable nutrition as an adjunct to the overall management of those with HIV disease (4). The current confusion about the role of effective micronutrients as adjuncts in the overall management of HIV disease often overlooks the value of supplementation with food-state or chelated minerals and vitamins. Evidence of clear benefit for such interventions has been shown across a number of trails conducted in both the developing and developed world. Selenium (5), zinc (6) and vitamin A (7) have been shown to have positive benefits on immune function, and viral load reduction.

Health Empowerment Through Nutrition (www.hetn.org), a small United Kingdom based NGO working in partnership with Southern African NGO's has shown that a bioavailable nutritional supplementation programme can improve the outcomes for those with TB and HIV co-infection. A programme was developed in collaboration with SANTA, the South Africa National Tuberculosis Association, which delivered a highly bioavailable micronutrient supplement in the form of an easy to prepare porridge. Monitoring and evaluation of these programmes has shown an improvement of the TB cure rates in some centres by as much as 39% (8).

Such wellbeing programmes contribute to the communities that they aim to serve. Observations from the past need to be remembered where Europe saw dramatic reductions in epidemic infections, not through the development of new and modern pharmacological agents, but through the application of strict public health and hygiene including the development of clean water supplies, proper public sanitation and isolation of infectious cases. These simple and cost effective public health interventions have been a great advantage to the improvements that have been seen in public health in the developed world. Surely it is therefore vital that any integrated healthcare intervention will also need to be applied across society and the environment as well as to the individual in order to see the greatest change and benefit for all.

HIV AND MENTAL HEALTH

There is a well recognised negative impact of the HIV virus on the mental health of the individual and evidence from the developed world indicates a direct viral impact on the cognitive function of the HIV positive individual with associated wider impact on those around the index patient particularly if he or she is the main source of income for the family unit. The consequences have been a shift of primary care givers to an older population of grandparents and also children becoming carers for dying parents with loss of educational opportunities and continued economic disenfranchisement of the next generation meaning that the longer term social ramifications could extend beyond the current youth generation We have already seen a dramatic decrease in the life expectancy of populations in the Southern African region.

It is now recognised that HIV impacts on mental health in a number of different domains including cognitive function with associated dementia due to direct viral infection of the brain; the nature of HIV disease is known to adversely affect mood and anxiety with associated problems with alcohol and substance misuse which can contribute to an increase in risk taking behaviours with a wider societal impact. It is also known that there are neuropsychiatric sequelea associated with anti-retro viral treatment regimes. These factors contribute to the poor social outcomes for those with HIV disease. Mental illness and specifically depression is associated with worse outcomes for those with HIV disease, but little is done to integrate physical and psychological health for those with HIV disease (9). Affective disorders are often the most commonly reported mental health problem in people with HIV infection. Depression has a significant impact on the individual's quality of life. This is increasingly recognised with negative outcomes for HIV disease, including progression to AIDS and mortality. Furthermore depression is associated with poor adherence to anti-retroviral regimes. This would suggest that more robust systems would ideally be evolved for the recognition and prompt treatment of co-morbid depression in those with HIV disease so improving adherence, quality of life and social functioning of those with HIV disease (10).

Health professionals and aid workers across the globe welcomed the advent of the "3 by 5" initiative, but the 2004 "3 by 5 and Mental Health" Meeting in Johannesburg recognised that significant numbers of people affected by HIV disease went onto develop mental health problems that had a negative impact on HIV treatment and adherence with worsening of psychosocial outcomes(11).This meeting recognised that there was limited evidence about the extent of mental health problems in those with HIV disease in the developing world and that there was ever greater paucity of access to mental health services that were able to contribute effectively to the integrated management of these problems in a developing world context.

The outcome of the meeting proposed that all HIV treatment programmes should ideally include a collaborative approach between mental health and physical health to manage the care of those who present with HIV disease. It was also suggested that more research was required into the mental health and social aspects of the epidemic. The group acknowledged that there was a limitation to the resource of mental health workers in such developing world environments, and suggested a widespread integration with primary care workers to further develop capacity. Others have argued that effectively contributing to improving the quality of life for those with HIV disease is particularly important given that HIV could progress to being a long term chronic condition even in a resource depleted setting such as sun-Saharan Africa. Sherbourne et al (12) argued that the utilization of sufficient numbers of mental health professionals may reduce "unnecessary utilization of other health services and improve health-related quality of life in persons with HIV infection". Whether or not this can transpire in a resource poor setting remains to be seen, but if such settings are to consider tackling the enormity of the task, then novel approaches that are culturally contiguous need to be considered. The Global Fund has identified that adequate capacity of a health system is needed for any successful implementation of major health interventions. There is recognition that capacity and human resource constraints are an issue in the frontline battle against HIV disease (13) in the developing world context.

INTEGRATED PSYCHOLOGICAL MEDICINE

An integrated approach would aim to address the physical, psychological, nutritional and spiritual consequences of such a devastating disease process. The sophisticated health and social care systems of the developed world have been able to evolve systems that aim to address the need for integrated physical, social and psychological care for those with HIV disease. These systems have long recognized the impact of HIV as a multi-factorial disorder, and in one service, based at the Chelsea and Westminster Hospital in London; there has been a Psychological Medicine Unit that works closely with the HIV Unit in the same hospital. This service has developed close liaison between mental health workers including psychiatrists and psychologists as well as specialist liaison psychiatric nurses, and the doctors and allied health care staff working on the HIV Medicine Unit. The unit aims to provide immediate assessment, triage and ongoing care to those who present with evidence of acute and chronic mental health conditions associated with HIV disease. The unit also provides a consultation – liaison psychiatry service to the acute hospital. An ongoing programme of internal audit and outcomes has shown long term benefit to those who have received mental health support in the context of their HIV disease. Staff on the unit also provide ongoing training and support to those who work with HIV positive patients in the acute medical environment as well as providing harm reduction programmes for patients and outlying non-governmental agencies that work with those who are HIV positive in the local community (14).

Unfortunately such systems in the developed world are often confined to a Newtonian – Cartesian paradigm which informs the modern biomedical approach to current evidence based medical practice. This paradigm makes it difficult to create an evidence base for integrating a psycho-spiritual aspect to integrated healthcare. Such an approach is by definition individual and patient focused rendering the gold standard randomized controlled trial ineffective as a reliable means of evaluating such interventions.

TRADITIONAL HEALERS

It is recognised that there are limitations to the provision of widespread allopathic medical services in the developing world. There are approximately 400,000 traditional healers currently practising in Southern Africa. This contrasts with approximately 40,000 qualified medical personal. The World Health Organization and other involved multinational organizations are now recognizing the potential role of traditional healers in the provision of primary care services in Southern Africa and other developing global regions where traditional medicine is widely practised. In a region where many are unable to access clinics and hospitals due to resource or actual physical constraints the role of the traditional healer is powerful and provides accessible services to the local community. It is estimated that approximately 70 to 80 % of people access traditional healers as primary care givers. It has even been argued that this system fulfils an idealized form of basic public health being effective, low budget, patient focused and culturally contiguous. There is increasing recognition of the role of traditional healers at a statutory level particularly in South Africa where formal organizations are being set up with associated regulatory structures which aim to provide a formalized system of training and accreditation (15,16). These structures are in their infancy and still have a journey to travel to overcome some of the stigma and prejudice that such health providers face.

In many cultures explanations of disease are often rooted in concepts of psychological and social disequilibrium that manifest in physical symptoms. The consequent disharmony may result from psychological or spiritual factors that often form part of the healing process in which traditional healers engage with their patients. Traditional healers are able to provide a client centred and personalized approach to a health problem that takes account of the cultural and spiritual elements that might not be present in a mainstream allopathic medical consultation at a medical clinic or hospital. Such integration of a psycho-spiritual and physical approach through the use of medicinal plants and herbal remedies brings about a healing process that is often lacking in allopathic medicine which maintains the basis of a mind – body duality to healing with an emphasis on medical and surgical interventions focused on alleviating suffering rather than bringing a return to health (16). The World Health Organization defines health as state of "complete physical, mental and social wellbeing and not just the absence of disease or infirmity" (17).

There is an emerging evidence base to support the role of traditional healers as health care providers in the HIV epidemic. Peltzer et al report that up to a third of people consult traditional healers for symptoms of sexually transmitted diseases (18) and it is now becoming increasingly accepted that traditional healers have a contributory role in the collaborative provision of health and social care for those with HIV disease. The relationship between traditional healer and patient also provides an opportunity for the promotion of behaviour change. The development of collaborative health systems can be of positive benefit to both the individual and the community. Peltzer developed a traditional healer training model to test if training would increase knowledge, reduce risk practises, improve HIV management strategies and improve referral pathways to allopathic healthcare providers. They found that training improved HIV and TB management strategies as well as improved risk reduction management, condom distribution, and community education (19).

Hoff in a review of traditional healers suggests that such practitioners are a valuable resource in communities where access to primary health care is scant. The review claims that community health resources would be strengthened by collaboration between traditional healers and allopathic medical services, with properly trained traditional healers being utilized to provide health promotion, prevention and primary care when appropriate. The review acknowledges that many traditional healing approaches have been marred by prejudice and the unscrupulous practises of some. Media focus on instances of witchcraft and malpractice serve to underlie the suspicion surrounding what is a potentially valuable and potent resource (20).

INTEGRATED APPROACH

Integrated health aims to bring about a more holistic concept of disease and begin to accommodate an understanding of the biology, environment, social position, and the role of the mind, culture, spirituality, race, and sex (21). It is well recognized that HIV and similar life threatening chronic health conditions are major psychological and physical stressors.

Psychoneuroimmunology continues to provide evidence of the underlying mechanisms linking stressful events and physical health outcomes. It is increasingly acknowledged that the interaction between behaviours, the central nervous system and the endocrine system can have a negative impact on the immune system. This knowledge has important implications for thinking about future integrated healthcare systems. Tosevki et al suggest that a multidimensional basis to diagnostics and treatment should be part of an integrated approach to healthcare delivery aimed at improving quality of life for patients (22).

CONCLUSION

The link between psychological and physical processes has long been understood by ancient healing traditions, but modern medicine with a Cartesian duality of mind and body has allowed this understanding to be diluted. Ultimately all healing processes incorporate an understanding of roles for the patient, and the healer with prescribed rituals of the healing process and place of healing. There are expected outcomes of efficacy and a return to social functioning and reintegration of the patient into the community.

African cosmology with a deep rooted understanding of spirituality and the potential of the collective conscious to bring about healing needs to be strengthened as part of a collaborative association between the traditional and modern worlds of healing and medicine. I have argued that a paucity of resources at the clinical coal face requires an urgent increase in human resources to meet the health challenges that Africa faces. There is an expanding and valid Cartesian – Newtonian based evidence which supports the role of the traditional healer at the primary care interface for the management of HIV disease and its associated mental health problems. It becomes a logical extension to argue for the greater integration of the healing paradigm between modern biomedicine and African traditional medicine.

Western developed-world medicine places great emphasis on understanding the patho-physiological processes that underpin disease such that the knowledge gained has been used to develop the complex pharmacological and surgical interventions which are the fundamental healing interventions of modern medical science. These interventions have been highly successful at improving the health of those in the developed world. However there is also an increasing search for alternative systems of healing that take account of the psychological, spiritual and physical aspects of disease. We seem to be approaching greater acceptance of culturally contiguous traditional healing disciplines but our scepticism, fear of lack of efficacy, and limited understanding of African traditional spirituality all contribute to the prejudices that prevent the evolution of novel and locally specific integrated approaches to health care.

REFERENCES

[1] Corbett EL, Watt CJ, Walker N, Maher D, Williams BG, Raviglione MC et al. The growing burden of tuberculosis: Global trends and interactions with the HIV epidemic. Arch Intern Med 2003;163;1009 - 21.

[2] Labadarios D, Swart R, Maunder EMW, Kruger HS, Gericke GJ, Kuzwayo PMN, et al., Executive summary 6 – South Africa National Food Consumption Survey. SA 2008 Nutritional Survey. S Afr J Clin Nutr 2008;21(3)(Suppl 2):245-300.

[3] Personal communication – Econocom Foods: www.epap.co.za

[4] Orr N, Patient D. Viral load reduction and primary HIV infection: The new frontiers of reducing HIV transmission? Unpublished, June 2010.

[5] Hurwitz BE, Klaus JR, Llabre MA, Gonzalez A, Lawrence PJ, Kevin J. Suppression of human immunodeficiency virus type 1 viral load with selenium. A randomised controlled trial. Arch Intern Med 2007;167:148-54.

[6] Baum MK, Lai S, Sales S, Page JB, Campa A. Randomized, controlled clinical trial of zinc supplementation to prevent immunological failure in HIV-infected adults. Clin Infect Dis 2010;50(12):1653-60.

[7] Patrick L. Nutrients and HIV Part 2: Vitamins A and E, zinc, B-vitamins and magnesium. Altern Med Rev 2000;5(1):39-51.

[8] Orr G, Douglas G. HETN HIV/TB and nutrition. Poster presented to AIDS IMPACT Conference, Gaborone, Botswana, September 2009.

[9] Hartzell JD, Janke IE, Weintrob AC. Impact of depression on HIV outcomes in the HAART era. J Antimicrobial Chemother 2008;62(2):246-55.

[10] Starace F, Ammassari A, Trotta MP, Murri R, De Lonqis P, Izzo C, et al. Depression is a risk factor for suboptimal adherence to highly active antiretroviral therapy. J Acquired Immune Defic Syndr 2002;31(Suppl 3):S136-9.

[11] Freeman MC, Patel V, Collins CY, Bertolote JM, et al. Integrating mental health in global initiatives for HIV/AIDS. Br J Psychiatry 2005;187:1-3.

[12] Sherbourne CD, Hays RD, Fleishman JA, Vitielo B, Magrunder KM, Bing EG, et al. Impact of psychiatric conditions on health-related quality of life in persons with HIV infection. Am J Psychiatry 2000;157:248–54.

[13] Dräger S, Gedik G, Dal Poz MR. Health workforce issues and the Global Fund to fight AIDS, tuberculosis and malaria: An analytical review. Hum Resour Health 2006;4:23.

[14] Author's personal experience – Honorary Consultant Psychiatrist, Department of Psychological Medicine, Chelsea and Westminster Hospital, London, United Kingdom 2007 – 2008.

[15] Morris K. Treating HIV in South Africa. A tale of two systems. Lancet 2001;357(9263):1190.

[16] Hewson MG. Traditional healers in Southern Africa. Ann Intern Med 1998;128(12 Pt 1):1029-34.

[17] http://www.who.int/about/definition/en/print.html/

[18] Peltzer K, Mngqundaniso N, Petros G. HIV/AIDS/STI/TB knowledge, beliefs and practices of traditional healers in KwaZulu-Natal, South Africa. AIDS Care 2006;18(6): 608-613.

[19]

[20] Peltzer K, Mngqundaniso N, Petros G. A controlled study of an HIV/AIDS/STI/TB intervention with traditional healers in KwaZulu-Natal, South Africa. AIDS Behav 2006;10(6):683-90.

[21] Hoff W. Traditional healers and community health. World Health Forum 1992;13:182-7.

[22] Engebretson J. Cultural constructions of health and illness. Recent cultural changes toward a holistic approach. J Holistic Nurs 2003;21(3):203-27.

[23] Tosevski DL, Milovancevic MP. Stressful life events and physical health. Curr Opin Psychiatry 2006;19(2):184-9.

Submitted: May 15, 2011.
Revised: June 29, 2011.
Accepted: July 01, 2011.

In: Alternative Medicine Research Yearbook 2012
Editors: Søren Ventegodt and Joav Merrick

ISBN: 978-1-62808-080-3
© 2013 Nova Science Publishers, Inc.

Chapter 12

THE TRADITIONAL HEALING SYSTEM IN SOUTH AFRICA

Nhlavana Maseko, TDr, Phephsile Maseko, THP and Jeanne Viall*

South African NGO Coalition, Africa Traditional Health Network, Traditional
Medicine Platform- Department of Science and Technology, Johannesburg, South Africa

ABSTRACT

The adoption of the modern-day healthcare delivery system has brought about a set-back
in the practice of traditional medicine in most societies of the world. Against all odds,
traditional medicine has continued its influence and has been found to play a prominent
role in the health of the people in most societies, without backing and sometimes without
approval from governments. This indicates that traditional therapeutic systems of care are
a significant component of health care delivery in most developing countries of the world
because they enjoy considerable support from the people.

Keywords: Medicine, alternative medicine, traditional healers

INTRODUCTION

The adoption of the modern-day healthcare delivery system has brought about a set-back in
the practice of traditional medicine in most societies of the world. Against all odds, traditional
medicine has continued its influence and has been found to play a prominent role in the health
of the people in most societies, without backing and sometimes without approval from
governments. This indicates that traditional therapeutic systems of care are a significant
component of health care delivery in most developing countries of the world because they

---

* Correspondence: Phephsile Maseko, THP, National Coordinator, Traditional Healers Organisation in South
Africa. P0Box 3722 Johannesburg 2000, South Africa. E-mail: phepmas@yahoo.co.uk; thohealth@gmail.com.

enjoy considerable support from the people. In other words, the health care delivery system is incomplete in Africa without the inclusion of traditional medicine.

The African indigenous health system dates back to ancient times. Only since the mid 1970s have a number of international resolutions been passed to promote the regulation of traditional healing practice and measures to regulate traditional medicine use. Recent research has shown that up to 80% of Africans depend on traditional medicine in Africa, while about 72% of South Africans make traditional medicine their health care of choice before seeking western health care advice from local clinics. Traditional medicine is part of people's culture and heritage in Africa. It occupies pride of place because it is affordable and easily accessible. The profile of traditional health practitioners needs to be raised, as well as the important role they play in the health care system (1).

Africa bears 24 percent of the world's disease burden and yet has only 3 percent of the world's health workers.

Africa simply does not have enough health care professionals or good quality basic services. Demand is high, because many people contract preventable killer diseases, but health workers and the health care system are struggling to cope. People are dying from avoidable deaths, even when they do eventually reach a hospital or clinic and get treated.

TRADITIONAL HEALTH PRACTITIONER ACT

The introduction of the Traditional Health Practitioner's Act (No. 22 of 2007) has affirmed these practitioners as a strong and readily available resource for health provision in all the provinces of the country. The Act stipulates the categories of practitioners that are covered under this Act. These include: diviners (izangoma), herbalists (iinyanga), traditional birth attendants (ababelethisi) and lastly the traditional surgeons (iingcibi). Using the word "sangoma" for all traditional healers is not only incorrect, but does not credit the rich diversity contained in traditional medicine. It is also important to notice that African traditional medicine comes from Africa, it was not imported, but developed in Africa. Today 600-million indigenous people worldwide practise their own traditional system of healing.

In South Africa systems work alongside each other: the traditional, which incorporates a greater spiritual element, the medical, the modern medicine and the integrative religious. Traditional healers fall into three groups: about 40% do their healing in a "possessed" state (ie by ancestral spirits); 36% are non-possessed and 20% use a combination of both traditional medicine and religion. These are called holy spiritualist faith healers. Like all other health care systems there are specialists such as wound healers, traditional obstetricians, dentists, bonesetters and traditional counsellors, and they make up the other 4%.

Diagnosing apparatus includes bones from animals, shells and other objects. Training to use these can take one and a half year to about three years, depending on your area of focus. Other methods include looking into the eyes, crystals, palmistry, even using the Bible. Sound, for example drums, is also used. The healer will look and see what your problem is, via your ancestral spirit. Some read personal problems through the stars. Sangomas form only one part of a group, those possessed by ancestral spirits. "I'm a witchhunter, an astrolger (among others)," stated TDr Maseko. "But everyone is called sangoma. When I'm asked, am I sangoma, I say yes. But that doesn't tell you everything, and the person still doesn't know who you are."

The "possessed" can be divided into the clairvoyants, the matron healers, the master healers, the spirit mediums, the fortune tellers, the witch hunters, the ancestral spiritualist diviner. "So when you say sangoma, who's that?" "If you talk about sangoma, what are you talking about? You do not know who's who." The respectful way to greet these healers is to kneel down, put your hands together, and say "thokoza". These people are called to their profession and can take three to six years to become operational. For you to qualify as a healer, your master healer or tutor should confirm that title after you have been assessed and deemed competent.

The non-possessed include the rainmaker, the medicine man or the herbalist, the mental health practitioner, the traditional birth attendant specialists, among others. These people go for training and often learn from their grandmothers, fathers or parents.

> "I grew at the feet of my grandfather, I got my training from the grandfather. At a young age I was a doctor's attendant, I would prepare the medication. The one who carries the medicine kit/bag on his shoulder is a herbalist, one who was taught by me, a trained practitioner. They collect leaves and plants for me and prepare them. The western health care system has to find a way to recognise and incorporate them as equal to the possesed, but they are only collectors of medicine. We have traditional birth specialists, child birth controllers, and traditional family planning specialists. These are specialists to help people space their children, a practice well known in our culture"

Calling birth specialists birth attendants was inadequate, as they were experienced and highly trained specialists, who do not only get involved in birthing but also in assisting the couple with planning the child and providing infertility interventions, until the baby grows into an adult. Traditional medicine also has surgeons who perform initiation work including circumcision; eye specialists, people who treated skin problems, indigenous nutritionists. Here is some case stories:

> He told the story of a client of his, an elderly woman in Germany, who had a wound which hadn't healed for seven years. With permission from his King (King Sobhuza the second of Swaziland) he flew the medicine over. "It was open, you could see the bone, and other wound specialists there couldn't heal it. Within 31 days it healed completely. The old lady cried with happiness."

> He also told of an accident he had in which he was badly injured. When western medical doctors told him he wouldn't walk again, and the foot may need to be amputated, he refused. "As a bonesetter myself I knew I had to take over and treat the leg. I then negotiated with the Principals of Rob Ferreira Hospital in Nelspruit to release me to take care of myself back at home. The doctors were worried that the legs would not work again, and as such I would not be able to walk. They were reluctant to release me, but in about five months I went back to them to show them how I was doing, and a lot of them were very impressed such that they requested that we share healing knowledge. But I refused because I knew my knowledge was not protected and as such I would not be given the compensation I deserved."

BACKGROUND HISTORY

For many decades African Traditional Medicine was not only marginalised, but also suppressed, in South Africa and elsewhere on the continent. Traditional medicine has been practised for centuries and remains the most common source of healthcare in rural Africa. An extensive pharmacopeia of medicinal plant and animal materials has been developed, and passed down from generation to generation.

In their history of missionary medicine, Benatar and Van Rensburg write how western medicine in Africa was largely pioneered by Christian missionaries during the last quarter of the 19th century and early 20th century, and hundreds of mission hospitals and dispensaries were established (2).

One result of this contact was the emergence of a relationship between western allopathic and African traditional medicine best described as one of "superiority–inferiority", symbolising the strengths of imperial and indigenous powers and the official superimposition of western values over African practices. In time, allopathic medicine enjoyed dominant official support over traditional medicine, which was relegated to an officially inferior and often covert position (2).

During the colonial period policies and legislation towards traditional medicine took two forms: herbalists were not forbidden to practise their medicine, but divination, witchcraft, sorcery, ordeals, and oaths were outlawed and prosecuted as criminal offences (the Witchcraft Suppression Acts). In general, colonial governments and early Christian missionaries despised and therefore discouraged or suppressed the use of traditional medicine.

Later, this rejection of traditional medicine was carried further by organised professions and councils in the western-scientific mold. "In time, however, four broad varieties of relationships crystallized: exclusive (monopolistic) systems, recognizing only scientific medicine; tolerant systems, characterized by laissez-faire policies which virtually ignore traditional medicine, yet allow its existence; inclusive (parallel) systems, recognizing traditional health systems alongside scientific medicine; and integrated systems, tending to unite allopathic and traditional medicine in both training and practice."

The first type of relationship prevails in the former French and Belgian colonies in Africa; the second was/is typical of the arrangement in former British colonies. Inclusive and integrated systems have not generally been encountered in Africa (2). In spite of suppression and lack of financial backing, traditional medicine has survived, and thrived. In most African countries, traditional healers have a much bigger following than western forms of medicine.

However, as the Traditional Healers Organisation website (3) states: "Due to decades of colonialism, cultural imperialism and the power of the multi-national pharmaceutical industry, traditional health practitioners and traditional medicine have been marginalised and our value to communities underplayed. "There is therefore a need for urgent investment and support of traditional health practitioners and traditional medicine – not only by government, but also by civil society and the private sector. "In the country, Traditional Health Practitioners are already a trusted source of health information and treatment. Given appropriate skills and means, they are well placed to play a bigger role in combating Africa's major diseases" (3).

REFERENCES

[1] African Traditional Medicine Conference, Johannesburg, 30 March 2004.
[2] Van Rensburg HJC, Benatar SR. Pre-modern Africa, missionary medicine and religious influences. Colonial Africa, benefits to medicine. Accessed 2011 Jun 30. URL: http://www.jrank.org/health/pages/32784/Africa-%E2%80%94-history.html
[3] Traditional Healers Organisation. Accessed 2011 Jun 30. URL: www.traditionalhealth.org.za.

Submitted: May 20, 2011.
Revised: June 25, 2011.
Accepted: July 01, 2011.

In: Alternative Medicine Research Yearbook 2012 ISBN: 978-1-62808-080-3
Editors: Søren Ventegodt and Joav Merrick © 2013 Nova Science Publishers, Inc.

Chapter 13

SOUTH AFRICAN HEALING VILLAGES

*Renee Usdin, MBChB**

Private Practice, Hout Bay, and City of Cape Town HIV Clinics Western Cape,
South Africa

ABSTRACT

South African Healing Villages is an NGO initiated in July 2009 by a group of medical
doctors, complementary therapists, community workers, counsellors and other health care
professionals who share a common vision of facilitating community based holistic
approaches to health care. It wishes to support innovative ways of approaching health and
illness holistically, helping to raise consciousness and facilitate healing. It is too early to
judge the success of the project but the goodwill of the community in response to the
initiative has been wonderful and people are attending the clinic in increasing numbers.
So far we have all been working voluntarily but are hoping to be able to source funding
to make the project sustainable in the long term.

Keywords: Medicine, alternative medicine, traditional healers, village

INTRODUCTION

In this paper I would like to reflect on two different elements: the first is my own personal
experience of the meeting in South Africa we had with the small professional group of
forward thinkers in the health arena. The other is a project in which I am personally involved
that reflects a practical implementation of the changing paradigm in health.

My experience from the meeting was the strong sense of the participants commitment
and enthusiasm to engage in many deep and sensitive issues around how and why we heal,
the way we do and how we in the West particularly, need to shift and expand our concept of
medicine and healing to a more inclusive one that takes into account so much more than just

---

* Correspondence: Renee Usdin, Private Practice, 8189 Orange Kloof Road, Hout Bay, Western Cape, South Africa.
E-mail: renusdin@gmail.com.

the physical body and its pathology. I really enjoyed how people came together with a wonderful respect for our work and each other, always with an ability to laugh and enjoy. In the context of the articles written by other participants in this special issue, it would seem that the model described below is a possible means of practically implementing some of the concepts discussed. It would in any event be interesting to see the feasibility and acceptability of such a project.

PROJECT DESCRIPTION

South African Healing Villages is an NGO initiated in July 2009 by a group of medical doctors, complementary therapists, community workers, counsellors and other health care professionals who share a common vision of facilitating community based holistic approaches to health care. It wishes to support innovative ways of approaching health and illness holistically, helping to raise consciousness and facilitate healing.

At the centre of our ethos are the principles of holistic health, viewing the human being as comprising body, mind and spirit in a symbiotic relationship with the environment. It is a world view that is inclusive, united and expansive. It involves an awareness of the interconnectedness of all creation. If we do something to someone else, we do it to ourselves; if we harm the earth we also harm ourselves.

Our vision is to create ecologically balanced healing villages to provide holistic health care and skills development, with special attention to disadvantaged communities and those affected by HIV/AIDS and chronic disorders, with a focus on raising consciousness and facilitating social transformation.

The HIV epidemic has reached cataclysmic proportions. The estimated number of deaths in South Africa in 2010 has reached the equivalent of two Boeing 747s crashing every day. Thousands of children are orphaned and the epidemic has placed a profound strain on the economy and health services. This comes on top of a huge burden of disease caused by poverty, as well as personal, family and community trauma, all of which compromises the immune system, creating fertile ground for the epidemic to spread.

Currently there are no options available through conventional health facilities until the patient's CD4 count falls to a critical level. We see the Healing Village providing opportunities for patients with HIV to maintain and strengthen their immune systems.

Various disciplines, including psycho neuroimmunology, have proven that the immune system and health in general can be powerfully influenced by reducing states of physiological and psychological stress. i.e. reducing levels of sympathetic arousal. Viral loads decrease and CD4 counts rise significantly by creating positive restorative psychological states such as hope, meaning, courage and adaptability; and re-orientating one's locus of control internally. Such states have also been shown to improve the overall immune system, compliance to medications, and physiological homeostasis (the body's balance) (1-3).

The role of nutrition in HIV and other immune disorders is well documented. It is of particular importance in HIV not only in relation to the immune system but also in preventing complications of the anti-viral medicines such as hyperlypidaemia, lipodystrophy and lipoatrophy and diabetes mellitus (4,5).

We see our work as complementary to that provided by the state health sector and not as an alternative option. The modalities we offer are regarded as a support and extension of the medical treatments currently available. It is an initiative which will make available to disadvantaged people treatment modalities that are normally only available for more affluent individuals. We have a four-tiered approach:

- *Health promotion and awareness*: this includes HIV counselling, testing and education, prevention measures and health maintenance
- *Integrative Medicine*: bringing together the best of Western medical practice with the best of traditional African and complementary healing modalities, including massage, traditional African use of potentised herbs for bathing and steaming and ritual practices of soul medicine to bring balance to communities and individuals, reflexology, homeopathy, acupuncture, counselling, story¬telling, drumming and many more.
- *Therapeutic Arts and Crafts*: giving expression to the inner and outer creative journey of the artist is a healing process. This healing is deepened through the production of items forged from earth's natural elements – minerals, metals, plants and animals - connecting and aligning the human being with nature.
- *Skills development:* training is offered in the various healing modalities of the Village and the development of arts and crafts enable people to both earn a living as well as to broaden the healing modalities to reach their families and communities.

Our broader vision sees the healing villages as operating from ecologically sensitive smallholdings where food and medicinal gardens complement healing spaces, and offering outreach programs to the hospitals and community clinics.

We have initiated the Amajoni Wellness Clinic pilot project in Hout Bay, Cape Town. It is an integrated medical clinic and operates one day of the week from the Hout Bay Cultural Community Centre.

The Xhosa name "Amajoni" means freedom fighter or warrior, and is used in HIV counseling to describe the principle immune cells (CD4) of the body. We have very good contact with the local HIV clinic, various youth organizations, church groups and civic structures.

Hout Bay is in many ways a microcosm of South Africa, consisting of a mix of neighborhoods from the very rich to the very poor and housing a diverse range of people of different race groups and nationalities, ranging from locals to refugees, and to immigrants from Africa and the rest of the world

In the spirit of non-discrimination The Village will be accessible to the whole community and to anyone wishing to strengthen their mind-body-spirit.

When a client first comes to the centre they are welcomed by one of the community workers, who sits them down, gets their details and offers them a cup of tea. If it is their first visit they will see the doctor who will work out an appropriate programme for them. This may entail HIV counseling and testing (HCT), or counseling if they decline testing, in the hope that talking about it will encourage them to consider testing in the future.

Depending on the diagnosis, the doctor may prescribe herbal or homeopathic medicine or refer the client to the clinic for ARVs or other medical treatments. Clients may also be referred for further investigations such as the exclusion of TB or measuring their CD4 count. They might be advised to complete a course of massage or Reiki energetic healing treatment or may be referred for in-depth counseling. Somebody touch work or quantum healing may be recommended, and everyone is encouraged to join the yoga and breath work sessions provided by the Village. While patients are waiting to see the doctor or counselors they are encouraged to try some of the complementary modalities on offer.

The clinic is open to anyone with an immune related or chronic disorder, although our primary focus is HIV positive individuals and their caregivers. The clinic is embryonic. As time progresses we hope to add many more dimensions to the programme.

Ideally we would like to operate out of the clinic premises so that it is very clear that our and the clinics work is integrated. Unfortunately the clinic barely has enough space for its own activities, hence our decision to use the community cultural centre.

We are including a research aspect to the project in an attempt to accurately document the impact of the programme. Lack of emphasis on research has meant that there is no empirical evidence showing the effectiveness of our techniques in prolonging the time needed before ARVs, or showing substantive improvements in CD4 counts or drops in viral loads. The onus is on ourselves to show, using independent funding, that the project does in fact have cost-benefit advantages.

It is too early to judge the success of the project but the goodwill of the community in response to the initiative has been wonderful and people are attending the clinic in increasing numbers. So far we have all been working voluntarily but are hoping to be able to source funding to make the project sustainable in the long term.

In the context of the discussions that took place at Stanford this type of project may go some way to making an integrative approach to healthcare more mainstream.

ACKNOWLEDGMENTS

Thank you to Dr Raoul Goldberg and Dr James LaPorta for their input.

REFERENCES

[1] Balbin EG, Ironson GH, Solomon GF. Stress and coping: The psychoneuroimmunology of HIV/AIDS. Best Pract Res Clin Endocrinol Metabol 1999;13(4):615-33.
[2] McDaniel S Gillenwater DR. Psychneuroimmunology and HIV disease progression. Psychiatric Times 1999;16(10):1-2.
[3] Godbout JP Glaser R. Stress induced immune dysregulation. Implications for wound healing, infectious disease and cancer, J Neuroimmune Pharmacol 2006;1(4):421-7.
[4]
[5] Anabwani G, Navario P. Nutrition and HIV/AIDS in sub-Saharan Africa: An overview. J Appl Basic Nutr Sci 2005;21(1):96-9.
[6] Roubenoff R Schmitz H. Reduction of abdominal obesity in lipodystrophy associated with HIV infection by means of diet and exercise. Clin Infect Dis 2002;34(3):390-3.

Submitted: May 28, 2011.
Revised: June 28, 2011.
Accepted: July 01, 2011.

In: Alternative Medicine Research Yearbook 2012
Editors: Søren Ventegodt and Joav Merrick

ISBN: 978-1-62808-080-3
© 2013 Nova Science Publishers, Inc.

Chapter 14

HEART MATTERS: THE ART OF HEALING

*Erna Oldenboom, MPhil**
Orakel BV, Cape Town, South Africa

ABSTRACT

In science the heart is more often seen as a physical technical instrument, a pump responsible for pumping the blood. I suppose that this function is well studied in medical sciences especially, but does that mean that we know about the heart? In our modern society we tend to believe that all discomfort immediately needs to be resolved. We search for instant solutions instead of knowing that our immune system can solve most of our diseases perfectly well over time. Alternatively we could know that certain reactions in the body, mind and spirit are "normal" fluctuations that keep us healthy. We know of illnesses, diseases, but do we know what health is? Health is not the absence of disease. Health is not a concept. What is health? Health is for most people the number one desirable state. What do we mean by health? In our mind we cannot find answers to what health really is. We can give definitions, but a definition is exactly what it says: It is a definition, but it does not tell us what health is. We cannot describe health. We are unable to fully understand what it is. It might be that this is one of the reasons that in medicine we are more focused on what health is not, namely: illness, tensions and diseases.

Keywords: Medicine, alternative medicine, mind and body

INTRODUCTION

We know by heart to position the heart in our bodies, but do we really know about the heart? I literally mean: do we know the heart? As we see in the word HEART – the following words can be derived: HEAR and EAR. Is the heart connected to (h)earing and listening?

---

* Correspondence: Erna Oldenboom, Jai Yoga Centre, 42 Hans Strijdom Avenue, Cape Town 8012, South Africa. E-mail: erna.oldenboom@gmail.com.

In science the heart is more often seen as a physical technical instrument, a pump responsible for pumping the blood. I suppose that this function is well studied in medical sciences especially, but does that mean that we know about the heart?

Do we know about the importance of knowing what is going on in our own heart besides the physical function? Are we aware of our heartbeat? Do we listen with our inner- and outer ear? Are we aware of the importance that our heart has in connection to the rest of the body?

The Institute of HeartMath, an international non-profit research and education organisation has found that the heart "possesses a far more developed communication system with the brain than do most of the body's organs" (1). The heart not only pumps blood, but also transmits complex patterns of information to the brain and the entire body. From literature we can learn that the heart has been for as long as we know highly connected to emotions, and feelings. We all know many expressions using "heart":

- A heart of gold
- A heart of stone
- A heart-to-heart relationship or conversation
- Home is where the heart is
- A broken heart
- Know by heart
- Learn by heart

Hopefully many of the (future) medical doctors will be "called" to their profession/vocation, "called" to a certain mission and the need to serve or to give meaning to a broader community. The word vocation is generally limited to a job or an occupation. However, the original meaning of the term extended well beyond the profession. The English word has its origins in the Latin "vocare", which means, "to call" or "calling" (2).

Gregg Levoy wrote in his book "Callings" (3) that vocations can be many things:

> They may be calls to do something (become self-employed, go back to school, leave or start a relationship, move to a country, change careers, have a child) or calls to be something (more creative, less judgmental, more loving, less fearful). They may be calls towards or away from something, calls to change something, review our commitment to something, or come back to it in an entirely new way; calls toward whatever we've dared ourselves to do for as long as we can remember... (3)

Unfortunately, we often simply tune out the longings we feel, rather than confront them and act on them. Perhaps we do not really forget our calls but we fear what they might demand of us in pursuing them. Anticipating the conniptions of change blocks us from acknowledging that we do know, and always have known, what our calls are.

PHYSICIANS AND SUFFERING

During the preparation of this assignment, in a "coincidence", my focus was directed to the following article: "Too many medical practitioners CHOOSE Death" (4). The authors of this article highly recommend cultural changes in the medical field, especially when it comes to suicides amongst medical doctors. Medical doctors who experience high levels of stress, frustration, irritation – and not just a few – often do not follow the advice they give to their own patients. The origin of this phenomenon is found in the medical professional culture. Isolation can result and is frequently the consequence of this cultural prevalence of ignorance of symptoms amongst themselves, and the deathly drugs are found close by in their direct environment. In one of the first lectures of the newly arrived medical students, a professor welcomes the newcomers as follows:

> Ladies and gentleman: Welcome to the medical studies, I have to warn you that you have chosen a very unhealthy profession. You run an increased risk of depression and addiction, especially for alcohol. Know that your chance of dying from suicide is much higher than that of a non-physician (4)

Serge Daneault (5) described the suffering of caregivers, which starts with overwork and the exhaustion it causes. This, in turn, results in feelings of helplessness and frustration, followed by strong feelings of guilt for not having done everything that could possibly be done. Caregivers also suffer because they feel trapped. The needs of their patients are often complex and sometimes contradictory. Grasping this complexity is difficult and takes time, time that physicians sorely lack. As the goal of caring well for patients becomes unreachable and has to be abandoned, physicians flee into the technicalities of the medical act. Their initial aspirations, hopes, and dreams for medicine are denied and repressed. In the process, physicians' work becomes devoid of meaning, and with this loss of meaning comes suffering that, if not recognised and if left untreated, can deteriorate into mental disorders that can lead to suicide. He continued addressing some answers to ancient questions:

> Does the idea of the wounded healer offer a way out of the suffering seen among health professionals?

The notion of the wounded healer dates back to antiquity. Plato (429–347 BCE), the father of Western philosophy, stated that the most skilful physicians, rather than being models of good health, are those who have suffered from all sorts of illnesses (6). Such physicians become eloquent examples of "the wounded healer".

The Greek myth of Chiron, the centaur from whose name chirurgie is derived in French, and surgery is derived in English, can help us to understand. The Greek Gods Apollo and Artemis taught medicine to Chiron. Chiron was wounded by an arrow from Heracles' bow. He did not die (because Gods are immortal); instead, he suffered excruciating pain for the rest of his eternal days. It was because of his grievous wound that Chiron became known as a legendary healer in ancient Greece. Chiron later took an orphaned child, Esculapius, into his care. The son of Apollo and a mortal, Coronis, Esculapius had been spared a certain death, when Apollo snatched him from his dead mother's breast just as she was about to burst into flames. The orphan was entrusted to Chiron, who taught him everything he knew about the healing arts. It was thus that Esculapius became one of the two founding fathers of Western medicine.

In 1951, Carl Gustav Jung (1875-1961), first used the term wounded healer (7). Jung believed that diseases of the soul could be the best possible form of training for a healer. In a book published days before his death (8) Jung wrote that only a wounded physician could heal effectively. In so doing, Jung drew upon the myth of Chiron, making it one of the most fundamental archetypes of human history and modern medicine.

In recent years, the work of Guggenbühl-Craig (9) has shed new light on this question. Guggenbühl-Craig wrote (9) that in the therapeutic encounter, there is the healer-physician and the wounded patient. In order to promote healing, the physician tries to activate the patient's own healing powers, for example, the patient's desire to make good lifestyle decisions or to follow the physician's advice. And yet, the healer-physician has wounds, too; this is the physician's own health story. The physician's experience of being wounded is what makes him a brother of the patient, rather than his master. This triggers a fundamental change in perspective. The suffering patient can be cared for by the physician and be instrumental in the physician's own healing. Each encounter between physician and patient can be transforming and creative for both people.

There is no reason for physicians to be ashamed of their suffering. Viktor Frankl (1905-1997) (10), a psychiatrist who survived the Nazi concentration camps, wrote that just like destiny or death, suffering is a fundamental human experience. For Frankl, if life has meaning, suffering must necessarily have meaning too. The way in which a person accepts his destiny and suffering provides his life with a profound sense of meaning.

The new focus on physicians, their health, and their suffering speaks in a profound and fundamental way about Western medicine in 2011. It offers the possibility that physicians' health is a function of the creative potential of medicine. This creative energy or force is based, in turn, on a humble acknowledgment of physicians' personal wounds and vulnerability. Eric Cassell wrote (11) in the preface to "Souffrance et médecine" that this acknowledgment of suffering is a notion that dates back to antiquity; throughout the world and regardless of the form it takes, medicine exists because of a universal recognition of the terrible suffering caused by disease. The act of acknowledging, owning that as physicians we are wounded healers could be a turning point for our profession. This primitive understanding of medicine would no doubt lead us to a new sense of solidarity with our patients, who stand beside us, struggling themselves to create a better world. This better world is not some Utopia in which everyone is always kind and constantly in perfect health, but the imperfect world in which we all find ourselves and which, as a result of our constant search for meaning, is evolving toward greater cohesion and solidarity. This process might bring us joy and will most certainly bring us greater peace of mind.

In Western medicine the focus is on disease, illness and on curing instead of healing. A radical shift is essential. Our immune system is overloaded; bacteria and viruses are becoming more and more resistant to medication (drugs) and healthcare costs us fortunes. Instead of searching for long- term solutions we tend to believe that our health highly depends on medication and on the pharmaceutical industry. Advertisements try to convince us that we cannot survive without Valium, Prozac, Viagra, antibiotics and painkillers.

PHARMACEUTICAL INDUSTRY

In our modern society we tend to believe that all discomfort immediately needs to be resolved. We search for instant solutions instead of knowing that our immune system can solve most of our diseases perfectly well over time. Alternatively we could know that certain reactions in the body, mind and spirit are "normal" fluctuations that keep us healthy.

We know of illnesses, diseases, but do we know what health is? Health is not the absence of disease. Health is not a concept. What is health? Health is for most people the number one desirable state. What do we mean by health? In our mind we cannot find answers to what health really is. We can give definitions, but a definition is exactly what it says: It is a definition, but it does not tell us what health is. We cannot describe health. We are unable to fully understand what it is.

It might be that this is one of the reasons that in medicine we are more focused on what health is not, namely: illness, tensions and diseases.

In ancient traditions such as in the Chinese tradition and in Ayurveda the focus is much more on health, wellbeing, and healthy lifestyles. Ayurveda translated from Sanskrit means "the science of life". The central philosophy is that the mind and body are one and the same, and that physical health can't be achieved without emotional, mental and spiritual health. Health is defined as: sama dosha samagnisca sama dhatu mala kriyaha. Translated from Vagbhat: "The person who always eats wholesome food, enjoys a regular lifestyle, remains unattached to the objects of the senses, gives and forgives, loves truth, and serves others, is without disease." The totality of body, mind and spirit, it includes physical health, mental health, emotional health, and social health.

SCIENCE OF LIFE

In science of life there is no imperfection
Here and there and everywhere
the answers are in nature's blossoms
connected trough all ocean rivers

Landscapes changing in the manifest illusions
Of the so called self-created world
Far beyond horizon in the cosmic field of Energy
Unbounded wisdom is smiling to be invited

Clearing processes of hidden consciousness
Finding what was never far away
Touching all our sentences
Still and patient waiting for an open door

Magnificent explanations existing in every
Single cell dancing in the radiant light
Of healing possibilities above all levels
Of emotions and repetitive thoughts

Dying is the end of living or
Living is the end of death
Serving well each other
Knowing there will be never any final end

Ancient mystics whisper silent in every hearing ear
Music in the empty space
Vibrating in tune with all forms of life
Truly an expression of unlimited intelligence

There is no need to believe all unspoken words
Laugh with gratitude all adventures
And experience the miracles of the present
The only state

Erna Oldenboom

To shift to another paradigm, it is in my opinion essential to (re)shape our mind. We have to re-learn, to unlearn old habits, mechanistic responses and try to shift to new, healthier approaches. We can do that by focusing on, giving attention to and consistently reflecting on the new way of thinking. Research has shown that neural changes accompanying learning are made as a result of repeated practice, and accurate and consistent feedback, and attention to the task to be learned.

Our "heart" can play an essential role. By focusing our attention into the heart with loving-kindness it will have an impact on our mind and thinking. We are not our thinking. Our ideas and thinking change over time. We can direct our thoughts into healthier directions by focusing on our heart. Once I read the following story:

A woman was brought into a circle of stones and a Shaman (Clay Miller) told her: "You have a beautiful strong mind" and he gave her a stone. "Your mind is strong as stone" and she received more stones. She received one after the other until the moment that she almost collapsed under the weight of her own "mind stones". "Feel what this strong mind does to you, how it has power over you. Your thoughts have taken over your life; you walk literally behind your thoughts. Let your soul speak. You are a strong woman, but do not protect yourself from your emotions. Feel your sadness, Feel disappointment. You do not have to be strong. Feel strong. Your mind works as glue, everything sticks to it. Love your fear and it cannot drive you. Push it away and it owns you. Try to experience your emotions, embrace them, that will move them. Emotions become e-motion, energy in movement" (12)

In most countries medical students are selected based on the highest grades, especially for mathematics, physics and chemistry. Indeed it is a wonderful foundation for diagnosing and learning analytical skills. If we would like to change the current paradigm we should also be focused on new medical students with a high level of emotional intelligence. We need students, future medical doctors, that are able to explain and to recognise in themselves stressful situations, and who are able to listen to their own body language and mental states.

The mind is a useful instrument and it enables us to discover new horizons, but we have to learn to recognise the mechanism between heart and mind. In our heart we are able to experience all feelings and emotions that we need to be aware of, to be mindful of what is going on in ourselves.

Our soul is guiding us in that direction when we feel connected to what I would like to call universal consciousness. It needs courage to change attitudes and behavior in a world that does not encourage expressions and feelings from the heart as mainstream. But we have no other choice.

Heart matters: The art of healing

Honor your soul's courage and know the path of the heart is the only path to be in
HH Sai Maa

CAREGIVERS WHO CARE

The doctor of the future will give no medicine, but will interest his patients in the care of the human frame and in the cause and prevention of disease

Thomas Edison (1847-1931)

I would highly recommend considering (re)introducing rituals and ceremonies in the medical sciences that are emanations of the new thinking, such as:

- Self-support groups
- Non-violent communication platforms
- Courses in mindfulness
- Dialogues about values and wellbeing
- Anti-stress courses
- Sport activities
- Art courses
- (Sound) Meditation
- An eye for emotional (im)balance

REFERENCES

[1]   Institute of HeartMath. Overview. Accessed 2011 May 15. URL: www.Heartmath.org.

[2]   Raybur CA. Vocation as calling. In: Bloch DP, Richmond LJ, eds. Connection Between spirit and work in career development. Palo Alto, CA: Davies-Black, 1997:162-83.

[3]   Levoy G. Callings: Finding and following an authentic life. New York: Three Rivers, 1997.

[4]   Van Schaik AM, Kleijn SA, Van der Veldt AAM, Van Tilburg W. Te veel dokters kiezen de dood. In: Medisch Contact, 2010. Accessed 2011 May 10. URL: http://medischcontact.artsennet.nl/Tijdschriftartikel/Te-veel-dokters-kiezen-de-dood.htm

[5]   Daneault S. The wounded healer. Can this idea be of use to family physicians? Can Fam Physician 2008;54(9):1218-9.

[6]   Plato. La république. In: Oeuvres complètes. Paris: Soissange et Frères, 1827.

[7]   Jung CG. Fundamental questions of psychotherapy. Princeton, NJ: Princeton University Press, 1951.

[8]   Jung CG. Ma vie: souvenirs, rêves et pensées recueillis et publiés par Aniéla Jaffé. Paris: Gallimard, 1967.

[9]   Guggenbühl-Craig A. Power in helping professions. Zurich: Spring Publ, 1976.

[10]   Frankl V. Man's search for meaning. New York: Simon Schuster, 1959.

[11]   Daneault S. Souffrance et médecine. Quebec: Les Presses de l'Université du Québec, 2006.

[12]   Aleh-zon. Accessed 2011 May 10. URL: http://www.arizonahealingtours.com/

Submitted: May 23, 2011.
Revised: June 29, 2011.
Accepted: July 01, 2011.

In: Alternative Medicine Research Yearbook 2012
Editors: Søren Ventegodt and Joav Merrick

ISBN: 978-1-62808-080-3
© 2013 Nova Science Publishers, Inc.

Chapter 15

THE THIRD WAY?

*Leslie Pleass, DO**
Quality of Life Centre,
Johannesburg, South Africa

ABSTRACT

The one thing that separates mankind from the rest of the living beings on this planet is choice. We have this blessing and/or curse, subject to a lot of internal and external parameters, of choice. Out of this surrendering to life emerged a science, philosophy and art of helping people which I use in my daily practice; of being of some use to man/woman kind. It has a Western bias with an Asian twist. I see people reacting to life's challenges through anxiety and fear. Choices are made to the benefit or detriment of themselves and others. In this, called or not called, the gods are present and bad things happen to good people; loss, grieving, sadness and feeling absolutely lost in the world. People consequently freeze their hearts and feel nothing, or they open their hearts up to more loss and hopefully gain, all the time making choices that are profoundly meaningful. People do not always realise the generational patterns placed on them consciously or unconsciously through their family, with cross-generational dynamics. The sins of the mother/father, and the rest are placed upon you. Now, this untidy explanation has roots in thousands of years of Asian medicine and Western evolutionary thoughts. That is how I treat the people who come to see me.

Keywords: Quality of life, medicine, alternative medicine

INTRODUCTION

I get my best ideas, visions and magnificent goals and outcomes in the bath. But I get the greatest hindsight, insight and foresight from my dreams. In this I take comfort from the Jungian analyst and psychiatrist Edward F Edinger (1922-1998) saying that the ego's view of itself and the world is totally subjective, while the psyche or unconscious, frequently

---

* Correspondence: Leslie Pleass, POBox 1156 Magaliessig 2067, South Africa. E-mail: leslie@foodstate.co.za.

expressed through dreams, is totally objective. Objectively dreaming oneself awake. The problem with the dream language is that it is not a language that we can clearly hear and see; rather it is loaded with deep ancient symbolic imagery, going back to man's first awakening from unconsciousness to some semblance of consciousness, culminating in this magnificent but deeply-flawed modern Homo sapiens. The one thing that separates mankind from the rest of the living beings on this planet is choice. We have this blessing and/or curse, subject to a lot of internal and external parameters, of choice.

So when I committed to writing an article on being part of the helping professions, I had made a choice. Which I immediately regretted. This led almost instantly to what I have battled with since I was in primary school, a mother of all headaches. After riding out this debilitating period, I then asked the psyche one night, the objective dream world, to give me some imagery from the omnipotent all-encompassing world of the great mystery. An imaginal, luminal image, which would allow me to at least start the article. As all writers know, our great fear is the blank page, or in the modern world the blank screen with the cursor winking at you in the upper left corner.

So I had a dream. I dreamt I was observing an old fashioned chicken run and a passageway between two chicken coops, a primitive first take on what is now a horrendous industry of battery chicken facilities. I was just observing this passageway with these two chicken-wired enclosed areas with a few chickens on either side. So, on awakening, I was frankly a little disappointed that it was not a grander dream. One of those big dreams you incubate for a longer time until they reveal a multi-faceted jewel of awareness. But that was it, a chicken coop. I then had a bath, hoping for some more insight from my rather miserable dream, writing, at times precariously, in the bath, images and thoughts that emerged from the dream and the bath.

These are the current delusions and illusions that I am working through: When I was in Stanford, a little town in the Western Cape, I had a dream and in the dream a woman in a most outraged way asked me what my "medicine name" was? In many indigenous cultures, when a person goes through a major healing and or initiation, they change their name to their medicine name. A new name for a new person. Later on, when I was back home, I had another dream where a women touched and held me in a totally present way to such an extent I almost lost consciousness, and she said, "this is the Third Way, the way you must work".

So the chicken coop dream with the passage between two enclosed ways felt like it was the confirmation of a Third Way; the middle way. Rather than being cooped up in one school of thought or an opposing other, there is a middle way, a Third Way. There is in addition a more modern interpretation of the chicken run, seeing who "chickens" out first in some game of risk. Like seeing who will swerve first when two cars race towards each other. A test of courage. And of course the root meaning of the word courage is "heart". To have enough courage to follow your heart, even perhaps at times recklessly. The relatively recent animation film called "Chicken run" centres on a band of chickens who seek a smooth-talking Rhode Island Red named Rocky as their only hope to escape from certain death when the owners of their farm decides to move from selling eggs to selling chicken pies. For a chicken, producing eggs requires effort, but creating chicken pies requires courage and commitment. In retrospect and fairness to my less than exciting dream, it appeared it had much more significance than I originally gave it.

How does one begin to discuss the life-changing decision of becoming someone who helps people? Why bother? Why does one not become an artist, a poet? Sean Haldane, a neuropsychologist who was recently on the shortlist to become the Professor of Poetry at Oxford University, said in an interview this year: "I don't have huge faith in the possibility of psychotherapy to change people as I used to. In fact I now think poetry has more capacity to change people than psychotherapy. If you read a poem and it gets to you, it can shift your perspective in quite a big way and writing a poem, even more so." Interesting...?

Within you lurks a way, a need to express itself in the act of helping another; helping and compassionately serving another, a stranger. A strange concept indeed. But out of it comes a story about who you are. We are story and pattern creators. If you want to enter the helping profession, it is possibly usual and most likely useful to have an aberrant childhood. The mythology of the wounded physician is quite possibly a requisite for becoming a caregiver. My late mother (I can speak a little bolder than when she was alive) was a full-blown narcissistic personality. When you are small and you have one mother, you obviously have the projection that she is the best, because you have no other comparative mechanism. She was the best, the greatest mother on this world. But ah, how sadly and slowly the delusions must be liberated from these firm, comforting attachments. It is truly as if our whole life is built strongly around delusions and illusions. Lately I have been imagining that we create this scaffolding we stand upon in order to be earthed and committed at a certain time of our lives. Then slowly we notice it dissolve under our feet, if we are aware, painfully or in a liberating way, to take us to another scaffolding. This in turn dissolves or breaks away. We need the scaffolds, but temporarily. Perhaps if we did not have them we would not exist at all. So emerging from a mother whose only reference was "what's in it for me?", with no innate ability to see her little boy as possibly needing and wanting something like love, was a difficult scaffolding to let go of. Not truly being seen or loved by your mother is a painful wound, and I have no reference on this because I do not know the inverse.

We most likely all suffer from what I consider the original wound. But again that is my illusion and delusion. One wonders what impact that kind of childhood has on the intra-psychic mechanisms of adaptation? Reductively one could say one would want to be helpful, liked, could I dare say, wanted?

If you have wisely or unwisely "chosen" to become part the helping professions, the problem as I see it is that however you enter the helping profession, you have to go through an initiation. This initiation almost has to be a form of propaganda, because all helping profession schools have to have a clear outcome they would like the student to achieve, otherwise its curriculum would be all over the place. It makes me think - if you were being trained to be a cab driver in London you would have to learn what they romantically call "the knowledge". That is, you need to know every street name in greater London. That would be the propaganda you would have to know, and not the streets of Berlin.

Belabouring an obverse pun, we may as well start with the Acupuncturist. As I frequently point out to my patients, if you go to an Acupuncturist don't be surprised that he might want to put a needle into you. If you go to a homoeopath don't be surprised that I might want to give you a remedy. An osteopath/chiropractor would examine your spine/body and find a restriction. The medical doctor would give you a drug or recommend surgery. The podiatrist an orthotic. The optometrist glasses. We could possibly go on forever. So is it possible we are all in a delusion and illusion? The propaganda that we have been taught or embraced at a undergraduate or postgraduate level has permeated all of our filters when we meet a person who needs to be helped.

Now the person who needs help is equally under the propaganda spell. If we use the Jungian model of the extrovert and introvert, and in addition his four functions of thinking, feeling, sensation and intuition, we then have a rich bag of possibilities, potential interactions and outcomes. If she is a deeply thinking logical individual, she lends herself perfectly to a very reductive helping model of evidence-based medicine with all its perceived logical surety. If though he is a feeling type who responds with a sense of deep emotional flavours to his outcomes and choices, his decisions are made from a non-logical basis. He just "felt right" with that treatment and person. Then there is the deeply sensating type, who functions from a physical awareness of their body, responding to how the individual physically touched them, how the environment, the total package had an influence on their physical being. Lastly, the most elusive of them all - thank heaven there are not a lot of them about - the deeply intuitive individual. She functions from a gestalt of the present moment, massively influenced by all aspects of her history. So anything could cure her or make her ill. These people have this massive sense of awareness of everything, good and bad. Exhausting for them, and you who treat them. In addition, as I mentioned in the beginning, you also have the Extroverted person who walks in and takes over the office while the Introverted will creep into the office and has to be coaxed into a dialogue with new and strange people.

So here we have two colliding worlds; the person who has a calling to be in the helping profession, and the individual who needs help.

I deliberately call it "a calling". It has to be a vocation, which in its original meaning is a calling from the divine to be a helper, a server, a compassionate giver of yourself to people in need. Otherwise don't do it. It needs to be an obsession, otherwise it is a hateful burden. You have to be a willing and able seller of help and care.

The individual who needs help is the willing and able buyer of help and care. They need the right person, with the right solution, in the right place at the right time. They personally need the right awareness and desire to recognise the possibilities of being relieved of some or all of these difficulties. It's a rich complex dance of possibilities that might or might not be fulfilled. Frequently too, our choices are not that rational. Simon Sinik in his book "Start with Why" points out the "why" a company or person does something is more important to the consumer than the "what" and "how". He argues most influentially that our decisions are made from the non-conscious parts of the brain, not our conscious parts. He uses the argument of brand and nationalistic loyalties. Try to argue with someone that their country is not the best. The 2010 soccer World Cup competition held in South Africa is an example of non-rational nationalistic fervour played out in a safe and fun environment of competitive sport. The support for your country and its team is almost irrational. The "why" we do something, coming from a deep inner commitment to something or someone, is non-rational. The "why" we feel something is difficult to articulate, it is a knowingness that transcends knowledge.

So our choices of why we do something, or submit ourselves to somebody to care for us, are often coming from a deep non-conscious place. It's the knowingness that supplants just head knowledge. If the individual has a deep knowingness of "why" they do or believe in something, they are often wildly successful. We in the helping profession all have a story to tell about the worst student academically in the class who, on barely graduating, does phenomenally well in the world. Possibly because he or she had an X-factor to them that transcended their poor intellectual qualities; the converse of that story is the brilliant student having a life post-academia of absolute mediocrity. It's the old story that having a high intellectual quotient does not imply you have a high emotional quotient. In an important aspect of my life I am a director and shareholder in a nutritional company. One of the great blessings in my life is that the chairman of our group of companies is an outstanding leader. He has an intangible quality about him that shifts and moves a meeting in extraordinary ways. Observing him for many years allows me to spot these intangible qualities in people I meet. I have also had the honour of serving on the Statutory Council that regulated the Allied Health Professionals for over twenty years. I was appointed by Ministers of Health from the apartheid and post-apartheid era. In that position I served on the executive for virtually all that time. Again, this offered me the chance to observe and interact with people from all spectrums of society, seeing qualities that are head-based or heart-based. Slowly and with great relief I am moving away to a more heart-based world view, trying to express love for myself and others.

I recently went through cancer and after exhausting what I perceived to be all alternative treatments I started to explore what orthodox care had to offer. I went through five specialists before I felt comfortable to submit and surrender to a particular surgeon's intervention. Why him? I can give you some tidy logical answers, but I noticed an intangible essence about him, an obsession with his craft, and an aesthetic priest-like commitment to his area of experience. I ticked all the logical head-stuff about him, but there was an intangible aspect to him and I knew I could allow him to do something radical (in my view) to me. To place some significance to this decision: I have never had surgery done to me, and never stayed in a hospital as a patient before. Never. So it required some deep surrendering on my part to allow this to happen.

Out of this surrendering to life emerged a science, philosophy and art of helping people which I use in my daily practice; of being of some use to man/woman kind. It has a Western bias with an Asian twist. I see people reacting to life's challenges through anxiety and fear. Choices are made to the benefit or detriment of themselves and others. In this, called or not called, the gods are present and bad things happen to good people; loss, grieving, sadness and feeling absolutely lost in the world. People consequently freeze their hearts and feel nothing, or they open their hearts up to more loss and hopefully gain, all the time making choices that are profoundly meaningful. People do not always realise the generational patterns placed on them consciously or unconsciously through their family, with cross-generational dynamics. The sins of the mother/father, and the rest are placed upon you. Now, this untidy explanation has roots in thousands of years of Asian medicine and Western evolutionary thoughts. That is how I treat the people who come to see me.

As an osteopath all I use are my hands, mind, intuition and words to attempt to align the body-mind-spirit. That is all I use, but what I did learn from my little sojourn in the little town of Stanford was this from a professor of Business at the local business school: research can be done to prove or disprove anything. However I also learnt that we are living in a synchronistic, non-causal world, and once anybody sees me, we are then entangled for the rest of our existence.

In closing, I would like to talk about the first night in Stanford. We were all warily sizing each other up. However, during dinner and afterwards over too much red wine, we discussed life. Yet death was present, people tenderly talking about people who had died, or were dying under their care. It has been for me a privilege, while only using my hands, mind, intuition and words, to comfort and be present as death became present in the people who seek me out for help. It helps to nudge us to living; as a dear friend calls it, dying to live.

Synchronistically, death had come that night to a family member of one of the delegates, and she had to leave the very next day for the funeral.

DEATH AND AWAKENING INTERWOVEN

That evening prompted me at the end of the time we had together to read my poem to Jackie to my fellow travellers on this road. Jackie was a beautiful soul who, when she was preparing to retire from a life time of work, was diagnosed with cancer of the stomach. During the last year of her life she bravely lived with an emerging lump growing menacingly in her stomach that felt like an incubating foetus. Using my hands, mind, intuition and words I worked with her; dying to live. It was a fulfilling yet emotionally exhausting time. As usual in paradise there is a caveat: her husband used to skulk in the corner as I treated her, at times I could feel my hair rise on the back of my neck as I spoke to him. He was the worst of "good" men. One day he had to do an errand and I worked with him not present. The room was so different that I boldly asked her if she felt comfortable with him present. She said not, with a look of relief on her face. He was sadly a major influence on her inner and outer dynamic. So from that day on, until she died, we worked on her living to die, dying to live. Appropriately I end this story with my poem to my beloved Jackie, who still brings tears to my eyes even when I write this.

THE FUNERAL OF JACKIE

At the funeral ceremony
I was thanked publicly
Even kissing my hands
With me weeping
At their pain
And my loss
Of a woman
Who I loved
Easily
Softly
What an honour
To have accompanied
Her to death, stillness
Of knowing I am of value
Benefitting, enriching
Not an apprentice
If I choose
To matter
At last
Easily
Softly

The third way? 135

Lovingly
Thought of my death
Don't want fake minister
One who jokes, drinks
Want people to read
Out aloud my words
To my music
My musings
I matter
Not organ wailing
Off key
Sadly wrong century
Wrong words
Myths not digested
Assimilated, embodied
All this from one funeral
Of a lady I briefly loved
Touched, blended with softly
Who I miss already, deeply
Epilogue
Many years later
The husband
Who sat crouched in corner
Who now I know
Sat
Enviously watching me
Just silently, lovingly, prepared her for death
Plotted my downfall

A betrayal cutting
To all my childhood fears
At Jackie's funeral
Should have been weeping at my loss
Coming

Submitted: May 25, 2011.
Revised: June 30, 2011.
Accepted: July 03, 2011.

In: Alternative Medicine Research Yearbook 2012
Editors: Søren Ventegodt and Joav Merrick

ISBN: 978-1-62808-080-3
© 2013 Nova Science Publishers, Inc.

Chapter 16

CONVERSATIONS: THE FIVE STAR DOCTOR

Saville N Furman, MBChB, FCFP(SA) *
Family Physician, Milnerton, South Africa

ABSTRACT

After graduating medical school I believed I would be a "knight in shining armour" and would "cure" all my patients with my knowledge of pharmacology. However, it did not take long to realize that this was an unrealistic expectation and joined a Balint Group. Here I learnt many new concepts and insights into the doctor-patient relationship and learnt that the doctor himself was the most potent drug. I learnt of concepts like the "door-handle syndrome" and a" mother presenting through the child." I began teaching undergraduates and started to adopt and incorporate the "biopsychosocial" model in the management of my patients in the family setting. I learnt of the three stage assessment and used the new techniques to the benefit of my patients. On a practical level there are everyday barriers that impede/inhibit me from being an effective five star doctor. These are imposed by the funders, ie medical aids that do not recognize "medications" needed for curative and preventative care of patients. I wish is that we could transmit the vibes of our conversations over the week-end and cross-pollinate with all health-care givers to provide excellent integrated care to our patients.

Keywords: Medicine, alternative medicine, family medicine

INTRODUCTION

When I was contacted to become part of a small select group of people to meet and discuss the current health issues, I became very excited at the prospect of meeting with other caregivers/healers. I was flattered to be included in a group of "wise" and "experienced" people to discuss the state of medicine and to give a focus and direction of where medicine

---

* Correspondence: Saville N Furman, MBChB, FCFP(SA), Family Physician, POBox 119, Milnerton 7435, South Africa. E-mail: savillef@iafrica.com.

should be going. I was intrigued at what format these "conversations" would take and curious to think what contribution, an 62 year old "old fashioned" general practioner could make.

I qualified at University of Cape Town in 1973 believing I would be a "knight in shining armour" and would "cure" all my patients with my knowledge of pharmacology. However, it did not take long to realize that this was an unrealistic expectation and joined a Balint Group in the late 1970's. Here I learnt many new concepts and insights into the doctor-patient relationship and learnt that the doctor himself was the most potent drug. I learnt of concepts like the "door-handle syndrome" and a" mother presenting through the child." I began teaching undergraduates in the early 1980's and started to adopt and incorporate the "biopsychosocial" model in the management of my patients in the family setting. I learnt of the three stage assessment and used the new techniques to the benefit of my patients.

However, there was still something "missing" as at medical school I learnt "it's a sin to miss" and you always have to make a diagnosis before you can successfully manage a patient. Due to the very nature of primary health care, we often see "undifferentiated" presentations and have to make rapid decisions.

During the early part of the new millennium, I had many personal losses and losses in my practice. I embarked on a new "journey" that I entitled from "synchronicity to serendipity." I realized that I needed to change and was exposed to other doctors who felt the same way. During this journey I met many wonderful people from other healing disciplines. I learnt new techniques such as mindfulness that I have incorporated into "healing techniques." I learnt to be more accepting of the role that complimentary medicine has to play in the holistic management of my patients.

REFLECTIONS OVER THE WEEK-END

I arrived on the friday very excited and pleased to escape the "crazy" frenetic world of my family practice. Personally I was in a bad space, as I had just admitted my 91 year old father, suffering from an acute dementia, to a frail-care facility with the realization that we would have to pack up his home. His message to me when I started my university education in 1967 was " to concentrate on my medical studies and leave politics to the politicians!!"

I have been to many workshops and congresses over the last 30 years, but have never experienced anything as incredible as the "conversations" and instant bonding with other caregivers/healers. From story-telling, dancing, the inside-out café, fireside chats, talking at meal-times, sitting on the grass, listening to other presentations or performing relaxation exercises, I felt safe, contained and did not even miss the television or reading the daily newspapers. Usually at medical meetings, doctors moan and whinge about medical aids, violence and negative aspects of our professional lives and practicing primary care in South Africa. I found every interaction and activity stimulating and left on a "high."

The next day, I tried to incorporate all I had learnt and experienced over the weekend into the management of my patients. I continually asked myself, "does this patient really need a drug?!!"

THE FIVE STAR DOCTOR

Recent years have seen a proliferation of interest in the role of the medical practitioner in today's society. A number of articles and opinions have appeared in journals and other publications devoted to a description of the ideal doctor and an analysis of his tasks and functions. There have been official pronouncements on the subject issued by health authorities, declarations made by professional associations, as well as statements made at expert meeting s and conferences. Quite apart from the volume of opinion expressed by the medical profession itself, there has been no shortage of opinions articulated by individuals and the community.

A review of this body of opinion shows that the profile of the ideal doctor would include five areas of expertise. A doctor with all five might be called a "five star doctor" (1). He would be expected to fulfill the following functions:

- Assess and improve the quality of care by responding to the patient's total health needs with integrated preventive, curative and rehabilitative services.
- Make optimal use of new technologies, bearing in mind ethical and financial considerations and the ultimate benefit of the consumer.
- Promote healthy lifestyles by means of communication skills and the empowerment of individuals and groups for their own health protection.
- Reconcile individual and community health requirements, striking a balance between patients' expectations and those of society at large, both short term and long term.
- Work efficiently in teams both within the health sector and across the health sector and other socio-economic sectors influencing health.

Peter Lee (2), the president of WONCA, responded to Bolen (2). He stated that it is becoming increasingly apparent that if doctors are to practice in an ideal way, not only do they need to be properly educated themselves, but society itself also needs to be educated to know what to expect of its health care services and doctors. It is sometimes the unrealistic expectations of the public and traditional health beliefs of individual patients which bring pressure to bear on the doctor to behave in a way which is not ideal. For example, in some societies the doctor is under continual pressure to prescribe more and more drugs, not just for curative purpose, or symptomatic relief, but for imagined or hear-say belief that the drug can do them good. The doctor who attempts to prescribe rationally runs the risk of his patients leaving him for doctors who will meet their unprofessional demands.

Therefore the family doctor has a sixth role: that of educating patients and the community to change their expectations to those that are consistent with good medical practice as we understand it today.

Lee (2) ends off by stating:

> So perhaps we should be adding a sixth star:" to educate individual patients and the community at large about the nature of health and illnesses, what medicine can and cannot do, the dangers of over-medication or self-medication, and the most cost –effective way of utilizing the community's health care resources.

After the weekend, I reflected on the barriers that are preventing me from becoming a five or six star doctor. There are two main ones. The first is communication skills that were not previously effectively taught at traditional medical schools. We need to learn to communicate with patients, colleagues and all members of the health care team. We have to be accepting, non-judgmental and non-condemnatory. Secondly, we as doctors need to learn tolerance and acknowledge that we don't own the exclusive rights to be the only recognized members of the health care team. We need to work more efficiently in teams.

On a practical level there are everyday barriers that impede/inhibit me from being an effective five star doctor. These are imposed by the funders, ie medical aids that do not recognize "medications" needed for curative and preventative care of patients. For example they will not pay for certain vaccines. They also refuse to pay for iron, vitamin B and omega 3 as they maintain there is no "scientific" evidence as to their efficacy. Psychiatric benefits are very limited. They will not fund a "suicide" patient's admission to a private hospital as it is considered a "self-induced" injury, yet do not blink an eyelid to pay benefits for cirrhosis of the liver caused by alcohol or lung cancer caused by excessive smoking! Some complimentary therapies like acupuncture, stress-relief are not recognized as therapeutic by some of the funders.

My wish is that we could transmit the vibes of our conversations and cross-pollinate with all health-care givers to provide excellent integrated care to our patients.

REFERENCES

[1]   Boelen C. The five star doctor. As I see it. Hong Kong Pract 1994;16(7):339-40.
[2]   Lee PCY. The five star doctor. As I see it. Hong Kong Pract 1994;16(7):338-9.

Submitted: May 30, 2011.
Revised: July 01, 2011.
Accepted: July 07, 2011.

SECTION TWO – FROM SLEEP TO HIPPOCRATES

In: Alternative Medicine Research Yearbook 2012
Editors: Søren Ventegodt and Joav Merrick

ISBN: 978-1-62808-080-3
© 2013 Nova Science Publishers, Inc.

Chapter 17

SLEEP DISORDERS AND SLEEP PATTERNS IN ADOLESCENTS

Donald E Greydanus, MD*
and Cynthia Feucht, PharmD

Department of Pediatrics and Human Development, Michigan State University College of Human Medicine, Kalamazoo Center for Medical Studies and Department of Pharmacy Practice, Ferris State University, Borgess Ambulatory Care, Kalamazoo, Michigan, US

ABSTRACT

Healthy sleep-awake cycles are essential for normal physical and psychological health in humans. There are a number of sleep disorders in adolescents including excessive daytime sleepiness, insomnia, narcolepsy, restless legs syndrome, parasomnias, nocturnal enuresis, and others. Behavioral management (including establishing proper sleep hygiene) is the key to many sleep problems in youth, though the judicious use of pharmacologic agents is helpful in some, as reviewed in this discussion. The prescription of sedative medications, particularly those with addictive qualities, should be used only with great caution and restraint by clinicians in patients with insomnia. There is no established role for the use of herbal products for insomnia except perhaps, for melatonin. Research in sleep medicine is expanding and promises more treatment options for sleep concerns and disorders in youth.

Keywords: Adolescence, sleep, sleep disorders, sleep pattern

---

[*] Correspondence: Professor Donald E. Greydanus MD, Dr. HC (ATHENS), Pediatrics and Human Development, Michigan State University College of Human Medicine, Pediatrics Program Director, Michigan State University/Kalamazoo Center for Medical Studies, Kalamazoo, MI 49008-1284 United States. E-mail: Greydanus@kcms.msu.edu.

INTRODUCTION

There are three basic stages of human consciousness that are identified as wake, non-REM (rapid eye movement) sleep, and REM sleep (see table 1) (1). Quality sleep is important for all humans to allow proper health and to function properly during waking hours (2-12). Those between 6 to 12 years of age generally need 10-11 hours per 24 hours and adolescents need an average of 9 hours per 24 hours, though there is some variation from individual to individual. Delta sleep (slow wave sleep or deep sleep) occurs in Stages 3 and 4 of non-REM sleep and is the most restorative sleep time as well as the sleep time that is most difficult to arouse someone. REM sleep ("dream sleep") is characterized by generalized atonia of muscles, bursts of rapid eye movement, dreaming along with inhibition of erections and diaphragmatic movements. In contrast to non-REM sleep, REM sleep involves increased cardiovascular and cerebrovascular activities along with irregular breathing.

Human beings need less total night sleep as they mature from infancy to late adolescence and a later sleep onset hour (bedtime) is characteristic of many adolescents along with a 40% reduction in REM sleep stage from ages 10 to 20 years. As the adolescent matures the non-REM to REM sleep ratios become 75% to 25% with a normal pattern of 4-6 cycles of change (i.e., every 90 minutes) from non-REM to REM sleep cycles with normal transient periods of arousals during night sleep. Daytime naps are not needed by adolescents unless night sleep is significantly interrupted. A number of factors regulate and influence sleep-wake cycles, especially the endogenous circadian rhythm or internal biologic clock mechanism. This internal clock mechanism is affected by light exposure that turns off the endogenous melatonin production while absence of light (dark) turns on melatonin production. Research in sleep medicine has identified a number of "zeitgebers" or external stimuli that affect the internal clock, such as meal timing, a ringing alarm clock or other environmental cues. The circadian pacemaker is located in the suprachiasmatic nucleus in the brain. Puberty initiates a normal circadian sleep delay in most adolescents that results in a later desired bedtime than notes in childhood. Sleep disorders and abnormal sleep patterns are found in as many as half of adolescents with potentially very negative impact on their mental and/or physical health.

A number of sleep disorders have been classified as listed in Table 2. Some adolescents are at increased risk for sleep problems, including those with chronic illnesses, psychiatric disorders, and developmental disorders, as noted in Table 3.

Table 1. Stages of Human Life*

1. Being awake
2. Non-REM sleep (rapid eye movement)
a.   Stage 1 Sleep (transition of wake and sleep): light sleep
b.   Stage 2 Sleep (starts true sleep state)
c.   Stage 3: first part of deep sleep (also called delta or slow wave sleep)
d.   Stage 4: second part of deep sleep
3. REM Sleep (rapid eye movement with generalized muscle atonia)

* Used with permission from: Greydanus DE: "Sleep disorders in children and adolescents" In: Pediatric and Adolescent Psychopharmacology. Eds: DE Greydanus, JL Calles JR, and DR Patel. Cambridge University Press: Cambridge, England, ch. 11, page 200, 2008.

Sleep disorders and sleep patterns in adolescents 145

Table 2. Sleep Disorders

1. Excessive Daytime Sleepiness
2. Insomnia
a.   Delayed Sleep Phase Disorder (Sleep Onset Association Disorder)
b.   Limit Setting Sleep Disorder
c.   Adjustment Sleep Disorder
d.   Psychophysiologic Insomnia
e.   Altitude insomnia
3. Post-traumatic hypersomnolence
4. Narcolepsy
5. Klein-Levin Syndrome
6. Sleep-disordered Breathing: OSAHS (Obstructive Sleep Apnea/hypopnea Syndrome
7. Parasomnias
a.   Sleep Talking
b.   Nightmares
c.   Sleep Terrors (pavor nocturnes)
d.   Nocturnal enuresis
e.   Others seen in childhood (Bruxism; Rhythm Movement Disorders (head banging, head rolling, body rocking)
8. Restless Legs Syndrome
9. Periodic Limb Movement Disorder

Table 3. Disorders with Increased Incidence of Sleep Disorders*

1. Chronic Medical Disorders
a. Asthma
b. Cystic fibrosis
c. Hyperthyroidism
d. Organ failure (i.e., liver, kidney)
e. Gastroesophageal reflux
2. Psychiatric Disorders
a. Attention-Deficit/Hyperactivity Disorder (ADHD)
b. Mood Disorders
c. Anxiety Disorders
d. Conduct Disorder
e. Oppositional Defiant Disorder
f. Schizophrenia
g. Others
3. Developmental Disorders
a. Autistic Spectrum Disorders
b. Severe Mental Retardation
c. Angelman's syndrome
d. Rett's syndrome
e. Smith-Magenis syndrome
f. Down syndrome
g. Prader-Willi syndrome
h. Others
4. Fatal Familial Insomnia (noted in adults)
5. Neuromuscular Disorders
a. Myotonic Dystrophy
b. Duchenne's Muscular Dystrophy
6. Medications (Prescription and Over-the-Counter) (see Table 5)

* Used with permission from: Greydanus DE: "Sleep disorders in children and adolescents" In: Pediatric and Adolescent Psychopharmacology. Eds: DE Greydanus, JL Calles JR, and DR Patel. Cambridge University Press: Cambridge, England, ch. 11, page 202, 2008.

Youth with chronic medical conditions may develop abnormal sleeping patterns due to the impact of pain, intermittent hospitalizations (with frequent awaking at night from staff), family dynamic issues, mental health problems (anxiety, depression, others), and consumption of various medications (over-the counter and prescription) that can cause sleep disruption (see table 4). Clinicians should always be cognizant of the side effects of medications they recommend including those that can lead to nocturnal arousals, daytime sleepiness, worsened obstructive sleep apnea or restless legs syndrome (see table 4).

Perhaps half of adolescents with attention deficit/hyperactivity disorder (ADHD) develop sleep problems that include insomnia, frequent night awakenings, and incomplete sleep that may be caused by or complicated by the stimulant effects of anti-ADHD stimulant medications and other ADHD co-morbidities, such as anxiety, depression, oppositional defiant disorder, and others. A variety of sedating medications are often used to improve insomnia in ADHD patients, include alpha-2 agonists, antihistamines, and antidepressants given at bedtime: clonidine (0.1 mg to 0.3 mg), imipramine (50 mg to 75 mg), trazodone (25 mg to 50 mg), exogenous melatonin (3 mg to 6 mg), paroxetine (20 mg to 30 mg), mirtazapine (7.5 mg to 15 mg), and others as noted in the section on Insomnia.

Table 4. Medications Interfering with Normal Sleep Patterns*

Drug	Sleep Effect
Alcohol	Insomnia due to delayed sleep onset
Anticonvulsants	Sedation during the day
Antihistamines (first-generation) • diphenhydramine • hydroxyzine • chlorpheniramine	Daytime sleepiness; lowers efficiency
Antidepressants • SSRI[1] • TCA[2] • Bupropion • Duloxetine (SNRI)	Activating effects with sleep interruption Sleepiness in the day due to slow wave sleep blunting
Caffeine	Insomnia due to delayed sleep onset
Corticosteroids	Stimulating effects leading to insomnia
Opioids	Daytime sleepiness, insomnia, nightmares, worsening of obstructive sleep apnea
Nicotine (tobacco)	Insomnia due to delayed sleep onset
Stimulants • methylphenidate • dextroamphetamine	Stimulant effects with insomnia (delayed sleep onset)
Theophylline	Delayed sleep onset, increased arousals during sleep

[1] SSRI: Selective Serotonin Reuptake Inhibitor
[2] TCA: Tricyclic Antidepressant

* Used with permission from: Greydanus DE: "Sleep disorders in children and adolescents" In: Pediatric and Adolescent Psychopharmacology. Eds: DE Greydanus, JL Calles JR, and DR Patel. Cambridge University Press: Cambridge, England, ch. 11, page 203, 2008.

Sleep evaluation

The careful medical history and physical examination is crucial to identifying the specific sleep abnormality of an adolescent (13-16). One should inquire about the regular time of sleep onset and waking up, nocturnal sleep duration, sleep awakening frequencies, and the presence of such issues as excessive snoring, daytime sleepiness, sleep walking, sleep talking, nightmares, and others. The examination may document the presence of enlarged tonsils, fatigue in the office during the day that suggests excessive daytime sleepiness, and others. It is very helpful to have the youth keep a sleep diary to record their sleep habits that can be used to diagnose various abnormal sleep-awake cycles.

Those with complicated sleep problems and/or those resistant to therapy should be referred to a local sleep center that can use such tools as actigraphy and a sleep lab study. The actigraphy involves use of a wrist or ankle device to record sleep and awake cycles while a sleep lab study provides a detailed recording of the youth while sleeping that involves an electrocardiogram, electroencephalogram, chin and tibial movements, oronasal flow, movements of chest and abdomen, oxyhemoglobin saturations, end-tidal carbon dioxide levels, and others. A careful evaluation of the youth's sleep problems allows a more accurate diagnosis with the ability to develop an effective management plan. Various sleep disorders are now considered with emphasis on pharmacologic management.

INSOMNIA

Insomnia is a term and not a specific diagnosis referring to acute or chronic difficulty in falling asleep due to many factors such as chronic poor sleep hygiene, obstructive sleep apnea, effects of medications (prescription, over-the-counter, or illict), and others (5). Sleep onset association disorder is described in infants or young children who normally awaken frequently that is complicated by parents who intervene on a frequent basis with rocking or feeding so that the infants learns to fall asleep only with some type of parental intervention.

Limit setting sleep disorder is described in those three years of age and older who refuse to go to bed because of various issues, such as parents who do not instill a regular bedtime hour, effects of medications, the development of primary sleep disorders, concomitant anxiety, and others. Adjustment setting sleep disorder may arise in a child who does not want to go to bed or wakes up frequently from normal nightmares often due to a traumatic event; the parents become worried and then the child becomes excessively worried leading to a chronic pattern of sleep dysfunction. Behavioral management that identifies and corrects the underlying mechanism is usually sufficient treatment for these three sleep disorders.

Sleep dysfunction may arise from high altitude exposure (Altitude Insomnia) with abnormal, intermittent breathing (Cheyne-Stokes) occurring in non-REM sleep, probably because of the combined effects of hypoxia and hypocapnia. Fortunately, this usually rapidly clears over a few days with acclimatization to the higher attitude. Acetazolamide has been used for severe and/or persistent situations.

An older child and an adolescent may develop psychophysiologic insomnia in which one is not able to fall asleep or remain asleep normally due to a wide variety of factors such as erratic bedtime schedules, medication effects (i.e., caffeine, ADHD stimulants, illict drugs, others), underlying disorders (medical and/or psychiatric), development of anxiety about sleep, and others. As noted, puberty alters the circadium rhythm for youth in which many prefer to stay up later yet need to arise early for school while still in a deep sleep stage.

This sleep dysfunction can evolve into an overt Delayed Sleep Phase Disorder (DSPD) complicated by daytime sleepiness, development of a school avoidant or refusal pattern, and/or anxiety or depression about school. This is a common problem for many adolescents that can range from mild to severe. A significant sleep debt may develop with the emergence of many times of transient, unconscious "microsleeps" that may be misdiagnosed as ADHD. Placing the youth on stimulant ADHD medications only makes the situation worse.

Management

Management of psychophysiologic insomnia or overt delayed sleep phase disorder is based on what underlying factors are present. The differential diagnosis includes psychiatric disorders, circadian preference, primary insomnia, and inadequate sleep hygiene. Youth with underlying psychiatric disorders can present with insomnia but usually not with delay in the sleep wake pattern. Those with circadian preference can conform to a normal sleep wake pattern if they are motivated to do so. Many youth sleep well when allowed to choose their sleep wake patterns distinguishing them from those with primary insomnia who have problems with falling asleep and staying sleep even when allowed to choose their own sleep wake patterns.

Management of such delayed sleep onset or delayed sleep phase disorder (DSPD) involves correction of underlying factors with behavioral management where possible. If there is poor sleep hygiene, education is required to correct the underlying disruptors. Thus, the clinician can seek to recommend a strict sleep schedule for going to bed and waking up 7 days a week (including weekends!), avoidance of daytime napping, and avoidance of drugs interfering with sleep (i.e., nicotine, caffeine, others). Chronotherapy is part of a behavioral therapy program that seeks to adjust the bedtime-awake schedule until the desired times are achieved. Bright light therapy utilizes light boxes that provide 10,000 lux of blue light (or exposing to bright sunlight) to take advantage of a major zeitgeber—light.

Melatonin

Melatonin (N-acetyl-5-methoxytryptamine) is a pineal gland hormone that is regulated by the suprachiasmatic nucleus and can be given 30-120 minutes before the attempted bedtime. Since melatonin is considered an herbal supplement, its production is unregulated by the FDA and thus there may be a lack of standardization and risk for impurities in the melatonin as well. Dosages range from 0.3 to 6 mg at a time given orally. If these treatments are not beneficial or if there are concomitant problems (sleep, psychiatric, or medical), consultation is recommended. See Table 5.

Table 5. Medications for insomnia

Drug class	Examples	Adult Dosages + Comments	Side effects
Alpha-2-agonists	Clonidine (Catapres)	Dosing typically starts at 0.05 mg at night with increases of 0.05 mg every 3-7 days to a maximum of 0.4 mg at bedtime. Its onset of action is 45 to 60 minutes, the half-life is 8 to 12 hours and its sedative effect peaks in 2 to 4 hours. Gradual tapering is recommended when stopping to avoid rebound hypertension. Effects include lowered latency to sleep and suppression of REM sleep. It is not FDA approved as a hypnotic drug. It is not a DEA controlled schedule drug.	Hypotension, dysphoria, dry mouth, irritability, bradycardia, dizziness, fatigue, tolerance.
Anti-depressants	Tricyclic Antidepressants Amitriptyline (Elavil) Doxepin (Silenor) Nortriptyline (Pamelor) Other Antidepressants Mirtazapine (Remeron) Trazodone (Desyrel)	Amitriptyline (25 to 100 mg) Doxepin (3-6 mg) Nortriptyline (25 to 100 mg) Mirtazapine (7.5 to 45 mg) Trazodone (25 to 100 mg) These are sedating antidepressants that are not FDA approved (except Silenor®) as sedative-hypnotic drugs. They are not DEA controlled schedule drugs. Tricyclics: acetylcholine antagonist, H1 antagonist Mirtazapine / trazodone: H1 antagonists	TCA: anticholinergic effects; agitation, arrhythmias, overdose with tricyclic antidepressants: tachycardia, arrhythmias, hypotension (orthostatic), death Trazodone: hangover effect, dry mouth, constipation, priapism (rare) Mirtazapine: dry mouth, constipation, abnormal dreams, increased appetite, dizziness
Anti-histamines	Diphenhydramine (Benadryl) Doxylamine (Unisom)	*Diphenhydramine:* Commonly used in children as a hypnotic agent despite confirmatory research; pediatric dose: 1 mg/kg up to 50 mg at night; sedation peaks at 1-3 hours & may last 4-7 hours; may lower latency to sleep onset and increase total sleep time; crosses blood-brain barrier & blocks histamine (H_1) receptors; FDA approved for insomnia age $\geq$ 12 years	Anticholinergic side effects: dry mouth, tachycardia, hypotension, irritability, urinary retention, daytime sedation; tolerance, can see paradoxic excitation in children; overdose: respiratory depression, seizures, hypotension, rhabdomyolysis.
Benzo-Diazepines (BZD)	Clonazepam (Klonopin) Estazolam (Prosom) (initial adult dose: 1 mg) Flurazepam (Dalmane) (Initial adult dose: 15 mg) Lorazepam (Ativan) (Initial adult dose: 1 mg) Quazepam (Doral) (Initial adult dose: 7.5 mg) Temazepam (Restoril) (Initial adult dose: 7.5-15 mg)	BZD are used for the treatment of anxiety, insomnia, and other conditions. These are DEA controlled schedule IV drugs; they are FDA approved drugs for adults with insomnia (except for clonazepam and lorazepam). They bind to several gamma-aminobutyric acid (GABA) type A receptor subtypes with resultant decreased sleep latency and delta sleep with increased total sleep time; increase stage N2 sleep and REM latency; reduce arousals (awakenings) between sleep-stage changes; have anxiolytic and anticonvulsant effects. Use with great caution in adolescents due to many side effects including dependence.	Dependence with chronic use; common cause of addiction; daytime sleepiness, memory impairment, depression, behavioral disinhibition, anterograde amnesia, rebound insomnia, withdrawal, tolerance, many others.

Table 5. (Continued)

Drug class	Examples	Adult Dosages + Comments	Side effects
	Triazolam (Halcion) (Initial adult dose: 0.125-0.25 mg)	Clonazepam is used in adolescents in disorders with severe partial arousal at doses of 0.25 to 0.5 mg at bedtime. All agents are hepatically metabolized and have active metabolites with potential for CYP 450 drug interactions except lorazepam and temazepam	Abuse of prescription medications has become a public health dilemma, such as seen in current abuse and misuse of BZDs.
Herbal Supplements	Melatonin Chamomile Lavender Kava-kava Valerian	*Melatonin*: see text. Half-life is 30 to 50 minutes & onset of action is ½ to 1 hour; widely used; formulation not standardized. Wide range of dosages: 0.3 mg to 10mg; may lower latency for sleep onset & increase sleep maintenance & total sleep time; *Others dietary supplements:* anecdotal reports of benefit only seen; no overt research and not FDA approved.	*Melatonin:* Common: fatigue, dizziness, headache and irritability. Long-term side effects unknown; may reduce seizure threshold; caution in patients with vascular disorders; avoid in immune disorders and those on immunosuppressants & cortico-steroids; not FDA approved or regulated. Avoid melatonin from animal sources due to risk for contamination.
Melatonin Agonist	.Ramelteon (Rozerem)	Half-life up to 5 hours; 8 mg given ½ hour before bedtime; onset within 30 minutes. Binds to melatonin receptors MT_1 and MT_2 in the suprachiasmatic nucleus; FDA approved in adults for insomnia; metabolized by cytochrome (CYP) 1A2 & use with caution if combined with 1A2 inhibitors; avoid fatty meal before taking. It is not a scheduled drug & is not limited to short term use. See the text.	Side effects include sedation, dizziness, fatigue, and headaches. Reports of overt dependence, tolerance, addiction, or rebound effects are not found in the literature.
Non-barbiturate hypnotic	Chloral hydrate (Somnote)	Formerly popular as hypnotic agent in children but not currently due to side effect profile; pediatric dosage: 25-50 mg/kg/24 hr (maximum: 1 gram); peaks at ½ to 1 hour & lasts 4-8 hours; see lowering of latency to sleep onset and increased total sleep time; not FDA approved. Should not be used long-term for sedation. Can see tolerance, dependence (if used over 2 weeks); withdrawal symptoms (delirium & seizures) can be seen if stopped suddenly after chronic use. Classified as a controlled substance schedule IV.	Nausea, emesis, malaise, disorientation, ataxia, hangover effect (due to long half-life), paradoxic excitement, drowsiness, gastric distress; avoid or very cautious use for those with severe organ dysfunction (cardiac, liver), renal insufficiency (CrCl < 50 ml/min), gastritis/ esophagitis, porphyria

Sleep disorders and sleep patterns in adolescents 151

Drug class	Examples	Adult Dosages + Comments	Side effects
Non-benzo-diazepines	Eszopiclone (Lunesta) Zalepon (Sonata) Zolpidem (Ambien)	*Zolpidem* has a half-life of 2.5 hours and an adult dosage of 5 to 10 mg (immediate release: IR) and 6.25 to 12.5 mg (controlled release [CR] formulation). Potential CYP 3A4 interactions. In adults use IR for sleep initiation concerns & CR for adults for sleep onset as well as sleep maintenance. *Zaleplon* has a half life of 1 hour and an adult dose of 10-20 mg. Use in adults for sleep onset problems or to maintain sleep during mid sleep awakenings (up to 4 hours before wake time). *Eszopiclone* has a half life of 6 hours and an adult dose of 2-3 mg. Reduce dose to 1mg with potent CYP 3A4 inhibitors. Use for adults to initiate sleep and maintain sleep. FDA approved for chronic insomnia in adults. Minimal risk for rebound insomnia, withdrawal symptoms and development of tolerance & dependence.	Controlled substance Schedule IV. Dizziness, amnesia (dose-dependent), excess sedation, fatigue, hyperexcitability, ataxia. Do not combine with CNS depressants. Can see sleepwalking, sleep-related eating disorders, sleep-driving, parasomnias; untreated sleep-disordered breathing problems can worsen; use with caution in hepatic impairment, overdose leads to respiratory depression. Also with eszopiclone: headache, nervousness, unpleasant taste, dry mouth

Reference (29).

Alpha-2-agonists

Clonidine is a centrally acting alpha-2 agonist used for its hypnotic effects, especially to combat the stimulant effects of anti-ADHD stimulant medications. It has not been approved as a sedative drug. See table 5.

Melatonin agonist

The use of melatonin receptor agonists such as ramelteon is controversial since it is best to utilize non-pharmacologic approaches for adolescents with delayed sleep phase disorder. Ramelteon is FDA-approved for adults with insomnia and pharmaceutical companies are marketing their sleep-inducing products directly to the general public as well as to clinicians. One advantage is it is the only non-scheduled (US DEA), prescription drug that is FDA approved as a sedative-hypnotic drug and is not limited to short-term use.

Ramelteon is a melatonin 1 and 2 receptor agonist and is called a chronohypnotic that is available as an 8 mg tablet; there is no dose response relationship and effective daily doses range from 4 mg to 8 mg orally. Introducing such medications to adolescents with their changing central nervous system and when other measures can be beneficial are issues clinicians should consider before starting youth off on such medications. Mechanisms of action include aiding sleep onset, improvement of circadian rhythm dysfunction, and increase

152   *Donald E Greydanus and Cynthia Feucht*

in the total sleep duration. Youth should be counseled to avoid mixing such medications with illict drugs. Other medications used for adults with insomnia are listed in Table 5.

Benzodiazepines

Several benzodiazepines are indicated for the short-term treatment of insomnia. They are associated with a decrease in sleep latency and an increase in total sleep time and alter sleep architecture by increasing Stage 2 sleep and decreasing Stage 4 or delta sleep. Benzodiazepines should be used very cautiously in youth to correct insomnia because of their side effects that include tolerance, dependence, and addiction (See chapter 9 and Table 5).

Non-benzodiazepine hypnotics

These include eszopiclone (Lunesta), zaleplon (Sonata), and zolpidem (Ambien). They are usually well accepted in adults for insomnia, as reviewed in Table 5. Nonbenzodiazepine hypnotics are associated with a decrease in sleep latency, increase in total sleep time (expect zaleplon due to its short half-life) and maintenance of sleep architecture. Zolpidem immediate release is beneficial for the short-term treatment of sleep-onset insomnia compared to zolpidem extended-release which is effective for both sleep-onset and sleep-maintenance insomnia and may be used for longer time periods. Zaleplon is beneficial for sleep onset and for situations such as jet lag where short sleep duration is the goal; it is FDA-approved for short term use in adult insomnia. Eszopiclone is FDA approved for adult insomnia and is beneficial for sleep onset and sleep maintenance with less nighttime awakening. It can be used for the long term treatment of insomnia. Nonbenzodiazepine hypnotics have been associated with minimal risk for rebound insomnia, withdrawal symptoms or development of tolerance and dependence. See table 5.

EXCESSIVE DAYTIME SLEEPINESS

As noted with insomnia, excessive daytime sleepiness is a symptom and not a specific diagnosis. Potential causes are noted in Table 6. Chronic daytime sleepiness can lead to many consequences including irritability, impulsivity, ADHD-like features, depression, academic problems, and even death and/or injury from motor vehicle accidents. As noted, puberty can stimulate circadian rhythm alteration with adolescents delaying bedtime, staying up later, and sleeping in until late morning or even the afternoon. If they get up early for school or other activities, a sleep debt develops.

Many adolescents develop poor sleep hygiene with trouble falling asleep due to many distractions even in their bedrooms such as watching television, playing video games (or other internet activities such as Facebook), and/or listening to music (CD players, MP3 players, radio, others).

This can lead to delayed sleep phase disorder (DSPD) as noted earlier. Additional complications include having too much light in the bedroom, having a room that is too cold or

Sleep disorders and sleep patterns in adolescents 153

hot, eating within a few hours of planned bedtime, consumption of caffeinated beverages, and others. Management is based on correction of the issues preventing the adolescent from getting to sleep on time, improving their sleep hygiene, and using behavioral management to establish regular, healthy sleep-awake cycles. Use of medication to correct this form of "insomnia" is discussed in the previous section. As noted, medication in these situations should only be used with great caution and only for a short amount of time in connection with behavioral management.

Medications used to management excessive daytime sleepiness as noted in narcolepsy include modafinil, methylphenidate, and amphetamines; these are reviewed in the next section.

Table 6. Causes of Excessive Daytime Sleepiness*

Poor sleep hygiene (see text)
Delayed Sleep Phase Disorder (see text)
Drug effects (alcohol, first generation antihistamines, anticonvulsants, others; see Table 4)
Psychiatric Disorders (see Table 3)
Medical Disorders
• hypothyroidism
• anemia
• infectious mononucleosis
• Lyme disease
• substance abuse disorder
• epilepsy
• central nervous system (CNS) tumor
• trauma to the paramedian thalamic areas of the CNS
Narcolepsy
Klein-Levin syndrome
Restless Leg syndrome
Parasomnias
Obstructive Sleep Apnea/ Hypopnea syndrome (OSAHS)
Jet Lag (Rapid Time-Zone Change) syndrome
Others

* Used with permission from: Greydanus DE: "Sleep disorders in children and adolescents" In: Pediatric and Adolescent Psychopharmacology. Eds: DE Greydanus, JL Calles JR, and DR Patel. Cambridge University Press: Cambridge, England, ch. 11, page 206, 2008.

NARCOLEPSY

Narcolepsy is a chronic neurological disorder with REM sleep dysfunction that has an incidence of approximately 0.1% (range of 0.02% to 0.18%) and a positive family history of about 25% with a prevalence that increases 40 times in first-degree relatives (5, 18,19). In some situations there is a history of CNS trauma. Those with narcolepsy usually have some but not all of the classic narcolepsy characteristics: excessive daytime sleepiness, cataplexy, hypnagogic hallucinations, and sleep paralysis. There can be frequent night awakenings, interrupted sleep, problems with initiating or maintaining sleep, and nightmares. Children with narcolepsy may be misdiagnosed as having ADHD.

A deficiency of hypocretin from the hypothalamus is found in some patients with narcolepsy; hypocretin is a neuropeptide transmitter that is part of the process in being awake and inhibiting REM sleep. Thus, it is a process of sleep intruding into wakefulness and wakefulness interrupting sleep. Narcolepsy has an association with two HLA class II antigens: DR2 and DQ1. DQA*0102 is found in narcolepsy as well while HLA DQB1*0602 is the most closely associated marker for narcolepsy, particularly for cataplexy.

Excessive daytime sleepiness

This is associated with REM-onset sleep and usually occurs while the youth is not in motion, such as when sitting down; however, it can be seen in other situations such as while standing or even eating. There are many causes for excessive daytime sleepiness as noted in Table 6 leading often to a delay in a diagnosis of narcolepsy that may not be made until adulthood though it may actually peak in incidence in adolescence.

Management of narcolepsy-based excessive daytime sedation includes behavior treatment reviewed earlier (i.e,, improve sleep hygiene, allow two 20-minute naps in the daytime, others) with the use of medications to help keep the patient awake (such as modafinil and psychostimulants; see Table 7).

Medication is for a lifetime to control symptoms and patients (as well as parents, guardians, school teachers) should be educated regarding this disorder. Repeated counseling is needed especially regarding the importance of having good sleep hygiene and sleep-wake patterns. Modafinil is a non-amphetamine medication that is FDA-approved for patients with narcolepsy who are over 16 years of age. iIt is a wakefulness-promoting drug and is considered a first-line medication for excessive daytime sleepiness for adults with narcolepsy. Its mechanism of action is linked to its effects on dopaminergic signaling. It is not FDA-approved as a pediatric drug for ADHD management.

MPH (methylphenidate) (see table 7) is a CNS stimulant used to treat ADHD but also for excessive daytime sleepiness in narcolepsy. See the chapter on ADHD. Its sympathomimetic effects and DEA Schedule II status makes it a second line drug after modafinil, at least for those over 16 years of age.

Amphetamine (dextroamphetamine) is another CNS stimulant that is an alternative to MPH for treatment of excessive daytime sleepiness; it is also used to treat ADHD. Patients on psychostimulants should have certain parameters periodically checked, such as the blood pressure, pulse, and weight.

Due to cardiovascular side effects, avoid use in patients with serious cardiovascular disease, including structural and rhythm abnormalities. Consider baseline ECG as part of a cardiovascular assessment prior to initiation of the medication.

These medications also have the potential for dependency and should be used with caution in individuals with a history of dependence. Avoid abrupt discontinuation after prolonged administration to prevent withdrawal.

Sleep disorders and sleep patterns in adolescents   155

Table 7. Medications Used to Manage Narcolepsy: Daytime Sleepiness*

Class	Agent	Dose	Side effects
Psychostimulants	Methylphenidate (MPH) Mixed amphetamines Dextroamphetamine	10-60 mg/d; start with 5-10 mg 2x/d; no more than 20 mg in a single dose or 60 mg/d; dosing can be a single AM dose (long-acting products) or 3x/d (immediate-release products). Dose similar to MPH dose	Both MPH and amphetamines: insomnia, reduced appetite, loss of weight. nausea, elevated blood pressure, headache, depression, rebound symptoms, FDA black box warning for potential of drug dependence (avoid abrupt d/c); tolerance; controlled Scheduled II substance with abuse risk; others, see ADHD chapter.
Wakefulness promoting agent (long-acting)	Modafinil	Start with 100-200 mg once a day in the morning; some need a morning and noon dose; maximum dose is 400 mg/d in divided doses. Avoid using after 2 PM (1400 hours) to avoid interference with night sleep; it has a long half-life (15 hrs).	Controlled substance Schedule IV due to potential for abuse; FDA approved for narcolepsy >16 years of age; headache, nervousness, hypertension, rhinitis, diarrhea, back pain, dry mouth, nausea, insomnia, dizziness, dyspepsia. Substrate for CYP 3A4; potential for drug interactions. Associated with life-threatening skin reactions and psychiatric symptoms (anxiety, mania, hallucinations)

* Used with permission from: Greydanus DE: "Sleep disorders in children and adolescents" In: Pediatric and Adolescent Psychopharmacology. Eds: DE Greydanus, JL Calles JR, and DR Patel. Cambridge University Press: Cambridge, England, ch. 11, page 208, 2008.
Reference (29).

Other narcolepsy features

Cataplexy is more a feature of adults with narcolepsy and involves a transient loss of tone in facial and extremity striated muscles without the development of unconsciousness; it may be precipitated by the individual becoming suddenly fearful, angry, or even having laughter.

The patient is conscious during the episode and it can last seconds to minutes. Patients with cataplexy may be misdiagnosed as having epilepsy.

Hypnagogic hallucinations refer to the development of dream-like states that are very real to the patient, involve various senses in these states, and occur either while falling asleep or waking up. The other classic feature of some patients with narcolepsy is sleep paralysis which is typically transient (under one minute) but can be frightening in that the patient cannot move during the time of waking up or falling asleep.

156 *Donald E Greydanus and Cynthia Feucht*

Table 8 reviews medications to manage cataplexy, sleep paralysis, and hypnagogic hallucinations; these drugs suppress REM sleep, deep delta sleep, and lower inter-sleep cycle arousals. These medications include antidepressants (i.e., SSRIs, [fluoxetine], venlafaxine, tricyclic antidepressants [imipramine, protriptyline, clomipramine], benzodiazepines [clonazepam], and sodium oxybate).

The clinician should use these drugs very cautiously keeping in mind their various side effects and the fact that they do not directly treat the underlying sleep disorder. The issues of overdose (as with tricyclic antidepressants and benzodiazepines) as well as tolerance and addiction (benzodiazepines) must be considered at all times (see chapter 9).

Rebound effect may occur when stopping these drugs. It is not known what the exact effect of chronic deep sleep wave suppression is on adolescents with maturing central nervous systems.

Table 8. Medications Used to Manage Narcolepsy: Cataplexy, Sleep Paralysis, Hypnagogic Hallucinations*

Class	Agent	Oral Dose	Side effects
SSRIs	Fluoxetine	10-20 mg/d (up to 60 mg/d)	Insomnia, headache, nausea. See Chapter 5.
SNRI	Venlafaxine ER	37.5 to 150 mg/d	Sedation, dry mouth, dizziness, headache, nausea, dose-dependent hypertension. See Chapter 5
Tricyclic antidepressants	Imipramine Protriptyline Clomipramine	25-200 mg/d 10-40 mg/d 25-150 mg/d	Confusion, constipation, dizziness, sedation, dry mouth, tremor, urinary retention, weight gain; see chapter 5. See Table 5
Benzodiazepines	Clonazepam	0.25 mg to 2 mg orally at night.	Adverse effects: sedation, ataxia, confusion; if stopped too soon: rebound reactions. Schedule IV controlled substance. See Table 5
Miscellaneous	Sodium Oxybate (gamma-hydroxy-butyrate)	Age ≥ 16: 4.5gm in 2 divided doses, maximum 9 gm/day; formulation is liquid.	FDA-approved for cataplexy; to prescribe, must enroll in Xyrem Patient Success Program; sedation, headache, nausea, dizziness, disorientation, death from overdose, high abuse potential. Schedule III controlled drug when used for narcolepsy; see text.

* Used with permission from: Greydanus DE: "Sleep disorders in children and adolescents" In: Pediatric and Adolescent Psychopharmacology. Eds: DE Greydanus, JL Calles JR, and DR Patel. Cambridge University Press: Cambridge, England, ch. 11, page 209, 2008.
Reference (29).

Gamma-hydroxybutyric acid (Sodium Oxybate) is a GABA metabolite and binds to GABA$_B$ and GHB receptors. It is approved for treatment of adults with narcolepsy with cataplexy and can improve both cataplexy and daytime sleepiness, though it may take up to 6 to 12 weeks for the latter. Its half-life is 30-60 minutes and is given in two doses—one at bedtime (after patient is in bed) and then 3 (range of 2.5 to 4) hours later.

Sodium oxybate is a DEA schedule III when used for narcolepsy and physicians must enroll in the Xyrem Patient Success Program in order to prescribe. Potential side effects can be severe including death from an overdose and a high risk for abuse. It should not be combined with other CNS depressants including alcohol.

RESTLESS LEGS SYNDROME (RLS)

RLS is a neurologic sensorimotor disorder that is better identified in adults versus children or teenagers and it is often not diagnosed until the adult years (5,20-24). It refers to extremity discomfort (lower > upper) that can be described as an aching sensation or "crawling-creeping." RLS is also associated with abnormal sleeping patterns. It may present with "growing pains in childhood" with sleep dysfunction. Movement of the affected extremities typically relieves the uncomfortable feeling until the next wave occurs. Any extremity can be affected and its unpleasant feeling may delay or interrupt sleep. A formal sleep study (polysomnography) may corroborate the history and note nocturnal intermittent foot dorsiflexion, first toe extensions, and periodic limb movements over 5 per hour. RLS implies the symptoms occur while the patient is awake and if occurring during sleep can be called periodic limb movement disorder (PLMD). At least 80% of people with RLS have PLMD but the reverse is not necessarily true. One can refer to RLS while awake or while asleep and the movements can be voluntary or involuntary. The mnemonic "URGE" can be used to identify RLS: U: urge to move legs due to unpleasant feelings or sensations; R: worsens during periods of rest; G: gets better with activity; E: worse in the evenings. RLS is associated with ADHD, depression, anxiety, and parasomnias. A 2% prevalence is noted in adolescents and a higher prevalence is noted in those with epilepsy and diabetes mellitus; a prevalence of 5% is noted in adults. One third of adults with RLS have a positive family history in a partial autosomal dominant pattern. Complicating this association is that those with RLS also have disturbed quality of sleep (i.e., prolonged sleep latency with disturbed night sleep) that can induce or worsen such associations, such as anxiety, depression, ADHD, and others. It is also noted that RLS can worsen under the following conditions: pregnancy, increasing sleep debt, iron deficiency anemia, diabetic neuropathy, malignancy, amyloidosis, renal failure, and under the influence of caffeine.

Management of RLS includes non-pharmacologic measures as noted in Table 9. Proposed underlying mechanisms include iron deficiency and hypofunction of the dopaminergic system. Thus, management strategies for RLS include iron supplementation (3 mg/kg/day of elemental iron) to maintain serum ferritin levels over 50 ng/mL as well as prescribing dopaminergic drugs (Table 10).

Iron absorption is enhanced if combined with vitamin C. Assess serum ferritin levels periodically, adjust the iron dose to the laboratory data, and avoid an iron overload. Calcium decreases iron absorption and should be avoided one to two hours before and 4-6 hours after the iron supplementation is given.

Only ropinirole and pramiprexole are FDA-approved for treatment of adults with moderate to severe RLS (23). Ropinirole (Requip; Ropark; Adartrel) is a non-ergot dopamine agonist approved by the FDA for use in adults with RLS; its initial adult dose is 0.25 mg 1-3 hours before bedtime and its daily dose is titrated over the next 7 to 8 weeks and should not exceed 4 mg per day. Side effects may include nausea, emesis, hallucinations, sedation, dizziness, fainting, peripheral edema and postural hypotension. It can also induce sleepiness during daytime activities and this may occur without any warning symptoms; it may, for example, occur during driving a motor vehicle even after chronic use. Dopamine agonists have also been associated with compulsive behaviors or loss of impulse control such as gambling, binge-eating and hypersexuality. Symptoms may improve with dose reduction or discontinuation of therapy.

Rebound of the RLS symptoms may occur usually in the early morning as determined by the drug's half-life. Augmentation can be can be treated by giving the medication earlier in the day, lowering the dose or using a different dopaminergic drug as pramiprexole (non-ergot dopamine agonist: Mirapex; Mirapexin; Sifrol) which is also FDA approved for adults with RLS. The initial dose of pramipexole is 0.125mg 2-3 hours before bedtime and a maximum dose of 0.5mg per day based on manufacturer recommendations. It has a similar side effect profile as ropinirole.

Another dopamineric agent, though not FDA-approved, is carbidopa/levodopa (Sinemet), a medication used primarily to treat Parkinson's and dopa-responsive dystonia in adults (24). It's initial adult dose is 25/100 mg of immediate release formulation ½ to 1 hour before bedtime. Carbidopa/levodopa has a higher augmentation and rebound profile than ropinirole and pramiprexole.

Adverse effects are similar to the dopamine agonists described above and include dry mouth, nasal congestion, nausea, emesis, constipation, anorexia, hypotension, dizziness, headache, daytime sedation, peripheral edema, abnormal dreams, and compulsive behaviors. Other medications used in RLS (though not FDA-approved) include benzodiazepines, anticonvulsants, and opioids (Table 10).

Table 9. Non-pharmacologic measures to manage Restless Legs Syndrome (RLS)

1. Avoid or reduce issues that make RLS worse:
    a. Nicotine
    b. Caffeine
    c. Alcohol
    d. Dopamine antagonists
    e. SSRIs
    f. Antihistamines
2. Establish a good sleep hygiene pattern and avoid a sleep debt
3. Massage the areas of unpleasant sensations
4. Apply hot or cold packs to areas of unpleasant sensations
5. Exercise
6. RLS support groups (www.RLS.org)

Table 10. Medications Used to Treat Adults with Restless Legs Syndrome (RLS)

1. Dopamine agonists
   a. Ropinirole (FDA-approved in adults; see text)
   b. Pramiprexole (FDA-approved in adults; see text)
   c. Levodopa-carbidopa (non-FDA-approved)
   d. Bromocriptine (limited use due to rare side effect of pleuropulmonary fibrosis and cardiac valvulopathy)
2. Opioids (Narcotics)
   a. Codeine
   b. Oxycodone
   c. Tramadol
3. Anticonvulsants
   a. Gabapentin
   b. Carbamazepine
4. Benzodiazepine
   a. Clonazepam
   b. Diazepam
5. Oral iron replacement

KLEIN-LEVIN SYNDROME

The Klein-Levin syndrome is a combination of hypersomnia (as much as 20 hours in a 24 hour period) with episodes of behavior characterized by hyperactive (augmented) sexuality and confusion (5). The increased sleeping can be followed by bulimic episodes with compulsive overeating in combination with hypersexuality (i.e., excessive masturbation), irritability, and sometimes, hallucinations.

This unique syndrome is typically noted in males in late adolescence and may be precipitated by stress-induced hypothalamic dysfunction, major central nervous system trauma, or even a viral illness. There may be 3-4 episodes of this cycle in a year and polysomnography may show short REM latency with heightened REM and non-REM sleep patterns.

During the work-up the clinician should consider a number of conditions in a differential diagnosis, including encephalitis, bipolar disorder, and temporal lobe epilepsy. There are no specific proven pharmacologic management protocols, though some clinicians have tried tricyclic antidepressants and anticonvulsant medications for severe situations. Some have also tried psychostimulants but without proven efficacy. The history in most cases is that there is gradual improvement and no further episodes are recorded in the adult years.

Post-traumatic hypersomnolence is a variation of this pattern in which there is excessive daytime lethargy or sleepiness and prolonged night sleeping noted within a few weeks of a history of major CNS trauma. The differential diagnosis includes depression, epilepsy, secondary narcolepsy, and encephalopathy. There is usually full resolution within 6 to 18 months.

SLEEP DISORDERED BREATHING

Sleep disordered breathing (SDB) may develop in adolescents because of upper airway obstruction and four basic types of SDB are noted: Snoring (with no gas exchange dysfunction), Upper Airway Resistance Syndrome (UARS), Obstructive Hypoventilation (OH), and Obstructive Sleep Apnea Syndrome (OSAS). There is a 10% incidence of snoring in adolescents versus a 2-5% incidence of OSAS and OH with an equal female to male ratio.

Table 11 notes risk factors for OSAS and the underlying pathophysiology consists of increased upper airway resistance due to abnormal anatomy or abnormal upper airway neuromuscular control (25).

In childhood the peak incidence is between ages 2 and 6 years in association with peak years for adenotonsillar hypertrophy.

Nocturnal airflow obstruction leads to hypoxemia, hypercarbia with negative intrathoracic pressure, and movements of the chest/abdomen that are paradoxical.

Table 11. Risk Factors for Obstructive Sleep Apnea Syndrome (OSAS)

Adenotonsillar Hypertrophy
Allergic Rhinitis
Arnold-Chiari malformation
Asthma
Being African-American
Cerebral Palsy
Chronic Sinus Disease
Craniofacial syndromes
Down syndrome
Gastroesophageal reflux (GERD)
Laryngeal masses
Laryngeal web
Laryngomalacia
Micrognathia
Mucopolysaccharidoses
Obesity
Positive family history
Prader-Willi syndrome
Prematurity
Smoke exposure
Ventilatory Muscle weakness (due to neuromuscular disorders)

Sleep is marked by snoring, sweating, enuresis, frequent arousals with choking and gasping along with severe sleep dysfunction. Severe obstruction leads to a number of problems as listed in table 12. The correct diagnosis is based on a careful history and physical examination aided by a sleep diary and nocturnal polysomnogram (one or more respiratory events per hour). The clinicians should rule out allergic rhinitis and an antihistamine trial can be useful to eliminate allergy as a cause (primary or secondary).

Principles of management are noted in table 13. Pharmacologic agents have a limited role in OSAS management at this time. Adenotonsillectomy is the major treatment for those with OSAS due to adenotonsillar hypertrophy. Nasal continuous positive airway pressure is recommended for patients with post-surgery sleep apnea, those who cannot have or refuse

Sleep disorders and sleep patterns in adolescents 161

surgery, or as a choice of management selected by the patient. Oxygen is a limited option as the only treatment and does not affect the apneic or arousal episodes. In addition oxygen does not improve excessive daytime sedation and can lead to hypercapnea as well as higher oxygen saturations. However, oxygen can be helpful to those in selective situations, such as unable to use nasal continuous positive airway pressure, continue to have major residual sleep apnea after surgery (adenotonsillectomy), and/or are not willing to have a recommended tracheostomy.

Table 12. Potential Consequences of OSAS

1. Excessive daytime sleepiness
2. Snoring, restlessness, perspiration, and apneic episodes during sleep
3. Diaphoresis, neck hyperextension during sleep
4. Inward rib-cage movement during inspiration (paradoxical)
5. Unusual sleeping positions
6. Morning headaches
7. Growth delay
8. Ventricular hypertrophy
9. Cor pulmonale
10. Aspiration
11. Secondary enuresis
12. Gastroesophageal reflux (GERD)
13. Hypertension,
14. Increased intracranial pressure
15. Parasomnias
16. Academic dysfunction (limited attention span, poor memory skills, cognitive dysfunction, and lowered reaction time)
17. Misdiagnosis of ADHD
18. Misdiagnosis of Learning Disorders
19. Others

Table 13. Principles of OSAS Management*

1. Rule out disorders noted in Table 11
2. Trial of antihistamine medication
3. Trial of protriptyline (REM-suppressant antidepressant)
4. Adenotonsillectomy for enlarged adenoids and tonsils (OSAS, UARS, OH, and select primary snorers)
5. Weight loss measures to treat obesity if present
6. Positive airway pressure to keep airways open while sleeping:
    a. CPAP (continuous positive airway pressure)
    b. Bi-PAP (bilevel positive airway pressure)
7. Uvulopalatopharyngoplasty (UPPP)
8. Tracheostomy
9. Rapid palatal expansion
10. Supplemental oxygen
11. Medication:
    a. Fluticasone nasal spray: reduce number of obstructions in mild disease
    b. Montelukast for those with obstruction with mild OSA and no allergic rhinitis/atopy

* Used with permission from: Greydanus DE: "Sleep disorders in children and adolescents" In: Pediatric and Adolescent Psychopharmacology. Eds: DE Greydanus, JL Calles JR, and DR Patel. Cambridge University Press: Cambridge, England, ch. 11, page 218, 2008.

Intranasal steroids and leukotriene modifiers cannot be used as the sole treatment for OSAS since they do not lead to full resolution of apnea and hypopnea; they may be useful as adjuvant treatment in mild to moderate disease while waiting for nasal positive airway pressure and/or adenotonsillectomy. More research is needed to more clearly establish the role of these medications in OSAS.

Table 14. Factors Associated with Primary Nocturnal Bedwetting*

Genetics (75% increased if 2 parents had childhood NB; 45% increase with 1 parent)
Being male
Small bladder
"Heavy sleeper"
Deficiency of nocturnal antidiuretic hormone surge
Chronic illness
Institutionalization
Poverty
Unstable bladder

** Used with permission from: Greydanus DE: "Sleep disorders in children and adolescents" In: Pediatric and Adolescent Psychopharmacology. Eds: DE Greydanus, JL Calles JR, and DR Patel. Cambridge University Press: Cambridge, England, ch. 11, page 213, 2008.

Table 15. Causes of Secondary Enuresis*

Diabetes mellitus or insipidus
Posterior water intoxication
Mental subnormality
Hinman-Allen syndrome (non-neurogenic neurogenic bladder)
Unstable bladder
Intake of too much fluid
Consumption of caffeinated beverages
Urinary tract infection
Urethral or bladder obstruction
Lumbosacral abnormality (spinal cord tumor, tethered spinal cord)
Sickle cell disorder (anemia or trait)
Obstructive sleep apnea syndrome (OSAS)
Renal disorders (as tubulointerstitial disease)
Constipation
Anterior labial frenulum displacement
Food allergies

* Used with permission from: Greydanus DE: "Sleep disorders in children and adolescents" In: Pediatric and Adolescent Psychopharmacology. Eds: DE Greydanus, JL Calles JR, and DR Patel. Cambridge University Press: Cambridge, England, ch. 11, page 213, 2008.

ENURESIS

Primary nocturnal enuresis is often considered a parasomnia (see next section) and refers to bedwetting at night after an age at which nocturnal bladder control is expected (i.e. 5-7 years

Sleep disorders and sleep patterns in adolescents 163

of age) and can occur at any sleep stage. The incidence falls precipitously from 3% to 4% at age 12 to less than 1% in 19 year old males.

Table 16. Pharmacologic Agents for Primary Nocturnal Enuresis*

Agent	Dose	Adverse Effects	Comments
Imipramine	25-75 mg orally at night. Age < 12: maximum 50 mg/day Age ≥ 12: maximum 75 mg/day	Anticholinergic and other tricyclic anti-depressant effects: sedation, restlessness, poor concentration, weight gain, syncope, dry mouth (decreased salivary flow and increased tooth decay), blurring of vision (including cycloplegia and mydriasis), confusion, dizziness, constipation, anxiety; urinary retention; drug interactions with SSRIs & MAOIs; EKG changes (sinus tachycardia, AV blocks, prolonged PR interval, increased QTc interval); overdose can be fatal with arrhythmias and respiratory depression.	Start with 25mg with gradual increase if necessary; 50% will respond; taken 60 minutes before bedtime. If helpful, use for 3-6 months. Avoid abrupt discontinuation.
Oxybutynin	5 mg orally at night; up to 5 mg, 3x/d. Extended release form available for treatment of overactive bladder and also detrussor overactivity due to neurological disorders.	Anticholinergic adverse effects including dry mouth, constipation, sedation, blurred vision, dizziness and flushing; avoid overheating on hot days.	Start with low dose and use for 3-6 months if beneficial before gradual weaning off; helps to suppress uninhibited bladder activity
Agent	Dose	Adverse effects	Comments
Desmopressin acetate) (synthetic analogue of anti-diuretic hormone (ADH)	0.2-0.6 mg orally	Anecdotal reports of hyponatremia in those with underlying liver and kidney disease; increased LFTs with oral formulation	First agent of choice for many clinicians. Start with low dose 20-30 minutes before bedtime; increase after 2-3 weeks to maximum of 0.6mg. The pills can be chewed if necessary. Use the most efficacious dose for 3-6 months before any attempts to wean off. Restrict fluid intake 1 hour prior to dose until the next morning or for at least 8 hr after dose; avoid in patients with hyponatremia, history of hyponatremia or renal insufficiency.

Factors associated with nocturnal enuresis are noted in table 14 while table 15 notes causes of secondary enuresis (26-28). Many cases of primary nocturnal enuresis can be managed with behavioral modification therapy, such using operant conditioning devices (wetting alarms), hypnosis, acupuncture, diet changes, and scheduled voiding programs. A number of medications are beneficial for primary nocturnal enuresis and they are reviewed in table 16.

PARASOMNIAS

Parasomnias (table 3) are arousal disorders (partial or full) along with dysfunction of sleep-wake transitioning involving CNS dysfunction and skeletal as well as autonomic muscular disturbances (2,5). Some are more common in children than adolescents. For example, Rhythmic movement disorders (i.e., head banging, head rolling, body rocking) refer to irregular movements that start during the first year of life at the sleep-wake transition in both normal and developmentally delayed infants. Parents can be reassured that this is a transient phenomenon that usually resolves before age 4, though bed padding may be necessary. Severe and refractory situations are usually associated with neuropsychiatric disorders and may be improved with the use of benzodiazepines or tricylic antidepressants.

Bruxism is frequent teeth grinding at night and found in half of infants as teeth begin to erupt. Approximately 20% of older children may have bruxism as well and this can lead to excessive dental surface wearing and temporomandibular joint pain. Children with persistent teeth grinding can be fitted for a mouth guard for night use in addition to analgesics and biofeedback therapy. Severe cases may improve with judicious use of benzodiazepines.

Sleep talking is a benign parasomnia characterized by talking while sleeping; the talking is purposeless to others hearing it and reassurance of its normal nature is usually all that is needed. Nightmares occur during the last phase of the night sleep, during REM sleep, and may be triggered by a number of issues, such as psychological factors (including sexual abuse, anxiety, depression, others) and withdrawal from alcohol as well as other illicit drugs. The youth can be reassured of the benign nature of nightmares and offered behavior management for underlying psychological factors.

Sleep walking (somnambulism) is a partial arousal parasomnia characterized by the person arising from sleep and walking, typically during the first part of sleeping as there is transitioning from slow wave Stage 4 sleep. There may be a positive family history of others with sleep walking. The youth and the parents can be reassured of the benign nature of this parasomnia, though injury can occur while sleep walking. The youth's living space should be safely guarded with alarms set to tell others in the house that sleep walking is occurring. Keep the walker safe is the key to management.

Night terrors (pavor nocturnus, sleep terrors) is a partial arousal parasomnia that usually occurs in non-REM sleep in one between 4 and 12 years of age; it can continue into the adolescent years in up to one-third while persistence into adulthood is uncommon. It begins with vivid vocalizations (i.e., loud crying, screaming) with tachycardia, tachpnea, and sweating. The night terror usually does not exceed 30 minutes, typically recurs at the same time each night, and the person does not have any recall for this event. There may be a positive family history of others with this phenomenon. There may be underlying issues

Sleep disorders and sleep patterns in adolescents 165

leading to prolonged slow wave sleep induced by sleep deprivation leading to an increase in pavor nocturnus. In the work-up clinicians should also consider temporal lobe epilepsy, complex partial seizure, confusional arousal, and nocturnal pain attack.

Sleep terror usually resolves in a year and reassurance is all that is needed in this situation. Some are helped if woken up ½ hour after falling asleep. If there is sleep deprivation, correct the underlying factors for this, such as medication effect or obstructive sleep apnea. Pharmacologic intervention for sleep terror is usually not needed. If the situation is severe and/or persistent, clinicians can prescribe medications that suppress slow wave sleep or change the non-REM to REM sleep transition. Examples include a trial of tricyclic antidepressants (such as imipramine), SSRI (such as sertraline), or a benzodiazepine (e.g., clonazepam—0.25 mg to 2 mg at night). Medication can be used for 3-6 months and then stopped to see if the sleep terrors return.

CONCLUSION

Healthy sleep-awake cycles are essential for normal physical and psychological health in humans (5). There are a number of sleep disorders in adolescents as noted in this chapter. The most common issue with youth is excessive daytime sleepiness due to various factors (table 6). A careful history and physical examination (including an otolaryngologic exam) are necessary to identify the nature of the sleep problem. Many medications can induce sedation and sleep problems can worsen existing medical and psychiatric disorders. Youth who are sleepy in the daytime may be misdiagnosed as having learning problems, ADHD, laziness, or depression. A sleep diary may be helpful and a polysomnogram is also useful in selective situations to identify such disorders as narcolepsy, restless legs syndrome (periodic limb movement disorder), sleep apnea, and others.

Behavioral management (including establishing proper sleep hygiene) is the key to many sleep problems in youth, though the judicious use of pharmacologic agents is helpful in some, as reviewed in this chapter. For example, modafinil and psychostimulants are useful for daytime sleepiness of narcolepsy and a number of medications (imipramine, oxybutynin, and DDAVP) are useful for nocturnal enuresis. The prescription of sedative medications (table 5), particularly those with addictive qualities, should be used only with great caution and restraint by clinicians in patients with insomnia (see chapter 9). Abuse of these medications, such as benzodiazepines, has reached epidemic proportions in the United States and many parts of the world. There is no established role for the use of herbal products for insomnia except perhaps for melatonin, though this and other popular agents (such as alpha-2-agonists in youth with ADHD) are not FDA-approved for insomnia (table 5).

ACKNOWLEDGMENTS

This paper is an adapted version of a chapter in the book "Adolescent medicine: Pharmacotherapeutics in general, mental and sexual health" edited by Donald E Greydanus, Dilip R Patel, Cynthia Feucht, Hatim A Omar, Joav Merrick and published with permission by Walter de Gruyter, Berlin and New York.

REFERENCES

[1]   American Academy of Sleep Medicine. The international classification of sleep disorders, 2nd ed. New York: Westchester American Academy Sleep Medicine, 2005:125-9.

[2]   Chhangani B, Greydanus DE, Patel DR, Feucht C. Pharmacology of sleep disorders in children and adolescents. Pediatr Clin North Am 2011;58(1):273-91.

[3]   Colrain IM. Sleep and the brain. Neuropsychol Rev 2011;21:1-4.

[4]   Gradisar M, Gardner G, Dohnt H. Recent worldwide sleep patterns and problems during adolescence: a review and meta-analysis of age, region, and sleep. Sleep Med 2011;12:110-8.

[5]   Greydanus DE. Sleep disorders in children and adolescents. In: Greydanus DE, Dilip DR, CallesJr JL, eds. Pediatric and adolescent psychopharmacology. Cambridge, UK: Cambridge University Press, 2008:199-222.

[6]   Harvey AG. Sleep and circadian functioning: critical mechanisms in the mood disorders? Annu Rev Clin Psychol 2011;7:297-319.

[7]   Lewandowski AS, Ward TM, Palermo TM. Sleep problems in children and adolescents with common medical conditions. Pediatr Clin North Am 2011;58:699-713.

[8]   Owens JA. Sleep disorders in children and adolescents. In: Greydanus DE, Patel DR, Pratt HD, eds. Behavioral pediatrics, 2nd ed. New York: iUniverse Publishers, 2006:236-64.

[9]   Pandi-Perumal SR, Kramer M, eds. Sleep and mental illness. Cambridge: Cambridge University Press, 2010.

[10] Brand S, Kirov R. Sleep and its importance in adolescence and common adolescent somatic psychiatric conditions. Int J Gen Med 2011;4:4235-42.

[11] Gregory AM, Sadeh A. Sleep, emotional and behavioral difficulties in children and adolescents. Sleep Med Rev 2011;13:23-30.

[12] Schuen JN.Sleep disorders in the adolescent. In: Greydanus DE, Patel DR, Pratt HD, eds. Essential adolescent medicine. New York: McGraw-Hill, 2006:281-297.

[13] Babcock DA. evaluating sleep and sleep disorders in the pediatric primary care setting. Pediatr Clin North Am 2011;58:543-54.

[14] Owens JA. Etiologies and evaluation of sleep disturbances in adolescence. Adolesc Med State Art Rev 2010;21:430-45.

[15] Roberts RE, Roberts CR, Xing Y. Restricted sleep among adolescents: prevalence, incidence, persistence, and associated factors. Behav Sleep Med 2011;9:18-30.

[16] Weiss SK, Garbutt A. Pharmacotherapy in pediatric sleep disorders. Adolesc Med State Art Rev 2010;21:508-21.

[17] Carrot B, Lecendreux M. Evaluation of excessive daytime sleepiness in child and adolescent psychopathology. Arch Pediatr 2011 Jun 14 [EPub ahead of print]

[18] Kanbayashi T, Sagawa Y, Takemura F, Ito SU, Tsutsui K, Hishikawa Y,, et al. The pathophysiologic basis of secondary narcolepsy and hypersomnia. Curr Neurol Neurosci Rep 2011;11:235-41.

[19] Sullivan SS. Narcolepsy in adolescents. Adolesc Med State Art Rev 2010;21:542-55.

[20] Durmer JS, Quraishi GH. Restless legs syndrome, periodic leg movements, and periodic limb movement disorder in children. Pediatr Clin North Am 2011;58:591-620.

[21] Mitchell UH. Nondrug-related aspect of treating Ekbom disease, formerly known as restless legs syndrome. Neuropsychiatr Dis Treat 2011;7:251-7.

[22] Picchietti DL, Stevens HE. Early manifestations of restless legs syndrome in children and adolescence. Sleep Med 2008;9(7): 770-781.

[23] Scholz H, Trenkwalder C, Kohnen R, Riemann D, Kriston L, Hornyak M. Dopamine agonists for restless legs syndrome. Cochrane Database Syst Rev 2011;3:CD006009.

[24] Scholz H, Trenkwalder C, Kohnen R, Riemann D, Kriston L, Hornyak M. Levodopa for restless legs syndrome. Cochrane Database Syst Rev 2011;2:CD005504.

[25] Burg CJ, Friedman NR. Diagnosis and treatment of sleep apnea in adolescents. Adolesc Med State Art Rev 2010;21:457-79.

[26] Greydanus DE, Torres AD, Wan JH. Genitourinary and renal disorders. In: Greydanus DE, Patel DR, Pratt HD, eds. Essential adolescent medicine. New York: McGraw-Hill, 2006:355-9.

Sleep disorders and sleep patterns in adolescents 167

[27] Kiddoo D. Nocturnal enuresis. Clin Evid (Online) 2011 Jan 31; pii:0305.
[28] Neveus T. Nocturnal enuresis-theoretic background and practical guidelines. Pediatr Nephrol 2011;26:1207-14.
[29] Lexi-Comp (Lexi-Drugs®). Lexi-Comp. Accessed June 30, 2011.

Submitted: October 15, 2011. *Revised:* November 25, 2011. *Accepted:* December 10, 2011.

In: Alternative Medicine Research Yearbook 2012
Editors: Søren Ventegodt and Joav Merrick

ISBN: 978-1-62808-080-3
© 2013 Nova Science Publishers, Inc.

Chapter 18

ADOLESCENCE AND HYPERTENSION

Alfonso D Torres, MD
and Donald E Greydanus, MD, Dr. HC (Athens)*

Pediatrics and Human Development, Michigan State University College of Human
Medicine, Michigan State University/Kalamazoo Center for Medical Studies,
Kalamazoo, MI, US

ABSTRACT

Hypertension is a major disorder in adolescents that has potentially severe consequences
in adult life with increased morbidity and mortality. This chapter considers important
concepts in high blood pressure including its definition, proper measurement,
classification, etiology, evaluation, and pharmacologic management. Proper recognition
and management of hypertension is youth will yield enormous dividends for health
during the adolescent and adult years of life.

Keywords: Adolescence, hypertension, blood pressure

INTRODUCTION

The consensus recommendations of the Fourth Report (US National Heart, Lung and Blood
Institute in Bethesda, Maryland) defines normal blood pressure in children and adolescents as
systolic and diastolic blood pressure (BP) below the 90th percentile for age, gender and
height, and hypertension is defined as systolic and/or diastolic BP that is equal or above the
95 percentile for age, sex and height (1). High normal blood pressure or "prehypertension" is
defined as BP between the 90 and the 95 percentile (see table 1).

---

* Correspondence: Professor Donald E Greydanus, MD, Dr. HC (ATHENS), Professor, Pediatrics and Human
Development, Michigan State University College of Human Medicine, Pediatrics Program Director, Michigan
State University/Kalamazoo Center for Medical Studies, 100 Oakland Drive, Kalamazoo, MI United States.
E-mail: Greydanus@kcms.msu.edu.

Measurement of blood pressure in children and adolescents

The measurement of BP in children and adolescents should be performed in a standardized manner by an experienced individual who utilizes the proper technique to prevent errors that result in misdiagnosis of hypertension. The most accurate results are obtained with mercury sphygmomanometers, but are no longer available because of concern of environmental toxicity.

Table 1. Classification of casual BP in adolescents (1)

HTN classification	2004 Working Group (percentile)
Normotensive	< 90th
Prehypertensive	90th to < 95 or if BP ≥ 120/80 mmHg even if < 90th
Stage 1 HTN	95th -99th + 5 mmHg at three separated visits
Stage 2 HTN	> 99th + 5 mmHg at three separated visits

Currently accepted methods include auscultation with standard aneroid sphygmomanometers; these instruments require frequent calibration to ensure accuracy of measurements. Automate oscillometric BP measurement devises are becoming more commonly use in the medical office setting, in home BP monitoring in the very young infants and children, and in the intensive care units of hospitals.

Finally ambulatory BP monitoring is becoming more frequently utilized in the outpatient clinical setting. Specific applications include circumstances when there is variability in BP values, in the evaluation of "white coat" hypertension, for the diagnosis of mask hypertension, for the measurement BP at night to determine the presence of non "night BP dipping," BP load, assessment of the effect of medication on BP, and other factors important in assessing the risk of chronic cardiovascular disease (2,3).

Accurate BP measurements require the appropriated BP cuff size for the specific patient with a cuff that is appropriated for the child size upper arm. In order to measure BP in children 3 year through adolescence, it requires BP cuffs of different size including the adult cuff. For obese adolescents and for measurement of leg BP, an oversize BP cuff may be necessary (4).

Elevated blood pressure in adolescents needs to be confirmed by at least three different visits before the categorization of the adolescent as hypertensive. In the measurement of BP, attention to details is important. Patient conditions include posture, equipment, technique, and measurement performance. Measurement of BP in the lower extremities is part of the evaluation of children and adolescents to exclude the possibility of aorta coarctation or mid aortic syndrome. Symptomatic hypertensive patients require rapid evaluation of target organ involvement and prompt pharmacologic treatment, even before a definitive diagnosis of the cause of the hypertension is known.

The development of hypertension in the adult is closely associated with risk factors for cardiovascular disease and associated complications including cerebrovascular diseases, retinopathy, heart failure, renal failure, and cognition. Hypertension is one of the leading causes for end stage renal disease. It is increasingly recognized that many of these factors begin early in life, many are genetically determined, and can result from intrauterine hypertension programming such as seen with intrauterine growth retardation, and preterm delivery, predisposing to hypertension and obesity. After birth, in childhood and adolescence, there is a mismatch between the conditions for what the fetus was programmed and the extra uterine conditions actually encountered (5,6).

The progression from normotensive males and females at 17 years of age to hypertensive young adults at 42 years of age (reaching a hazard ratio of 2.5 [95% CI: 1.75 to 3.57] for boys and 2.3 [95% CI: 0.71 to 7.60] for girls in the group with BP at 130 to 139/85 to 89 mmHg) correlates with BMI at 17 years of age and sex hormones. Longitudinal studies in young adolescent males from different ethnic groups in the United Kingdom indicate no difference in systolic blood pressure at 12 years of age, but greater difference with increased systolic BP in the adolescent years; this is also noted in African-American males at 16 years of age as compared with Caucasians (9+2.9 mmHg). The blood pressure differences in girls were not significantly different at any age. The diastolic BP differences in girls were more significant, with socioeconomic disadvantages having a greater effect in girls in minority groups (7).

Primary hypertension (PH) or essential hypertension has been considered to result from accelerated maturation in children and adolescents. The degree of maturation can objectively be assessed by determination of bone age using dual energy x-ray absorptiometry (DEXA). Recently these observations have been validated by researchers in a group of newly diagnosed non treated adolescent patients (8).

Causes of hypertension in children and adolescents

Essential hypertension in adolescents has dramatically increased in the last twenty years from 2.7 percent to 5% of school children defined by an average of systolic or diastolic blood pressure > than the 95th percentile corrected for age, gender, and height. This increase in blood pressure correlates with increase in overweight and obesity, hyperlipidemia, and insulin resistance; these factors are particularly evident in certain ethnic groups in which hypertension and obesity is observed in up to 50 % these populations (9,10).

Essential hypertension has become the most common cause of hypertension in adolescents. Criteria for the diagnosis of essential hypertension in adolescents include inability to identify a known secondary cause of hypertension, a positive family history of hypertension, heightened response to emotional stress, and stage 1 hypertension at presentation in most cases. Determination of plasma renin activity may not be useful for the diagnosis of essential hypertension. However, very low plasma renin activity may indicate other, rare causes (monogenic causes) of hypertension (11).

Essential hypertension is considered to be a multifactorial and polygenic condition involving environmental, developmental, and genetic factors. Currently in the United States, the diagnosis of hypertension in children and adolescents is based on recent research (1). As noted, hypertension is defined as an average systolic blood pressure (SBP) and/or diastolic blood pressure (DBP) = 95th percentile for gender, age, and height on = 3 occasions. Prehypertension in children is defined as average SBP or DBP levels that are = 90th percentile but <95th percentile.

Adolescents with blood pressure levels =120/80 mm Hg should be considered prehypertensive, and preventive life style modifications should be recommended. A patient that is hypertensive at the physician's office or clinic, but normotensive outside a clinical setting has "white-coat hypertension". Mask hypertension is diagnosed when the blood pressure measured in the office is normal, but is elevated in other settings. Mask hypertension is not a benign condition as it may be associated with left ventricular hypertrophy.

Ambulatory blood pressure monitoring (ABPM) is often necessary for the diagnosis of these conditions and is also useful for evaluation of adolescents with stage 2 hypertension. Left ventricular hypertrophy is found in 5.7 percent in normotensive adolescents, 9.4 percent in white-coat hypertensive adolescents, 22.2 percent in mask hypertension, 18 percent in stage 1 hypertension and 32.4 percent is observed in stage 2 hypertension (12,13). Other markers for cardiovascular risk that have been demonstrated in adolescents include carotid intima-media thickness. Obese hypertensive patients have higher cholesterol and higher insulin levels.

Secondary causes of hypertension continue to be the most frequent form of hypertension observed in children less than 12 years of age and can be characterized by the acuity and duration of the hypertension. Acute and transient forms of hypertension are seen with renal parenchymal diseases, vasculitis, tumoral diseases, trauma, neurologic, and other causes (see Table 2). These forms of acute transient hypertension usually respond well to treatment with antihypertensive medication with complete or partial resolution after the acute kidney injury. Table 3 lists causes of secondary chronic hypertension.

As noted in the research on adults, there is a correlation between the severity of hypertension and evidence of organ damage, if appropriate markers are utilized, such as left ventricular hypertrophy (LVH), retinopathy, microalbuminuria, and others. The existence of comorbidity issues, such as diabetes mellitus, renal disease, cardiovascular disease, and positive family history are important considerations in the decision to intervene therapeutically. Common causes of hypertension in adolescent are indicated in table 3.

Table 2. Acute and transients forms of secondary hypertension (4)

Renal parenchymal diseases:
    Acute post infectious glomerulonephritis
    Interstitial nephritis
    Hemolytic uremic syndrome
    Acute renal failure of any cause
    Acute urinary tract obstruction
Iatrogenic:
    Fluid overload in acute renal failure
    Hormone treatment: corticosteroids
	Vascular:
	    Renal vein and renal artery thrombosis
	    Embolic diseases
	    Vasculitis: Henoch-Schoenlein purpura
	    Renal tumor, renal compression
	    Renal trauma/surgery

Neurologic:
    Increased intracranial pressure
    Guillain-Barre´
    Poliomyelitis
    Dysautonomy
	Drugs:
	    Oral contraceptives
	    Sympathomimetic drugs
	    Erythropoietin
	    Stimulants
	    NSAIDs

Illicit drugs:
    Cocaine
    Amphetamines
	Diet mediated:
	    Alcohol
	    Licorice

Evaluation of the hypertensive adolescent

The evaluation of the hypertensive adolescent requires the confirmation that hypertension exist, utilizing objective measurements at the office, at home or school and if possible with the use of ABPM. A complete personal history provides important clues about use of medication, and other substances able to cause hypertension; these drugs include those used for ADHD, anti-depressives, medication use for treatment of asthma, nonsteroidal anti-inflammatory medications (NSAIDs) and others. Use of substances of abuse such as alcohol, tobacco and illicit drugs are also associated with hypertension. The family history is important given the observation that predisposing factors for hypertension (such as cardiovascular diseases, diabetes mellitus and obesity) accumulates in families. Adolescents with mild to moderate hypertension and a positive family history of primary hypertension as a general rule, have the diagnosis of primary hypertension.

Table 3. Secondary causes of chronic hypertension (4,11)

Renal
Congenital abnormalities of the kidneys and urinary tract (CAKUT)
Hydronephrosis
Hypoplastic/dysplastic kidney
Chronic glomerulonephritis
Polycystic kidney diseases
Medullary cystic disease
Interstitial nephritis
Other parenchymal kidney diseases
After an acute kidney injury
Reflux nephropathy
	Reno vascular disease:
	   Renal artery stenosis:
	   Fibromuscular dysplasia
	   Mid aortic syndrome
	   Coarctation of the aorta
	   Takayasu arteritis

Chronic kidney disease with worsening renal failure of multiple causes	Endocrine causes:
	   Hyperthyroidism
	   Catecholamine excess:
	   Pheochromocytomas
	   Paragangliomas
	   Corticosteroid excess:
	   Iatrogenic
	   Cushing's disease
	   Conn's syndrome
	   Monogenic forms of hypertension

Tumors:
   Wilms tumor
   Neuroblastoma	

Drugs:
   Corticosteroids
   Alcohol, nicotine
   Appetite suppressants
   Anabolic steroids
   Oral contraceptive
	Syndromes:
	   Alport's syndrome
	   Williams syndrome
	   Turner's syndrome
	   Neurofibromatosis

The physical examination provides information regarding the growth and development of the individual patient that can be affected by chronic diseases of the renal, cardiovascular, endocrine, and other systems resulting in hypertension. Ophthalmoscopic examination, may give clues in terms of the chronicity and/ or severity of the hypertension. The existence of a bruit in the flanks may be the clue for renovascular hypertension. Blood pressure measurement of the four extremities is the most important finding for the diagnosis of aortic coarctation or mid aortic syndrome.

Basic laboratory screening that is common to all hypertensive patients includes a CBC, electrolytes (sodium, potassium, chloride, bicarbonate), glucose, BUN, creatinine, uric acid, and urinalysis. Serum uric acid elevation is a frequent finding in patients with primary hypertension and should be measured as well as a fasting lipid profile. Echocardiographic examination is also indicated.

Ambulatory blood pressure monitoring (ABPM) is now considered the preferred method to diagnose and provide therapeutic monitoring of arterial hypertension in children and adults. It allows the determination of several blood pressure patterns that are difficult to assess in the clinical setting, such as mean blood pressure, diurnal blood pressure rhythm (including dipping, morning surges, and variability), as well response and duration of drug effects. The recommendation for the use of ABPM in clinical practice include white coat hypertension, labile hypertension, resistant hypertension, hypotension episodes, mask hypertension, postural hypertension, and for monitoring treatment response (2).

An effort should be made to obtain important laboratory tests that may be altered by administration of certain medications, such as plasma catecholamines after the administration of labetalol or plasma rennin levels after administration of ACE inhibitors, angiotensin receptor blockers (ARBs) or diuretics. The history, physical examination, basic laboratory data, and renal ultrasound results, guides the clinical decision for more specific testing needed for the evaluation of secondary forms of hypertension in these adolescents.

The type of imaging studies for the identification of anatomical abnormalities will be dictated by the information obtained from the history, physical examination, and basic laboratory results. Given the predominance of renal diseases in the secondary causes of hypertension, a bilateral retroperitoneal renal ultrasound with Doppler is indicated. When there is a history of recurrent febrile urinary tract infections, a VCUG (voiding cystourethrogram) will be useful to confirm or exclude reflux nephropathy. DMSA (dimercaptosuccinic acid) scan is a valuable nuclear medicine scan study to identify the presence of renal scars frequently associated with hypertension. MRI angiography may be indicated when there is significant difference in renal size that may suggest renal artery stenosis (RAS), or when the captopril scan is suggestive of RAS.

Management of hypertension in adolescents

Patients with symptomatic severe hypertension, regardless of their age, need to rapidly be treated in order to bring their blood pressure down to safer levels to prevent further target organ damage; this should be done even before a definitive diagnosis is established. Pharmacologic intervention is not the first step in the management of adolescents with pre-hypertension and stage 1 hypertension. The recommended approach is therapeutic life changes. This implies a lifelong-lasting commitment in lifestyle that includes modifications in diet, exercise, avoidance and treatment of obesity, and cigarette smoking avoidance or cessation (14).

Adolescents with mild to moderate hypertension will benefit from regular, moderate aerobic exercise. An increase in fruits and vegetables, as part of normal nutrition, is associated with demonstrable decrease in systolic and diastolic blood pressure; also, reduction in salt intake to less than 100 mmol (less than 3 g of Na) a day causes reduction of blood pressure (15,16). Weight reduction in obese individuals decreases systolic and diastolic blood pressure (17). Aerobic exercise of moderate intensity 3–5 times a week is associated with moderated reduction in blood pressure. The effect of resistance exercise in blood pressure is less clear.

Table 4. Non diuretic antihypertensive drugs class

Drug class	Mechanism of Action	Side Effects
Angiotensin-Converting Enzyme (ACE) Inhibitors; some class members: Benazepril, Captopril, Enalapril, Fosinopril, Lisinopril	Decreases angiotensin II-induced-vasoconstriction	Cough, dizziness, hyperkalemia, rash, acute renal failure (particularly in patients with bilateral renal artery stenosis or hypovolemia). Contraindicated in pregnancy
Angiotensin II type 1 Receptor Antagonists; some class members: Candesartan, Eprosartan, Irbesartan, Losartan, Olmesartan, Telmilsartan, Valsartan	Decreases angiotensin II-induced vasoconstriction by blocking angiotensin II Type-1 receptors	Cough (less than ACE inhibitors), dizziness, angioedema (rare), hyperkalemia, acute renal failure (particularly in patients with bilateral renal artery stenosis or hypovolemia). Contraindicated in pregnancy
Renin Inhibitors: Class member: Aliskiren	Decreases vasoconstriction by inhibition of renin formation necessary for transformation of angiotensinogen into angiotensin-I the precursor of angiotensin-II. High dose causes diarrhea.	Cough (less than ACE inhibitors), dizziness, angioedema (rare), hyperkalemia, acute renal failure (particularly in patients with bilateral renal artery stenosis or hypovolemia). Contraindicated in pregnancy
Calcium Antagonists; Some class members (dihydropyridines): Amlodipine, Felodipine, Isradipine, Nifedipine ER, and others.	Attenuation of cellular calcium uptake or its mobilization from intracellular stores. Direct acting-vasodilators. They lower peripheral vascular resistance in all patients.	Dizziness, headache, peripheral edema, tachycardia, flushing, nausea
β-Adrenergic Antagonists; There are many members of these class of antihypertensive agents.	Competitive inhibition of catecholamines at the β-adrenergic receptor. They reduce cardiac contractility and peripheral vascular resistance. Labetalol, Carvedilol and Celiprolol also inhibit α-adrenergic receptors. Pindolol, acebutolol, penbutolol & carteolol have intrinsic sympathomimetic activity	Bradycardia, fatigue, dizziness, depression, insomnia, erectile dysfunction, decreased exercise tolerance, may mask symptoms of hypoglycemia, worsen peripheral arterial insufficiency, may worsen allergic reactions, bronchospasm (caution in patients with bronchospastic disease), increased serum triglycerides, decreased HDL Avoid abrupt withdrawal; taper over 1-2 weeks.
Central Adrenergic α_2-agonist and I_1 Imidazoline receptors; class members Clonidine, α-Methyldopa. Rimenidine and Moxomidine act on $I_1 > \alpha_2$ receptors (Not FDA-approved)	Cross the brain barrier and have a direct agonist effect on the α-agonist receptors in the midbrain and the brainstem &/or the I_1-imidazoline receptors by decreasing total sympathetic outflow, resulting in vasodilatation of the resistance vessels.	Sedation, dizziness, dry mouth, fatigue, orthostatic hypotension, rash (clonidine patch), rebound hypertension with abrupt withdrawal (clonidine), urine discoloration (methyldopa)

Table 4. (Continued)

Drug class	Mechanism of Action	Side Effects
		Methyldopa (rare reactions): Coombs-positive hemolytic anemia, hepatitis, hepatic necrosis, lupus-like syndrome
Central and Peripheral Adrenergic Neuronal Blocking Agents, class member Reserpine	Reduces blood pressure by depleting catecholamines in CNS and organ tissues, reduces cardiac output heart rate and peripheral vascular resistance.	Dizziness, headache, depression, nightmares, sedation, GI upset, bradycardia, nasal congestion Use with caution in patients with a history of depression & discontinue if depression occurs
Direct-Acting Vasodilators; class members Hydralazine and Minoxidil	The direct acting vasodilators reduce systolic and diastolic blood pressure by decreasing peripheral vascular resistance acting directly in vascular smooth muscle cells. They have no significant effect in the venous capacitance vessels.	Tachycardia, headache, dizziness, aggravate angina, peripheral edema Hydralazine: lupus-like syndrome(dose-related), hepatitis Minoxidil: hair growth on face & body, pericardial effusion (may progress to tamponade)
Moderately Selective peripheral α1-Adrenergic Antagonists; class member Phenoxybenzamine	Antihypertensive effect results for the irreversible binding to the α-receptors; long-acting. Only used for treatment of Pheochromocytoma	Orthostatic hypotension, tachycardia, sedation, fatigue, GI irritation, nasal congestion
Peripheral α1- Adrenergic Antagonists; some class members: Doxazosin, Prazosin Terazosin	These drugs are selective competitive inhibitors of the post synaptic α-1 receptor blunt the increased vessel tone mediated by the release of norepinephrine release causing vasodilatation and decreasing BP	Headache, dizziness, vertigo, fatigue, orthostatic hypotension, syncope (especially with first dose), tachycardia, fluid retention, sedation

These changes in lifestyle are the foundation for risk reduction of hypertension-related cardiovascular events later in life. Those individuals with more severe, stage 2 hypertension and those that are symptomatic or with evidence of end organ target damage require prompt evaluation and pharmacologic treatment.

Pharmacologic treatment of hypertension in adolescents

Blood pressure is determined by the interrelationship of two independent variables: cardiac output and peripheral vascular resistance. Pharmacologic treatment of hypertension is based on the ability of a medication to modify either cardiac output and/or peripheral vascular resistance. Currently, there are many therapeutic agents available to the clinician for the management of hypertension particularly in adults (see tables 4-8). Fortunately there is new information regarding the indication in the use of new pharmacologic agents for the treatment of hypertension in children and adolescents (3,18-22).

Adolescence and hypertension

Table 5. Diuretics class and site of action in the nephron

Distal Convoluted Tubule Diuretics, Hydrochlorothiazide, Chlorthalidone
Loop Diuretics: Furosemide, Bumetanide, torsemide

Distal potassium sparing diuretics:
   Epithelial sodium channel blockers: Amiloride, Triamterene
   Aldosterone antagonists: Spironolactone, Eplerenone

Table 6. Dosing of Antihypertensive medication in children adolescents and adults

Drug	Pediatric dose/adolescent dose	Adult dose	Formulation
ACE inhibitors			
Benazepril	Start: 0.2 mg/kg/day Max: 0.6mg//kg/day or 40mg/day	Initial: 10 mg/day Max: 80 mg/day	T: 5/10/20/40mg Extemp: 2mg/ml.
Captopril	Start: 0.2-0.5mg/kg/dose Q12h or 12.5 mg to 25 mg dose 2-3x/day Max: 6 mg/kg/day	Initial: 12.5mg 2-3x/day Max 450 mg a day	T: 12.5/25/ 50/100mg Extemp: 1mg/ml
Enalapril	Start: 0.08 mg/kg/day, up to 5mg Max 0.6 mg/kg/day, up to 40mg/day	Initial: 2.5-5mg daily Max: 40 mg/day	T: 2.5/5/10/20mg Extemp1mg/ml
Fosinopril	Start (≥ 6yrs & 50kg): 5-10mg/day Max: 40mg daily	Initial: 10 mg/day Max: 80mg/day	T: 10/20/40mg
Lisinopril	Start (≥ 6yrs): 0.07 mg/kg/day, up to 5mg/day MAX: 0.6mg/kg/day or 40 mg/day	Initial: 10 mg/day Max 40mg/day	T:2.5/5/10/20/30/40mg Extemp: 1mg/ml
Quinapril	Start: 0.1-0.2 mg/kg/day	Initial: 10 mg/day Max: 80 mg/day	T: 5/10/20/40mg
AT II receptor-1 antagonists			
Candesartan	Start 0.13mg/kg	Initial 8 mg/day Max: 32 mg/day	T 4/8/16/32mg
Irbesartan	Start (≥6-12 yrs): 75 mg/day Max: 150 mg/day	Initial: 150 mg/day Max: 300 mg/day	T: 75/150/300mg
Losartan	Start (6-16 yrs): 0.7 mg/kg/day Max: 50 mg/day	Initial: 25-50 mg/day Max: 100 mg/day	T: 25/50/100mg
Valsartan	Start (6-16 yrs): 1.3 mg/kg/day, up to 40mg/day Max: 2.7 mg/kg/day, up to 160 mg/day	Initial: 80 mg/day Max: 320 mg/day	T: 40/80/160/320mg Extemp: 4 mg/ml
Calcium channel Blockers			
Amlodipine	Start (6-17 yrs): 0.1-0.2 mg/kg/day, up to 2.5-5 mg/day Max: 0.6 mg/kg/day, up to 10 mg/day	Initial: 5 mg/day Max: 10mg/day	T: 2.5/5/10mg Extemp:1mg/ml
Isradipine	Start: 0.15-0.2 mg/kg/day divided in 2-3 doses (CR in 1-2 doses) Max: 0.8 mg/kg/day, up to 20 mg/day	Initial: C 2.5 mg 2x/day CR: 5 mg/day Max: 20 mg a day	C: 2.5/5mg CR: 5/10mg Extemp: 1 mg//ml
Beta-adrenergic antagonists			
Atenolol	Start: 0.5 -1 mg kg/day Max: 2 mg/kg/day, up to 100 mg/day	Initial: 25-50 mg/day Max: 100 mg/day	T:25/50/100mg Extemp: 2 mg/ml
Metoprolol	Start (≥ 6yrs): 1mg/kg/day, up to 50 mg/day (ER) Max: 2 mg/kg/day, up to 200 mg/ day (ER)	Initial: 25-50 mg/day (ER) Max: 400 mg/day	T: (ER): 25/50/100/200mg Extemp: 10 mg/ml
Propranolol	Start: 0.5-1 mg/kg/day in 2-3 divided doses Max: 16 mg kg/day	Initial: 40 mg 2x/day; LA: 80 mg/day Max: 640 mg/day	T:10/20/40/60/80mg C (ER): 60/80/120/160mg Solution: 4/8 mg/ml

Table 6. (Continued)

Drug	Pediatric dose/adolescent dose	Adult dose	Formulation
Labetalol (alpha, beta1, and beta-2 adrenergic receptors site blocker)	Start: 1-3 mg/kg/day in 2 divided doses Max: 10-20 mg/kg/day, up to 1200 mg/day	Initial: 100 mg 2x/day Max: 2400 mg/day	T: 100/200/300mg Extemp: 40 mg/ml
Central alpha-2 adrenergic agonists			
Clonidine	Start: (<12 yrs): 5 to 10 mcg/kg/day in 2-3 divided doses Start (≥12 yrs): 0.2 mg/ day in 2 divided doses Max: (<12 yrs): 25 mcg/kg/day, up to 0.9 mg/day Max: (≥ 12 yrs): 2.4 mg/day	Initial: 0.1 mg 2x/day Max (oral): 2.4 mg/day Max (patch): 0.3 mg/week	T: 0.1/0.2/0.3mg Transdermal: 0.1/0.2/0.3 mg
Alpha-adrenergic antagonists			
Doxazosin	Start: 1mg/day Max: 4mg/day	Initial: 1 mg/day Max: 16 mg/day	T: 1/2/4/8mg
Prazosin	Start: 0.05-0.1mg/kg/day in 3 divided doses Max: 0.5 mg/kg/day	Initial: 1mg 2-3x/day Max: 20mg/day	C: 1/2/5mg
Terazosin	No data	Initial: 1mg/day Max: 20 mg/day	C: 1/2/5/10mg
Vasodilators			
Hydralazine	Start: 0.75-1mg/kg/day in 2-4 divided doses Max: 7.5 mg/kg/day, up to 200mg/day	Initial: 10mg 4x/day Max: 300 mg/day	T: 10/25/50/100mg Extemp: 20 mg/5 ml
Minoxidil	Start (<12 yrs): 0.1-0.2 mg/kg/day divided in 1-2 doses, up to 5mg/day Max: 50 mg/day	Initial: 2.5-5 mg/day Max: 100 mg/day	T: 2.5/10mg Extemp: 2 mg/ml

It is important for the clinician assuming the responsibility of prescribing these antihypertensive medications to be certain that the selected medications have been found to be safe and effective in studies of children and adolescents; if this is not possible, or at a minimal that there is abundant experience of their use in this population. The use of ACE (angiotensin-converting enzyme) inhibitors and ARB (angiotensin receptor blockers) in women in the reproductive age, requires special attention for the association of the teratogenic effects of these medications as they are clearly contraindicated in any stage of pregnancy. In sexually active female adolescents these medications should be avoided unless the female adolescent is on an effective contraceptive agent. In order to improve compliance, the number of doses should be once or twice a day in an easy to take regimen. Another consideration of increasing importance for families and clinicians is the cost factor, as in many instances patients and families are not able to afford the new and more expensive medications.

Beneficial changes in target organ damage can be seen within a few months of pharmacologic treatment. For example, left ventricular hypertrophy may regress within 6 months with effective treatment of hypertension. Normalization of blood pressure seems to be more important than the type of medication used in decreasing the risks of development of cardiovascular events and strokes particularly in adults, as demonstrated in meta-analysis studies involving large number of patients (23). This meta-analysis indicated that ß-blockers are protective from recurrence of coronary events by 30%, when initiated immediately after a myocardial infarction; this effect lasts a few years as compared with other antihypertensive drugs (23). Only calcium channel blockers provide slight benefit in prevention of strokes as compared with other antihypertensive drugs. The study also indicates that blood pressure lowering drugs should be provided to all patients at high risk of cardiovascular events (23). Long term studies are clearly necessary in hypertensive children and adolescents.

Table 7. Diuretics use in the treatment of hypertension. Suggested Dosing of antihypertensive Medications in Children, Adolescents and Adults (4,18,19,23)

Diuretics	Pediatric dosing	Adult dosing	Formulation	Comments / Side effects
Amiloride	Start: 0.4-0625 mg/kg/day Max: 20 mg/day	Initial: 5-10 mg/day Max: 20 mg/day	T: 5 mg	Specific epithelial channel blocker is a potassium sparing diuretic; monitor potassium levels Side effects: hyperkalemia, GI upset, rash, headache
Chlorothiazide	Start: 10-20 mg/kg/day in 1-2 divided doses Max: <2 yrs: 375mg/day; 2-12 yrs: 1000 mg/day	Initial: 125-500mg/day in 1-2 divided doses Max: 2 gm/day	T: 250/500mg Susp:250 mg/5ml	Side effects: electrolytes disturbances: hypokalemia, hyponatremia, hypercalcemia and metabolic alkalosis. Long term use is associated with increase uric acid levels. May cause hypoglycemia, elevated cholesterol & triglycerides, rash & photosensitivity reactions Avoid in renal insufficiency.
Chlorthalidone	Start: 0.3 mg/kg/day Max: 2 mg/kg/day, up to 50 mg/day	Initial: 25 mg/day Max: 100 mg/day	T: 25/50/100g	
Hydrochlorothiazide	Start (2-17 yrs): 1mg/kg/day in 1-2 divided doses Max: 3 mg/kg/day, up to 50 mg/day	Initial: 12.5-25 mg/day Max: 50mg/day	C:12.5 mg T: 25/50mg	
Spironolactone	Start: 1mg/kg/day in 1-2 divided doses Max: 3 mg/kg/day, up to 100 mg/day	Initial: 25 mg 1-2x/day Max: 100 mg/day	T: 25/50/100m g Extemp: 25mg/ml	Spironolactone an aldosterone antagonist is a potassium spearing diuretic, anti-fibrosis effects. Spironolactone side effects: hyperkalemia, hyponatremia, gynecomastia, menstrual irregularities, GI upset, rash Triamterene is an epithelial sodium channel blocker and a potassium sparing diuretic. Triamterene side effects: Hyperkalemia, GI upset, nephrolithiasis Avoid in renal insufficiency.
Triamterene	Start: 1-2 mg/kg/ day in 2 divided doses Max: 3-4 mg/kg/day, up to 300 mg/day	Initial:50-100 mg/day in 1-2 divided doses Max: 300 mg/day	C: 50/100mg	

It is now accepted that for diabetic hypertensive patients, particularly with albuminuria, ACEs and/or ARBs offer advantages over other anti-hypertensive drugs. Similar observations have been made in hypertensive patients with chronic kidney diseases and proteinuria. During randomized therapy beneficial effects of antihypertensive medications in decreasing the frequency and severity of cardiovascular diseases and death has been observed, as compare with the control group. These beneficial effects persist in the actively treated group even after discontinuation of blinded therapy, when all the study patients were advised to take the same therapy. This observation indicates a legacy effect of early intervention that will result in improved outcomes in patients whose blood pressure is controlled earlier (24).

The clinician prescribing antihypertensive medications needs to become familiar with the indications, contraindications, and side effects of these therapeutic agents. The different antihypertensive medications are listed in tables 4-7.

Antihypertensive medications are divided in two groups: non diuretics and diuretics; the most common non diuretic and diuretics are listed in table 4 and 5. Pharmacologic treatment of hypertension is indicated in adolescents with primary hypertension and evidence of end-organ damage, with blood pressure consistently over the 99th percentile, in those that do not respond to or are unable to comply with life style modifications, and in patients with secondary forms of hypertension.

Pharmacologic treatment needs to be individualized (25). Some of the factors to keep in mind include the effects of medication on electrolytes disturbances, glucose and lipid metabolism, and renal as well as cardiovascular function. Medication can also interfere with physical and intellectual activities, and interact with other medications.

Table 8. Fixed combinations of antihypertensive drugs (23)

Fixed-Dose Combination Therapy	
Class	Combination
ß-Adrenergic blockers and diuretics	Atenolol 50-100 mg/chlorthalidone 25 mg
	Bisoprolol 2.5; mg; 5; 10mg /HCTZ 6.25
	Metoprolol 50-100 mg/HCTZ 25-50 mg
	Propranolol 40-80 mg/HCTZ 25 mg
	Nadolol 40-80 mg/bendroflumethiazide 5mg
ACEIs and diuretics	Benazepril 5-20 mg/HCTZ 6.25 mg-25 mg
	Captopril 25-50 mg/HCTZ 15-25 mg
	Enalapril 5-10 mg/HCTZ 12.5-25 mg
	Lisinopril 10-20 mg/HCTZ 12.5-25 mg
Fixed- Dose Combination Therapy (continuation)	
Class	combination
Angiotensin II receptor blocker and diruetic	Losartan 50-100 mg/HCTZ 12.5-25 mg
	Valsartan 80-320 mg/HCTZ 12.5-25 mg
	Eprosartan 600 mg/HCTZ 12.5-25 mg
	Irbesartan 150-300 mg/HCTZ 12.5-25 mg
	Telmisartan 40-80 mg/HCTZ 12.5-25 mg
	Candesartan 16-32 mg/HCTZ 12.5-25 mg
	Olmesartan 20-40 mg/HCTZ 12.5-25 mg
Renin inhibitor and diuretic	Aliskiren 150mg – 300mg/HCTZ 12.5 mg-25 mg
Calcium antagonists and ACEIs	Amlodipine 2.5-10 mg/benazepril 10-40 mg
	Verapamil ER 180-240 mg/trandolapril 1-4 mg
Calcium antagonists and angiotensin II receptor blockers	Amlodipine 5-10 mg/valsartan 160-320 mg
	Amlodipine 5-10 mg/olmesartan 20-40 mg

Additional factors to consider include preexisting conditions, patient compliance with taking medications, and medication costs. Adolescents with hypertension requiring pharmacologic intervention should be under the supervision of consultants in nephrology or cardiology who are familiar with hypertension in adolescents. Table 6 lists the most commonly used drugs for the management of hypertension in children, adolescents and adults. Table 7 reviews diuretic medications and table 8 lists fixed dose combinations.

Pregnancy

Pregnancy in adolescents deserves special consideration in view of the high risk of the development of hypertension in pregnant teens with the potential for complications threatening the well being of the mother and the infant.

Severe hypertension in the mother increases the risk for hypertensive encephalopathy, intracranial bleeding, and renal insufficiency (26,27). In the fetus, the risk of premature delivery increases, with all its consequences. Preterm and small-for-gestational-infants are born with decreased number of nephrons and are at risk of developing hypertension.

The evaluation of the hypertensive mother is complicated. Common radiologic or nuclear scans are contraindicated. The use of angiotensin converting enzyme inhibitors, and angiotensin II receptor antagonists are teratogenic and are contraindicated in pregnancy. These patients are better served when follow by a team that includes an obstetrician, perinatologist, and a nephrologist.

CONCLUSION

Hypertension is a major disorder in adolescents that has potentially severe consequences in adult life with increased morbidity and mortality.

This chapter considers important concepts in high blood pressure including its definition, proper measurement, classification, etiology, evaluation, and pharmacologic management (28). Proper recognition and management of hypertension in youth will yield enormous dividends for health during the adolescent and adult years of life.

ACKNOWLEDGMENTS

This paper is an adapted version of a chapter in the book "Adolescent medicine: Pharmacotherapeutics in general, mental and sexual health" edited by Donald E Greydanus, Dilip R Patel, Cynthia Feucht, Hatim A Omar, Joav Merrick and published with permission by Walter de Gruyter, Berlin and New York.

REFERENCES

[1] National High Blood Pressure Education Program Working Group on High Blood Pressure in Children and Adolescents. The fourth report on the diagnosis evaluation and treatment in children and adolescents. National Heart, Lung and Blood Institute, Bethesda, Maryland. Pediatrics 2004;114:555-76.

[2] Wühl E. Ambulatory blood pressure monitoring methodology and norms in children. In: Flynn JT, Ingelfinger JR, Portman RJ, eds. Pediatric hypertension, Second ed. New York: Humana Press, 2011:161-78.

[3] De Moraes AC, de Carvalho HB. Evaluating risk factors in hypertension screening in children and adolescents. Hyperten Res 2011 Jun 9. [Epub ahead of print]

[4] Falkner B. Hypertension in children. In: Oparril S, Weber MA, eds. Hypertension companion of Brenner and Rector's The Kidney, Second ed. Philadelphia, PA: Elsevier Saunders, 2005:603-15.

[5] Lurbe E, Carvajal E, Torro I, Aguilar F, Alvarez J, Redon J. Influence of concurrent obesity and low birth weight on blood pressure phenotype in youth. Hypertension 2009;53:912-7.

[6] Dionne JM, Abitbol CL, Flynn JT. Hypertension in infancy: diagnosis, management and outcome. Pediatr Nephrol 2001 Jan 22. Epub ahead of print]

[7] Harding S, Whitrow M, Lenguerrand E, Maynard M, Teyhan A, Cruickshank JK, et al. Emergence of ethnic differences in blood pressure in adolescence. The determinants of adolescent social well-being and health study. Hypertension 2010;55:1063-9.

[8] Pludoski P, Litwin MK, Niemirska A, Jaworski M, Sladowska J, Kryskiewicz E, et al. Accelerated skeletal maturation in children with primary hypertension. Hypertension 2009;54:1234-9.

[9] Feber J, Ahmed M. Hypertension in children: new trends and challenges. Clin Sci (Lond) 2010;119(4):151-61.

[10] Kamboj M, Torres A, Patel D. Endocrine causes of systemic hypertension in children and adolescents: a clinical review. Pediatr Health Med Ther 2011:239-47.

[11] McNiece KL, Gupta-Malhotra M, Samuels J, Bell C, Garcia K, Poffenbarger T, et al. Left ventricular hypertension in hypertensive adolescent analysis of risk by 2004 National High Blood Pressure Education Program Working Group Staging Criteria. Hypertension 2007;50:392-5.

[12] Brady TM, Fivus B, Flynn FT, Parekh R. Lability of blood pressure adolescents Pediatr 2008; 152:73-8.

[13] Sorof JM, Alexandrov AV, Garami Z, Turmner JL, Grafe AE, Lai D, et al. Carotid ultrasonography for detection of vascular abnormalities in hypertensive children Pediatr Nephrol 2003;18:1020-102.

[14] Siklar Z, Berberoglu M, Erdeve SS, Hacihamdioglu B, Ocal G, Egin Y, et al. Contribution of clinical, metabolic, and genetic factors on hypertension in obese children and adolescents. J Pediatr Endocrinol Metabol 2011;24:21-4.

[15] Stabouli S, Papakatsika S, Kotsis V. The role of obesity, salt and exercise on blood pressure in children and adolescents. Expert Rev Cardiovasc Ther 2011;9:753-61.

[16] Centers for Disease Control and Prevention. Vital signs: prevalence, treatment, and control of hypertension. United States, 1999-2002 and 2005-2008. MMWR 2011;60:103-8. Flynn JT, Falkner BE. Obesity hypertension in adolescents: epidemiology, evaluation, and management. J Clin Hypertension 2011;13:323-31.

[17] Flynn JT. Successes and shortcomings of the Drug and Food Modernization Act. Am J Hypertension 2003;16910):889-91.

[18] Blowey DL. Pharmacotherapy of pediatric hypertension. In: Flynn JT, Ingelfinger JR, Portman RJ, eds. Pediatric hypertension, Second ed. New York: Humana Press, 2011:537-58.

[19] Listernick R. A 15-year girl with hypertension. Pediatr Ann 2011; 40:235-8.

[20] Yoon SS, Ostchega Y, Louis T. Recent trends in the prevention of high blood pressure and its treatment and control, 1999-2008. NCHS Data Brief 2010;48:1-8.

[21] Tocci G, Volpe M. Olmesartan medoxomil for the treatment of hypertension in children and adolescents. Vasc Health Risk Manag 2011;7:177-81.

[22] Weir MR, Hanes DS, Klassen DK. Antihypertensive drugs. In: Brenner BM, ed. Brenner and Rector's The Kidney, eight ed. Philadelphia, PA: Saunders Elsevier, 2008:222-34.

Adolescence and hypertension

183

[23] Law MR, Morris JK, Wald NJ. Use of blood pressure lowering drugs in the prevention of cardiovascular disease: meta-analysis of 147 randomized trials in the context of expectations from prospective epidemiological studies BMJ 2009;338:1665.

[24] Drugs for Hypertension. Treatment guidelines. Med Letter 2009;7(77):1-10.

[25] Duley L. Pre-eclampsia, eclampsia, and hypertension. Clin Evid (Online) 2011;2011. pii:1402.

[26] Cifkova R. Why is the treatment of hypertension in pregnancy still so difficult? Expert Rev Cardiovasc Ther 2011;9:647-9.

[27] Kostis WJ, Thijs L, Richart T, Kostis JB, Staessen JA. Persistence of mortality reduction after the end of randomized therapy in clinical trials of blood pressure-lowering medications. Hypertension 2010;56:1060-8.

Submitted: October 18, 2011. *Revised:* November 27, 2011. *Accepted:* December 10, 2011.

In: Alternative Medicine Research Yearbook 2012
Editors: Søren Ventegodt and Joav Merrick

ISBN: 978-1-62808-080-3
© 2013 Nova Science Publishers, Inc.

Chapter 19

BREATH-MEDITATION: PRANA-DHYANA

Vinod D Deshmukh, MD, PhD*
University of Florida, Jacksonville, Florida, US

ABSTRACT

This short article is for reporting a novel method that I use to combine effectively a daily practice of disciplined breathing or Prāṇāyāma प्राणायाम and Presence meditation or Dhyāna ध्यान. Because this new technique is such a helpful and meaningful combination, I call it "Breath-Meditation or Prāna-Dhyāna प्राणध्यान. It is different from the traditional techniques of breath-control or awareness and focused or mindfulness meditation. This breath-meditation method is simple, effective and easy to learn. It is described in details in this article for anyone to learn and practice regularly during their busy schedule. One can really appreciate a gradual self-transformation with frequent insightful moments. The usual restless body, a talkative and wandering mind, and a self-centered ego are transformed into a more calm, content, silent, serene, creative, and blissful being, called Sat~Cit~Ānanda सच्चिदानन्द in vedānta. That is our essential nature and a true potential for full personal growth and maturity. We just have to understand and uncover this great wonder within each one of us.

Keywords: Breath-meditation, Prāna-dhyāna, Prāṇāyāma, Meditation, Mindfulness, Yoga, Vedānta

INTRODUCTION

This is a simple, direct and novel method that I use to combine the practices of disciplined breathing or Prāṇāyāma and Presence or Mindfulness Meditation or Dhyāna, in a meaningful and effective way. That is why I have called this new technique, "Breath-Meditation or Prāna-

---

* Correspondence: Vinod D Deshmukh, MD, PhD, 3600 Rustic Lane, Jacksonville, Florida 32217 United States. E-mail: vinod38@aol.com.

Dhyāna प्राणध्यान." It is different from the traditional techniques of disciplined breathing or Prānāyāma (1-3), yoga therapy (4-8), and meditation or dhyāna (9-13). It is also different from the breath-awareness and mindfulness meditation practices (14-17). However, it does contain some elements of all of these Yogic and Buddhist meditative and breathing practices. A general reference by the author on the Neuroscientific and Vedāntic perspectives of our astonishing brain and holistic consciousness or one energy~being~awareness Cidātma-Śaktih चिदात्मशक्ति: or Ekam Jyotih एकंज्योति: will provide further details and references (18).

This is how I practice breath-meditation on a daily basis. Usually, as a first thing in the morning, I sit erect in a vertical chair, with both hands interlocked or folded and tips of both thumbs touching each other, in front of my lower abdomen. Both index fingers and thumbs form a complete circle, as if I am holding a sphere of empty space in my hands. An empty sphere of space symbolizes both the quantum, holistic reality as well as an empty conscious cognitive space-time. It is infinite space or sky or Gaganam गगनं in Sanskrit.

I use seven full breaths with nineteen key words for directing my attentive awareness, and contemplation, during Breath-Meditation, as shown in the table below. For all seven breaths, the first column in the table is associated with full inhalation; the second column is with full exhalation, and the third column represents post-exhalational pause or rest.

During the first breath, I extend my neck, inhale fully and think of the word "Full or पूर्ण Pūrna" and experience the state of fullness of my lungs and body~mind~being. When I flex my neck and exhale completely, I think of the word "Empty or शून्य Śūnya" and experience the state of overall emptiness of my being, letting go of everything; I hold on to nothing. When I calmly pause at the end of exhalation, I think of the word "Pulse or स्पन्द Spanda" and feel the pulse at the tips of my thumbs and also in between my fingers. I clearly experience the pulsatile nature of my body~mind~being at that particular moment, which is quite revealing.

It is very important to actually experience the state of one's body~mind~being, as it is present, at each stage of this Breath-Meditation. This completes the observation of the first breath. This technique is participatory, self-calming and self-healing. It is simple, direct and easy to do. One may repeat these meaningful key words with breathing as many times as one thinks it is necessary to satisfactorily achieve different states of specific energy~awareness~being with related feelings or qualia.

Qualia is what it feels like to be in a particular conscious state, for instance, when one thinks of the word "Wordless, Nishabda निशब्द," one should actually know and feel that the mind is silent and free of words, speech or thoughts. In such a state, one usually hears the spontaneous sound of silence or Anāhata Nāda अनाहत नाद. However, this may take some time before one's habitual inner chatter, the residual subconscious memories and conflicts are resolved. Then, the mind spontaneously comes to a state of serene and restful vigor. It is a unique experience of a truly silent mind listening to the great silence – a nondual holistic state, advaita sthiti अद्वैत स्थिति.

During the remaining six breaths, I pay attention to other meaningful words from the three columns, as listed in the table. I am fully present and attentive to the reality of my body~mind~being at each moment, during the whole procedure. Once, one learns to be in

Breath-Meditation: *Prana-Dhyana* 187

such an attentive state realistically, without any distractions, there is no need to repeat any words. One should just breathe naturally and stay fully present and at-ease with one's energy~being in a quiet and peaceful environment. I call it the holistic presence.

In the second phase, I move my folded hands just above the umbilicus and breathe slowly at half-maximum depth, without thinking of any words. I usually count quietly up to 10-20 breaths. I am fully aware of the abdominal breathing movement and also other nonverbal cues like my pulse, breath-flow and sounds, the moist sweetness on tongue, and especially the spontaneous sound of silence, the Anāhata Nāda. Such silence is ever present in reality, but one can only appreciate it, if one has developed the necessary skill of quiet attentive listening and when one is free of the internal verbal chatter and mental rumination.

In the third phase, I move my folded hands over the upper abdomen and the lower chest. I breathe minimally, almost like the slow waves on a quiet lake. I usually count quietly up to 10-20 breaths. This helps me remain internally still, silent and serene, and gives me a feeling of blissful abidance in my spiritual heart हृदयम् Hridayam, as described by Śri Raman Maharshi (19). In the fourth phase, I rest both of my hands, palms-down, on my thighs with thumb and index finger touching each other and the rest of my fingers relaxed in a curvilinear fashion. This position is comfortable and restful. I breathe quietly and stay fully present and at-ease with myself, for about 50 breaths or 5 minutes. This completes the formal sitting session of Breath-Meditation or Prāna-Dhyāna.

Table. English and Sanskrit terms with their transliteration and translation

	Inhalation	Exhalation	Pause
1.	FULL	EMPTY	PULSE
2.	BREATH	TASTE	NECTAR
3.	STILL	SILENT	SERENE
4.	INFINITE	UNDIVIDED	BLISS
5.	WORLD-ENERGY	INTERNAL-ENERGY	ONE-ENERGY
6.	WORLD-PEACE	INTERNAL-PEACE	ONE-PEACE
7.	OUM	OUM	OUM
१.	पूर्ण	शून्य	स्पन्द
२.	प्राण	रस	अमृत
३.	निश्चल	निःशब्द	निरीच्छ
४.	अनन्त	अखण्ड	आनन्द
५.	बहिर्ज्योतिः	अन्तर्ज्योतिः	एकंज्योतिः
६.	बहिःशान्तिः	अन्तःशान्तिः	शान्तिःशान्तिः
७.	ॐ	ॐ	ॐ

TRANSLITERATION AND TRANSLATION OF THE KEY SANSKRIT WORDS

1. पूर्ण, Pūrṇa: Full, Complete, Holistic, Unitive, Existential Creative Matrix.

2. शून्य, Śūnya: Zero, Empty, Clear, Transparent, Spacious, Sky-Like.

3. स्पन्द, Spanda: Spontaneous pulsating, Neuro-Behavioral Impulse, Pulsatile Consciousness.

4. प्राण, Prāna: Breath-Energy, Life-Energy, Limbic-Autonomic Arousal.

5. रस, Rasa: Taste and Smell, Chemo-sensorium, Visceral Awareness.

6. अमृत, Amrita: Nectar, Sweet Water, Saliva, Immortal, Unending, Self-Renewing.

7. निश्चल, Nishchala: At-ease with self~energy~being, Still, Effortless, Unmoving, Existential.

8. नि:शब्द, Nihshabda: Wordless, Speechless, Silent, Thought-Free, Presence, Calm essential awareness with spontaneous Anāhata Nāda or spontaneous sound of silence.

9. निरीच्छ, Niriccha: Free of desires and subtle motivations.

10. अखण्ड, Akhanda: Uninterrupted, Undivided by Space-Form-Time, Timeless Continuum of Reality.

11. आनन्द, Ānanda: Unconditional Joy, Bliss, Self-Content, Self-Ease.

12. अनन्त, Ananta: Infinite, Endless, Unlimited, Unified field of experience, Reality.

13. अन्तर्ज्योति: Antar-Jyotih: Inner flame, Conscious Arousal~awareness~attention.

14. बहिर्ज्योति: Bahir-Jyotih: Environmental energies, Light-Energy, Sound-Energy, Bio-Energy.

15. एकंज्योति: Ekam-Jyotih: One energy~being~awareness.

16. बहि:शान्ति: Bahih-Shantih: Outer or World Peace.

17. अन्तःशान्तिः Antah-Shantih: Internal or intrinsic peace, calmness or serenity.

18. शान्तिःशान्तिः Shantih-Shantih: Peace of peace or profound peace. Blissful serenity.

19. ॐ OUM: Vedic symbol for the Absolute Reality or Ātman~Brahman.

Breath-Meditation with seven breaths and contemplation on these key words may be performed in any sequence, and repeated in any position, such as sitting, standing, walking or lying down. It is a simple reminder for anyone to remain in a serene, silent and restful state, during most of one's daily activity.

Throughout the day, I try to remain in presence, being present-minded or mindful. I take frequent mental breaks or pauses between physical activity and conversations. This is to appreciate some of the most wonderful and peaceful moments during our daily lives. Many of these moments can be insightful and inspiring, only if we are truly present, calm and receptive to the present reality. Any conscious moment has such a potential to spark an inspiring insight in us. However, it is difficult to remain fully present and attentive all the time. But, I keep trying, and every now and then, I clearly feel these precious moments of great insight, serenity, self-understanding, natural wonder, awe, and creativity.

We should just enjoy and appreciate within us, this infinite, silent and blissful energy~being~awareness. This is our intrinsic, essential nature and our conscious ground state - an infinite, holistic field of one energy~being~awareness. एकंज्योतिः बहुधा विभाति | Ekam jyotih bahudhā vibhāti, "One flame, one energy~being~awareness shines in infinite ways, in many forms and processes."

Some of the Sanskrit Ślokas or verses that I recite and find them helpful to remember before or after Breath-Meditation are listed below:

देहो देवालयः प्रोक्तः स जीवः केवलः शिवः |
त्यजेत् अज्ञाननिर्माल्यं सोऽहंभावेन पूजयेत् ||

This body is the temple. The living being is sacred. Let us discard the old flowers of self-ignorance and worship the self as the Divine. Skandopaniṣad स्कन्दोपनिषद् 10.

देहभावेन दासोऽस्मि | जीवभावेन त्वदंशकः ||
आत्मभावेन त्वमेवाहं | इति मे निश्चिता मतिः ||

When I consider myself as the physical body, Dehabhāva देहभाव, I am your servant; when I consider myself as a living person, Jīvabhāva जीवभाव, I am an integral part of you; but, when I consider myself as the self-existent, essential, holistic Being, Ātmabhāva आत्मभाव, I am You. This is my firm conviction.

अपाणि पादोः अहं अचिन्त्यशक्तिः |
पश्यामि अचक्षुः स शृणोम्यकर्णः||
अहं विजानामि विविक्त रूपो |
न च अस्ति वेत्ता मम चित्सदाहं ||२१||

I am that incomprehensible holistic energy that acts without hands or feet that can see without eyes and hear without ears. I can comprehend various forms, but, no one knows me as the timeless subjective awareness. Kaivalyopanisad (21).

अन्तर्ज्योतिः बहिर्ज्योतिः
प्रत्यक्ज्योतिः परात्परः |
ज्योतिर्ज्योतिः स्वयंज्योतिः
आत्मज्योतिः शिवोऽस्मिहम् ||१९||

I am the intrinsic energy, the extrinsic energy, the existential energy, the transcendental energy. I am the energy of energy, the self-effulgent energy, and the self-energy. I am Lord Śiva, the God of absolute auspiciousness and perfect goodness. Ādi Śaṅkarāchāryā's Brahmajñānāvali.

प्रकाशमानं न पृथक् प्रकाशात् |
स च प्रकाशो न पृथक् विमर्शात् ||
नान्योविमर्शोऽहमितिस्वरूपात्| अहंविमर्शोऽस्मि चिदेकरुपः ||

All conscious experience is not separate from the conscious energy~being. The conscious being is not different from the existential energy~being~awareness. I am that energy~being~awareness, which is my true nature. I am the energy~being~awareness, the holistic consciousness. Vijñānbhairava.

हृदय कुहर मध्ये केवलं ब्रह्ममात्रं |
हिअहमहम् इति साक्षात् आत्मरूपेण भाति||
हृदि विश मनसा स्वं चिन्वता मज्जता वा|
पवन चलन रोधातात्मनिष्ठो भव त्वं||

Within the sanctum of the *heart, Brahman* alone exists. "I…I"-feeling pulsates and shines *as* the *Ātman* itself. Enter your *"heart"* yourself, *by* self-inquiry, or *ego-mergence.* By *quieting* breathing, *(and mentation), a*bide *blissfully* in your *true Being~Self." Śri Raman Maharshi.*

ठेविले अनन्तेतैसेचि रहावे|

चित्ती असो द्यावे समाधान॥

वाहिल्या उद्वेग दुःखचि केवळ।

भोगणे ते फळ संचिताचे॥

तुका म्हणे घालू तयावरी भार। वाहू हा संसार देवापायी॥

One should live, in the way the "Infinite Being" intended for us to live. Let the "*heart*" always be content. Carrying the burden of anger, fear, conflicts and worries, makes one suffer even more. In life, one has to endure the fruits of one's own actions and thoughts. Tukaram says it is better to surrender and lay down the burden of this worldly life, at the feet of God.

प्राणायामं प्रत्याहारं।

नित्यानित्यविवेकविचारं ॥

जाप्यसमेत समाधिविधानं।

कुरु अवधानं महत् अवधानम् ॥

One should self-discipline breathing and sensory-motor activities. One should always discriminate between the ever-changing transient events from the changeless continuum. One should contemplate on meaningful words with a clear understanding and meditate whole-heartedly. Always be attentive and ever vigilant. From Bhaja Govindam of Adi Shankaracharya.

प्रसन्न मन गगनी शिरतां।

गगनरूप होतें सर्वथा ॥

त्या गगनाचाहि द्रष्टा मी ऐसें भाविता ।

उन्मनावस्था अनुभवा ये ॥

When a cheerful mind enters the infinite sky of consciousness, it becomes the infinite space itself. When one realizes that one is the witness even of that infinite space, then one experiences the mind-free conscious state. Swāmi Swarūpānanda.

DISCUSSION

One can really appreciate the gradual self-transformation, from the usual restless body, a talkative and wandering mind, and a self-centered ego, to a silent, serene, creative, mindful and blissful being. That is our true nature. We just have to understand and uncover this potential wonder within all of us.

Initially, Breath-Meditation involves a deliberate effort to self-regulate one's physiological functions and habitual behaviors. One tries to shift one's mindset from habitual verbal mode to a quieter nonverbal mode of functioning. One's basal feeling shifts from stressful agitation, anger, greed and fear to a more silent and serene mode of blissful energy~being. The autonomic nervous system is no longer dominated and driven by the stress-related sympathetic hyperactivity, but it nicely settles in a high energy-high control, equilibrium state.

I think the development and evolution of our biophysical and conscious energy and its self-conscious control goes through four phases: i) low energy – low control in infants, ii) high energy – low control in children and adolescents, iii) low energy – high control in stressed and exhausted adults and finally, iv) high energy – high control or the optimal state of conscious equanimity in expert meditators.

Patanjali described Yoga as a skill in action, as an art of living. योगः कर्मसु कौशलम् | Yoga, karmasu kouśalam. An acquisition of any new mental skill requires an initial effortful self-regulation followed by progressive competence till one reaches a stage of expertise. Finally, one may reach a masterly stage, when one's behavior and the way of life become natural, spontaneous, peaceful and effortless. One can live a life of full presence, mindfulness, creativity, kindness and wisdom.

The initial stages of learning Breath-Meditation require full attention, which is mediated by the Prefrontal-Parietal, multimodal network. This Prefrontal network is known to have both excitatory and inhibitory controls on human behavior and mentation. The prefrontal cortex is linked to the subcortical structures by three neural networks, which are involved in the executive control of attention and cognition. These functions include intention, response initiation, inhibition, persistence, and switching. These processes are central to the planning and generation of goal-directed behavior.

The dorsolateral prefrontal cortical network is involved in working memory, temporal sequencing of information, generating and maintaining response flexibility. The orbitomedial prefrontal network modulates impulses, mood, and working memory. The anterior cingulate network plays a major role in drive and motivation. With proficiency in Breath-Meditation, the prefrontal executive functions and the Default-Mode network activity may be enhanced.

This "default mode network" has been functionally linked to the stream of thoughts occurring automatically in the absence of goal-directed activity. A set of brain regions that are metabolically active during wakeful 'rest' are consistently deactivated during the performance of a variety of demanding tasks. Zen meditation is traditionally associated with a mental state of full awareness with reduced conceptual contents. Zen practitioners displayed a reduced duration of the neural responses linked to conceptual processing in the default network. This suggests that meditative training may foster the ability to control the automatic cascade of semantic associations triggered by a stimulus and to voluntarily regulate the flow of spontaneous mentation (20).

The inhibitory self-regulation during Yoga session was studied by MRI spectroscopy. The changes in the brain's inhibitory neurotransmitter, gamma-amino-butyric acid (GABA) were studied during a session of yoga versus a reading session. The GABA-to-Creatine ratios that were measured in a 2 cm axial slab using MRI spectroscopic imaging, immediately prior to and immediately after interventions. The study showed a 27% increase in GABA levels in the yoga practitioner group, but no change in the reading group (21).

Increased default mode network connectivity even during rest periods, was demonstrated recently in a group of meditators, when compared to a non-meditators control group. The difference was statistically significant in the medial prefrontal cortex (22).

It seems that yogic practices like the disciplined breathing or Prāṇāyāma and meditation or Dhyāna are associated with skillful self-regulation of behavior, attention and mentation.

Breath-Meditation: Prana-Dhyana 193

Well controlled, double-blind studies using this new Breath-Meditation method will provide new and interesting information for all of us.

REFERENCES

[1]   Nāgendra HR. Prānāyāma: The art and science. Bangalore, India: Vivekānanda Kendra Yoga Prakāśana, 1998.

[2]   Rāmdev S. Prānāyāma: Its philosophy and practice. Haridwar, India: Divya Prakāśan, 2005.

[3]   Kuvalayānanda S. Prānāyāma. Mumbai, India: Popular Prakaśan, 1966.

[4]   Leggett T. Śankara on the yoga sūtrās. Delhi, India: Motilal Banārasidāss Publishers, 1992.

[5]   Taimni IK. The science of yoga: The yoga sūtrās of Pātañjali. Wheaton, IL: Theosophical Publishing House, 1961.

[6]   Vivekānanda S, Translation and commentary. The yoga sūtrās of Pātañjali. London, UK: Watkins Publishing; 2007.

[7]   Gunde DG. Yoga and health (in Marathi). Kolhapur, India: GJG Yoga Academy, 1988.

[8]   Shannahoff-Khalsa DS. Kualini yoga meditation: Techniques specific for psychiatric disorders, couple therapy and personal growth. New York: WW Norton, 2006.

[9]   Ādiśwarānanda S. Meditation and its practices: A definitive guide to tachniques and traditions of meditation in yoga and vedānta. Mayavati, Champwat, India: Advaita Ashram, 2004.

[10]   Chinmayānanda S. Meditation and life. Chennai, India: Govindass Parekh for Chinmaya Publication Trust, 1962.

[11]   Tejomayānada S, Śantānanda S, eds. Living in the present. Langhorne, PA: Chinmaya Publications, 2008.

[12]   Krishnamurti J. The meditative mind. Ojai, CA: Krishnamurti Foundation of America, 1989.

[13]   Deshmukh VD. Neuroscience of meditation. Sceinetific World Journal 2006;6:275-89.

[14]   Tolle E. The power of now: A guide to spiritual enlightenment. Vancouver, Canada: Namaste Publishing, 2004.

[15]   Siegel DJ. The mindful brain: Reflection and attunement in the cultivation of well-being. New York: WW Norton, 2007.

[16]   Gunaratana BH. Mindfulness in plain English. Boston, MA: Wisdom Publications, 2002.

[17]   Rosenberg L. Breath by breath: The liberating practice of insight meditation. Boston, MA: Shambhala, 1999.

[18]   Deshmukh VD. The astonishing brain and holistic consciousness: Neuroscience and vedanta perspectives. New York: Nova Science, 2012.

[19]   Śri Ramana Maharni. Talks with Śri Ramaṇn Maharni. Tiruvannamalai, India: Śri Rama āshramam; 2010.

[20]   Pagnoni G, Cekic M, Guo Y. Thinking about not-thinking: Neural correlates of conceptual processing during Zen meditation. PLoS One 2008;3(9):e3083.

[21]   Streeter CC, Jensen JE, Perlmutter RM, Cabral HJ, Tian H, Terhune DB, et al. Yoga asana sessions increase brain GABA levels: a pilot study. J Altern Complement Med 2007;13(4):419-26.

[22]   Jang JH, Jung WH, Kang DH, Byun MS, Kwon SJ, Choi CH, and Kwon JS. Increased default mode network connectivity associated with meditation. Neuroscience Letters 2011:358-362.

Submitted: October 03, 2011. *Revised:* December 01, 2011. *Accepted:*December 12, 2011.

In: Alternative Medicine Research Yearbook 2012
Editors: Søren Ventegodt and Joav Merrick

ISBN: 978-1-62808-080-3
© 2013 Nova Science Publishers, Inc.

Chapter 20

ANTIDIABETIC EFFECT OF CAMEL MILK ON ALLOXANE DIABETES: COMPARISON WITH INSULIN

Amel Sboui[*], PhD[1,2], Touhami Khorchani, PhD[1], Mongi Djegham, PhD[3] and Omrane Belhadj, PhD[2]

[1]Arid Land Institute, Livestock and Wildlife Laboratory, Medenine Tunisia
[2]College of Sciences, Biochemistry and Technobiology Laboratory,Tunis and
[3]Veterinary School, Physiology and Therapeutic Laboratory, Sidi Thabet, Tunisia

ABSTRACT

This study was performed to evaluate the efficacy of camel milk on alloxan-induced diabetic dogs and to follow this effect in addition to Can-insulin®. Four groups, composed of four diabetic dogs each, were used as follow: group 1 was getting camel milk, and group 2 treated simultaneous with camel milk and Can-insulin®, and group 3 received cow milk simultaneous with Can-insulin®. Group 4 contained clinically healthy animals and was used as control. Each dog received 500 ml of milk/day during five weeks. After three weeks, group 1 showed a significant decline on blood glucose levels from 10.33 ± 0.55 to 6.22 ± 0.5 mmol/L, this improvement on glycemic control was accompanied to a significant decrease on total proteins concentrations (from 79.66 ± 2.11 to 63.63 ± 4.43 g/L). A significant decline of cholesterol levels (from 6.84 ± 1.2 to 4.9 ± 0.5 mmol/L) was shown after only two weeks of treatment. The same result was illustrated on group 2 treated simultaneous with camel milk and Can-Insulin. In group 3 the effect of Can-insulin was well shown only on blood glucose levels during the treatment. The investigation in this research was the beneficial effect of camel milk on diabetic dogs and its independence to the treatment with Can-insulin®.

Keywords: Camel milk, cow milk, alloxan, diabetes, dog

---

[*] Correspondence: Amel Sboui, PhD; Arid Land Institute, Livestock and Wildlife Laboratory; Route Edjorf, Elfgè 4119, Medenine, Tunisia. Tel: +216.75.633.005; Fax: +216.75.633.006; E-mail: amelsb6@yahoo.fr.

INTRODUCTION

Diabetes mellitus is one of the gland endocrine diseases in Human and animal which involves the blood circulatory system. About 6.3% of world population lives with diabetes (1). Diabetes mellitus is a chronic disorder of metabolism caused by an absolute or relative lack of insulin. It is characterized by hyperglycemia in the postprandial and or fasting state and in its severe form is accompanied by ketosis and protein wasting (2). This metabolic disorder can be caused chemically using alloxan, streptozotocine; alloxan diabetes is caused by the selective pancreatic beta cell toxicity of this composite (3,4).

Several species were sensitive to alloxan toxicity such as rats, rabbit and dogs (5,6). In modern medicine, no satisfactory effective therapy is available to cure diabetes mellitus, although it can be managed by insulin treatment. However, the pharmaceutical drugs used in diabetic therapy are either too expensive or have undesirable side-effects or contraindications (7). Therefore the search for more effective and safer hypoglycaemic agents has continued to be an area of active research (8).

In arid regions and in the wilderness, camel milk is known for its usefulness to treat diabetes mellitus. For example, an Indian study reported a hypoglycemic effect of camel milk on diabetic rats (9).

In this context this research was conducted to study the effect of camel milk added or no with Caninsulin® on alloxan – induced diabetic dogs. Alloxan-diabetic dog was used because it is a model of insulin deficiency and insulin resistance while simulating postprandial conditions in diabetic patients (1,10). This animal model can be useful to study the diabetic deficiencies and helpful to veterinary and medical researches (1).

METHODS

Twenty clinically normal adult mixed-breed dogs were prepared for this experiment. These dogs were housed individually in the Tunisian Veterinary Medicine School, Sidi Thabet. Animals were fed once daily with 350-400 g of commercial dry chow and 300 g of beef. This food was given to all dogs daily in the morning after drinking milk. All animal were controlled when drinking milk to be sure that all the quantity given was consumed by the dogs. Water was available ad libitum for dogs throughout the duration of the experiment.

Induction of diabetes

After fasting for an overnight, dogs were injected by an intravenous administration of 65 mg of alloxan monohydrate (Sigma, Aldrich, Germany)/Kg of body weight (10).

Milk samples

Camel milk used during this study was obtained from a camel herd (camelus dromedarius) belonging the Arid Land Institute and cow milk was given from a Tunisian breed of cow housed in the Veterinary School of Medecine.The two types of milk were used fresh without any treatment or dilution.

Before distribution of raw milk to the animal, the pH and acidity of the milk sample was checked to monitor the freshness of milk. The gross composition of the two types of milk was determined (fat, total proteins and total solids). Fat content was measured using the neusol method as indicated by Farah, 1996 (11) and the total proteins concentration was determined by the Kjeldahl method using a nitrogen conversion factor of 6.36 (12). Total solids were evaluated after drying at 105°C until a steady weight was achieved.

Experimental design

Five groups composed of four dogs each were used in this stage; group 1: diabetic dogs treated with camel milk, group 2: diabetic dogs treated simultaneous with camel milk and Can-insulin®, and group 3: diabetic dogs treated with Can-insulin® in addition to cow milk, and group 4 consisted of diabetic dogs no treated and group 5 composed of healthy dogs used as control. Five hundred ml of milk was given to each dog daily during five weeks. Can-insulin® (Intervet, Nederland B.V) was injected subcutaneously with (1IE/kg of body weight + 3IE) at drinking milk (500 mL for each dog daily). The experiment was divided into two periods: the first consisted of four weeks in which, the animals were treated with milk and/or Can-insulin® and the second period lasting three weeks (weeks 5, and 6 and 7) to follow the variations of all analyzed parameters after stopping the milk / and or Can-insulin® treatment.

Blood samples and serum analysis

Blood samples were drawn three times per week from the radial vein with catheter system; these samples were divided in two tubes: one for blood glucose assay (enclose oxalate fluorure), the other for cholesterol, Triglycerides (TG) and total proteins measures.

Blood glucose concentration was measured by a glucose oxidase method (Biomaghreb®) using a spectrophotometer CECIL (CE 2041) at 505 nm. Cholesterol and triglycerides concentrations were determined by enzymatic methods (Biomaghreb®) using spectrophotometer at 505 nm. Total proteins levels were measured at 546 nm.

Urine analysis

A urine sample from each animal was analyzed- weekly during the trial- using Bayer reagent strips for urine analysis. The parameters followed in our study were: Glucosuria, and proteinuria and ketones.

Statistical analysis

The data were expressed as the mean ± SEM and represent the average values for the animals in the same group. Each analysis was repeated three times and the average was used to compare between treatments.

These data were subjected to statistical analysis using SAS computer software (SAS institute, 1998) and the data were compared between and within the experimental groups. This test combines ANOVA with comparison of differences between the means of the treatments at the significance level of $p < 0.05$.

RESULTS

The pH and acidity of the camel milk provided to the animals were respectively 6.41 ± 0.18 and 16.87 ± 1.035°Dornic. These characteristics for the cow milk were as follows: 6.61 ± 0.24 for pH and 17.12 ± 0.64°Dornic. The camel milk used during this study was rich in total protein (34.15 ± 3.11 g/L) and in total solids (119.43 ± 1.84 g/L) compared with bovine milk (30.5 ± 1.95 g/L for total proteins and 104.88 ± 4.39 g/L for total solid amounts). There was no significant difference in fat among the camel and cow milk used (34.5 ± 3.1 g/L in camel milk and 32.5 ± 2.12 g/L in bovine milk).

Effect of milk and/ or Can-insulin treatment on diabetic dogs

Blood glucose levels

After drinking camel milk for four weeks, group 1 showed statistically significant decrease in blood glucose levels (from 10.33 ± 0.55 to 6.22 ± 0.5 mmol/L; p=0.028; figure 1), The hypoglycemic effect of camel milk on this group was significantly observed after 3 weeks of treatment illustrated by a non significant difference in comparison with the healthy group (figure 1).

The same result was shown on dogs from group 2 (figure 1) and a non significant difference between groups 1 and 2 was revealed. During the trial, diabetic dogs from group 3 (treated with cow milk in addition to Can-insulin®) showed a significant decrease of blood glucose levels during the Can-Insulin treatment (from 10 ± 0.72 mmol/L to 6.66 ± 1.27 mmol/L, figure 1).

Once the Can-insulin® treatment was stopped (weeks 5, and 6 and 7), weekly variations of blood glucose levels showed a significant increase of this parameter (from 6.66 ± 1.27 to 9.72 ± 0.58 mmol/L). During the period of testing, blood glucose levels in the healthy dogs (group 4) were within the normal range (3.33 – 6 mmol/L) (figure 1).

Total proteins, cholesterol and TG variations

Only TG concentrations did not show any variations for all treatments during the experiment (table 1). In group 1, the improvement of glycemic balance after three weeks of camel milk treatment was accompanied to a significant decrease in total proteins concentrations (from 79.66 ± 2.11 g/L to 63.93 ± 2.61 g/L, table 2).

A fast decline on cholesterol levels was shown after 2 weeks on this group (from 6.84 ± 1.2 mmol/L to 4.35 ± 0.61 mmol/L, table 1).

Table 1. Weekly variations of cholesterol and TG levels in groups 1, 2, 3 and 4 during the trial

	Cholesterol (Mmol/L)				TG (Mmol/L)			
	Group1	Group2	Group 3	Group4	Group 1	Group2	Group 3	Group 4
Day 0	$6.84^a \pm 1.2$	$6.94^a \pm 0.5$	$6.7^a \pm 0.5$	$4.17^b \pm 1.2$	$1.19^a \pm 0.27$	$1.03^a \pm 0.17$	$1.03^a \pm 0.27$	$0.95^a \pm 0.27$
Week 1	$6.9^a \pm 0.25$	$6.58^a \pm 0.85$	$6.9^A \pm 0.15$	$3.98^b \pm 0.25$	$1.21^a \pm 0.2$	$0.97^b \pm 0.19$	$0.82^a \pm 0.22$	$0.64^a \pm 0.22$
Week 2	$4.9^b \pm 0.5$	$5.23^b \pm 0.5$	$7.75^a \pm 0.07$	$4.7^b \pm 0.07$	$1.13^a \pm 0.1$	$0.9^{a,B} \pm .63$	$0.85^a \pm 0.15$	$0.66^a \pm 0.18$
Week 3	$4.92^b \pm 0.36$	$5.03^b \pm 0.4$	$6.95^a \pm 0.1$	$4.82^b \pm 0.54$	$1.12^a \pm 0.1$	$0.94^a \pm 0.07$	$0.9^a \pm 0.15$	$0.74^a \pm 0.15$
Week 4	$4.4^B \pm 0.62$	$4.08^b \pm 0.6$	$7.82^a \pm 0.46$	$4.21^b \pm 0.46$	$1.17^a \pm 0.1$	$0.97^b \pm 0.25$	$1.1^A \pm 0.08$	$0.92^a \pm 0.83$
Week 5	$4.35^b \pm 0.61$	$4.33^b \pm 0.6$	$7.13^a \pm 0.33$	$4.08^b \pm 0.33$	$0.99^A \pm 0.3$	$0.94^a \pm 0.33$	$1.03^A \pm 0.3$	$0.9^a \pm 0.32$
Week 6	$4.27^b \pm 0.5$	$4.44^b \pm 0.6$	$7.34^a \pm 0.56$	$4.11^b \pm 0.62$	$1.05^a \pm 0.4$	$0.99^a \pm 0.52$	$1.01^a \pm 0.38$	$1^A \pm 0.42$
Week 7	$4.11^b \pm 0.42$	$4.48^b \pm 0.7$	$7.26^a \pm 0.36$	$4.6^B \pm 0.56$	$1.02^a \pm 0.4$	$1.13^a \pm 0.64$	$0.98^a \pm 0.62$	0.97 ± 0.33

For each analyzed parameter: Means with the same letter in each line are not significantly different.
Group 1: diabetic dogs receiving camel milk.
Group 2: Diabetic dogs treated simultaneous with camel milk and Caninsulin®.
Group 3: Diabetic dogs treated simultaneous with cow milk and Caninsulin®.
Group 4: Healthy group receiving camel milk and used as control
Week 1 to week 4: during the treatment.
Weeks 5 + 6 + 7: After stopping to drink milk and injection of Caninsulin®.

It was the same for the animal from group 2 (treated with camel milk and Caninsulin®); the weekly variations of these parameters demonstrated a non significant difference between groups 1 and 2.

Animals treated with cow milk in addition to Can-Insulin (group 3) showed a steady high cholesterol and total proteins concentrations during and after stopping of the treatment (about 7.23 ± 0.32 mmol/L for cholesterol and 81.49 ± 4.56 g/L for total proteins levels, table 1 and table 2).

Table 2. Weekly variations of Total Proteins concentrations in groups 1, 2, 3 and 4 during the experiment

	Total proteins (g/l)			
	Group 1	Group 2	Group 3	Group 4
Day 0	$79.66^a \pm 2.11$	$80.36^a \pm 0.9$	$79.18^a \pm 2.11$	$68.48^b \pm 2.01$
Week 1	$74.35^a \pm 7.25$	$71,93^a \pm 5.5$	$81.56^a \pm 7.25$	$68.8^b \pm 3.25$
Week 2	$67.06^{a,b} \pm 9.91$	$67.35^{a,b} \pm 7.13$	$82.45^a \pm 9.91$	$67.06^b \pm 2.27$
Week 3	$63.63^b \pm 4.43$	$66.05^b \pm 2.47$	$85.2^a \pm 4.43$	$65.75^b \pm 2.27$
Week 4	$64.58^b \pm 3.16$	$65.98^b \pm 1.77$	$74.76^a \pm 3.16$	$64.82^b \pm 2.11$
Week 5	$63.93^b \pm 2.61$	$63.14^b \pm 1.21$	$84.33^a \pm 2.61$	$65.45^b \pm 1.03$
Week 6	$66.57^b \pm 2$	$62.46^b \pm 2.35$	$82.09^a \pm 3.49$	$66^b \pm 1.77$
Week 7	$64.63^b \pm 1.04$	$62.63^b \pm 3.14$	$82.36^a \pm 3.67$	$66.63^b \pm 0.53$

For each analyzed parameter: Means with the same letter in each line are not significantly different.
Group 1: diabetic dogs receiving camel milk.
Group 2: Diabetic dogs treated simultaneous with camel milk and Caninsulin®.
Group 3: Diabetic dogs treated simultaneous with cow milk and Caninsulin®.
Group 4: Healthy group receiving camel milk and used as control.
Week 1 to week 4: during the treatment.
Weeks 5 + 6 + 7: After stopping to drink milk and injection of Caninsulin®.

The effectiveness of the treatment with camel milk supplemented or no with Caninsulin® (groups 1 and 2) was investigated on blood glucose, total proteins and cholesterol concentrations after the dogs stopped drinking milk (weeks 5, and 6 and 7); no significant differences were noted in outcomes analyzed (figure 1, table 1 and table 2) and all dogs showed a clinical healthy state by the end of the trial.

The non diabetic state was demonstrated in groups 1 and 2, firstly: by a normal range of fast blood glucose (5.66 ± 1.11 mmol/L), total proteins (64.63 ± 1.04 g/L), TG (1.02 ± 0.37 mmol/L) and cholesterol (4.11 ± 0.42 mmol/L) levels. Secondly: by the end of camel milk treatment all animal from groups 1 and 2 illustrated absence of glucose, proteins and ketones in urine sample which were well detected in urine sample after induction of diabetes.

DISCUSSION

This study was performed to evaluate the efficacy of camel milk (supplemented or no with Caninsulin®) in achieving glycemic control on Alloxan – induced diabetic dogs; Alloxan injection causes a toxic effect on kidney and liver in addition to the pancreas as investigated by other study on alloxan induced- diabetes in (13,14). Diabetes in dogs is generally associated, in addition to high blood glucose levels, to an increase of total proteins concentrations (4) which are illustrated in our study especially in dogs treated with cow milk (group 3) (82.83 ± 3.83 g/L).

Some hypothesis (9 and 15) reported that the hypoglycemic effect of camel milk may be due to the high level of insulin in comparison with cow milk.

But in this assay our results cannot be due to this particularity because the effect of camel milk on glycemic control, proteins and lipids profile was observed also by the end of treatment (groups 1 and 2).

Hypoglycemic effect of Caninsulin was shown when it was injected with cow milk to the diabetic animals (figure 1). This effect was not illustrated when Caninsulin was injected to the diabetic animals treated simultaneous with camel milk. Caninsulin doesn't have any supplementary effect on the glycemic balance when added to camel milk (non significant difference compared with the effect of camel milk only). Camel milk may be able to eliminate the alloxan toxicity on pancreas or has a regenerative effect on beta cells and could be used as a curative treatment of diabetes in dogs.

High mineral content (Sodium, Potassium, Copper and Magnesium) as well as a high vitamin C intake (16) may act as antioxidant there by removing free radicals, which may provide an additional benefit to the animals treated with camel milk (17) It may be explained by the particularity and properties of camel milk in comparison with milk from other species, such as the absence of ß-lactoglobulin, the high amount of polyunsaturated fatty acids (C18:1-C18: 3), and the high amount of vitamin B3(18 and 19) and also some particularities of camel immunoglobulin, such as their small size and weight which offers enormous potential to camel milk. Also camel milk immunoglobulins, of relatively small size and weight, might offer interplay with host cell protein leading to an induction of regulatory cells and finally leading to a downward regulation of immune system and ß-cell salvage (20, 21).

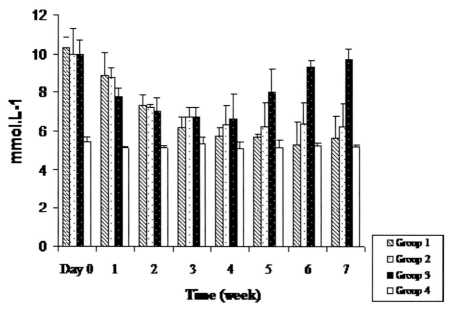

p1: period 1: Treatment with milk and / or Caninsulin®.
p2: period 2: After the end of the treatment (milk and/or Caninsulin®).
Group 1: Diabetic dogs treated with camel milk.
Group 2: Diabetic dogs treated with camel milk and Caninsulin®.
Group 3: Diabetic dogs treated with cow milk and Caninsulin®.
Group 4: Healthy group.

Figure 1. Weekly variations of blood glucose levels in groups 1, 2, 3 and 4 during the experiment.

From the results offered in our study, a therapeutic efficacy of camel milk on alloxan induced diabetes is showed. This may have important implication for the clinical management of diabetes mellitus in humans. But further studies are warranted to fractionate the active principle and to find out its exact mode of action.

REFERENCES

[1] Valilou M, Sohrabi HI, Mohamednejad D, Soleimani RJ. Histopathological and ultrastructural lesions study of kidneys of alloxan induced diabetes mellitus in German Shephered dogs. J Animal Vet Adv 2007;6(8):1012-6.
[2] Tyberg B, Anderson A, Hakan Borg LA. Species differences in susceptibility of transplanted and cultured pancreatic islets to the ß- cell. Gen Comparat Endocrinology 2001;122:238-51.
[3] Rerup CC. Drugs producing diabetes through damage of the insulin secreting cells. Pharmacol Rev 1970;2:485-518.
[4] Toulon F. Le diabète sucré du chien, maladie chronique. Le Point Vétérinaire 1986;17(94):681- 91. [French]
[5] Sakudelski T. Mechanism of alloxan and streptozotocin action in beta cells of the rat pancreas. Physiol Res 2001;50:537-46.
[6] Stanely-Prince P, Kamalakkannan N, Menon VP. Antidiabetic and antihyperlipidaemic effect of alcoholic Syzigium cumini seeds in alloxan induced diabetic albino rats. J. Ethnopharmacol 2004;91: 209–13.

[7] Lemhadri A, Zeggwagh NA, Maghrani M, Jouad H, Eddouks M. Anti-hyperglycaemic activity of the aqueous extract of Origanum vulgare growing wild in Tafilalet region. J Ethnopharmacol 2004; 92:251–6.
[8] Bell GI, Molecular defects in diabetes mellitus. Diabetes 1991;40: 413-7.
[9] Agrawal RP, Sahani MS, Tuteja FC, Ghouri SK, Sena DS, Gupta R, Kochar DK. Hypoglycemic activity of camel milk in chemically pancreatectomized rats. An experimental study. Int J Diab Dev Countries 2005;25(3):75-9.
[10] Matsuhisa M, Shi ZQ, Wan C. The effect of pioglitazone on hepatic glucose uptake measured with indirect and direct methods in alloxan – induced diabetic dogs. Diabetes 1997;46:224-31.
[11] Farah Z. Camel milk: Properties and products, 3rd ed. St Gallen, Switzerland: Swiss Centre Dev Cooperation Technol Manage, 1996.
[12] Association française de normalisation. Contrôle de la qualité des produits alimentaires. Lait et produits laitiers. Paris: AFNOR, 1993.
[13] Kim JM, Chung JY, Lee SY, Choi EW, Kim M.K, Hwang CY, Youn HY. Hypoglycemic effects of vanadium on alloxan monohydrate induced - diabetic dogs. J Vet Sci 2006;7(4):391–5.
[14] Pari L, Satheesh MA. Antidiabetic activity of Boerhaavia diffusa L: Effect on hepatic key enzymes in experimental diabetes. J Ethnopharmacol 2004;91:109–13.
[15] Agrawal R., Swami SC, Beniwal R. Effect of camel milk on glycemic control, risk factors and diabetes quality of life in type 1 diabetes: A randomized prospective controlled study. J Camel Pract Res 2003;10(1):45-50.
[16] Stahl HP, Sallmann R, Duehlmeir U, Wernery U. Selected vitamins and fatty acid patterns in dromedary milk and colostrums. J Camel Res Pract 2006;13(1):53-7.
[17] Elsner M, Tiedge M, Lenzen S. Mechanism underlying resistance of human pancreatic beta cells against streptozotocin and alloxan. Diabetologia 2003;46:1713-4.
[18] Farah Z. Composition and characteristics of camel milk. J Dairy Res 1993;60:603-6.
[19] Zhang H, Yao J, Zaho D, Liu H, Guo M. Changes in chemical composition of Alxa Bactrian camel milk during lactation. J Dairy Sci 2005;88:3402-10.
[20] Hamers-Casterman C, Atarbouch, T, Muyldermans S, Robinsonn G, Songa EB, Hamers R. Naturally occurring antibodies devoid of light chains. Nature 1993;363:446-8.
[21] Rajendra P, Agrawal SS, Poornima S, Rajendra PG, Kochara DK, Mohan SS. Effect of camel milk on residual ß-cell function in recent onset type 1 diabetes. Diab Res Clin Pract 2007;77(3):494-5.

Submitted: January 15, 2011. *Revised:* March 18, 2011. *Accepted:* March 30, 2011.

In: Alternative Medicine Research Yearbook 2012
Editors: Søren Ventegodt and Joav Merrick

ISBN: 978-1-62808-080-3
© 2013 Nova Science Publishers, Inc.

Chapter 21

TRANSFER OF EFFECT OF HEAT SHOCK AND DRUG TREATMENT FROM ONE PLANT TO ANOTHER THROUGH WATER

Sandhimita Mondal, MSc, Soma Sukul, MSc, PhD and Nirmal C Sukul, MSc, PhD*

Department of Botany, Visva-Bharati University, Santiniketan, West Bengal, India

ABSTRACT

Cowpea plants, *Vigna unguiculata* (L) Walp, grown in pots, were kept in two pairs of rows, each containing 10 plants. Plants in each pair were connected by water filled polythene tubes, the open ends of which were dipped into water in two beakers. In each beaker a mature leaf of a plant was immersed. Plants in one row of a pair were given heat stress through hot water while the corresponding water connected row of the same pair remained unstressed. Plants in one row of the second pair were treated with *Cantharis* 200c, a homeopathy potency used for the treatment of burns. The corresponding water connected row of this pair remained untreated. Another single row of plants served as the unstressed and untreated control. After a fixed time leaves of all the plants were harvested and homogenized. Leaf proteins of the plants in each row were separated by fast protein liquid chromatography (FPLC).Leaf protein profile of the heat stressed plants showed similarity with that of unstressed but water connected plants. *Cantharis* -treated plants and the corresponding untreated but water-connected ones showed similarity in the leaf protein profile. Leaf protein profile of the control plants was different from that of the two groups. It appears that an external stimulus to a plant brings about a change in the water structure in the plant which is transmitted through the global molecular network(GMN) of water connecting the two plants.

Keywords: Homeopathic potency, Cantharis, heat-shock, inter individual transfer, water network

---

* Correspondence: Professor Nirmal C Sukul, Department of Botany, Visva - Bharati University, Santiniketan - 731235, West Bengal, India. E-mail: nimal@sukulhomeopathy.com, ncsukul@gmail.com.

INTRODUCTION

New-born babies are very often treated by potentized homeopathic medicines through their nursing mothers. Potencies thus produce therapeutic effect on the babies through their mother's milk during breast feeding. Many allopathic drugs, taken by mothers, are known to be transferred to the breast milk and from there to the sucking babies (1).Here the allopathic drug molecules are directly transferred from the nursing mother to the baby. Homeopathic potencies above 12c do not contain any drug molecule.

A potentized homeopathic drug in aqueous ethanol is thought to carry the structural information of the molecules of the drug, from which it has been prepared, through the process of successive dilution and succussion. Water can form an innumerable variety of structural configuration through hydrogen bonding strengthened by succussion and preserved by ethanol. Thus water serves as informational molecules through specific three-dimensional structures of water polymers (2). It has been hypothesized that a homeopathic potency initially interacts with and modulates the water structure over the plasma membrane thereby bringing about a conformational change of protein domains in contact with the membrane. The local change is propagated to all parts of the organism through the global molecular network (GMN) of proteins and water. A homeopathic potency may act through the global water structure and protein network of an organism (3). If this is so, then the effect produced on an organism could be transferred to another through a column of water connecting the two individuals.

We have devised an experiment to verify this hypothesis. Here cowpea plants were grown on pots and connected by polythene tubes containing sterile water. The effect of heat shock on one plant was observed on another plant connected by water column in the form of heat shock proteins in leaves. Similarly, the effect of treatment of one plant with a homeopathic potency, *Cantharis* 200c was observed on another plant connected by water column in terms of the leaf protein profile. Sukul *et al.* (4) has demonstrated that *Cantharis* 200c could induce expression of heat-shock-like proteins in plants. *Cantharis* is a homeopathic drug used for the treatment of burn injuries. In plants the effect of infection with a parasite or of treatment with a drug at one part is transferred to the distant parts. The effect here relates to the expression of pathogenesis related proteins (5-7).

METHODS

Earthen pots, 22.5cm in diameter at upper edge and 22.5 cm in depth, were filled with a mixture of loam soil and cow dung manure in the proportion of 1:1 v/v. The soil filled pots were treated with boiling water twice to remove soil-borne plant pathogens. Seeds of cowpea were surface sterilized with 0.1% mercuric chloride, allowed to germinate on moist filter paper and sown, one seed/pot, in all the 50 pots. The pots were divided into 5 batches and kept individually over bricks. Four batches were arranged in two pairs (Set I and II) and kept side by side. Pots of each pair were 60 cm apart. There were two sets of pairs, each set containing 10 plants. One mature leaf of each plant of the two sets of pairs was immersed in sterile tap water in a glass beaker. A soft polythene tube 2 mm in diameter and 90 cm in length was filled with sterile tap water and their open ends immersed into water in a pair of beakers in which leaves of the partners of each pair of plants were also immersed. This arrangement is shown in a diagram (Figure 1).

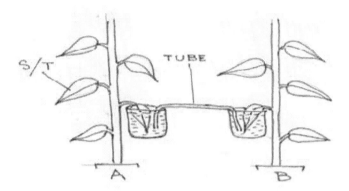

Figure 1. Diagram showing connection between two plants A, B by a water –filled tube with its ends dipped in two beakers containing water. While one beaker has one leaf of heat-stressed or *Cantharis 200c* treated plant (A), the other has a leaf of unstressed and untreated plant (B). Stress(S) or treatment (T) is given to a leaf different from that immersed in water.

In set no. I, one plant in each pair was given heat shock by immersing a mature leaf in hot water at 61^0 to 54^0C for 5 min. In case of set no. II one plant in each pair was treated with *Cantharis 200c*. The drug, obtained from Seth Dey and Co. Kolkata, was diluted with sterile distilled water in the proportion of 1:500 in order to minimize the effect of ethanol. A piece of filter paper was soaked in the dilution and gently placed on a mature leaf covering an area of 1cm diameter. The treatment was given on both sides of the leaf in the same spot for 1 min. Heat shock or drug treatment was given 60 min after the plant pairs in each set were connected by water filled tubes. The purpose was to equilibrate the plants in each pair in the connected state.

Separation of proteins

Leaves were harvested one hour after heat shock, and one hour after *Cantharis* treatment. Treated leaves and those immersed in water were not harvested. Leaves of the control plants were also harvested at the same time. These leaves were homogenized in a chilled extraction buffer. Protein extraction buffer was added at a rate of $4cm^3$ of buffer/g of tissue. The extraction buffer was composed of 50mM Tris-HCl, 2% β-mercaptoethanol, 1mM ethylene diamine tetraacetic acid disodium salt (EDTA-Na_2), 5% sucrose, 1.5% PVPP, 1mM phenyl methyl sulfonyl fluoride (PMSF) at a pH adjusted to 8.0 with 1M HCl. The mixture was centrifuged at 15,000g for 20 min at 4^0C. Supernatant of each sample was kept at -80^0 C until further analysis. Each sample of 1ml of extract was injected into the column Superdex 75071. Protein separation was done by Fast Protein Liquid Chromatography (FPLC) using the mobile phase of 0.5M Tris –HCl buffer (pH 7.5) with protease inhibitors at a flow rate 0.5 ml/min at $25\ ^0$C with UV detector fixed at the wave length of 280nm. The instrument was of GE healthcare, AKta purifier, model 10. Leaf extract and buffer were filtered through Millipore filter (0.45μm) to remove any suspended particles before FPLC run. The chromatograms were monitored and printed. Gel electrophoresis was not done in this case because the quantity of proteins extracted from cowpea leaves was very low.

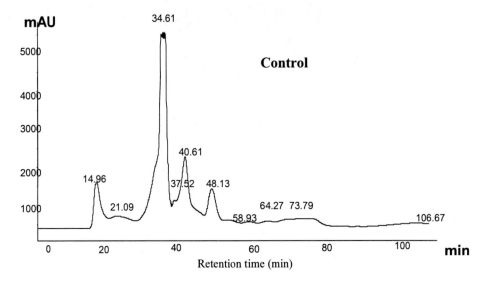

Figure 2. Leaf proteins separated by FPLC of cowpea plants, unstressed and untreated (Control). N=10 plants.

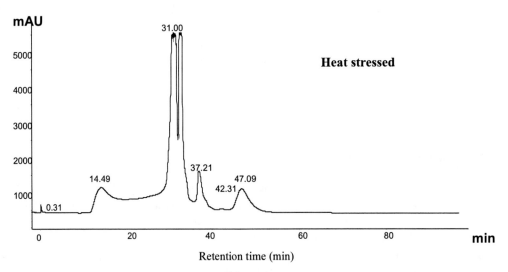

Figure 3a. Leaf proteins separated by FPLC of cowpea plants given heat stress through hot water (61-54 ^{0}C for 5min) to one leaf in each plant. N=10 plants.

RESULTS

Leaf protein profile of the control plants is given in figure 2, of heat-stressed plants in figure 3a, of unstressed but connected to heat stressed plants by water column in figure 3b, of *Cantharis* treated plants in figure 4a, and of corresponding untreated but connected plants in figure 4b.

Transfer of effect of heat shock and drug treatment ... 207

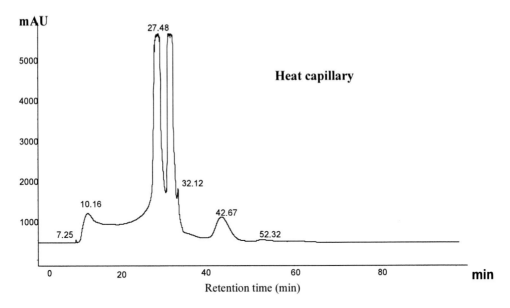

Figure 3b. Leaf proteins separated by FPLC of unstressed cowpea plants connected by water to heat stressed plants. N=10 plants.

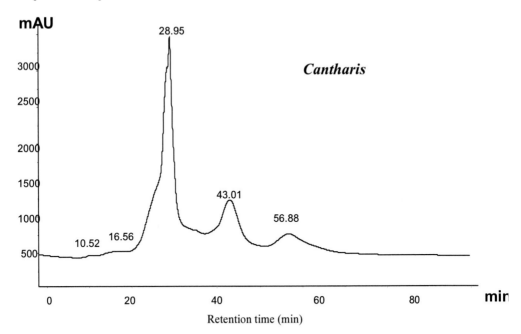

Figure 4a. Leaf proteins separated by FPLC of cowpea plants treated by *Cantharis* 200c. The drug was diluted with mili Q water 1:100, soaked in a sterile filter paper and applied by gentle touch to one leaf in each plant. N=10 plants.

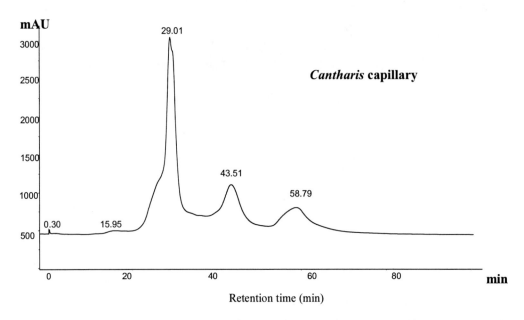

Figure 4b. Leaf proteins separated by FPLC of untreated cowpea plants connected by water to treated plants. N=10 plants.

There was a marked similarity between the heat stressed plants and the water connected unstressed plants in the leaf protein profile. *Cantharis*-treated plants and untreated but connected plants showed similarity in the leaf protein profile.

Both heat-stressed plants and their unstressed but water connected counterparts show a protein peak around the retention time (RT) of 30-31min which is absent in the control (figure 3a, 3b, 2).The unstressed but connected plants show a new protein peak around the RT of 27 min which is absent in both heat stressed and control plants (figure 3a, 3b, 2). Both *Cantharis* treated plants and their untreated but water connected counterparts show protein peaks around the RT 29 min and 43 min which are absent in the control plants (figure 4a, 4b, 2). However, these two protein peaks show very close similarity in the RT's with those of plants connected to heat-stressed ones (4a, 4b, 3b).Three protein peaks around RT's 14 min, 33-34 min and 47-48 min were common to both the control and heat-stressed plants (figure 2, 3a).The control protein peak around RT 40 min is absent in all the stressed, treated and connected plants (figure 2, 3ab, 4ab).

Discussion

Protein peak at RT 30-31 min appears to have been induced directly by heat shock (figure 3a) and indirectly through water connection (figure 3b). Protein peaks at 28-29 min might have been induced directly by *Cantharis* 200c (figure 4a) and indirectly by water connection (figure 4b). These proteins may have protective effect against heat shock as is evident in their expression in plants connected to heat-stressed ones (figure 3b). Protein peak at RT 40 min, found in the control (figure 2) might have been repressed due to heat shock and *Cantharis* treatment (figure 3ab, 4ab).

The results demonstrate that the effect of any treatment on a plant can be transmitted to another plant of the same species through water. This suggests the role of water as informational molecules, and strengthens the assumed physical basis of a homeopathic potency. Living cells in an organism are dynamic reactive structures formed by membranes surrounding a singular fluid mixture. The existence of global metabolic structure was verified for some organisms and that the self-organized enzymatic configuration appears to be common to all cellular organisms (8-9). The metabolic network is a dynamic complex superstructure which integrates different dynamic systems, the metabolic subsystems. The transmission of information between the metabolic subsystems forces them to be interlocked between themselves (10). A stimulus in the form of heat shock or drug treatment in an area of a leaf would bring about a local change in the metabolic activity in that area. This change is dissipated through the global metabolic network to all parts of the plant. Here the change occurs in the form of expression of new proteins.

Experimental studies have shown that enzymes may form functional catalytic associations in which molecular oscillations may occur spontaneously. When the oscillations are periodical the metabolic intermediaries oscillate with the same frequency but different amplitudes (11). Chabot *et al* (12) reported spontaneous emergence of molecular oscillations in experimental studies on several fundamental metabolic processes including gene expression. It is quite possible that molecular oscillations also involve water structure covering the surface of integral membrane proteins. A homeopathic potency, which is specifically structured water with characteristic molecular oscillation, may act on water structure over macromolecules of cells and change their pattern of oscillations. The local change is dissipated through GMN to all parts of the treated plants and from there to the untreated plants connected by water column. The oscillatory pattern in the untreated plant is reorganized corresponding to the treated plant resulting in the expression of similar proteins in both the plants connected to each other by water. Hydrogen bond network controls water dynamics. There exist intermittent molecular motions associated with the rearrangement of the hydrogen bond network and concomitant fluctuation and relaxation in water (13). Wen *et al* (14) observed that upon vibrational excitation there was conversion of highly coordinated strongly hydrogen bonded water structures to less ordered water structures with weaker hydrogen bonding as recorded by femtosecond X-ray spectroscopy. Since the preparation of homeopathic potencies involves succussion or mechanical agitation through successive steps, the hydrogen bonds become stronger and more coordinated (2). This specific coordination and H-bond strength in the H-bond network in a potency may induce corresponding changes in the water structure and oscillations over macromolecules of the cell membrane resulting in expression of specific proteins.

ACKNOWLEDGMENTS

We thank The Asiatic Society, Kolkata for providing financial support to the work described here. We also thank the Director, Bose Institute, Kolkata for providing instrumentation facility relating to FPLC. A special word of thanks to Mr. Samir Mukherjee of the Bose Institute for his help in the operation of the FPLC instrument. This paper was presented at an

International conference held at Kolkata, West Bengal, India on 10-12 December, 2010 and published in the form of an abstract.

REFERENCES

[1] American Academy of Pediatrics. The transfer of drugs and other chemicals into human milk. Pediatrics 2001;108:776-80.

[2] Sukul NC, Sukul A. High dilution effects: physical and biochemical basis. Dordrecht: Kluwer Academic Publishers, 2004.

[3] Sukul NC, Sukul A. Molecular mechanism of action of homeopathic potencies with references to holism. Environ Ecol 2009; 27:71-7.

[4] Sukul NC, Mondal S, Sukul S. *Cantharis* 200 C may induce expression of small heat shock –like proteins in *Adhatoda vasica* leaves. Sci Cult 2010;240-3.

[5] Bowels D. Local and systemic signaling during a plant defense response. In: Callow JASA, Green J R, eds. Society for experimental biology seminar series 48: perspectives in plant cell recognition. Cambridge: Cambridge University Press, 1992:123-35.

[6] Roy D, Sinhababu S P, Sukul NC. Root-knot nematode extract increases growth of plants and reduces nematode infection. Environ Ecol 1995;13:775-9.

[7] Nandi B, Sukul NC, Banerjee N, Sinhababu SP. Salicylic acid reduces Meloidogyne incignita infestation of cowpea. Proc Zoo Soc Calcutta 2000;53:93-95.

[8] Almas E, Kovacs B, Vicse K T, Oltvai ZN, Barabasi A L. Global organization of metabolic fluxes in the bacterium *Escherichia coli*. Nature 2004;427:839-43.

[9] Almas E. Biological impacts and context of network theory. J Exp Biol 2007; 210:1548-58.

[10] Fuente I M De la, Vadillo F, Pirez-Samartin A L, Pirez –Pinilla M-B, Bidaurrazaga J, Vera – Lopez.2010. Global self-regulation of the cellular metabolic structure. PLoS One 2010;5-3:e9484.

[11] Goldbeter A. Rythmes et chaosdans les systemes biochimiques et cellulaires. Paris: Masson, 1990.

[12] Chabot J R, Pedraza J M, Luitel P, Van Qudenaarden A. A stochastic gene expression out of steady state in the cyanobacterial circadian clock. Nature 2007; 450:1249-52.

[13] Ohmine I, Saito S. Water dynamics: fluctuation, relaxation and chemical reactions in hydrogen bond network rearrangement. Acc Chem Res 1999; 32:741-9.

[14] Wen H, Huse N, Schoenlein R W, Lindenberg A M. Ultra fast conversions between hydrogen bonded structures in liquid water observed by femtosecond x-ray spectroscopy. J Chem Phys 2009; 132:234-9.

Submitted: April 22, 2011. *Revised:* July 01, 2011. *Accepted:* July 25, 2011.

In: Alternative Medicine Research Yearbook 2012
Editors: Søren Ventegodt and Joav Merrick

ISBN: 978-1-62808-080-3
© 2013 Nova Science Publishers, Inc.

Chapter 22

THE CAPABILITIES OF NEW CHINESE ENTREPRENEURS IN CHINA

Jing Sun, PhD[1], Nicholas Buys, PhD[2] and Xinchao Wang, PhD[3]*

[1]School of Public Health and Griffith Health Institute. Griffith University,
Gold Coast campus, Parkland, Australia,
[2]School of Human Services and Social Work and Griffith Health Institute,
Griffith University, Gold Coast campus, Parkland, Australia,
[3]Guanghua Graduate School of Management, Peking University, Beijing, China

ABSTRACT

This paper explores the clusters of capabilities in Chinese entrepreneurs and the relationships between entrepreneurial capability and regional socio-economic and GDP level in terms of the development of the new enterprise. In October 2007, 38,875 participants from a randomly selected sample of 50,000 entrepreneurs (response rate of 77.8%) from 31 provinces in China completed a survey on entrepreneurial capability. Eight major areas of entrepreneurial capabilities were measured, including opportunity identification, interpersonal skills, conceptualisation, organising, strategies, commitment, learning and emotional control. Cluster analysis was used to classify the entrepreneurs into three types: learning based, basic capability based and opportunity focused. Multilevel analysis was used to analyse further the relationship between clustered capabilities, area socioeconomic and GDP level, while other variables were controlled in the analysis. The findings suggest that learning-based entrepreneurs have higher abilities in emotional control, learning, organising and conceptual skills than do opportunity-focused or basic capability-based entrepreneurs. Opportunity-focused entrepreneurs were found to be stronger in opportunity taking, interpersonal skills, commitment and strategic capabilities than the other entrepreneurial types. Basic capability-based entrepreneurs were found to have the lowest capabilities across all measures. The significant differences in capabilities between the three clusters of entrepreneurs highlight the

---

* Correspondence: Jing Sun, PhD, School of Public Health, Griffith University and Griffith Health Institute, Griffith University, Logan campus, Meadowbrook Q4131, Australia. E-mail: j.sun@griffith.edu.au.

importance of the desire to learn and seize opportunities as success factors in start-up businesses, and the need for education and training for a comprehensive range of capabilities to run businesses successfully. The capabilities were found to be significantly related to area socioeconomic and GDP level.

Keywords: Entrepreneur, capabilities, Chinese, Small to Medium Size Enterprises

INTRODUCTION

By 30 December 2009, China's registered small- and medium-sized enterprises (SMEs) exceeded 43 million (1). Among them, 38 millions are private companies. China's SMEs play an important role in employment and economic development. SEMs account for more than 99.8% of the total number of businesses in China, and contribute to 58.5% of total annual GDP, 50% of taxation revenues, 68% of exports and 75% of new jobs. SMEs employ more than 80% of the labour force (1). In terms of high-tech and innovation, only 3% of the SMEs are hi-tech related, 92% of which are privately owned enterprises. These high-tech enterprises are owners of 65% of the patents and 80% of new products (2).

Private enterprises have become a major driving force in the contemporary Chinese economy and the emergence of entrepreneurs as a new social class has now attracted enormous interest from Chinese and international researchers (3-6). In February 2010, the Chinese economy was confirmed as the second largest in the world, having overtaken Japan (7). In light of these trends, it is not surprising to find strong recognition for the opportunities afforded by entrepreneurship in China.

Entrepreneurs show strong orientation in experiential learning and opportunity identification. Numerous studies show that experiential learning is essential to entrepreneurs (8). Deakins and Freel (8) found that the process of experiential learning includes feedback from clients and customers, problem identification and problem solving. Rae and Carswell (9) further explored how people learn entrepreneurial behaviour. They found entrepreneurs develop their capabilities in the 'process of recognizing and acting on opportunities, and from organizing and managing ventures'. Politis (10) further argues that entrepreneurial leaning is an experiential transfer. This includes entrepreneurial, management and industry experience.

This learning process can shape and develop entrepreneurs' capabilities by changing their perceptions and intentions to be an entrepreneur.

Entrepreneurs have strong intention in opportunity identification and information search and this may reflect entrepreneurs' capability to handle complex information and their experience and knowledge (11). Information search plays a crucial role in improving entrepreneurs capabilities in relation to innovation and strategies in start-up business (12).

Rauch's meta-analysis on entrepreneurial traits found that when the measured entrepreneurial traits were specific traits instead of general ones, the relationships between entrepreneurs' personality traits and entrepreneurial success are more significant. Many researchers noticed the problem and began to turn their research topics to specific traits.

In this context, the concept of capabilities, which is discussed below, has emerged as a factor that suggests some entrepreneurs are more successful than others (13, 14). To date, few studies have examined capabilities among the entrepreneurs in a representative national sample in China.

The concept of capabilities

Capabilities are conceptualised based on a process or personality perspective (15,16). The terms 'capabilities' and 'competencies' are often used interchangeably in literature: 'Entrepreneurial competencies are considered a high level ability encompassing personality traits, skills and knowledge, and therefore can be seen as the total ability of the entrepreneur to perform a job role successfully' (17). Eight entrepreneurial capabilities were identified based on the previous studies (12,17) and these include opportunity identifying, interpersonal skills, concept, organising, strategy and commitment.

These capabilities were found to be influenced by the entrepreneurs' experience, education, family background and other demographic variables (18,19). We hypothesise that hidden opportunities can be uncovered with stronger conceptual competencies, sufficient skills in emotional control, strategy, commitment, interpersonal skills and organising abilities. Entrepreneurs having strong capabilities and being successful in start-up business is significantly related to an area's economic performance. However, the intertwining relationship between types of entrepreneurs and capabilities is not clear in Chinese entrepreneurs at both individual and area levels.

The proposed study aimed to identify the types of entrepreneurs based on the clustered capabilities, and the relationship between types of entrepreneurs and capabilities, and its contribution to area economic performance including GPD level, area income and area socio-economic level.

METHODS

A cross-sectional study design was used for the study, which was undertaken in China in 2007. The study sample was identified from a list of entrepreneurs provided by China Central Television (CCTV). Entrepreneurial businesses (SMEs) included in the sample were those who had more than seven employees, with a business manager aged 18 years or older. The sample consisted of businesses in sectors that included computer and software operations, retail and trade, real estate services, culture, sport and entertainment, education, health and agriculture. To minimise bias, candidates for the survey were selected from both genders and all occupations. As entrepreneurs are unequally distributed across China (e.g. over 25% of entrepreneurs are located in Beijing and Shanghai compared to 11% in Guangzhou), a proportional cluster random sampling technique was employed to approach some 50,000 entrepreneurs from 31 provinces. Of these, 38,870 responded to the invitation to participate and complete the survey, representing a high response rate of 78%. Forty prizes ranging from RMB 400,000 (USD\$50,000) to RMB 100,000 (USD\$12,500) each were offered as business start-up funds to encourage entrepreneurs' participation in the study.

Measurement

A survey with two sections was used to collect the data. The first section comprised questions to collect information on demographic variables that included age, gender, education, profession, entrepreneurial experience and marital status.

These were included as confounding factors in the survey. The second section of the survey consisted of questions regarding capabilities as the dependent variable for the study, and it measured 40 items on scales that measured the following components: opportunity identification, interpersonal skills, conceptualisation, organising, strategies, commitment, learning and emotional control. For the current study, the measurements of emotional control (20) and learning (10,21) were adopted based on previous studies. Other components, including strategy, commitment, interpersonal skills, opportunity identification, conceptualisation and organising ability, were developed for the current study based on a pilot test for a small sample of entrepreneurs. The questions were divided into 'yes' or 'no' answers, and respondents were asked to choose one answer in each given statement. More 'yes' answers indicated higher capabilities.

For the current study, these items went through expert review for face validity and were incorporated into the survey. The reliability for the eight components ranges from 0.92 to 0.75. The reliability for the questionnaire with 40 items is 0.93. GDP was measured by GDP number per 10 million; area socioeconomic level was measured as high, medium-high, medium-low and low level. Income level was measured by the ranking of area incomes at city level.

Data analysis

For the eight components of capabilities, cluster analysis was used to identify types of entrepreneurs who are likely to cluster around capabilities that are related to each other. One-way analysis of variance was used to compare the difference among types of entrepreneurs in the different clusters of capabilities, and thirdly, multiple linear regression was used to analyse the relationship between capabilities and background characteristics including age, gender, and education.

Finally, the relationship between capabilities and area economic level was analysed by multilevel analysis. The multi-level models took into account the two-level hierarchical structure of the data for entrepreneurs (Level 1), sampled within cities (Level 2). Multi-level modelling was preferred for entrepreneurs sampled within cities because it was likely that there was some standardisation in urban environmental factors. Thus, the clustering effect of entrepreneurs within cities, which may generate improper estimates of standard errors, was adjusted.

RESULTS

Table 1 shows the patterns of capabilities that entrepreneurs have using cluster analysis.

Cluster 1 contains entrepreneurs who have strong learning orientation in the sense that they have a strong desire to learn through entrepreneurial experience in addition to their general capabilities including ability to control emotion, strategy, commitment, interpersonal abilities and entrepreneurial concept. Cluster 1 entrepreneurs are weak in business opportunity identification and organising abilities.

Cluster 2 is dominated by the general capability component. The entrepreneurs have capabilities including ability to control emotion, strategy, commitment, interpersonal abilities and entrepreneurial concept. They are generally weak in learning orientation, opportunity identification and organising capabilities.

Cluster 3 has a strongly positive opportunity identification component. Entrepreneurs in this cluster base their company on the opportunity of possible business development. This type of opportunity is addition to other general capabilities but it seems to be a very powerful asset for an entrepreneur. They are weak in experiential learning and organising capabilities.

Table 1. Results of cluster analysis

Capabilities	Cluster1	Cluster2	Cluster3
Emotion	**3.39**	**2.56**	**2.95**
Learning	**2.96**	1.50	1.89
Strategies	**2.74**	**2.58**	**2.86**
Commitment	**2.84**	**2.48**	**2.95**
Interpersonal	**2.49**	**2.41**	**2.62**
Opportunity	1.97	1.49	**3.50**
Organisation	1.84	1.26	1.84
Concept	**3.12**	**2.28**	**2.35**
Total	12309	13527	13034

Table 2. Differences between three types of entrepreneurs in learning-based capability, general capability and opportunity-based capability

	Cluster 1 (n=12309) M(SD) A	Cluster 2 (n=13527) M(SD) B	Cluster 3 (n=13034) M(SD) C	F	Post hoc
Learning based	2.77 (0.34)	2.15 (0.36)	2.49 (0.38)	10448***	**A>B***** **A>C***** **C>B*****
General capability	2.91 (0.47)	2.46 (0.48)	2.74 (0.48)	5090***	**A>B***** **A>C***** **C>B*****
Opportunity	2.75 (0.41)	2.30 (0.40)	2.87 (0.41)	9875***	**C>B***** **C>A*****

$*p < 0.05$, *** $p<0.001$; M is mean, SD is standard deviation. To ease the comparison among three types of cabilities, letters of A, B, C were used to represent each type of capability clusters.

Table 3. Multilevel analysis of effects of learning capability on GDP, areas' SES and income level

		GDP	Area SES	Income
Learning	Estimate (SE)	-127.66 (57.3)	0.001(0.002) 1.00	0.005 (0.021) 0.23
	t	**-2.22***		
Experience	Estimate (SE)	-147.66 (50.78)	0.003 (0.002)	0.027 (0.019)
	t	**-2.90***	1.5	1.42
Random	Estimate (SE)	6506662 (48409)	0.043 (0.01)	3.11 (0.02)
	t-value	**134.41*****	**43*** **	**135.22*** **
	Variance	**8.16%**	**4.9%**	**5.62%**
Fixed	Estimate (SE)	84485568 (6464540)	0.841 (0.064)	52.25 (3.96)
	t-value	**13.06*****	**13.14*** **	**13.21*****
	Variance	**92.84%**	**95.10%**	**94.38%**

Notes: Significance level: * $p<0.05$, ** $p<0.01$, *** $p<0.001$. Estimate refers to parameter estimate, SE refers to standard error, and t-value refers to the ratio of the Estimate to its standard error. A t-value greater than or equal to 2 indicates significant effect. ES refers to estimate, experi refers to entrepreneur experience. Learn refers to learning-based capability.
Figures in bold indicate statistically significant efffect.

Table 4. Multilevel analysis of effects of general capability on GDP, areas' SES and income level

		GDP	Area SES	Income
General	Estimate (SE) t	**-103.47 (49.24)** **-2.10** **	**0.004 (0.002)** **-2** **	0.021 (0.018) 1.17
Experience	Estimate (SE)	**146.94** **(50.79)**	0.003 (0.002)	0.027 (0.019)
	t	**2.95** **	1.5	1.42
Random	Estimate (SE)	22609280 (168253)	0.043 (0.01)	3.11 (0.02)
	t	**134.37*** **	**43*** **	**135.22*** **
	Variance	**13.18%**	**4.9%**	**5.62%**
Fixed	Estimate (SE) t Variance	148908944 (11543382) **12.90***** **86.82%**	0.841 (0.064) **13.14*** ** **95.10%**	52.25 (3.96) **13.21***** **94.38%**

Notes: Significance level: * $p<0.05$, ** $p<0.01$, *** $p<0.001$. Estimate refers to parameter estimate, SE refers to standard error, and t-value refers to the ratio of the Estimate to its standard error. A t-value greater than or equal to 2 indicates significant effect. General refers to general capability.
Figures in bold indicate statistically significant efffect.

The capabilities of new Chinese entrepreneurs in China   217

Table 2 demonstrates that there are progressive decreasing scores in both learning capability and general capability from the order of Cluster 1 to Cluster 3 and then to Cluster 2, and Cluster 2 had the lowest score among the three clusters. In opportunity capability, Cluster 3 had the highest score among the three clusters and Cluster 2 had the lowest score. All of these differences have reached statistical significance at $P < 0.01$ level.

Multiple linear regression was used to analyse the relationship between capabilities and background characteristics including age, gender, and education.

The variance explained by these demographic variables had nearly negligible level, suggesting entrepreneurial capabilities are not related to these background variables. These variables were therefore not added to the subsequent multilevel analyses in relation to the relationship between capabilities and area socio-economic, GDP level, and area income ranking.

Tables 3, 4 and 5 show the result of the multilevel regression effect of capability and entrepreneurial experience on the GDP level, areas' SES and income level. Low GDP level at a regional level is significantly related to a high level of learning, general and opportunity-based capabilities, suggesting areas with low GDP contribution in China mostly need entrepreneurs with a high level of capabilities for start-up ventures.

The probability of having a higher area socioeconomic largely depends on having a higher level of general capabilities, and opportunity-based capability, but not learning-based capability. Area income is not related to any of the capabilities of entrepreneurs.

Having entrepreneurial experience is significantly related to area GDP when it is combined with learning-based capability and opportunity-based capability, and is significantly related to areas' SES level when it is combined with general capability.

Table 5. Multilevel analysis of effects of general capability on GDP, areas' SES and income level

		GDP	Area SES	Income
Opportunity	Estimate	-136.06	0.004	0.024
	(SE)	(52.69)	(0.002)	(0.020)
	t	-2.59*	-2*	1.20
Experience	Estimate	-147.07	0.003	0.027
	(SE)	(50.78)	(0.002)	(0.019)
	t	-2.90*	1.50	1.42
Random	Estimate	22608148 (168244)	0.043	3.11
	(SE)		(0.01)	(0.02)
	t	134.41***	43***	135.22***
	Variance	13.2%	4.9%	5.62%
Fixed	Estimate	148904176 (11549238)	0.841	52.26
	(SE)	12.89***	(0.064) 13.14***	(3.96) 13.21***
	t-	86.80%	95.10%	94.38%
	Variance			

Notes: Significance level: * p<0.05, ** p<0.01, *** p<0.001. Estimate refers to parameter estimate, SE refers to standard error, and t-value refers to the ratio of the estimate to its standard error. A t-value greater than or equal to 2 indicates significant effect. Experience refers to entrepreneur experience, Opportunity refers to opportunity-based capability.
Figures in bold indicate statistically significant efffect.

The area effect (random effect) for learning-based, general and opportunity-based capability is significant and explains 8–13% of variances. This suggests that the capabilities and entrepreneurial experience of entrepreneurs varies from area to area.

Individual level capability and entrepreneurial experience explain 86 to 92% of variances, indicating the effects of capability at individual level explains the larger variance than the area level.

DISCUSSION

This study addresses the types of entrepreneurs and difference among three types of entrepreneurs. There is a learning component, general capability component, and finally an opportunity-based capability. The three components of capability encompass all aspects of capabilities required to start a business. Based on the three components, several types of entrepreneurs can be distinguished. First, there is a group of entrepreneurs that rely heavily on learning and knowledge gained in previous employment. This type of entrepreneurs mainly transfer experience to their new firm from experiential learning through problem identification and problem solving. The second group of entrepreneurs has general capability. Finally, the third group of entrepreneurs rely on opportunity identification and information search. These entrepreneurs normally have good knowledge of the product, the organising and the market. Having market knowledge and the identification of suitable market and clients is an important characteristic of a entrepreneur (22). A good understanding of the possible market can be highly beneficial for an entrepreneur's success in start-up business.

Differences between types of entrepreneurs demonstrated that the first type of entrepreneurs has a higher level of learning capability, general entrepreneur capabilities, and the third group has the highest level of opportunity identification and information search capability. The learning-based and opportunity-focused entrepreneurs run business types requiring resources and skills, and showed stronger capabilities than did entrepreneurs who run their businesses through risk taking and application of theory and knowledge. The significant differences between the three clusters of entrepreneurs in capabilities highlight the importance of the desire to learn and seize opportunities as success factors in start-up businesses and the need for education and training for a comprehensive range of capabilities to run businesses successfully.

This study also addresses the relationships between capability and area, and individual level characteristics. In many studies, entrepreneurs with high level of capabilities are needed to set up a new firm when the regional economy is in the developing stage. However, it is unclear what area characteristics are related to entrepreneurial capability. This study takes the area socioeconomic GDP level and percentage of urban population as outcome performance measure and it is shown that all the types of entrepreneurial capacities are significantly related to the area's socioeconomic status and GDP level. This finding is important and suggests that the areas with developing economy need all types of entrepreneurial capabilities to set up businesses, and the socioeconomic level of the area is significantly related to high level of capabilities of entrepreneurs. This has an impact on more opportunity identification and information search in relation to venture start-up. The effects of capabilities and entrepreneurial experiences of entrepreneurs have both area- and individual-level effects. This has significant implication that capability and entrepreneurial experience are important factors to determine areas' socioeconomic performance in relation to GDP level and socioeconomic level. This is also important to individual entrepreneur's start up business' success.

REFERENCES

[1] China Small and Medium Enterprise Association. Accessed 2011Apr 10. URL: http://www.ca-sme.org/consult_view.asp?id=5

[2] Liang FG. The Chinese innovative SMEs and entrepreneurship in global context. Beijing, China: Ministry Science Technology China, 2005.

[3] Gibb A, Li J. Organizing for enterprise in China: What can we learn from the Chinese micro, small, and medium enterprise development experience. Futures 2003;35(4):403-21.

[4] Liao D, Sohmen P. The development of modern entrepreneurship in China. Stanford J East Asian Aff 2001;1:27-33.

[5] Pun KF, Chin KS, Lau H. A review of the Chinese cultural influences on China's enterprise management. Int J Manage Rev 2000;2(4):38-325.

[6] Sebora T, Li W. The effects of economic tansition on Chinese entrepreneurship. J asia Entrepreneurship Sustainability 2008;2(3):1-20.

[7] BBC News Business. China overtakes Japan as world's second-biggest economy. In: Ee SF, ed. BBC News, 2011.

[8] Deakins D, Freel M. Entrepreneurial learning and the growth process in SMEs. Learning Organ Int J 1998;5(3):144-55.

[9] Ray JJ. A behavior inventory to measure achievement motivation. J Soc Psychol 1975;95:135-6.

[10] Politis D. The process of entrepreneurial learning: a conceptual framework. Entrepreneurship Theory Pract 2005;29(4):399-424.

[11] Shane S, Venkataraman S. The promise of entrepreneurship as a field of research. Acad Manage Rev 2000;25:217-26.

[12] Jiao H, Ogilvie D, Cui Y. An empirical study of mechanisms to enhance entrepreneurs' capabilities through entrepreneurial learning in an emerging market. J Chinese Entrepreneurship 2010;2(2):196-217.

[13] Chen G, Gully SM, Eden D. Validation of a new general self-efficacy scale. Organ Res Methods 2001;4:62-83.

[14] Karra N, Phillips N, Tracey P. Building the born global firm developing entrepreneurial capabilities for international new venture success. Long Range Plann 2008;41:440-58.

[15] McCelland DC. The Achieving Society. Princeton, NJ: Van-Nostrand, 1961.

[16] McCelland DC. Characteristics of successful entrepreneurs. Keys to the future of American business. Proceedings Third Creativity, Innovation and Entrepreneurship Symposium; US. Small Business Administration and the National Center for Research in Vocational Education, Framingham, MA,1986:1-14.

[17] Man TWY, Lau T, Chan KF. The competitiveness of small and medium enterprises A conceptualization with focus on entrepreneurial competencies. J Bus Venturing 2002;17:123-42.

[18] Timmons J. Growing up big-entrepreneurship and the creation of high potential ventures. In: Sexton DL, Smilor RM, eds. Art and science of entrepreneurship. Cambridge, MA: Ballinger; 1986:223-39.

[19] Willard GE, Kruger DA, Feeser HR. In order to grow, must the founder go: A comparison between founder and non-founder managed high growth manufacturing firms. J Bus Venturing 2002;7(3):181-94.

[20] Rosenbaum M. A schedule for assessing self-control behaviour. Preliminary finding. Behav Ther 1980;11:109-21.

[21] Rae D. Entrepreneurial learning: a practical model from the creative industries. Educ Training 2004;46(8/9):492-500.

[22] Geenhuizen MV. How can we reap the fruits of academic research in biotechnology? In search of critical success factors in policies for new-firm formation. Environ Plann 2003;21:139-55.

Submitted: August 05, 2011. *Revised:* October 02, 2011. *Accepted:* October 20, 2011.

In: Alternative Medicine Research Yearbook 2012 ISBN: 978-1-62808-080-3
Editors: Søren Ventegodt and Joav Merrick © 2013 Nova Science Publishers, Inc.

Chapter 23

MENTAL INFLUENCING OF THE GROWTH OF MUNG BEAN SEEDLINGS: A PILOT STUDY

Andrea Leitner[1,2], Caroline Weckerle[2], Wolfgang Matzer[1] and Christiane W Geelhaar[1]*

[1]Interuniversity College for Health and Development, Graz/Castle of Seggau, Austria and [2]University of Zürich, Institute of Systematic Botany, Zürich, Switzerland

ABSTRACT

The purpose of this study was to determine whether the growth of seedlings can be influenced mentally. Mung beans (Vigna radiata) underwent a standardized shamanistic growth and development ritual performed by a Swiss spiritual healer. Untreated seeds were used as control. An initial trial and a repeat trial were each performed on 84 test seeds and 84 control seeds (altogether 336 seeds). In both trials the group of seedlings that had undergone mental treatment achieved significantly greater length than the group of untreated seedlings. On the seventh day the test seedlings were 26% longer (i.e. 126% as long as) than the control seedlings (100%) ($p < 0.01$). Effect strength (d) was in the medium range at the level of seedlings and in the high range at the level of germination pots. Further research with refined experimental designs is needed to be able to judge the value of these results.

Keywords: Mung beans, spiritual healer, mental influencing, shamanism, fundamental research

INTRODUCTION

Jahn et al (1), Princeton researchers on consciousness-related physical anomalies, have performed meticulous experiments on mind/matter interactions over 25 years. The authors describe a relative insensitivity of such effects to physical correlates, including distance and

---

* Correspondence: Wolfgang Matzer, Interuniversity College for Health and Development, Graz / Castle of Seggau, Austria. E-mail: college@inter-uni.net.

time, discrepancies between male and female testers, and in many cases statistically consistent reproducibility. They conclude that "theoretical requisites include better understanding of the information dialogue between conscious and unconscious aspects of mind; more pragmatic formulations of the relations between tangible and intangible physical processes; and most importantly, cogent representation of the merging of mental and material dimensions into indistinguishability at their deepest levels" (2). It is believed that quantum physics may offer a theoretical basis for explaining such phenomena (3,4). Persons who are able to facilitate mind/matter interaction, i.e. "enable experiential realities that are responsive to intention, desire, or need" (5) are described as being open to alternative perspectives, including the use of transdisciplinary metaphors, self-sacrificially resonant, tolerant of uncertainty, and as inclined towards mental complementarity rather than dualistic rigor (5).

Our interest in this sphere of inquiry stems for one part from our previous involvement in conventional biological research and for another from reports on "subtle" plant communication (6-8). The possibility of plants showing differential growth behaviour in response to subtle influences is also indicated by research carried out by Baumgartner et al (9) and Geelhaar (10). According to the teachings of anthroposophy the interplay between the spiritual and the material world can be observed more clearly in plants than in any other class of biological systems (11).

Reports on "high dilution" effects (12-15) might also be counted among the body of scientific research on phenomena of mind/matter-interaction. A recent bibliometric analysis on "Repetitions of fundamental research models for homeopathically prepared dilutions beyond 10^{-23}", i.e. beyond Avogadro's limit of 0-molarity, by Endler et al (12) identified 24 laboratory bio-assays that have up to now been investigated by the international research community in 107 controlled, blinded studies (of which 30 involved initial and 77 repeat studies). Considering the 77 repeat studies alone, 69% reported effects similar to that of the initial study. Aside from publication bias and different degrees of handling know-how, experimental outcomes in ultra high dilution research are also interpreted as possibly representing an instance of mind-matter interaction (16).

Our interest in phenomena of mind-matter interaction was further inspired by research on "distance healing" and "hands-on healing". In a systematic review of clinical and laboratory studies on hands-on and distance healing, Crawford et al (17) identified 90 randomized, controlled trials of spiritual healing performed in clinical and laboratory settings and published in peer reviewed journals included in MEDLINE, PSYCH LIT, EMBASE, CISCOM or the Cochrane Library from their inceptions to 2001. 66% of these studies reported positive and 21% reported negative results. Among the major methodological problems mentioned by the authors were inadequacy of blinding, dropped data, lacking reliability of outcome measures, rare use of power estimations and lack of independent replication. When assessed in terms of internal validity, laboratory studies fared better than clinical studies. At the same time, the latter accounted for 62% of all positive and 33% of all negative outcomes (17). "Healing Touch" has been researched upon so extensively that it has had a systematic review dedicated to it (18).

The present pilot trials form part of a larger study on the senstivity of plants to mental influences. For the initial stages of this project a point was made of investigating situations as close to everyday life as possible ("talking to plants", "green thumb"). Further research based on more refined expermental designs is under preparation. The specific question under investigation here was whether mentally influenced mung bean seedlings differ in growth from control seedlings.

METHODS

Mung beans underwent a standardized shamanistic growth and development ritual performed by a Swiss spiritual healer. Untreated seeds were used as control. An initial trial was performed in February 2010 and a repeat trial in February 2011. In either trial 84 test und 84 control seeds (totalling 336) were observed in subgroups of 12 seeds per germination pot. Seedling length was measured daily over a period of 7 days.

The trials were performed on mung beans (Vigna radiata [Phaseolus radiatus], which had been produced without the use of herbicides or pesticides (Mauser company, Winterthur, Schweiz). Approximately 10% of all seeds were found to be damaged and removed prior to the start of the trial. Both trials (February 2010 und February 2011) were performed with seeds of the 2009 harvest.

The trials were carried out in Adliswil near Zürich. They were coordinated and supervised by C Weckele (Institute for Systematic Botany, Zürich) and PC Endler (Graz Inter-University College).

Brand-new clay pots (11 cm top diameter, procured from a garden dealer) were used as germination pots. Each was filled with 193 g of all-purpose soil (Mioplant, Swiss garden quality) and the soil was then saturated with Zürich tap water. Excess water was allowed to drain for 15 minutes.

The "mental influencing" of the mung bean seeds was performed by a Swiss spiritual healer (AL) following a standardized shamanistic ritual (8). During the ritual the healer held a disposable plastic bag (18x20cm) containing the test seeds for 4 minutes between the palms of her hands. In a frame of mind inviting the dissolution of boundaries between subject and object she offered the seeds information enabling them to manifest their fastest possible growth (8). The control seeds were kept in a disposable plastic bag at body temperature for 4 minutes without any attempt at influencing them mentally.

After having undergone treatment by the healer or mock treatment the seeds were placed on the moist soil at a distance of 1 cm from the edge of the pot (see figure 1, left). The pots were placed in clay saucers and sealed in airtight plastic storage bags (18 x 20cm) (Figure 1, right). Room temperature was 21 ± 1 °C in both trials. All pots were exposed to natural indirect light.

In either of the trials in February 2010 und 2011 84 test and 84 control seelings (totalling 336) were grown and monitored in subgroups of 12 seedlings per pot (28 pots in total). Seedling length was measured daily over a period of 7 days. For this purpose all plastic bags were opened at approx. 7 p.m. and, after the seedlings had been measured with a ruler, closed again in the same order in which they had been opened.

The arithmetic mean and S.D. of stalk length were calculated by pot (12 seedlings) and by treatment group (84 seedlings), and the results were compared by one way analysis of variance. Effect sizes (Cohen's d, standardized difference of means = absolute difference between means of verum and control group, divided by S.D.) were also calculated. An effect size > 0.2 is regarded as small, > 0.5 as medium and > 0.8 as large.

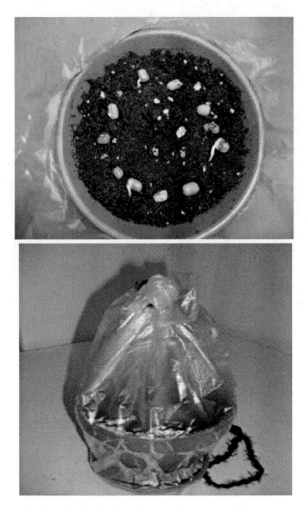

Figure 1. Pots used for raising mung bean seedlings. See text for further explanations.

Homogeneity of stalk length within the verum group and within the control group was investigated by one way analysis of variance with post-hoc pairwise comparison by means of the Tukey HSD test. Evaluation of data was done blindly, i.e. the statistician (HL) was not aware of the meaning of the codes used.

RESULTS

Both in the initial trial in 2010 and in the repeat trial in 2011 the group that had undergone treatment by the healer showed significantly greater seedling length than the group of untreated seedlings. In the 2010 trial (N = 84+84) the difference at day seven was 10.3±4.8 versus 8.0±4.4 (mean ± standard deviation) p<0.01), while in the 2011 trial (N = 84+84) it was 15.2±3.3 versus 12.4±4.8 (N = 84+84) (p<0.01). In the 2010 trial the test seedlings were 28.8% longer than (i.e. 128.8% as long as) the control seedlings (100%) at day seven, while in the 2011 trial they were 23.2% longer than (i.e. 123.2% as long as) the control seedlings

(100%) at this point in time. Effect sizes were d = 0.48 (2010) and 0.71 (2011), i.e. both in the medium range. Figure 2 shows the pooled data of the 2010 and the 2011 trial. Calculating standard deviations for day seven at pot level (i.e. from N = 7 + 7 values for either year, giving SD (2010) = 1.4 and SD (2011) = 2.0), yielded effect sizes in the *high* range, with d (2010) = 2.0 and d (2011) = 1.6.

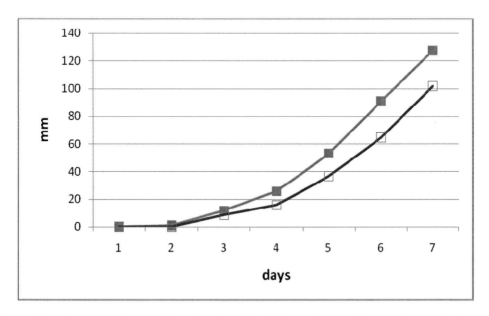

Figure 2. Length of mung bean seedlings in a "mentally influenced" group (blue) and in a control group (red): pooled data of 2010 and 2011. The differences are significant on days 4, 5, 6, 7 (p<0.01).

Thus, in both trials a significant difference in seedling length was observed between the "mentally influenced" and the control group. At the same time the values within each of the groups were statistically homogenous.

DISCUSSION

Both in the initial 2010 trial and in the repeat trial in 2011 mung bean seedlings that had undergone a standardized shamanistic growth and development ritual performed by a Swiss spiritual healer achieved a significantly greater length than did untreated seedlings. At day seven the treated seedlings of the 2010 trial (N = 84) were 28.8% longer than the control seedlings, while those of the 2011 trial (N = 84) were 23.2% longer than control (N = 84 in either trial).

The present pilot trials form part of a larger study on the sensitivity of plants to mental influences. For the initial stages of this project a point was made of investigating situations as close to everyday life as possible ("talking to plants", "green thumb"). It was also decided to start with experimental designs without blinding. Thus, the following work has been performed up to now:

226   *Andrea Leitner, Caroline Weckerl, Wolfgang Matzer et al.*

- An initial trial including a control group performed by one person
- A repeat trial including a control group performed by the same person

The following steps are now needed to be able to draw further conclusions and bring this research within the domain of modern scientific inquiry:

- Blinded repeat trials and
- Multiple trials performed independently by different persons

CONCLUSION

The treatment given to the mung bean seedlings may have influenced their growth behaviour. Further research using refined experimental designs is needed to be able to judge the value of these results and discuss them in the context of the relevant literature (1-18).

CONFLICTS OF INTEREST

None.

REFERENCES

[1] Jahn RG, Dunne BJ, The PEAR proposition. Explore 2007;3(3):205-26,340-1.
[2] Jahn RG, Dunne BJ. A modular model of mind/matter manifestations (M5). Explore 2007;3(3):311-24, 344-5.
[3] Jahn RG, Dunne BJ, Sensors, filters, and the source of reality. Explore 2007;3(3): 326-37, 345.
[4] Schrödinger E., Was ist wirklich? Die Gründe für das Aufgeben des Dualismus von Denken und Sein oder von Geist und Materie. In: Dürr H-P. Physik und Transzendenz. Die grossen Physiker unserer Zeit über ihre Begegnung mit dem Wunderbaren. München: Driediger Verlag, 2010:141. [German]
[5] Görnitz T., Quanten sind anders. Die verborgene Einheit der Welt. Heidelberg: Spektrum Verlag, 2008:93. [German]
[6] Narby J. Intelligenz in der Natur. Eine Spurensuche an den Grenzen des Wissens. Baden: AT Verlag, 2006. [German]
[7] Storl W. Mit Pflanzen verbunden. Meine Erlebnisse mit Heilkräutern und Zauberpflanzen. Stuttgart: Kosmos Verlag, Stuttgart 2005:13. [German]
[8] Scheppach J. Das geheime Bewusstsein der Pflanzen. Botschaften aus einer unbekannten Welt. München: Droemer Verlag, 2009:29.
[9] Baumgartner T, Baumgartner S. Eurythmische Bildkraftfelder. Ätherisch-energetische Wirkung auf Lebewesen. Auftakt. Fachzeitschrift Eurythmie Verband Schweiz und Berufsverband der Eurythmisten in Deutschland Sonderdruck April 2007:1-12. [German]
[10] Geelhaar CW. Biosensibilität. Zur Wirkung von Wasser das mit Infrarostrahlung beaufschlagt wurde auf die Keimung von Mungobohnen. Graz: Interuniversity College Health Development, 2004.
[11] Volkamer K., Feinstoffliche Erweiterung unseres Weltbildes. Berlin: Weissensee Verlag, 2009:149-50. [German]

Mental influencing of the growth of mung bean seedlings 227

[12] Endler PC, Thieves K, Reich C, Matthiessen P, Bonamin L, Scherr C and Baumgartner S. Repetitions of fundamental research models for homeopathically prepared dilutions beyond 10^{-23}. Homeopathy 2010;99:25-36.

[13] Marschollek B, Nelle M, Wolf M, Baumgartner S, Heusser P, Wolf U. Effects of exposure to physical factors on homeopathic preparations as determined by Ultraviolet light spectroscopy. ScientificWorldJournal 2010;10:49–61.

[14] Jäger T, Scherr C, Simon M, Heusser P, Baumgartner S. Effects of homeopathic arsenicum album, nosode and gibberellic acid preparations on the growth rate of arsenic-impaired duckweed (lemna gibba L). ScientificWorld Journal 2010;10:2112-29.

[15] Endler PC, Matzer W, Reich C, Reischl T, Hartmann AM, Thieves K, et al. Seasonal variation of the effect of extremely diluted agitated gibberellic acid (10e-30) on wheat stalk growth – a multi researcher study. ScientificWorldJournal, in press.

[16] Endler PC. Homeopathy research. An expedition report. An old healing system gains plausibility. Graz: Interuniversity College Health Development, 2006.

[17] Crawford CC, Sparber AG, Jonas WB. A systematic review of the quality of research on hands-on and distance healing: clinical and laboratory studies Altern Ther Health Med 2003;9(Suppl 3):A96-104.

[18] Anderson JG, Taylor AG. Effects of healing touch in clinical practice: A systematic review of randomized clinical trials. J Holist Nurs 2011;12. [Epub ahead of print]

Submitted: October 07, 2011. *Revised:* November 27, 2011. *Accepted:* December 08, 2011.

In: Alternative Medicine Research Yearbook 2012 ISBN: 978-1-62808-080-3
Editors: Søren Ventegodt and Joav Merrick © 2013 Nova Science Publishers, Inc.

Chapter 24

GENDER EFFECTS IN MASSAGE THERAPY

Thomas Edward Smith, PhD, Pamela Valentine, PhD and Bruce A Thyer, PhD*

Southeastern Research Institute, Tallahassee, Florida and College of Social Work,
Florida State University, Tallahassee, Florida, US

ABSTRACT

Massage therapy is a widely used alternative therapy whose outcomes and mediating processes are under-researched. Objective: To examine the possible role client and therapist gender played in the outcomes of massage therapy. Study group: Gender effects on massage therapy were examined in this study of 45 male and 125 female clients treated by 51 male and 119 female massage therapists. Methods: The clients provided ratings of pain and range of movement before and after a 60 minute session of massage therapy. Results: Clients had significant pain relief and improved range of motion after treatment and that these effects were not mediated by gender. Improvements were experienced equally among the male and female clients, and obtained equally from the male and female massage therapists. Conclusions: The beneficial effects of massage therapy appear to transcend gender factors, which argues for the robustness of their positive impact.

Keywords: Massage therapy, gender effects, client-therapist matching, wellness, pain

INTRODUCTION

Within our culture, society, and inherent nature, gender provides a predisposition upon which we act and how others react to us. Because gender roles affect us in everyday life, it is not surprising that the same effects are reproduced in therapy. Gender often moderates the treatment effects of therapeutic relationships and interventions (1). In the psychotherapeutic

---

* Correspondence: Thomas E. Smith, PhD, Southeastern Research Institute, 1328 Avondale Way, Tallahassee, FL 32317 United States. E-mail: thomassmith558@gmail.com.

process, clients learn ways to perceive and understand their behaviors, beliefs, and thoughts in the context of their environment. (2). Because of ubiquitous effects of gender in many aspects of life, this study examined whether the effects of massage therapy are mediated by the gender of the client, of the therapist, or by the interaction of the two factors. Studies point towards sex-dependent reactions to situations that are closely linked to therapeutic processes. Baumeister and Sommer (3) reported that women generally oriented themselves to close dyadic relationships, whereas men direct themselves to larger groups. In a meta-analysis, Feingold (4) found that men are more assertive and have higher self-esteem than women who are more extroverted, anxious, and nurturing. These gender roles are also often present during the therapeutic encounters. Because of their socialization, men are less likely to seek out therapy and, if they do so, are less likely to disclose personal details than are women (5). Heatherington and Allen (6) found that communication patterns involving male clients, regardless of the therapist's gender tended to be short, abrupt, and quick. The exchanges in answers and questions were rapid and labeled as though the male clients were trying to gain some edge or control during the session. This style of communication was explained by inferring that male clients were trying to protect or reduce a perceived threat to their self-esteem. Carli (7) also found that men are more assertive toward other men and women, and that women tend to be more assertive with other women, but tentative with men.

Kirshner, Genack, and Hauser (8) focused on gender interactions in therapy outcomes and demonstrated that selected areas of the therapeutic outcome were dependent on gender. Female clients improved more than male clients in attitudes toward careers, academic motivation, academic performance, and relationships with family members. More so than male therapists, their female counterparts reported having their clients improve more with major problems, self-esteem, and overall greater satisfaction with therapy. Jones and Zoppel (9) found that the clients of female therapists rated their therapy as more successful than clients of male therapists. This study found that these same clients of female therapists perceived that them as more effective, attentive, accepting, and as having formed a stronger therapeutic relationship than male therapists. Finally, Cottone, Drucker, and Javier (10) conducted a large study to assess gender effects in psychotherapeutic dyads involving 163 clients (43 men and 120 women) and 113 therapists (49 men and 64 women). With gender distribution equivalent to normal intake percentages and involving an ethnically diverse sample, possible gender effects were evaluated on the dimensions of treatment length, depression and anxiety. It was found that female clients were more likely to advance in treatment and complete treatment, relative to male clients. More male clients reported having lower anxiety scores with female therapists than the female-female dyads or the female client to male therapist dyad. Female therapist dyads showed lower anxiety scores overall, while male clients with the female therapists improved the most. While there were no male-male dyad interactions reported, this may have been caused by small sample size for this dyad.

MASSAGE THERAPY

Massage therapy is an ancient form of medical treatment that can be seen in such texts as the Ayur-Veda from India around 1800 B.C. that lists massage therapy as necessary for health along with proper diet and exercise (11). Today, massage therapy is being used to treat a number of maladies including dropsy, mental illness, torpor, spasm, stomach pain, heart disease, muscular and skeletal disorders and diabetes (12).

In an address to the Massage Research Agenda Workgroup, Kahn (13) expressed the need for massage therapy to define its own techniques, to study what comprises best practices for specific problems, and then compare optimal massage therapies to other fields and forms of treatment. She went on to exhort practitioners to study both the process and outcome of massage therapy. One key recommendation was to manualize massage therapy because of the inconsistency in treatment protocols. With manualized, replicable treatments, massage therapy will be more amenable to systematic outcomes research and process studies. Not surprisingly, she called for better collaboration between researchers and practitioners. More recently, Moyer (14) urged massage therapy practitioners and researchers to conduct research on this healing practice under clinically representative conditions, so that the external validity of findings may be enhanced.

Marjorie (15) published a case study of a client who suffered from atrial fibrillation. During an episode of acute arrhythmia, hypertension, and erratic pulse rate, Marjorie massaged the client along the spine, neck, and rib cage. The heart rate and blood pressure were lowered and most importantly the client relaxed and the arrhythmia subsided. While informative, this case study, it could be definitively shown that massage therapy per se produced these improvements. Beeken et al (16) conducted a study with 5 individuals who suffer from chronic obstructive lung disease (COLD), where the goal was to improve lung function. Beeken et al (16) employed neuromuscular release massage therapy (NRMT) in which pressure is applied to muscle groups to increase blood flow, to release fluid and accumulated wastes, and to support healing. The four male clients and one female client received 24 weeks of NRMT and were tested and evaluated on measures that assessed respiratory functioning. Beeken et al. concluded that this form of massage therapy was effective in increasing respiratory functioning. Once again, the results showed improvement but could not clearly isolate what was responsible for the positive results. Soft tissue manipulation, the psychosocial support, a mixture of the two interventions, the passage of time, simple physical contact, placebo influences are all plausible explanations for client improvements?

Hammer (17) studied the treatment of chronic hip and shoulder bursitis by using transverse friction massage. This case study involved a 55 year-old female with hip bursitis and a 40 year-old man with shoulder bursitis. In utilizing this massage treatment, both were relieved from joint inflammation of the bursae in their respective joints. Bursae are closed sacs composed of connective tissue inside the joint. Transverse friction massage also helped to remove scar tissue and essentially helped the healing process. Hammer (17) suggested that this mode of treatment be studied in controlled clinical setting along with a larger randomized sample. Although the need for well controlled trials is persuasive, it may not be clear what about the intervention was responsible for change. An example of a methodologically rigorous study involved massage therapy focused on the area of tension headaches. Puustjavir, Airaksinen and Potinen (18) studied 21 female patients with chronic tension headaches. Upper body massages which manipulated deep tissue were used during 10 sessions over two and a half weeks. Evaluation of the massage therapy included measures on range of motion, an EMG muscular test, and self reports of pain intensity. Puustjavir et al (18) found that this massage therapy increased range of motion, decreased muscular tightness and shortening, lessened perceived pain, and improved the subjects' mental state. Still not certain is the therapeutic mechanism underlying the effectiveness of the massage therapy.

Other studies have also reported positive results of case studies of massage therapy applied to different presenting problems, and in general the evidentiary foundations of the positive effects of massage therapy are modest but growing (19). One important step in defining a treatment model is to determine what moderates its effects. Massage therapists have many characteristics found in psychotherapists such as the use of highly honed skills to assist clients resolve pain, ability to create trusting and professional relationship, and a commitment to provide the best practices of their profession. Although massage therapists focus on kneading muscles, there is also a distinct emotional component to doing so. One well documented moderator of psychotherapy is gender. Given the similarities between psychotherapy and massage therapy, an intuitively reasonable speculation is that may be distinct gender effects in both modalities. In this study, we examined the potential effects of client/therapist gender on massage therapy outcomes. In a factorial design, we studied four pairings: male therapist/female client, male therapist/male client, female therapist/female client, and female therapist/male client.

METHOD

Clients were recruited from three clinics located in massage therapy training institutes in the state of Florida. After giving informed consent to receive massage therapy and to participate in the study, clients completed a demographic data sheet, health history questionnaire, and pain and wellness checklists. The intake procedure was designed to establish rapport, trust, and comfort. The health history questionnaire was administered to rule out contraindications and to facilitate the design of the massage treatment.

A licensed massage therapy instructor screened clients for the study and excluded those who had medical and health concerns.

Only experienced massage therapy trainees were recruited to participate in the study. After being identified by clinic administrators, trainees were asked whether they wished to participate in the study. All trainees were supervised by a licensed massage therapy instructor.

After receiving the massage, clients completed post-treatment pain and range of motion. The supervisor reviewed the massage procedures checklist to ensure that comparable massages had been given. The conduct of this study adhered to the principles of the Declaration of Helsinki.

Two methods of administration of the massage were given using similar techniques, consisting of a 60 minute table massage protocol and a 15 minute chair massage. The table massage protocol included manipulation on the face and neck, the hands and arms, anterior legs and feet, the abdomen (as requested), the posterior legs and feet, and the back. The chair massage protocol focuses on the upper back and shoulders, the neck, scalp, arms and hands, and the upper and lower back.

The techniques that are included in the sequence include effeurage, petrissage, friction, myofascial spreading, and trigger-point therapy. Although each treatment was structured, the goal was to replicate what actually occurs in the clinical practice of massage therapy. For the

Gender effects in massage therapy

purpose of generalizability, the therapists were instructed to design the treatment as if it were "real world" situation.

Client needs, desires, indications, and contraindications were used by each therapist in the design of the treatment session. The focus of the clinic treatments was "relaxation," and the clients were informed that the type of massage was a relaxation massage.

The post-treatment feedback session had two phases. First, clients provided their massage therapist with feedback about their administrative and technical proficiency. Second, participants completed post-treatment measures to describe treatment effects.

RESULTS

A pretest/posttest design was used to measure the possible impact of massage therapy on clients. Clients' experience of 1) pain 2) well-being, and 3) head and neck range of motion before and after massage was analyzed using paired t-tests.

After a Chi-square test was used to assess the effects of gender distribution of therapists across the gender of clients, analyses of covariance (ANCOVAs) were employed to determine the possible effects of client and therapist gender on the change in the pretest-posttest scores made by the clients.

The final sample consisted of 51 female and 119 male therapists and 125 female and 51 male clients. Chi-square analyses showed that the distribution of gender in both clients and therapists were not significantly different ($X2 = 32.45$; $p < .57$). See table 1 for the distribution of gender in therapists and clients.

The first analysis consisted of paired t-tests that measured gains on client-rated perceived pain, perceived wellbeing, and perceived range of motion of the head and neck, collapsed across gender, from pretest to posttest.

The results demonstrated that clients experience relief from their presenting concerns following massage therapy. Clients (collapsed across gender) reported a significantly pain as a result of massage therapy ($t = 15.75$; $p < .01$, df = 190). On perceived well-being ($t = 14.42$; $p < .01$, df = 194), clients showed a significant improvement. On the third outcome measure, perceived range of motion, clients also showed significant improvement ($t = 16.41$; $p < .01$, df = 194).

Separate paired t-tests were conducted for each gender across the three outcome variables. They also revealed significant differences from before to after treatment. Table 2 provides a breakdown of analyses by gender. Although gains from pretest to posttest were significant for both genders across the three outcome variables, an ANOVA showed that there was no interaction effect of gender (e.g., male therapist/female client; female therapist/female client).

Table 1. Therapist by client counts

		Therapist Gender		Total
		Male	Female	
Client	Male	15	30	45
Gender	Female	36	89	125
Total		51	119	170

Table 2. Effects of Massage Therapy by Client Gender

		Female (n=125)			Male (n=51)		
		Means	Standard Deviations	t-test (df)	Means	Standard Deviations	t-test (df)
Perceived Pain	Pretest	5.36	2.049	13.39	5.51	2.361	7.14
	Posttest	7.76	1.789	(124)**	7.66	2.219	(50)**
Perceived Well-Being	Pretest	6.07	2.135	11.82	6.76	2.016	7.17
	Posttest	8.01	1.793	(126)**	8.45	1.747	(51)**
Perceived Range of Motion	Pretest	5.50	1.816	14.34	5.80	2.324	7.65
	Posttest	7.61	1.619	(126)**	7.96	1.788	(51)**

*p<.05.
**p<.01.

DISCUSSION

The results showed that clients experienced a significant relief from pain and significantly increased their range of movement. These results were not unexpected. When done properly, immediate relief of muscular pain is a common benefit from massage therapy. More important than the outcomes on pain relief and enhanced range of motion was the lack of gender effects. This finding was unexpected. All four permutations of the therapist-client failed to show statistical significance. The practical implication is that gender makes no difference in massage therapy and that its beneficial effects transcend client or therapist gender. Because gender is a critical variable in psychotherapy and nearly every other aspect of life, this finding was not anticipate.

One possible reason for the lack of gender differences is that relaxation engendered positive attitudes regardless of the therapist, with gender influences being overshadowed by symptomatic relief, at least in the short run. Another possibility is that once a massage session has begun, clients typically close their eyes and become deeply relaxed, and in doing so become relatively oblivious to the gender of their therapist, indeed often oblivious to their surroundings as whole. Massage therapists themselves are taught to treat all clients similarly and in a respectful and non-sexual manner. This professional pattern of studied neutrality, similar to that taught within the practice of psychoanalysis, may also attenuate the influence of the therapists gender with the client.

Our concluding that the effects of massage therapy are not mediated by client/therapist gender must be tempered by the recognition that this was not a truly experimental study, with clients and therapists randomly assigned to the various combinations of gender. We used a quasi-experimental method, with client/therapist matching being dictated more by the convenience of the clinical setting. A true experiment would be needed to see if our quasi-experimental results regarding an apparent lack of gender effects in massage therapy practice can be replicated and corroborated.

We did not examine the related factors of race or of the physical attractiveness of clients and therapists. These would be other variables useful to examine in future studies of the processes and outcomes of massage therapy. To our knowledge this is the first large scale study of the possible role of gender in mediating the effects of massage therapy. Our failure to find any unilateral or factorial effects of client/therapist gender may be seen as a positive feature of massage therapy, indicating the robustness of its therapeutic benefits which appear to transcend nonspecific influences in treatment. This study could be consisted analogous to a Phase One clinical trial, an open-label, uncontrolled evaluation of the possible benefits of a treatment (20), involving subgroup analyses. Experimental replications involving the random assignment of clients and therapists to gender dyads would be a logical next step in investigating the possible mediating role of gender influencing the outcomes of therapeutic massage.

REFERENCES

[1]   Kaplan AG. Toward an analysis of sex-role related issues in the therapeutic relationship. Psychiatry 1979;43:112-20.

[2]   Orlinsky DE, Howard KI. The psychological interior of psychotherapy: Explorations with the therapy session report. In: Greenberg LS, Pinsolf WM, eds. The psychotherapeutic process: A research handbook. New York: Guilford. 1986:477-502.

[3]   Baumeister RF, Sommer KL. What do men want? Gender differences and two spheres of belongingness: Comments on Cross and Madison. Psychol Bull 1997;122:38-44.

[4]   Feingold A. Gender differences in personality: A meta-analysis. Psychol Bull 1994;116:429-56.

[5]   Carlson N. Woman therapist: Male client. In: Scher M, Stevens M, Good G, Eichenfield GA, eds. Handbook of counseling and psychotherapy with men. Newbury Park, CA: Sage, 1987:39-50.

[6]   Heatherington L, Allen GJ. Sex and relational communication patterns in counseling. J Couns Psychol 1984;31:287-94.

[7]   Carli LL. Gender, language and influence. J Pers Soc Psychol 1990;38:941-51.

[8]   Kirshner LA, Genack A, Hauser ST. Effects of gender on short-term psychotherapy. Psychother 1978;15:158-67.

[9]   Jones EE, Zoppel CL. Impact of client and therapist gender on psychotherapy process and outcome. J Consult Clin Psychol 1982;50:259-72.

[10]   Cottone JG, Drucker P, Javier RA. Gender differences in psychotherapy dyads: Changes in psychological symptoms and responsiveness to treatment during 3 months of therapy. Psychother 2002;39:297-308.

[11]   Field T. Massage therapy fore infants and children. Dev Behav Pediatr 1995;16:105-11.

[12]   Edwards BG, Palmer J. Effects of massage therapy on African Americans with Type 2 diabetes mellitus: A pilot study. Complement Health Pract Rev 2010;15:149-55.

[13]   Kahn JR. A new era for massage research. J Am Massage Ther Assoc 2001;40:104-11.

[14]   Moyer CA. Practitioner-generated massage therapy research. Int J Ther Massage Bodywork, 2011;4:3.

[15]   Marjorie C. The use of massage therapy in restoring cardiac rhythm. Nurs Times 1994;90(38):36-7.

[16]   Beeken JE, Parks D, Cory J, Montopoli G. The effectiveness of neuromuscular release massage therapy in five individuals with chronic obstructive lung disease. Clin Nurs Res 1998;7:309-25.

[17]   Hammer WI. The use of transverse friction massage in the management of chronic bursitis of the hip or shoulder. J Manipul Physiol Ther 1993;16:107-11.

[18]   Puustjarvi K, Airaksinen O, Pontinen PJ. The effects of massage in patients with chronic tension headache. Acupunct Electro-Ther Res 1990;15:159-62.

[19]   Ernst E, Pittler MH, Wider B, Boddy K. Massage therapy: Is the evidence-based getting stronger? Complement Health Pract Rev 2007;12:179-83.

[20]   Meinert CL, Tonascia S. Clinical trials: Design, conduct, and analysis. New York: Oxford University Press, 1986.

Submitted: October 26, 2011. *Revised:* November 26, 2011. *Accepted:* December 09, 2011.

In: Alternative Medicine Research Yearbook 2012   ISBN: 978-1-62808-080-3
Editors: Søren Ventegodt and Joav Merrick   © 2013 Nova Science Publishers, Inc.

Chapter 25

A FOLLOW-UP STUDY ON THE MORPHOLOGY OF ISOLATED RAT CORTICAL NEURONS AND INFORMATION TRANSFERRED VIA A "BIOPHOTON DEVICE"

Dietrich Vastenburg[1,2] and Sjoerd Pet[1,2]*

[1]Interuniversity College for Health and Development, Graz, Castle of Seggau, Austria and [2]Institute of Biophoton Research, Drammen, Norway

ABSTRACT

The purpose of this study was to determine whether information of the homeopathic remedy "Cerebrum Compositum", transferred via a "biophoton therapy device", exerts an effect on isolated rat cortical neurons when tested versus untreated control. 60 x 10^3 neurons were used per group according to treatment in each of 4 experiments. Viability after 10 days was defined by a) synaptic size, b) the number of synaptic contacts and c) by longevity. S*ynaptic size* in the test group was 63% greater (i.e. equal to 163% of) as compared to control W0 (100%) (p<0.01). *The number of synaptic contacts* in the test group was 49% greater (i.e. equal to 149% of) than W0 (p<0.01). These trends could also be observed in the four sub experiments separately. There was no difference between the groups respecting longevity. Data are in line with previous findings on information transfer via the biophoton therapy device.

Keywords: Rat, cortical, neurons, biophotons, biophoton therapy

INTRODUCTION

Previous studies aimed to transfer information from molecules via technical devices, using electronic circuits (1), amplifiers connected to single individual wires (2,3) or a "biophoton

---

* Correspondence: Dietrich Vastenburg, Interuniversity College for Health and Development, Graz, Castle of Seggau, Austria. E-mail: college@inter-uni.net.

238   *Dietrich Vastenburg and Sjoerd Pet*

therapy device". A pilote study (4) aimed to transfer information from "Cerebrum Compositum", a homeopathic remedy directed towards improving cerebral function (5), via a "biophoton therapy device", on isolated rat cortical neuron viability.

Isolated rat cortical neurons are a well-standardised bioassay widely used to test external influences on neuronal systems. This is due to the fact that neurons in culture retain their ability to form (extensive) physiological neuronal networks that are sensitive to subtle changes in their environment and show defined and well-regulated inter-neuron communication. These characteristics make *in vitro*-cultured isolated neurons a significant neuroscience research tool (6,7)

Thus, in a pilot study (4), isolated rat cortical neurons were either not treated (W0 = control) or treatment was attempted with information from a standard "harmonizing" program of a "biophoton therapy device" (8) (BTH = a program normally used for treatment of babies 0-2a, with an all frequencies pass and a duration of 1 min), or with information from the homeopathic remedy "Cerebrum Compositum", transferred with the BTH-program (BTH-CC).

Neurons were seeded with a density of 20 x 10^3 neurons per dish, and three dishes (i.e. 60 x 10^3 neurons) were used per group according to treatment in each of four experiments. Viability after 10 days was defined by a) synaptic size, i.e. the degree of synaptic clustering due to neural growth developed, b) the number of synaptic contacts and c) by longevity.

Synaptic size in the BTH-CC-group was 58% greater (i.e. equal to 158% of) and in the BTH-group it was 19% greater (i.e. equal to 119% of) as compared to the control group W0 (100%). SEM was about $\pm$ 20%. These differences are statistically significant (p<0.01). Differences in the number of synaptic contacts were significant only between BTH-CC (123%) and W0 (100%) (p<0.01), there were no significant differences concerning longevity.

These pilot data on isolated rat cortical neuron synapse development under the influence of information transferred via a "biophoton therapy device" (8) seemed to be in line with previous findings (9-11), i.e. as confirmation that such information *can influence* biological systems. However, a follow-up study was performed in order to verify or falsify the data on treatment of neurons. In the following, with the kind permission of the journal *"explore!"*, we have used text elements from our first publication (4) as the frame to present data from the follow-up study.

As is generally known, a photon is a particle of light, but all the same is equivalent to an electromagnetic oscillation. According to Popp (12), "biophotons" are weak emissions of light radiated from the cells of all living systems.

All organisms constantly emit photons as part of their vital activities. Plants, animals and humans have an intensity of emission from some hundreds up to one thousand photons/second/cm², and an almost continuous spectrum within the optical range of at least 200 - 800 nm (13). The light of the photon is too faint to be seen by the naked eye, its intensity comparable to that of a candle's light seen at a distance of 20 km.

Biophoton physics says that coherent photon patterns within structures of the organism are primary steering elements of all biochemical and biological interaction. Biophotons are said to create a dynamic, coherent web of light.

This could be responsible for the chemical reactions within the cells, the cellular communication throughout the organism, and the overall regulation of the biological system, including embryonic development. Balanced structures are said to emit phase coherent, unbalanced structures phase chaotic light (14,15).

A follow-up study on the morphology of isolated rat cortical neurons ... 239

According to Popp (12), a chemical cell reaction can only happen when the molecules are excited by photons. It has been reported that photon emissions vary according to differences in growth processes (13), and are elevated by environmental stresses (15) and disease response induced by pathogen attack (16).

Our intention was to approach the issue from a phenomenological point of view, i.e. to set up an experiment that would or would not yield significant results, regardless of whether or not we understood the principles underlying the "biophoton therapy device". However, some information on the manufacturer's assumptions may be of interest.

Biophoton physics says that photon patterns within structures of the organism are primary steering elements of all biochemical and biological interaction. Balanced structures are said to emit phase coherent, unbalanced structures phase chaotic light (17,18). According to J. Boswinkel, such photon patterns may be scanned by devices containing one-way glass fiber cables, filters, amplifiers and elements for phase correction, and may be fed (or fed back) to the biological system (8).

The objective of this study was to perform follow-up experiments on the isolated rat cortical neuron bioassay with and without the information of the homeopathic remedy "Cerebrum Compositum" transferred via the "biophoton therapy device", tested versus control. Alternations to the original protocol should help to optimize information transfer.

METHODS

The study was performed in the Neuroscience Laboratory of the University of Zürich, Switzerland. Experiments were performed in a sterile tissue culture hood area under standard culture conditions (temperature 37 °C $\pm$ 0.1°; 7.5 % CO_2; relative humidity 100%). All tissue culture ware used was of disposable nature.

Laboratory researchers were Dietrich Vastenburg and a supervision assistant from the Laboratory.

Experiments were performed on cortical neurons, isolated from rats according to the standard dissection protocol as described by Almeida and Medina. Briefly, brains from rat pups at postnatal day 0 were dissected, the meninges carefully removed and the cortices separated from white matter, hippocampus and cerebellum. The cortices were minced, digested and triturated in respective buffered media to obtain a single cell suspension. Neurons were seeded on glass cover slips (about 20 x 10^3 neurons / cover slip) in Poly-L-Lysine coated 60 mm cell culture dishes at a density of 60 x 10^3 cells / Petri dish. Poly-L-lysine was purchased from Invitrogen, Basel, Switzerland. 6 ml neuronal culture medium (Neurobasal™ cat. no. 21103, GIBCO, Switzerland supplemented with B27) was used per Petri dish which reflects and mimics the physiological cerebral environment to create optimal growth conditions and long-term survival of rat embryonic neurons. Neurons were kept in culture for the duration of the entire study.

In study phase 1 (see Introduction), the influence of a standard "harmonizing" program of the biophoton therapy device (J. Boswinkel) (a program normally used for treatment of babies 0-2a, with an all frequencies pass and a duration of 1 min) was tested with or without aiming to transfer information from the remedy Cerebrum Compositum.

240 *Dietrich Vastenburg and Sjoerd Pet*

In study phase 2, that standard program including the use of Cerebrum Compositum was modified by

- longer or shorter duration (> or < 1 min)
- using frequency passes (< 1000 Hz, < 500 Hz, < 200 Hz).

In study phase 3, according to the results of phase 2, the standard biophoton therapy programme was applied for 56 sec and a frequency pass < 200 Hz was used, aiming to transfer information from Cerebrum Compositum ("BT-CC"). Before exposure ("information transfer") the glass fibre cables of the device were ethanol-sterilised and subsequently thoroughly dried after which they were immersed into the neuronal culture medium. The procedure of immersing the glass fibre cables into the neuronal culture medium was similar for the control group, i.e. the untreated neurons ("W0").

Data base: In study 2, neurons were seeded with a density of 20×10^3 neurons per dish, and 1 dish (i.e. 20×10^3 neurons) were used per group according to treatment. In study 3, neurons were seeded with a density of 20×10^3 neurons per dish, and 3 dishes (i.e. 60×10^3 neurons) were used per group W0 and BT-CC in each of 4 experiments.

Viability after 10 days was defined by a) synaptic size, i.e. the degree of synaptic clustering due to neural growth developed, b) the number of synaptic contacts and c) by longevity, assessed by measuring the ratio of adhered compared to floating (i.e. dead) neurons.

Visual analysis of neuronal morphology and viability after fixation of neurons with 4% paraformaldehyde in phosphate buffered saline was performed using a bright field microscope with attached camera (Leica DMI RE2, Heerbrugg, Switzerland) at the terminal endpoint of the experiments, i.e., day 10 of culturing. The microscopy pictures represent the average morphological status of the neurons.

Digital assessment of change in neuronal morphology using ImageJ Imaging Software allowed for unbiased sample measurements.

The obtained microscopy images were analysed using the imaging software ImageJ (version 1.40g, National Institutes of Health, USA). Means, SD and, SEM were given for each group (sample size = number of dishes multiplied by the number of repetitions SEM = standard error of the mean = standard deviation SD divided by sample size). Groups were compared using Student's t-test (analysis using SD showed a comparable degree of significance as compared to using SEM). Synaptic size was calculated using the particle size tool of the ImageJ software (in the region of interest (ROI) the specific shape distribution of synapses was recognised and automatically counted by the software).

RESULTS

In study 2, neuron development under the standard programme, when applied for 56 sec with a frequency pass < 200 Hz, aiming to transfer information from Cerebrum Compositum (BT-CC) showed the biggest differences compared to control W0. In study 3, synaptic size in the BT-CC-group was 63% greater (i.e. equal to 163% of) as compared to the control group W0

(100%). SEM was about ± 9%. These differences are statistically significant (p<0.01). This trend could also be observed for the 4 experiments separately (figure 1).

The number of synaptic contacts in the BT-CC-group was 49% greater (i.e. equal to 149% of) than W0 (100%) (p<0.01). SEM was about ± 6%. This trend could also be observed for the 4 experiments separately (figure 1).

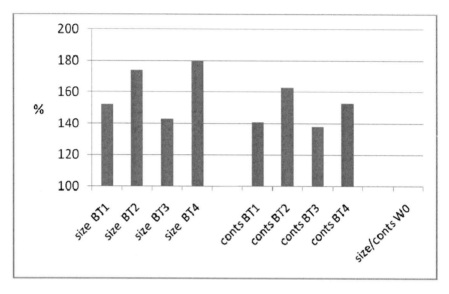

Figure 1. Relative differences in synaptic size ("size") and number of synaptic contacts ("conts") between BT-CC groups ("BT") in experiments 1-4 and W0 groups (zeroed) in per cent (ordinate). See text for further explanations.

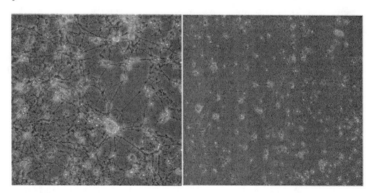

Figure 2. An example of the morphologic picture of neurons treated with BT-CC (left) and W0 (right) after 10 days. See text for explanation.

Longevity, assessed by measuring the ratio of adhered compared to floating (i.e. dead) neurons in the BT-CC-group was equal to 99% of W0 (100%) (p>0.05). SEM was about ± 4%.

Figure 2, *left and middle,* shows the morphologic picture of neurons treated with BT-CC, compared to W0 (*right*). Cultures showed an increase in neuronal branching with sustained dendrite length and an increase in synaptic contacts. The area of each photo covers about 2000 neurons.

242   *Dietrich Vastenburg and Sjoerd Pet*

In other words, there was a significant increase in synaptic size and in the number of synaptic contacts in the groups treated with BT-CC compared to control. There was no difference between the groups respecting longevity.

DISCUSSION

In this follow-up study, isolated rat cortical neurons were observed under the influence of information from the homeopathic remedy "Cerebrum Compositum", transferred via a "biophoton therapy device" ("BT-CC"). Neurons were grown in standard culture medium. Untreated neurons ("W0") were used as control.

Synaptic size in the test group was 63% greater (i.e. equal to 163% of) as compared to control W0 (100%) ($p<0.01$). The number of synaptic contacts in the test group was 49% greater (i.e. equal to 149% of) than W0 ($p<0.01$). These trends could also be observed in the 4 sub experiments separately. There was no difference between the groups respecting longevity.

Data are in line with the findings of a pilot study (4), where synaptic size in the BT-CC-group was 58% greater (i.e. equal to 158% of) as compared to control W0 ($p<0.01$). The number of synaptic contacts in the test group was 23% greater (i.e. equal to 123% of) than W0 ($p<0.01$), there was no significant difference respecting longevity. Data have recently been confirmed in another follow-up study (unpublished material) of similar size, where the number of synaptic contacts in the test group was 33% greater (i.e. equal to 133% of) than W0 ($p<0.01$).

Interestingly, when only the "standardized harmonizing programme" was applied ("BTH") without aiming to transfer information of the homeopathic remedy, the number of synaptic contacts was 39% greater as compared to control W0 in the study presented here, 19% greater in the pilot study (4) and 11% greater in the follow-up study (unpublished material).

These data on isolated rat cortical neuron synapse development under the influence of information transferred via a "biophoton therapy device" are in line with further previous findings. A botanical study aimed at transferring information from a "harmonizing" program of a "biophoton device" to wheat seedlings. Suitable control was used. 1440 grains were used per group according to treatment. Germination rate in the group treated with the "harmonizing" program was 17% *stronger* than (i.e. equal to 117% of) control germination rate (100%). This difference is statistically significant ($p<0.01$) (9).

A study on milk ageing (souring) aimed at transferring information from the harmonizing program to milk. Suitable control was used. 50 samples of fresh cow milk were used per group. Souring of milk in the group treated with the "harmonizing" program was 16,7% *less strong* than (i.e. equal to 83% of) souring of control (100%). This difference is statistically significant ($p<0.01$) (10).

A study on aggregation of erythrocytes (red blood cells) aimed at transferring information from the harmonizing program to volunteers, from whom blood samples were taken before and after treatment. Suitable control was used. 20 or 10 volunteers were included in a test- and in a control group. Aggregation of erythrocytes in the group treated with the

A follow-up study on the morphology of isolated rat cortical neurons ... 243

"harmonizing" program was 98% (!) *less* marked than (i.e. 2% of) aggregation of control (100%). This difference is statistically significant (p<0.01) (11).

The authors conclude that information produced by or transferred via the biophoton device *can influence* biological systems. It goes without saying that beneficial effects of information of the homeopathic remedy Cerebrum Compositum (5) or of a harmonizing program of biophoton treatment, or of the combination of both, on neuron synapses may have interesting practical medical aspects.

Further repetitive studies will have to be performed before these findings can be generally accepted, and further research will have to be done on the technical, physiologic and psychological backgrounds of such effects, including biophoton biology, before findings can be fully explained.

We are inclined to believe that the theoretical explanation of these phenomena will in future be inspired by de Broglie's concept of the wave nature of particles and the particle nature of waves (19) and by Montagniers biophysical concepts (20).

This paper is part of a doctoral thesis.

REFERENCES

[1]   Aissa J, Litime MH, Attias E, Benveniste J. Molecular signalling at high dilution or by means of electronic circuitry. J Immunol 1993;150:146A.

[2]   Citro M, Endler PC, Pongratz W, Vinattieri C, Smith CW, Schulte J. Hormone effects by electronic transmission. FASEB J 1995;9/3:392A.

[3]   Pongratz W, Endler PC, Lauppert E, Senekowitsch F, Citro M. Saatgut-Entwicklung und Information von Silbernitrat. In: Endler PC, Schulte J, eds. Homöopathie-Bioresonanztherapie. Physiologische und physikalische Voraussetzungen – Grundlagenforschung. Vienna: Maudrich Verlag, 1996. [German]

[4]   Vastenburg D, Pet S. Morphology of isolated rat cortical neurons and information transferred via a "biophoton device" – a pilot study. Explore 2011, in press.

[5]   Biologische Heilmittel Heel. Biotherapeutic Index, Ordinatio Antihomotoxica et Materia Medica. Baden-Baden 1986. [German]

[6]   Ramakers GJA, De Wit C, Wolters PS, Corner MA. A developmental decrease in NMDA-mediated spontaneous firing in cultured rat cerebral cortex. Int J Dev Neurosci 1993;11(1):25-32.

[7]   Tapia-Arancibia L, Rage F, Récasens M, Pin J-P. NMDA receptor activation stimulates phospholipase A2 and somatostatin release from rat cortical neurons in primary cultures. Eur J Pharmacol 1992;225(3):253-56.

[8]   Boswinkel J. Energetic anatomy, physiology and pathology. Drammen: Edition Health Angel Academy, 2008.

[9]   Boswinkel W, Muller J, Baars W, Lely B, Mikx B, Wassenberg GEM, et al. Wheat germination and information from a plant hormone and a herbicide, transferred via a „biophoton device" – a pilot study. Explore 2011;20(4):17-26.

[10] Mak P, Vastenburg D, Reich C. Milk aging and information from a „biophoton device" – a pilot study. Explore 2011;20(4):4-13.

[11] Pet S, Pet M, Vastenburg D. Human blood under the dark field microscope and information from a "biophotone device" – a pilot study. Expore! 2011, in press.

[12] Popp FA, Li KH, Gu Q. Recent advances in biophoton research and its applications, Singapore: World Scientific Publishing, 1992.

[13] Bischof M. Das Licht in unseren Zellen. Berlin: Verlag Zweitausendeins, 1995. [German]

[14] Kai T, Mitani M, Fujikawa M. Morphogenesis and bioluminescence in germination of red bean. Physica A (Amsterdam) 1994;210:391-402.

[15] Ohya T, Kurashige H, Okabe H, Kai S. Early detection of salt stress damage by biophotons in red been seedling, Jpn J Appl Phys 2000;39:3696-3700.

[16] Makino T, Kato K, Honzawa H, Tachiiri Y, Hiramatsu M. Ultraweak luminescence generated by sweet potato and Fusarium oxysporum interactions associated with a defence response. Photochem Photobiol 1996;64:953-6.

[17] Popp F.A. About the coherence of biophotons. Macroscopic Quantum Coherence Proceedings, Boston University and MIT. Boston: World Scientific Publishing, 1999.

[18] Zhang C.L., Popp F.A. Log-normal distribution of physiological parameters and the coherence of biological systems. Med Hypothesis 1994;43:11-6.

[19] Schulte J. Bio-Information between quantum and continuum physics. The mesoscopic picture. In: Schulte J, Endler PC. Fundamental research in ultra high dilution and homeopathy. Dordrecht: Kluwer Academic, 1998.

[20] Enserink M. Newsmaker interview: Luc Montagnier. Science 2010;330,1732.

Submitted: October 15, 2011. *Revised:* December 02, 2011. *Accepted:* December 15, 2011.

In: Alternative Medicine Research Yearbook 2012
Editors: Søren Ventegodt and Joav Merrick

ISBN: 978-1-62808-080-3
© 2013 Nova Science Publishers, Inc.

Chapter 26

HOLISTIC MEDICINE V:
ONE SESSION HEALING OF RAPE AND INCEST TRAUMAS IN A GROUP SETTING

Søren Ventegodt*, MD, MMedSci, EU-MSc-CAM[1,2,3,4,5],
Andrew Young MD[6], and Joav Merrick, MD, MMedSci, DMSc[5,7,8,]

[1]Quality of Life Research Center, Copenhagen, Denmark; [2]Research Clinic for Holistic Medicine and [3]Nordic School of Holistic Medicine, Copenhagen, Denmark; [4]Scandinavian Foundation for Holistic Medicine, Sandvika, Norway; [5]Interuniversity College, Graz, Austria; [6]Student Wellness Center, University of Cape Town; [7]National Institute of Child Health and Human Development, [8]Office of the Medical Director, Division for Intellectual and Developmental Disabilities, Ministry of Social Affairs, Jerusalem, Israel and [9]Kentucky Children's Hospital, University of Kentucky, Lexington, US

ABSTRACT

An intensive healing seminar with eight hours of mind-body medicine was constructed to help victims of rape, incest and other kinds of sexual abuse in South Africa. It was tested on five volunteer participants. In the beginning of the seminar a therapeutic goal for the day was defined, and this goal had to be sufficiently large to make a significant improvement in quality of life and sexual functioning. Four of the five participants reached their defined therapeutic goal and found the seminar very useful. The obtained goals were: A: I want to get rid of my hate and disgust with sex (incest victim, physically, psychologically and sexually abused by her father). B: I want to live life in an open and relaxed way and to let go of my hatred [of men] (rape victim). C: I want to let go of the victim role and blaming myself always so I need to fight to get out of my bed every

---

* Correspondence: Søren Ventegodt, MD, MMedSci, EU-MSc-CAM, Director, Quality of Life Research Center, Frederiksberg Alle 13A, 2.t.v., DK-1807 Copenhagen V, Denmark. Tel: +45-33-141113; Fax: +45-33-141123; E-mail: ventegodt@livskvalitet.org.

246 *Søren Ventegodt, Andrew Young and Joav Merrick*

morning (date rape victim – raped by her date and his friend). D: I want to get rid of this all consuming shame and self-disgust I live with (sexual abuse, abused by 7 year older step brother). For future research more participants, quantitative measurement of outcomes (quality of life, sexual functioning and self-reported mental and physical health), and long time follow up are recommended.

Keywords: Mind-body medicine, holistic therapy, rape, incest, sexual abuse, one-session healing, shamanistic healing, sexual trauma, intensive short term psychotherapy, sexology

INTRODUCTION

Sexual violence and abuse is one of the greatest threats to female quality of life and sexual functioning in our time. One in seven females have been sexually abused in the western world (1) and in less developed countries like South Africa the rate might be as high as one in four. The high incident of rape, incest and other kinds of sexual abuse makes it necessary to develop fast, safe and efficient cures for healing traumas after sexual violence and abuse. The traditional shamanistic one-day healing ritual used by many premodern cultures like the Native American medicine men (2) might be a useful model for modern holistic therapeutic practice.

These rituals have often been like the mitote, where the participants are using hallucinogenic plants and mushrooms like peyote (3) and "magic mushrooms" (Psilosybe Mexicana) (4), but in the European healing tradition going back to Hippocrates and his students, drugs and medical plants were rarely used for interior use, as there were considered too harmful (5).

Instead the physician used therapeutic touch, conversation and good intent – basically positive philosophy of life combined with tender, loving care and acceptance - to induce the process of existential healing (6), which we often now call "salutogenesis" (7,8). Recent reviews have documented holistic mind-body medicine (non-drug medicine) to be completely safe and efficient with most clinical conditions (9,10).

METHODS

We designed a one day healing seminar for victims of rape and sexual abuse in Cape Town. It was successfully run the May 4th 2010 at the Medi-Spa in Kloof Street. Participants were informed by two public lectures in Cape Talk with Soli Filander: Thursday April 27th on Sexuality and mental and physical health" and Monday May 3rd on "The horror of sexual violence and abuse and the gift of therapy". Søren Ventegodt presented the project.

The seminar was lead by Andy Young and Søren Ventegodt, and five victims of rape, incest or sexual abuse participated.

The participants were from 20-60 years, most around 30 years; three of these were Caucasian, and two were Colored.

The prize for the course was 500 Rand (45 EUROs), paid by the participants. The timeline of the seminar was the following:

Holistic medicine V

13.00-13.30 Welcome – Therapists and participants introduce themselves. Wow of confidentiality.

13.30-14.30 Theory of sexuality and sexual violence and abuse, including the scientific findings of *paradoxal post-traumatic growth* – the fact that many rape victims are doing exceptionally well after end therapy (11-14).

14.30-14.45 Defining the therapeutic goal for the day.

14.45-15.30 Sharing the content of the traumatic events in small groups. Every little detail is being told to the partner: What happened, what did you feel, what happened then etc.

15.30-16.00 Tea break.

15.30-18.00 Sharing in the group and processing the difficult feelings. Exploring what happened and the effect of it to understand the nature and dynamics of sexuality and sexual traumas. Letting go of negative attitudes and beliefs.

18.00-19.00 Dinner

19.00 – 19.45. Sessions with therapeutic touch to two participants who could not process traumas only by talking. Everybody participated in the physical holding. A healing group field was created.

19.45-20.15 Time line therapy: From conception to present time: See all that happened in your life and understand the greater picture: You were destroyed and you are now coming back to life. This is the story for everybody.

Everybody gets the challenge they need to grow and develop on their spiritual journey.

20.15-20.50 Sharing in the group: What happened. What did you learn? Did you reach your goal?

20.50-21.00 Documenting the results – tell what happened on paper

21.00 Holding hands in a circle to acknowledge the gifts received and saying good bye to the group.

RESULTS

The outcome of the day's eight intensive hours of therapy was the participants reaching their therapeutic goals.

All participants were encouraged to define a goal that they would see as a significant improvement and which would improve their general quality of life as well as their sexual functioning. The therapeutic goals obtained were the following:

A. I want to get rid of my hate and disgust with sex (incest victim, physically, psychologically and sexually abused by her father)

B. I want to life live in an open and relaxed way and to let go of my hatred [of men] (rape victim)

C. I want to let go of the victim role and blaming myself always so I need to fight to get out of my bed every morning (date rape victim – raped by her date and his friend)

D. I want to get rid of this all consuming shame and self-disgust I live with (sexual abuse by 7 year older step brother).

One participant left the course as she was not able to define her therapeutic goal: "I am not ready for this". She explained that she was so angry about being raped and not ready to let go of the hatred and forgive her perpetrator.

The remaining four of the participants were successfully helped, according to their own evaluation of the course and the healing process they had been though in the end of the day. Both therapists agreed on this.

Two of the participants reported that they had tried to process the trauma in psychological standard treatment, but has left the treatment as one hour of therapy a week just seemed to make things worse; it opened up to the trauma and gave them some very difficult days after the therapy. They were happy to learn that they felt very good in the end of the seminar, as they have had the time they needed to process the contacted traumas. One participant had a long record of psychiatric treatment without getting rid of the traumas of early sexual abuse by her father. She shared that she had been sexually abused regularly from she was 6-13 years old, in spite of the family knowing of the abuse. She felt that this day had helped her to let go of the little victimized girl inside of her.

DISCUSSION

The research design has several weaknesses. Firstly there were few participants. Secondly there was only qualitative evaluation by the participants and the two therapists. A questionnaire about health, quality of life and sexual functioning like the QOL10 (15) given before and after the seminar could have been helpful. A follow up study is needed to document that the effect of the healing seminar is lasting and that the therapeutic goals actually reached.

The findings are in accordance with earlier studies of holistic mind body medicine in a group setting (16) and the number of hours of therapy (8 hours) has earlier been found to be sufficient to heal even severe traumas (17,18-23).

As one in five of the participants were not able to state her goal with the therapy it seems that this approach is not useful for everybody; in the early phase where strong emotions of anger is prevalent it might be better to use individual therapy to help the rape victim confront her trauma.

Another possibility is that patients who are not ready to formulate their goal of therapy is taken directly into a session with bodywork so that they do not have to assume responsibility for healing their sexual trauma, as this might be too difficult for them emotionally.

CONCLUSION

It is possible to give eight hours of intensive mind-body therapy in a group setting, allowing victims of rape, incest and other sexual abuse to heal even severe traumas in one day. The therapy seems to be safe and highly efficient. This way of healing patients might be cost-effective in areas of the world, where sexual violence is occurring often and resources for therapy are limited.

ACKNOWLEDGMENTS

The research was carried out in accordance with the Open Source protocol for Clinical Holistic Medicine (24) and it followed the ethical standards of International Society for Holistic Health (25). The Danish Quality of Life Survey, Quality of Life Research Center and the Research Clinic for Holistic Medicine, Copenhagen, was from 1987 till today supported by grants from the 1991 Pharmacy Foundation, the Goodwill-fonden, the JL-Foundation, E Danielsen and Wife's Foundation, Emmerick Meyer's Trust, the Frimodt-Heineken Foundation, the Hede Nielsen Family Foundation, Petrus Andersens Fond, Wholesaler CP Frederiksens Study Trust, Else and Mogens Wedell-Wedellsborg's Foundation and IMK Almene Fond. The research in quality of life and scientific complementary and holistic medicine was approved by the Copenhagen Scientific Ethical Committee under the numbers (KF)V. 100.1762-90, (KF)V. 100.2123/91, (KF)V. 01-502/93, (KF)V. 01-026/97, (KF)V. 01-162/97, (KF)V. 01-198/97, and further correspondence. We declare no conflicts of interest.

REFERENCES

[1] Green A. Childhood sexual and physical abuse. In: Wilson JP, Raphael B. International handbook of traumatic stress syndromes. New York: Plenum, 1993.
[2] Luna E, White, S. Ayahuasca reader. Santa Fe, NM: Synergetic Press, 2000.
[3] Anderson EF. Peyote. The divine cactus. Tucson, AZ: Univ Arizona Press, 1996.
[4] Grof S. The great awakening: Psychology, philosophy, and spirituality in LSD psychotherapy. Albany, NY: State University of New York Press, 2003.
[5] Jones WHS. Hippocrates. Vol. I–IV. London: William Heinemann, 1923-1931.
[6] Ventegodt S, Andersen NJ, Merrick J. Holistic Medicine III: The holistic process theory of healing. ScientificWorldJournal 2003;3:1138-46.
[7] Antonovsky A. Health, stress and coping. London: Jossey-Bass, 1985.
[8] Antonovsky A. Unravelling the mystery of health. How people manage stress and stay well. San Francisco: Jossey-Bass, 1987.
[9] Ventegodt S, Merrick J. A review of side effects and adverse events of non-drug medicine (nonpharmaceutical complementary and alternative medicine): Psychotherapy, mind-body medicine and clinical holistic medicine. J Complement Integr Med 2009;6(1):16.
[10] Ventegodt S, Andersen NJ, Kandel I, Merrick J. Effect, side effects and adverse events of non-pharmaceutical medicine. A review. Int J Disabil Hum Dev 2009;8(3):227-35.
[11] Grubaugh AL, Resick PA. Posttraumatic growth in treatment-seeking female assault victims. Psychiatr Q 2007;78(2):145-55.
[12] Frazier P, Conlon A, Glaser T. Positive and negative life changes following sexual assault. J Consult Clin Psychol 2001;69(6):1048-55.
[13] Frazier P, Tashiro T, Berman M, Steger M, Long J. Correlates of levels and patterns of positive life changes following sexual assault. J Consult Clin Psychol 2004;72(1):19-30.
[14] Linley PA, Joseph S. Positive change following trauma and adversity: a review. J Trauma Stress 2004;17(1):11-21.

250   *Søren Ventegodt, Andrew Young and Joav Merrick*

[15]   Ventegodt S, Andersen NJ, Merrick J. QOL10 for clinical quality-assurance and research in treatment-efficacy: Ten key questions for measuring the global quality of life, self-rated physical and mental health, and self-rated social-, sexual and working ability. J Altern Med Res 2009;1(2):113-22.

[16]   Ventegodt S, Clausen B, Langhorn M, Kroman M, Andersen NJ, Merrick J. Quality of Life as Medicine III. A qualitative analysis of the effect of a five days intervention with existential holistic group therapy or a quality of life course as a modern rite of passage. ScientificWorldJournal 2004;4:124-33.

[17]   Ventegodt S, Kandel I, Neikrug S, Merric J. Clinical holistic medicine: holistic treatment of rape and incest trauma. ScientificWorldJournal 2005;5:288-97.

[18]   Ventegodt S, Thegler S, Andreasen T, Struve F, Enevoldsen L, Bassaine L, Torp M, Merrick J. Self-reported low self-esteem. Intervention and follow-up in a clinical setting. ScientificWorldJournal 2007;7:299-305.

[19]   Ventegodt S, Thegler S, Andreasen T, Struve F, Enevoldsen L, Bassaine L, Torp M, Merrick J. Clinical holistic medicine (mindful, short-term psychodynamic psychotherapy complemented with bodywork) in the treatment of experienced mental illness. ScientificWorldJournal 2007;7:306-9.

[20]   Ventegodt S, Thegler S, Andreasen T, Struve F, Enevoldsen L, Bassaine L, Torp M, Merrick J. Clinical holistic medicine (mindful, short-term psychodynamic psychotherapy complemented with bodywork) in the treatment of experienced physical illness and chronic pain. ScientificWorldJournal 2007;7:310-16.

[21]   Ventegodt S, Thegler S, Andreasen T, Struve F, Enevoldsen L, Bassaine L, Torp M, Merrick J. Clinical holistic medicine (mindful, short-term psychodynamic psychotherapy complemented with bodywork) improves quality of life, health and ability by induction of Antonovsky-Salutogenesis. ScientificWorldJournal 2007;7:317-23.

[22]   Ventegodt S, Andersen NJ, Kandel I, Merrick J. The open source protocol of clinical holistic medicine. J Altern Med Res 2009;1(2), 129-44.

[23]   Ventegodt S, Thegler S, Andreasen T, Struve F, Enevoldsen L, Bassaine L, Torp M, Merrick J. Clinical holistic medicine (mindful, short-term psychodynamic psychotherapy complemented with bodywork) in the treatment of experienced impaired sexual functioning. ScientificWorldJournal 2007;7:324-9.

[24]   Ventegodt S, Clausen B, Merrick J. Clinical holistic medicine: pilot study on the effect of vaginal acupressure (Hippocratic pelvic massage). ScientificWorldJournal 2006;6:2100-16.

[25]   de Vibe M, Bell E, Merrick J, Omar HA, Ventegodt S. Ethics and holistic healthcare practice. Int J Child Health Human Dev 2008;1(1):23-8.

Submitted: October 20, 2011. *Revised:* December 03, 2011. *Accepted:* December 15, 2011.

In: Alternative Medicine Research Yearbook 2012
Editors: Søren Ventegodt and Joav Merrick

ISBN: 978-1-62808-080-3
© 2013 Nova Science Publishers, Inc.

Chapter 27

REFLECTIONS FROM A STUDY TOUR TO HIPPOCRATES' ASKLEPIEION ON THE ISLAND OF KOS

Søren Ventegodt, MD, MMedSci, EU-MSc-CAM[1,2,3,4,5] and Joav Merrick, MD, MMedSci, DMSc[5,6,7,8,9]*

[1]Quality of Life Research Center, Copenhagen, Denmark
[2]Research Clinic for Holistic Medicine and
[3]Nordic School of Holistic Medicine, Copenhagen, Denmark
[4]Scandinavian Foundation for Holistic Medicine, Sandvika, Norway
[5]Interuniversity College, Graz, Austria
[6]National Institute of Child Health and Human Development, Jerusalem,
[7]Division of Pediatrics, Hadassah Hebrew University Medical Centers, Mt Scopus
Campus, Jerusalem, Israel
[8]Office of the Medical Director, Health Services, Division for Intellectual and
Developmental Disabilities, Ministry of Social Affairs and Social Services,
Jerusalem, Israel
[9]Kentucky Children's Hospital, University of Kentucky, Lexington, US

ABSTRACT

Hippocrates (460-377 BCE) was the leading priest-healer at the Aklepieion of Kos and we have today knowledge of about 500 Asklepieia (priest healers) that existed around that time and working in a large hospital complex, that later as destroyed by large natural disasters 554-551 BCE. Even with the destruction the Hippocratic mind body medicine has been described in the Corpus Hippocraticum and maybe it is time once again to build large holistic hospitals in the classical tradition, which without doubt could help so many patients to realise their divine Self and in that way heal body, mind and spirit ad modum Hippocrates.

---

* Correspondence: Søren Ventegodt, MD, MMedSci, EU-MSc-CAM, Director, Quality of Life Research Center, Frederiksberg Alle 13A, 2tv, DK-1661 Copenhagen V, Denmark. E-mail: ventegodt@livskvalitet.org.

252   *Søren Ventegodt and Joav Merrick*

Keywords: Alternative medicine, Hippocrates, Kos

INTRODUCTION

The famous physician Hippocrates (460-377 BCE) came from a well established tradition of priest-healers, his grandfather, also called Hippocrates, was the leading priest-healer at the Aklepieion of Kos around 500 BC (1,2).

The knowledge of the about 500 Asklepieia (priest healers) that existed around this time (1,2) comes from several sources:

1. The archaeological findings, like the excavation of the great Asklepieion on Kos, where the building covering an area of about 10,000 square meters (1,2).
2. The ancient written sources
3. Toponymic (names of places often still in use today)

Strabo (67-23 AD), the main geographer of ancient times, wrote about the Asklepieia and explained in detail about the Asklepieion of Kos and the Roman plundering of it. Strabo's information about its exact location helped the re-discovery of Hippocrates' Asklepieion by the German archaeologist Rudolf Herzog (1871-1953) in 1902, after 1350 years of burial and oblivion as the result of devastating earthquakes in the region around Kos in 554-551 AD and the oppression of the local authorities of Kos by the Romans.

About 70 books from the Hippocratic physicians of Kos, the Corpus Hippocraticum (3), has been preserved in many different languages from that time, and we also know that Platon praised Hippocrates for his wisdom and skills as a doctor. Many of the known 500 Asklepieia have been located and excavated by archaeologists during the last two centuries. Coins, statues, and rings have been found with motives from the Asklepieion, including quite accurate pictures of Hippocrates himself.

Many of the ancient names of cities and places are still used today. All this gives us a fair knowledge about the hospitals and their doctors in the civilised world of 500 BCE, but many mysteries still remains, when it comes to the actual processes of the healing.

What therapy was used?

It is obvious from the sources that the therapy was talk and touch therapy. Massage played a major role as did conversation that according to the sources had one primary aim: To support the patient's inner exploration of body, mind and soul. Hippocrates also recommended physical exercise, mostly in the form of walking: "Walking is the best medicine" (3).

The Asclepiads were priest-healers, and their function was to help the patient connect to the Divine and this way heal. All disease, disorders and problems of this world was seen as symptoms of lack of connection or oneness with the Divine. Hippocrates is often quoted for putting much more emphasis on the person having a disease that on the diseases the person had: "It is far more important to know what person the disease has than what disease the person has" (3). Only if you understand that the "person" itself is the problem, that this person creates a distance to the "inner soul" and thus to the divine can one understand the foundation of the Hippocratic medicine.

The role of the Asclepiad is to remind the patient that he or she is already connected to the God(s) and deep down, the patient is one with the universe – the patient has a divine nature – and only by this realization can true healing happen. That Hippocrates and the Asclepiads really believed everybody to be Divine themselves is clear from famous quotations on oneness like the following: "The soul is the same in all living creatures although the body of each is different" (3).

When it comes to the practical ceremonies of the healing there are lots of guessing, and unfortunately surprisingly little support from the written sources. A number of temples to a long series of Gods in the Asklepieion in Kos reveals that all aspects of life, represented by each God, has been involved in the process of healing, indicating that the cure was truly holistic. But how these temples were used is not well described; some researchers has guessed that they were for animal sacrifice, while others have speculated that they were for the patient's or the priest's meditation (1,2).

How many patients were treated?

The success of the healing system of the Asclepiads is clear from the number of known hospitals from that time, but it is quite impossible to say how many patients one Asklepieion could treat. The Hippocratic hospital was expanded three times, before is was buried in the ashes for more than a millennium. The number of beds was likely to be counted in hundreds judged from the size of the buildings and the 10,000 square meter was known to employ a large staff of priest-healers, physiotherapists and nurses. Judged from the continued large expansions of the hospital the patient flow to the Asklepieion of Kos could easily have been many thousands a year. The 500 Asklepieia could thus have been providing cure, healing and health to a large number of patients around 500 BCE. We often think that large numbers of patients could only be managed by modern-day medicine and hospitals, but it seems that the ancient world had a highly developed system of holistic hospitals that offered healing to a large fraction of citizens in the civilised world of that time. It is also possible that the Asklepieia was only for the chosen few with citizen rights and not for a large number of people in those days, who were slaves and other categories of people in the bottom of the social hierarchy, which might explain why Hippocrates so often stressed that the physician should treat rich and poor, slave and free man in the same way. This was at the core of the famous Hippocratic ethics, included in the Hippocratic Oath. With this said it is worth remembering that the beginning of the oath is devoted to the Gods: Apollo, the healer, Asclepius, Hygieia, and Panacea, and all the other gods and goddesses.

Hippocrates' hospital on Kos and his drug-free mind-body medicine - which in spite of rich medical gardens according to the Corpus Hippocraticum only used medical herbs for external purposes - was famous and known in the civilised world at that time. Many patients came travelling from far away to realize their inner Self, the soul that is one with all other souls, and thus they were healed on the island of Kos.

The Roman conquerors did not appreciate the priest-healers and the fine art of the Asklepieion was stolen and brought to Rome and after a complete destruction of the Asklepieion by large natural disasters 554-551 BCE, it was never brought back into function.

Its thousands of artistically decorated marble blocks were later used for building the churches and mosques of Kos, and hardly a stone was left, when Herzog finally established its original location in 1902, and today the sad remains of the once so famous Asklepieion of Kos is hardly worth a visit.

Luckily we still have the Hippocratic mind body medicine so well described in the Corpus Hippocraticum (3) and maybe it is time once again to build large holistic hospitals in the classical tradition, which without doubt could help so many patients to realise their divine Self and in that way heal body, mind and spirit ad modum Hippocrates.

REFERENCES

[1]   Hatzivassiliou VS. The Asklepieion of Kos. Kos: M Georvassakis JSC Publishing, 2008.
[2]   Vlakouli P. The Asklepieion of Kos. Athens: Davaris Advertising Publishing, 2005.
[3]   Jones WHS. Hippocrates, Vol. I–IV. London: William Heinemann, 1923-1931.

Received: September 01, 2011. *Revised:* October 03, 2011. *Accepted:* October 14, 2011.

SECTION THREE – LIFE SATISFACTION

In: Alternative Medicine Research Yearbook 2012
Editors: Søren Ventegodt and Joav Merrick

ISBN: 978-1-62808-080-3
© 2013 Nova Science Publishers, Inc.

Chapter 28

AGING AND QUALITY OF LIFE IN TAIWAN

Luo Lu, PhD[*]

Department of Business Adminstration,
National Taiwan University, Taipei, Taiwan

ABSTRACT

The purpose of this paper is two-fold: to explore older people's attitudes towards aging as a subjective aspect of quality of life (QOL), and to further examine whether leisure pursuits in later years are associated with QOL in a Chinese society (Taiwan). We will review recent evidence to show that in general Taiwanese older people possessed positive attitudes towards aging. This reveals that aging in Taiwan can be experienced favorably and meaningfully. We will then review emerging evidence to show that leisure pursuits in older age are related to emotional well-being (depressive symptoms), even after controlling for effects of demographics, physical health/disability, and social support. Also, for Taiwanese older people, positive (life satisfaction) and negative (depression) aspects of QOL are mutually linked over and beyond known factors of health, financial security, and social embeddedness. We purport that health care, financial planning, social integration and active participation in life are all integral aspects to ensure a high quality of life in later years.

Keywords: Adulthood, aging, quality of life

INTRODUCTION

Aging is a pressing problem for many countries in this century, especially for a developing country such as Taiwan. In Taiwan, advances in medical science and technology, successful promotion of health care, material prosperity, coupled with the gradual demise of Chinese family values and lifestyle (e.g., large extended family living together), have sent the birth rate in a steady decline, but the life expectancy in a steady increase. Consequently, as early as

---

[*] Correspondence: Luo Lu, Department of Business Adminstration, National Taiwan University, No. 1, Sec. 4, Roosevelt Rd., Da'an Dist., Taipei City 106, Taiwan. E-mail: luolu@ntu.edu.tw.

in September 1993, Taiwan was officially an aging society as the proportion of those aged over 65 had exceeded 7% of the country's population (1). However, systematic research on aging topics in Taiwan is still in its infancy, and relies heavily upon Western theories and findings. Furthermore, most research efforts have been devoted to medical gerontology and other aging-related medical care topics, while psychosocial issues of normative aging are generally overlooked. Although there has been some research pointing out the beneficial effects of social support for the Chinese older people in Taiwan (2,3), other psychosocial correlates of quality of life (QOL) in later years, such as leisure, have been largely overlooked. Furthermore, older people's self-definition and perception of aging have been ignored. The purpose of this paper, therefore, was twofold: first, to explore a basic issue in social gerontology from the older people's point of view: Can aging be a positive experience for older people living in a collectivist but socially and economically fast changing society? If yes, are positive attitudes towards aging beneficial for personal well-being, over and beyond effects of known protectors such as social support and social embeddedness? Second, in addition to the above known protectors of QOL in older age, does leisure have a role to play in ensuring a successful aging?

Is it possible to experience aging as a positive process?

Quality of life defined in ethical, theological, political, economic, and psychological terms has been studied in a large number of disciplines over many centuries, and has generated increasing interest among researchers and practitioners involved in caring for older people (4). QOL is the result of one's comprehensive appraisal of life against individual and social goals, and four sectors comprising "the good life" have been purported: behavioral competence, psychological well-being, perceived quality of life, and objective environment (5). This demarcation of sectors is in broad agreement with the objective/subjective distinction in the tradition of QOL research (4,6-8). Objective indicators of QOL are those that exist outside the body of the person, such as economic resources, health functioning, and social contact (6), while subjective indicators of QOL are those that are perceived, experienced, and evaluated by the human mind, such as life satisfaction, happiness, morale, and positive outlook (4). Mirroring the trend in earlier generic well-being research, far more efforts have been expanded on looking for "objective" external rather than subjective psychological indicators of QOL for older people, as the former is relatively easy to define and assess (6). Another characteristic of the QOL research is its focus on sick and frail older people rather than normal and healthy community older adults (5). As noted by Bowling and Gabriel, people of different age, health status, and residence arrangement may have different priorities when judging their QOL (7). Fry further suggested that personal mastery, autonomy, self-sufficiency, life style choices and privacy are the most important indicators of QOL for community-residing older people (9). All of these are subjective indicators. A recent Taiwanese study corroborates the above Western view, validating that a healthy body, a sense of self-worth, companionship, residential environment and leisure facilities, social contacts with friends and relatives, and joy are all important aspects of QOL for older people in Taiwan (10). The fact that even for disabled older people involved in this study subjective QOL is as relevant as objective indictors, serves to underline the necessity of emphasizing more on psychological aspects of QOL in gerontological research. So far, positive outlook of older age is a largely neglected topic in the QOL research.

As stated earlier, for many years, gerontological research was concerned nearly exclusively with problems of aging and older age, and has contributed to the problematization of older age and the negative image of the aging process. However, work in social gerontology has endeavored to deconstruct prevailing negative aging stereotypes, i.e., ageism in the society (11), to further promote educational interventions aiming at fostering positive attitudes towards older people (12) and the aging process (13).

Among older people, researchers have also recently found that the experience of aging is neither uniform nor necessarily negative. As part of the Berlin Aging Study, Freund and Smith collected spontaneous self-definition in a heterogeneous sample of 516 participants (aged 70-103 years) (14). The content of the self-definition revealed that these older adults still view themselves as active and present-oriented, and overall, there were more positive than negative self-evaluations. More importantly perhaps, positive emotional well-being was associated with naming more and richer self-defining domains. Another study found that when defining "old", older people focused less on appearance or body image, more on health status and psychological factors such as loss of autonomy (15).

In Taiwan, social gerontological research on self-perception of older people or normative aging experiences is very rare. Two notable exceptions are a large scale survey of young, middle-aged and older adults (16), and a study of older adults with medical conditions (17). Lee's study (16) focused on the general impression of life in middle to late adulthood, and found that Taiwanese people tended to perceive old age rather negatively, including losses in health, status, relationships, and work. Furthermore, more negative and undesirable traits and behaviors were attributed to older people than to middle aged people. These findings largely corroborate other studies in Taiwan showing that people of different age groups all possessed generally negative attitudes towards older people (18,19). Apparently, ageism is still prevalent in the Taiwanese society.

Although the above mentioned empirical results seem to depict a general negative image of the old age and older people held by a wide range of Taiwanese people, a finer grained analysis did reveal that some positive aspects of aging were acknowledged both by the older people themselves (19), and by members of other age groups (16,20). Specifically, positive attitudes and traits pertaining to psychological and cognitive aspects of aging, such as rich experiences, wisdom, and authoritative status, were attributed to older persons in aforementioned studies.

What about older people's own experience of aging then? Lu and Chang (17) argued that aging is not an inevitably negative experience, even for those with compromised health. They found that older age, male, living alone, and being financially-dependent were risk factors of worsened health, while female, living alone, and being financially-dependent were risk factors of lowered life satisfaction in a sample of community older adults (aged 65-90 years). Although participants in that study all had at least one chronic medical condition, authors observed that they nonetheless maintained good functioning in daily activities, perceived little interference of illnesses with their normal life, reported fairly good psychological health and optimistic outlooks in life. Such more encouraging positive experiences with aging corroborate Lu and Kao's most recent finding that older people indeed possessed more positive attitudes regarding cognitive and psychological aspects of aging than non-old adults in Taiwan (19). It needs to be noted though that the sample of older persons included in the study was rather small (N = 30), as the researchers were aiming at a wide spectrum of the general population.

One recently published study fortunately targeted community older people and assessed their perception of aging, using the same attitudinal measurement as that reported in the above study (21). Face-to-face interviews were conducted to collect data from a random sample of community older people in all regions of Taiwan (N = 316). The authors found that older people possessed positive attitudes towards aging in general, but there were some group attitudinal differences. Specifically, males were not different from females, the "young old" (aged 60-74 years) were not different from the "old old" (aged 75 years and above), and those living with family were not different from those living alone in their overall aging attitudes. However, education and urban residence had advantages of projecting a more positive outlook for the old age: those who were educated above elementary school level and living in urban areas avowed more overall positive attitudes towards aging.

It is worth mentioning that the "older people scale" (OPS) (19) used in both of the above mentioned studies, is the first standardized scale developed specifically for the Chinese people, assessing attitudes towards older people in general. When responding to the same items, young and older adults may base their opinions on different information. Specifically, older respondents are more likely to draw information from their own aging experiences, thus scale scores may thus reflect their attitudes towards aging itself. Using OPS as a measure of attitudes towards older people (when young people responding) and attitudes towards aging (when older people responding), empirical evidence can be compared across different demographic groups from different studies. Lu and Kao (19,22) have provided evidence of reliability, structural validity of a four-factor model, convergent validity with an existing Western scale (Aging Semantic Differential) (11), criterion validity in predicting intentions of interacting with older people in daily life, as well as college students' career choices of working in older people-related jobs. The OPS uses a stem "In general, older people are..." to assess four aspects of attitudes: Appearance and physical characteristics, Psychological and cognitive characteristics, Interpersonal relations and social participation, and Work and economic safety. Each item was rated on a 7-point scale (1 = strongly disagree, 7 = strongly agree). A higher score indicated more positive attitudes towards older people/aging. Older people reported high item means for the aggregated score on OPS (4.74) and those of its four subscales (4.61, 4.81, 4.72, 4.89). All five mean scores were not only in the positive ranges of the scale, but also statistically significant from the mid-point of 4 on the 1-7 scale. Furthermore, older people's own perception of aging was significantly more positive than the projections of them by a broad section of population in Taiwan (19), college students (22), company managers (23) and workers (24). These results are encouraging when interpreted as one indicator of QOL in old age: Taiwanese older people not only view aging more positively than their younger counterparts, they remain optimistic in all aspects of the aging process, physical, psychological, social, and financial.

Adopting a different research paradigm, a rare qualitative research reported 22 in-depth interviews with community older adults in Taiwan (25). Researchers noted that many of their interviewees held positive attitudes towards their family roles in later life. Such positive self-perceptions for the old age was rooted in the rich life experiences, in the belief that they can teach, guide and help their children and grandchildren, and in the prevailing societal value of respecting the old and ascribing authority to the old in family. From these rich personal accounts of aging in the family, researchers concluded that given adequate health and financial assurance, Taiwanese older people generally held positive attitudes towards the impending aging and were able to adapt to the family role transition with optimism.

Synthesizing these strands of research, we argue that aging can be experienced positively in a Chinese culture. At the society level, the prevailing social value of filial piety and social norm of respecting the old in a Chinese society help to strengthen status and prestige of older people both in and beyond the family domain (25). At the individual level, the possibility of maintaining a positive outlook for the old age and experiencing aging positively is supported by a theoretical perspective emphasizing life course development (26). As one negotiates with specific developmental tasks through the course of life, the process of aging should not necessarily be detrimental to well-being; instead there even exists possibilities for positive change and personal growth. This is exactly what has been revealed in a recent Taiwanese study: for community older people, less positive attitudes towards aging were related to more depressive symptoms while more positive attitudes were related to higher happiness (21). Furthermore, the associations of aging attitudes with well-being persisted even after controlling for the effects of social support and community participation.

Leisure: The incremental value beyond other social resources for successful aging

As stated earlier, most research efforts have been devoted to medical gerontology and other aging-related medical care topics both in the West and in Taiwan, some psychosocial factors has been proven beneficial for normative aging as well as maintaining certain quality of life among the frail. These protective factors are social support (2,3), family role participation (25), and positive attitudes towards aging (21). However, other domains of active participation in life such as leisure, especially subjective experiences of leisure have largely been ignored so far.

Research on leisure with Chinese people in general and with older people in particular is in the rarity, partly because hardworking has always been a highly regarded Confucius virtue. However, with economic development, material abundance, and the shortening of statutory working hour (now 40 per week), Taiwanese people are learning to "improve life with leisure" (27). Thus, against this transition of cultural mandate on a "good way of life", understanding the subjective experiences of leisure of older Chinese people will not only shed light on some interesting issues in leisure research, but also contribute to better leisure policies and management to promote successful ageing. Below we will theorize possible mechanisms linking meaningful leisure experiences in older age to psychological well-being, and present empirical evidence supporting the beneficial effects of leisure over and beyond those of known protectors such as physical health, financial security, and social embeddedness.

In a recent study, Bowling interviewed 337 British home-living older adults, and found that 43% regarded having/maintaining physical health and 34% regarded participating in leisure and social activities as elements of active ageing (28). It is rather encouraging to note that a third rated themselves as ageing "very actively" and almost half as "fairly actively". This research provides empirical basis for the notion of successful ageing as "engagement with life", including role participation with work, family, friends, community, and leisure (29).

In Taiwan, 65 is the statuary retirement age, and a recent nationwide survey noted only 5.9% of those aged 65 and above still held paid jobs (including part-time work) (24). This finding corroborates the popular image and commonly held expectation of older age in Chinese societies being a time of leisure and retreat into family life with grandchildren (25). Instead, active role participation with family, friends, and community has been repeatedly found pivotal to older people's well-being in Taiwanese studies (2,3,25). However, leisure in older age seems to be largely overlooked in existing Taiwanese studies. Time being one of the most available assets in older age, leisure can serve a key role in the successful ageing process, and can be a constructive way of engagement with life. One recent study found that Australian older people spent 4.5 h/day on solitary leisure and 2.7 h/day on social leisure (30). Although there is no data on time use of Taiwanese older adults, Chen did found that participation in various leisure activities was positively related to increased life satisfaction for older people (31).

More striking evidence came from a 10-year follow-up study with a nationally representative sample of Swedish older people (32). Researchers found that those increasing their leisure activity participation across domains tended to perceive an improvement in their life conditions. Another study found that for Japanese older men, less interaction with neighbors, society, and friends was highly associated with depressed mood, while for women engaging in various types of activities relating to society, leisure and children/grandchildren was associated with less depressed mood (33).

Various leisure theories have provided us with frameworks to understand the benefits of leisure. For instance, Beard and Ragheb purported that leisure could gratify basic human needs and generate satisfaction pertaining to six aspects: psychological (e.g., interesting activities), social (e.g., getting to know people), physical (e.g., getting exercise, keeping fit), educational (e.g., learning new things), relaxation (e.g., relaxed, rewind), and aesthetic (e.g., beautiful surrounding) (34). Existing leisure research has confirmed that various leisure activities could indeed generate short-term benefits including positive mood, physical fitness and immediate satisfaction, as well as long-term effects of happiness, mental health, physical health, and social integration (35,36). One in-depth interview study with Taiwanese college students further revealed that leisure also served an important function of structuring time (25), which should be more important for older adults with ample time to spend. It may be for this reason, previous Western research has found that leisure is especially important for older people (35).

A recent study (37) has shown that among a large sample of American adults (N = 1,399, 19-89 years), leisure participation in aggregate was associated with lower blood pressure, total cortisol, waist circumference, body mass index, and perceptions of better physical function. These associations withstood controlling for demographic measures. Leisure participation also correlated with higher levels of positive psychosocial states and lower levels of depression and negative effect. It seems that leisure activities are associated with both psychological and physical outcomes. A large-scale Taiwanese study with a national representative sample (N = 2,147, 20-96 years) found that leisure participation in aggregate across 13 common activities was associated with high leisure satisfaction (19). There is thus empirical evidence that Taiwanese people generally feel happy about their leisure and may indeed gain benefits from this particular aspect of life.

However, it is not clear whether some social aspects of leisure confound with social support, which is a known protector against distress and illness. This is particularly so for

Aging and quality of life in Taiwan

Taiwanese people. The above mentioned national survey in Taiwan revealed six most popular leisure activities: watching TV/DVDs/videos, listening to music, taking part in physical activities, spending time on the internet/PC, reading books, and getting together with friends, in that order (38). All these activities involve different degrees of socialization, especially for older people living in community with their families, except perhaps listening to music and reading books. As social embeddedness along with support received in social networks has been well-established as a protector of well-being in Taiwanese studies with older people (2,3,39,40), we need more solid evidence to tease out the incremental value of leisure participation over and beyond such known correlates of QOL.

One possible mechanism of leisure participation on enhancing successful ageing may indeed be through social support and social engagement, as many activities are conducted with family and friends (33,38). Joining in activities with others reflects the social organization of leisure, strengthens interpersonal relationships, and enhances a sense of belonging among the participants (41). Leisure-related social support has indeed been found to buffer the stress-illness relationship for the Americans (42).

Moreover, leisure has the potential to go beyond social engagement or social support. The aforementioned Swedish study (32) revealed that the beneficial effects of increased leisure participation was particularly strong among older adults who became widowed, developed functional impairments, and had relatively low contact with family. These results suggest that maximizing leisure activity participation is an adaptive strategy taken by older adults to compensate for social and physical deficits in later life.

Yet another possible mechanism of leisure participation on enhancing successful ageing may be through cognitive stimulation of the brain. Leisure activities may help brain function and protect against cognitive deterioration. The recent availability of longitudinal data on the possible association of different lifestyles with dementia and Alzheimer's disease (AD) allowed for exploration of the effects of social network, physical leisure, and non-physical activity on cognition and dementia. For all three lifestyle components (social, mental, and physical), a beneficial effect on cognition and a protective effect against dementia are suggested (43). However, a distinction should be drawn between activities that are "cognitive" and those that are "passive", as evidence showed leisure activities that do not involve social engagement but are cognitively stimulating are protective against cognitive decline in older people (29). However, such a salutogenic effect does not apply to watching TV, which is in fact a risk factor for cognitive decline (29).

So far, it seems that participation in leisure activities may facilitate successful aging partly via its instrumental gains in enabling people to join and maintain social networks, to stimulate brain function, and partly via enjoyment of leisure per se (36). Research in Western societies has shown that leisure activities per se may enhance reported physical and subjective well-being among older adults, but the sociability aspect of such activities makes a more substantial difference (44-46). It thus would be interesting to see if leisure activities not connected with social engagement had the same relationship with depression as those connected with social engagement.

Finally, leisure participation of older people, whether in aggregate or in individual activity, has received research attention in the West, subjective experiences of leisure have been understated. A recent study (47) probed into the significance of experiential components in leisure and found that for Australian older people, relaxation and engrossment were commonly expressed experiences. Such subjective experiences were different from yet complimentary to those derived from social support, such as care and respect.

One pioneering Taiwanese study (48) explored older people's subjective leisure experiences, and further examined associations of such experiences with their depressive symptoms in a national representative sample of community older people (N = 1,308, aged 65+). Known correlates of depression such as demographics, physical health, and social support, were taken into account. Face-to-face interviews were conducted to collect high quality data. A checklist of 10 types of leisure activities was provided, including TV/radio, reading newspaper/magazine, playing chess/board games/cards, visiting relatives/friends/neighbors, PC/internet, gardening/plants, interests/hobbies, attending concerts/plays, movies/shopping, and walking/exercising. Participants checked yes/no (1 = yes, 0 = no) for participation in each category of activities.

Results showed that being female, older, single, less educated, and had lower family income were demographic risk factors of depression. Worse physical health, lack of independent functioning in everyday life, and disability were found to relate to more depressive symptoms. Greater social support was once again confirmed to reduce depressive symptoms. Finally, having controlled for effects of demographics, physical health, and social support, positive leisure experiences, i.e. leisure meaningfulness tapping aspects of psychological, social, physical, educational, and relaxation experiences, were independently related to fewer depressive symptoms. However, neither aggregate leisure participation nor participation in each of the 10 activities could predict depressive symptoms in multivariate analysis. Thus, evidence from this large scale national survey seems to suggest that participation per se in leisure activities (whether individually or in aggregate) may not help reducing depressive symptoms, but positive experiences generated through leisure will. The benefits of meaningful leisure pursuits as a subjective human experience for successful ageing were thus clearly demonstrated over and beyond known QOL protectors for Taiwanese older people living in community.

This emerging evidence in Taiwan compliments Western findings of benefits of leisure on enhancing quality of life in older age (32), constructing the subjective experiences of active ageing (28), and reducing risks of dementia in older age (43). More importantly, while existing studies focused on benefits of leisure or life style per se on dementia, AD, physical and mental health, the above reported results were obtained after controlling for effects of social support, thus taking out any potential confound between leisure as a means of sociability (38) and social support as a function of social embeddedness (49). In other words, these results revealed a "cleaner" effect of leisure experiences on depressive symptomatology. Together, existing evidence from the West and Taiwan serves to underline the importance of including leisure as a means of engagement with life, along with social participation in the promotion of successful aging and QOL in older age (50).

Although research in Taiwan fails to find direct evidence linking specific activities to reduced depressive symptoms in the regression analysis, an inspection of the rank order of leisure pursuits in a nationwide sample of older people may still help us to understand why positive leisure experiences in the form of overall leisure satisfaction and subjective experiences of meaningfulness could protect older adults against depressive symptoms. As reported in Lu (48), the most popular leisure engagement for Taiwanese older people was TV/radio (90%), a solitary leisure that tops the list of leisure pursuits for the general population in Taiwan in another recent national survey (38). Although watching TV has been found to be a low arousal and sometimes boring activity (51), and may even be harmful for brain functioning in older age (29), reading newspaper/magazines which ranked the third popular leisure (25.6%) in Lu's study (48) and the 5th in Fu et al., is more cognitively engaging and challenging. Indeed this cognitive activity had the strongest correlation with depressive symptoms (r = -.21) in Lu's study. Its role within the active life style and potential function as a brain stimulus against depression deserve further exploration.

The second popular leisure pursuit for older people in Lu's study (48) was social in nature: visiting relatives/friends/neighbors (47.9%), which ranked the 6th in Fu et al (38). This is in agreement with the Australian finding that older people spent 2.7h/day on social leisure (30). In a close-knit Chinese society, older people tend to have relatives and friends living nearby. In Taiwanese rural areas, older people habitually get together in front of the village temple to chat and drink tea. Such casual social gatherings help to strengthen community bonds and satisfy social needs. Indeed this social activity correlated with lower levels of depressive symptoms (r = -.16).

Gardening (20.8%) was the fourth popular leisure pursuit for older people and the only one involving physical exertion in Lu's study. Physical activities can protect against dementia and AD for older people (43). Gardening is also regarded as a hobby which can generate a strong sense of achievement (52) and aesthetical enjoyment (35). Taken together, it is understandable that older adults who engaged in these popular leisure pursuits may harvest diverse benefits gratifying psychological, educational, social, physical, relaxation, and aesthetic needs. Such gratified needs thus are expressed in reported meaningfulness of and satisfaction with one's leisure life as-a-whole. To promote active engagement with life and successful ageing, these meaningful leisure pursuits may play an integral part.

Further evidence pertaining to psychosocial correlates of QOL in older age came from the latest national survey, Taiwan Social Change Survey (TSCS). TSCS is the largest nationwide social survey in Taiwan (also incorporated into the International Social Survey Program, ISSP, which involves 40 countries in the world). The TSCS series is operated by the Academia Sinica Taiwan, which has conducted 41 surveys as of 2008. With more than 80,000 interviews over the past 24 years, the TSCS has become the largest survey series among all of the general social surveys in the world in terms of the accumulated sample size (53). Highly reputed for its methodological rigor (e.g., nationwide three-stage stratified proportion-to-population size (PPS) sampling using household registration data, well-trained interviewers making home visits, strict supervision, post-interview verification and data checking), its high quality database is widely used for academic research and cross-cultural comparisons under the banner of the ISSP. The 2010 survey includes a full scale of depression symptoms (CES-D), and a comprehensive measure of QOL (global and domain satisfaction), as well as an index of social embeddedness, which is unprecedented in the TSCS/ISSP series. The following results were obtained using data from those aged above 60 years (60-93 years) in the survey sample.

When predicting depression in older age, female sex, impairing sickness, and financial insecurity were all significant risk factors. Physical ill-health had the gravest effect on mental well-being. On the other hand, when predicting life satisfaction in older age, staying married, not having impairing sickness, financial security, social embeddedness, and lack of depressive symptoms were all significant booster factors. Mental ill-health (depression) had the gravest impact damping life satisfaction. Interestingly, the three leisure activities included in the survey, namely visiting museums/galleries, physical exercises/sports, traveling, did not have any effects on either depression or life satisfaction. As TSCS is designed as a national survey for all age groups, the three listed leisure pursuits this time are not the most popular among older people (48). Thus, the lack of significant results involving leisure needs to be interpreted with caution.

Nonetheless, TSCS 2010 is ground-breaking in the sense that it is the first time a national survey includes both positive and negative indicators of QOL, namely, life satisfaction and depression. Furthermore, unlike large-scale social surveys, both indicators of QOL are measured with multiple items reflecting well upon their latent constructs: both CES-D and life satisfaction scales conformed to a one-factor structure, with all items highly loaded as they should be. The combined conceptual, psychometric, and methodological rigor renders us more confidence in claiming that health, finance, social integration and active participation in life are all integral aspects of a high quality of life in older age for Taiwanese adults.

DISCUSSION

The purpose of this paper was two-fold: to explore older people's attitudes towards aging as a subjective aspect of QOL, and to further examine whether leisure pursuits in later years are associated with QOL in a Chinese society--Taiwan. On the first front, we have presented unequivocal evidence from a recent series of studies assessing Taiwanese people's general attitudes towards older people, and older people's own projection of aging. What is consistently found is that in general Taiwanese older people possessed positive attitudes towards aging, confirming that aging can be experienced favorably and meaningfully. The limited existing Taiwanese research also noted that the preponderance of positive attitudes towards aging is most prominent in psychological and cognitive aspects, both viewed by older people themselves (19) and by other age groups (16,20). In other words, old age along with its rich life experiences, wisdom, and social prestige is to a certain extent represented in a positive light. Even more encouraging is the finding that from older people's perspective, positive attitudes are not restricted to any one aspect of the aging process—they remain optimistic for aging in physical, psychological, social, and financial aspects (21). These latest findings were consistent with Western studies showing overall positive self-evaluations among older people (14), and generally more favorable aging perceptions among older than younger people (54). In this respect, ample Western studies have demonstrated the beneficial effects of education programs on dismantling negative stereotypes and ageism (12,13), we in Taiwan need to be more rigorous in promoting and implementing such programs at school and in the community. Positive aging needs not remain an ideal; it is humanly possible and politically correct. More concerted research and practical efforts should be invested to ensure and enhance this subjective aspect of QOL for older adults in Taiwan.

On the second front, we have also presented unequivocal evidence from several large scale studies examining leisure as a psychosocial correlate of QOL for Taiwanese older people, along with other known factors. The most striking evidence presented is that leisure pursuits in older age are related to emotional well-being (depressive symptoms), even after controlling for effects of demographics, physical health/disability, and social support. Although leisure experiences were not the strongest predictors of depression, their contributions were greater than the often-studied social support and independent from those of physical health/disability and social support. Previous social gerontological research has firmly established the protective effects of social resources (49,55-57). We have extended the list of protectors to include leisure, which is so far largely overlooked in Chinese studies of older age. Last but not the least, for Taiwanese older people, positive (life satisfaction) and negative (depression) aspects of QOL are mutually linked over and beyond known factors of health, financial security, and social embeddedness. Looking ahead, in a fast changing developing society, health care, financial planning, social integration and active participation in life are all integral aspects of a high quality of life in later years. Individuals, family, organizations, and society at large need to join hands to ensure positive experiences in the above aspects of objective and subjective quality of living.

ACKNOWLEDGMENTS

In writing up this paper, the author was supported by a grant from the Ministry of Education, Taiwan, 10R706181B..

REFERENCES

[1] Lin WY. Family changes and family policy in Taiwan. J NTU Soc Work 2002;6:35-88.
[2] Hu YH. Gender and caring for the old. Q J Community Dev 1992;58:170-83.
[3] Lu L, Hsieh YH. Demographic variables, control, stress, support and health among the elderly. J Health Psychol 1997;2:97-106.
[4] Gentile KM. A review of the literature on interventions and quality of life in the frail elderly. In: Birren JE, Lubben JE, Rowe JC, Deutchman DE. The concept and measurement and quality of life in the frail elderly. San Diego, CA: Academic Press, 1991:75-90.
[5] Lawton MP. Environment and other determinants of well-being in older People. Gerontologist 1983;23:349-57.
[6] Arnold SB. The measurement of quality of life in the frail elderly. In: Birren JE, Lubben JE, Rowe JC, Deutchman DE. The concept and measurement and quality of life in the frail elderly. San Diego, CA:Academic Press, 1991:50-74.
[7] Bowling A, Gabriel Z. An integrational model of quality of life in older age. Soc Indic Res 2004;69(1):1-36.
[8] Rioux L. The well-being of aging people living in their own homes. J Environ Psychol 2005;25:231-43.
[9] Fry PS. Aging and quality of life (QOL)-The continuing search for quality of life indicators. Int J Aging Hum Dev 2000;50:245-61.
[10] Hsieh MO. Related factors of living arrangements and quality of life among disabled elderly: A quantitative exploration. Soc Policy Soc Work 2004; 8:1-49.
[11] Polizzi KG, Millikin RJ. Attitudes toward the elderly: identifying problematic usage of ageist and overextended terminology in research instructions. Educ Gerontol 2002;28:367-77.
[12] Funderburk B, Damron-Rodriguez J, Storms LL, Solomon DH. Endurance of undergraduate attitudes toward older adults. Educ Gerontol 2006;32:447-62.
[13] Harris LA, Dollinger S. Participation in a course on aging: Knowledge, attitudes, and anxiety about aging in oneself and others. Educ Gerontol 2001; 27:657-67.
[14] Freund AM, Smith J. Content and function of the self-definition in old and very old age. J Gerontol 1999;54B:55-67.
[15] Logan JR, Ward W, Spitze G. As old as you feel: Identity in middle and later life. Soc Forces 1992;71:451-67.

[16] Lee LJ. Adults' perceived images of life experience and personaliy traits of middle-aged and older adults. Bull Natl Chengchi Univ 1999;78:1-54.

[17] Lu L, Chang CJ. Health and satisfaction among the elderly with chronic conditions: Demographic differentials. Kaohsiung J Med Sci 1998; 14:139-49.

[18] Lin MJ. Children's attitudes toward elderly. J Educ Psychol 1987; 10:85-104.

[19] Lu L, Kao SF. Attitudes towards older people in Taiwan: Scale development and preliminary evidence of reliability and validity. J Educ Psychol 2009;32: 147-71.

[20] Lin MJ. College students' attitudes toward elderly. J Educ Psychol 1993;16: 349-84.

[21] Lu L, Kao SF, Hsieh YH. Positive attitudes toward older people and well-being among Chinese community older adult. J Appl Gerontol 2010; 29(5): 622-39.

[22] Lu L, Kao SF. Attitudes towards old people and their relation to career choices among Taiwanese university students. J. Educ Psychol 2010;33:33-54.

[23] Lu L, Kao SF, Hsieh YH. Attitudes towards older people and managers' intention to hire older workers: A Taiwanese study. Educ Gerontol 2011; 37(10):835-53.

[24] Lu L. Employment among older workers and inequality of gender and education: Evidence from a Taiwanese national survey. Int J Ageing Hum Dev 2010;70:145-62.

[25] Lu L, Chen HH. An exploratory study on role adjustment and intergenerational relationships among the elderly in the changing Taiwan. Res Appl Psychol 2002;14:221-49.

[26] Erikson EH. The life circle completed. New York: Norton, 1982.

[27] Lu L, Hu CH. Experiencing leisure: The case of Chinese university students. Fu Jen Stud Sci Engineering 2002;36:1-21.

[28] Bowling A. Enhancing later life: How older people perceive active ageing? Aging Ment Health 2008;12: 293-301.

[29] Rundek T, Bennett DA. Cognitive leisure activities, but not watching TV, for future brain benefits. Neurol 2006;66:794-95.

[30] McKenna K, Broome K, Liddle J. What older people do: Time use and exploring the link between role participation and life satisfaction in people aged 65 years and over. Aust Occup Ther J 2007;54:273-84.

[31] Chen CN. Older people's leisure and quality of life in Taiwan. J Popul 2003; 26:96-136.

[32] Silverstein M, Parker MG. Leisure activities and quality of life among the oldest old in Sweden. Res Aging 2002;24:528-47.

[33] Arai A, Ishida K, Tomimori M, Katsumata Y, Grove JS, Tamashiro H. Association between lifestyle activity and depressed mood among home-dwelling older people: A community-based study in Japan. Aging Ment Health 2007;11:547-55.

[34] Beard JG, Ragheb MG. Measuring leisure satisfaction. J Leis Res 1980;12: 20-33.

[35] Argyle M. The social psychology of leisure. London: Penguin Books, 1996.

[36] Lu L, Hu CH. Personality, leisure experiences and happiness. J Happiness Stud 2005;6:325-42.

[37] Pressman SD, Matthews KA, Cohen S, Martire LM, Scheier M, Baum A, Schulz R. Association of enjoyable leisure activities with psychological and physical well-being. Psychosom Med 2009;71: 725-32.

[38] Fu YC, Lu L, Chen SY. Differentiating personal facilitators of leisure participation: Socio-demographics, personality traits, and the need for sociability. J Tour Leis Stud 2009;15:187-212.

[39] Huang LH. A path analysis of correlates of the life satisfaction among the elderly. J Nurs 1992;39: 37-47.

[40] Lu L, Chang CJ. Support, health and satisfaction among the elderly with chronic conditions in Taiwan. J Health Psychol 1997;2:471-80.

[41] Cheek NH, Burch WR. The social organization of leisure in human society. New York: Harper Row, 1976.

[42] Iso-Ahola SE, Park CJ. Leisure-related social support and self-determination as buffers of stress-illness relationship. J Leis Res 1996;28:169-87.

[43] Fratiglioni L, Paillard-Borg S, Winblad B. An active and socially integrated lifestyle in late life might protect against dementia. Lancet Neurol 2004;3: 343-53.

[44] Litwin H. Activity, social network, and well-being: An empirical examination. Can J Aging 2000;19:343-62.

Aging and quality of life in Taiwan 269

[45] Duay D, Bryan V. Senior adults' perceptions of successful aging. Educ Gerontol 2006;32:423-45.

[46] Harahousou Y. Leisure and ageing. In: Rojek C, Shaw SM, Veal AJ. A Handbook of Leisure Studies. New York: Palgrave Macmillan, 2006:231-49.

[47] Sellar B, Boshoff K. Subjective leisure experiences of older Australians. Aust Occup Ther J 2006;53:211-19.

[48] Lu L. Leisure experiences and depressive symptoms among Chinese older people: A national survey in Taiwan. Educ Gerontol 2011;37:753-71.

[49] Hanson BS, Isacsson S, Janzon L, Lindell S. Social network and social support influence mortality in elderly men. Am J Epidemiol 1989:130(1): 100-11.

[50] Rowe J, Kahn R. Successful ageing. New York: Random House, 1998.

[51] Lu L, Argyle M. TV watching, soap opera and happiness. Kaohsiung J Med Sci 1993;9:350-60.

[52] Lu L, Argyle M. Leisure satisfaction and happiness as a function of leisure activity. Kaohsiung J Med Sci 1994;10:89-96.

[53] Smith TW, Kim J, Koch A, Park A. Social-science research and the General Social Surveys. ZUMA-Nachr 2005;56:68-77.

[54] Laditka SB, Fischer M, Laditka JK, Segal DR. Attitudes about aging and gender among young, middle age, and older college-based students. Educ Gerontol 2004;30:403-21.

[55] Antonucci TC, Jackson JS. Social support, interpersonal efficacy, and health: A life course perspective. In: Carstensen LL, Edelstein, AA. Handbook of clinical gerontology. New York: Pergamon Press, 1987:291-311.

[56] Holahan CJ, Moos RH. Personality, coping, and family resources in stress resistance: A longitudinal analysis. J Pers Soc Psychol 1986;51:389-95.

[57] Kahn RL, Antonucci TC. Convoys over the life course: Attachment, roles, and social support. In: Baltes PB, Brim JOG. Life-span development and behavior. New York: Academic Press 1980:253-86.

Submitted: October 12, 2011. *Revised:* November 26, 2011. *Accepted:*December 06, 2011.

In: Alternative Medicine Research Yearbook 2012
Editors: Søren Ventegodt and Joav Merrick

ISBN: 978-1-62808-080-3
© 2013 Nova Science Publishers, Inc.

Chapter 29

INTERPLAY BETWEEN MOOD AND PHYSICAL ACTIVITY AND THEIR EFFECT ON LIFE SATISFACTION IN LATER LIFE

Jessica Jones, MD*
and Natalie Wakefield, MD
Department of Psychiatry, University of Oklahoma, Tulsa, Oklahoma, US

ABSTRACT

The aging of the baby boomer generation predicts a significant growth in the American geriatric population. Caring for this population will continue to be a challenge in the coming years for healthcare providers. The aim of this paper is to explore the relationship between life satisfaction, mood, and exercise. Depressive symptoms increase with age and are underdiagnosed due to multiple factors. Depressed mood leads to difficulty in achieving developmental tasks and impacts life satisfaction. Using exercise as treatment and prevention of depression approaches a complex problem in several ways including physical health benefits, social interaction, improvement in mental health, and providing opportunities for mentorship. This approach from a biological, psychological, and social model aims to help older adults age well and live with improved life satisfaction.

Keywords: Mental health, quality of life, life satisfaction, mood, public health

INTRODUCTION

The aging of the baby boomer generation predicts a significant growth in the American geriatric population. Older adults face many challenges in late life including physical and mental health problems, role transitions, and a changing social environment. Almost 20% of older adults will experience mental illness, with depressive disorders being common. For

---

* Correspondence: Jessica Jones, MD, Department of Psychiatry, University of Oklahoma,Tulsa, Oklahoma, United States of America. E-mail: Jessica-Jones@ouhsc.edu.

some, this represents reactivation of previously controlled depressive symptoms. For others, new symptoms may emerge. It is thus imperative for those in the healthcare field to understand how they can best mitigate the challenges of aging and promote life satisfaction among our elders. The goal of this chapter is to explore the relationship between life satisfaction, mood, and exercise, in the older adult. In understanding the connection between mood and exercise, the goal is to outline the role of exercise in the treatment and prevention of depression to improve life satisfaction in older adults.

Life satisfaction, or the subjective assessment of one's well-being, can be measured in a variety of ways. This can include cognitive aspects as well as affective aspects of one's life (1).There are many theories about what constitutes life satisfaction. Trait theorists contend that one's life satisfaction is stable and independent of an individual's current situation but is closely linked to personality. However, need theorists propose that well-being is linked to having one's needs met. In Maslow's hierarchical needs model, individuals cannot focus on higher level needs if basic needs are not met (2). Thus, if activities of daily living such as bathing, toileting, and dressing cannot be accomplished independently, life satisfaction is likely to be negatively impacted. Activity theorists suggest that satisfaction is obtained through engaging in activities and making progress towards a new goal. In later life, the opportunity for new goals and activities may be seen as limited or difficult to integrate into one's routine.

Not only is life satisfaction influenced by environment, but also by genetics. It is important to consider the genetic influence of one's view of the world and his or her place in it (1). Evidence shows that people have a genetic disposition to be happy or unhappy. This genetic influence shades how he or she perceives experiences throughout the lifetime. In addition, life events appear to have a role in life satisfaction. Some theorists have shown that there appears to be a set point that is likely biologically determined. Although life events such as illness may skew one's life satisfaction, with time a person will gravitate back to this predetermined point (1). However, this set point is not absolute throughout life. Drastic changes in life such as a spinal cord injury or winning the lottery can alter the set point to a new level. In the later years of life, challenges of chronic illness and loss of a spouse may alter the set point to a lower level of life satisfaction. Thus, it appears that genetics, personality, basic needs, life experiences, and new activities interplay to produce life satisfaction at any given point in time.

In older adults, depression can have a large impact on affect and cognition and,therefore, on life satisfaction. Depressive symptoms such as lack of motivation and energy can make it difficult to engage in activities and set new goals. Significant life events in older age such as loss of a spouse, chronic illnesses, and loss of functioning not only confers risk of depression, but also can skew the set point of life satisfaction to a lower point. Depression can also impact one's ability to attend to basic needs which in turn hinders life satisfaction. In conceptualizing life satisfaction in the older adults, there are several points of intervention that can improve one's subjective assessment of well-being. This chapter focuses on exercise as the vehicle to address these points of intervention.

Both physical and mental health are important in understanding life satisfaction in the older adults. Quality of life is influenced by one's physical health status. In those between ages of 65-84, the prevalence of chronic health conditions ranges from 40% to 70% (2). There is a substantial body of evidencethat suggest physical health is a key determinant in life satisfaction. However, Deeg showed that while physical health is important to older men and women, there are other aspects such as faith, family, and relationships that influence quality of life (2). Health- related quality of life measures do not often take these other aspects into consideration. In addition to physical health, marriage was ranked second in life satisfaction and mental health was ranked as third most important in overall well-being. Among those who had few physical health problems, good mental health was considered more important. Research also suggests that older adults feel that the loss of physical health was bearable if their mental health remained well (2). Therefore, physical health appears to be one aspect of the global assessment of life satisfaction in older adults. Other aspects of life satisfaction such as marriage, family, and mental health are also important.

It is imperative to explore the aspects of life satisfaction in older adults as the rate of growth in this population is quickly rising and the impact of this population is great. By 2030, the number of older Americans is expected to double from 35 million to 70 million. The percentage of the total population that is aged 65 or older is expected to grow from 12% in 2000 to 20% in 2030 (3). By 2030, the American population will spend 25% more on health care than it does today. According to the Agency for Healthcare Research and Quality2009 report, total healthcare expenses for Americans age 45 to 64 in 2006 were $370 billion (4). This represents a doubling of the healthcare expenditures over just 10 years. Chronic conditions are responsible for half of all healthcare spending for non-institutionalized persons. Expenditures for chronic conditions increased from 31.7% for persons 0-17 years of age to more than 50% for those aged 45 and over (5).

Physical exercise plays a crucial role in maintaining health in older adults, by preventing and managing chronic illnesses and indirectly controlling healthcare expenditures. In a study conducted by King et al. between 1988 and 2006, 7,340 adults from 89 communities across the US, 40-74 years of age were surveyed regarding five healthy habits (6). Over time, adherence to healthy habits, including maintaining a healthy body weight, eating recommended fruits and vegetables, abstaining from tobacco, using alcohol moderately, and exercising regularly, decreased significantly. Particularly, participation in regular physical exercise fell significantly across ethnicity and gender from 1988 to 2006. Over this period, obesity rates and chronic disease rates increased significantly. Despite evidence and widespread dissemination of information across mainstream media that these healthy habits can reduce morbidity and mortality in chronic illnesses like diabetes, cardiovascular disease, hypertension, and hyperlipidemia across mainstream media, participation in healthy habits significantly decreased in individuals with these chronic diseases during the study's 24-year period. In a 1993 study, 14% of all deaths in the United States were attributed to insufficient activity and inadequate nutrition (7). Data from the Centers for Disease Control and Prevention (CDC) indicate that about up to 34% of adults aged 65 to 74 and up 44% of adults ages 75 or older are inactive, meaning they engage in no leisure-time physical activity. Inactivity is more common in older adults than their middle-aged counterparts and women are more likely than men to report no leisure-time activity (3). The cardiac risk of being inactive is comparable to the risk from smoking cigarettes (3). Clearly, the evidence is robust for the physical and mental health benefits of exercise; however, translating that data into an intervention to help improve quality of life presents a challenge. By understanding the complexities of the relationships among exercise, mental health and life satisfaction in older adults and recognizing the barriers that impede participation in activities that promote well-being, health care professionals may be more effective in promoting positive behavior change and thereby improve life satisfaction in older adults.

DEPRESSION

In older adults, mental illness is underreported and undertreated. Almost 20% of individuals 55 years or older experience mental disorders that are not a normal part of the aging process. The American Association for Geriatric Psychiatry lists the most common disorders in older adults as anxiety disorders, severe cognitive impairment, and mood disorders. The rate of utilization for mental health is lower in the elderly population than other adult age groups (8). It is estimated that half of older adults who acknowledge mental health problems receive treatment from a health care provider. Moreover, an even smaller number of individuals who acknowledge mental health problems receive specialty mental health services (8). The lack of adequate recognition and treatment of mental illness in older adults presents a large public health problem, as these illnesses have a significant impact not only on the patient and caregiver, but also on society.

As stated previously, depression can be a major determinant in the level of life satisfaction a person has with his or her life. This chapter focuses on unipolar depression in older adults. Bipolar depression and mania, while important, are outside the scope of this discussion. Unipolar depression has high comorbidity, high disability and high lethality. The suicide rate for the elderly is higher that of any other age group. For those individuals 85 and older, the suicide rate is the highest at twice the national average (8). Although the rate of major depression declines with age, depressive symptoms increase. It is estimated that 6% of Americans 65 years of age and older in a given year have a diagnosable depressive illness. A study by Katon showed that 11% of depressed patients in primary care settings receive adequate antidepressant treatment, 34% received inadequate treatment and 55% received no treatment (9). Several studies have shown that older adults visit a primary care physician very close to the time they commit suicide (10). It appears that older adults seek help from health care providers prior to suicide; however, clinicians fail to recognize the severity of the patient's symptoms. Therefore, understanding the biological, psychological, and social factors that leads to depression in later life helps identify points of recognition, intervention and prevention.

BIOLOGICAL FACTORS

Biological aspects of depression are quite significant in older adults. While the genetic predisposition for mental illness remains constant over a lifetime, one's physical health can change dramatically. Physical illness is a major risk factor for depression. The overlap in symptoms of physical illness and the neurovegetative symptoms of depression has made research of depression in older adults difficult. Moreover, there is evidence to suggest that some illnesses confer more biological etiology such as congestive heart failure and others such as chronic pulmonary disease appears to have more psychological etiology (11). This suggests that specific co-morbid illnesses are important to consider when tailoring treatment. Some co-morbid illness may require a biological approach while others will require a more psychological approach. Physical illness has been shown to be a major predictor of poorer outcomes and non-response to treatment as well (12).

Adding to the challenge of identifying depression in the older adults is the different presentation they may have compared to younger adults. While younger age groups may present with initial complaint of low mood or anhedonia, older adults typically report a lack of emotions (13). Other symptoms of depression in older adults are more prominent than in younger populations includes somatic complaints and psychomotor changes. These symptoms also have overlap with chronic medical illness, which again makes recognition difficult (13). Moreover, the presence of pain in older adults also contributes to depressive symptoms and may delay the diagnosis of depression. A systematic review by Cole and Dendukuri found five risk factors for depression in the elderly: bereavement, sleep disturbance, disability, prior depression and female gender (12). Bereavement, sleep disturbance, and disability are modifiable risk factors and should be considered points of treatment and prevention for depression. Bereavement can be addressed through social interventions and therapy. Sleep disturbance and disability have overlap with chronic co-morbid illness, and may be modifiable with physical activity interventions as discussed in the later part of this paper.

PSYCHOLOGICAL FACTORS

Psychological aspects of depression in the elderly are also important to consider. Numerous theories have been outlined regarding adult development and it is not the goal of this chapter to comprehensively review these; rather, this chapter focuses on several aspects that may illustrate the concepts that relate to aging. Jose' Ortega y Gasset, a Spanish historian-philosopher, wrote the bookMan and Crisisthat outlined human developmental stages from a combined individual and generational perspective (14). The stages were childhood (age 0 to 15 years), youth (age 15 to 30), initiation (age 30-45), dominant (age 45-60), and old age (age 60 +). These roughly correspond to Erikson's stages of development, discussed in his work Childhood and Society (15). Old age corresponds to Erikson's stage eight, "integrity versus despair." Initiation and dominant stages corresponds to Erikson's"generativity versus stagnation."

Some of the developmental issues particularly relevant to the older population and highlighted by these two developmental theorists are the movement into generativity rather than stagnation; the transition from a junior member of society (initiation) with little influence and power, to more a senior member (dominant) having influence and more responsibility for mentorship. Some of the central tasks of this stage transition include adjusting to physical changes of middle adulthood, achieving civic, social responsibilities, and using leisure time creatively. The next transition, from dominant to old age, represented by the Erikson stage ego integrity versusdespair describes a person's final developmental stage. The central task of this stage is to reflect on life and use wisdom to integrate life's events into a narrative from which to draw satisfaction. In each of the transitions to dominant and old age, there is a need to redefine roles, participate in new role, and interact socially with the younger generation. The biological changes that occur through this period of life also play a significant part in development. Finding ways to be physically active through and during these transitions and participating with those in one's current phase as well as those in other phases, can promote healthy transition and participation in development. Those who fail to transition well are at risk for depressive symptoms. Moreover, those who failed to successfully navigate earlier development are at a higher risk for not successfully navigating these transitions. When depressive symptoms arise, it is important to consider the psychological areas of life or developmental stage that could be contributing to one's current symptoms. Exercise groups can be a point of intervention in the development of one's life narrative.

SOCIAL FACTORS

Considering the social aspect of one's environment is also essential when formulating and designing treatment for depression in older adults. Factors of social isolation and stressful life events confer a high risk of depression in older adults (16). The complex interplay between social interaction and its benefits to health and cognition are difficult to study. Although the mechanism of social interactions on the brain is not entirely clear, three possible mechanism of protection have been proposed (16). First, social interactions may have effects on multiple bodily systems, including cognition, endocrine, and neuromuscular. Contact and collaboration with others confers positive changes in the brain and body. Moreover, some social interactions can also be integrated with exercise leading to increased health benefits. Secondly, social interaction may be a marker for helpful coping skills. Those individuals who are able to maintain relationships through social interaction likely have positive ways of dealing with stress. Thirdly, social interaction could reinforce patterns of attachment. The need to form loving, secure relationships with others is fundamental. Social interaction could be reinforcing those attachments or giving opportunity for a new pattern of more adaptive attachment. As discussed previously, older adults have a developmental need to create relationships for mentorship. Social interaction may provide older adults the avenue to work out this role transition. These domains may also reinforce one another (16). As it relates to depression, social interaction can provide support, encouragement, new perspective, and give opportunity for pleasurable activities. Given that part of the symptomatology of depression is reduction in social interaction, and that older adults are at risk for social isolation, it is imperative to consider this modality in treatment and prevention. Barriers to social interaction in older adults include sensory decline and transportation (17). Thus, being creative in the approach to increased social interaction is important. Although disability can be a barrier for social interaction, studies have shown social activity to decrease risk of further disability in older adults (17). In considering points of intervention to prevent depression, social activity is a modifiable risk factor that could not only improve mental health, but disability status as well.

TREATMENT

Treatment of depression in the older adults requires a different approach than in younger populations. As outlined previously, co-morbid illness, pain, social support, nutrition, and sleep are important aspects to consider for intervention alongside pharmacotherapy. Treatment of depression starts with education for the patient so that they can be involved in their own recovery. Increasing coping skills and understanding the triggers that lead to negative thought patterns can improve insight and depressive symptoms (13). Alongside education and lifestyle modification, treatment options include pharmacotherapy, interpersonal therapy, cognitive-behavioral therapy, and electroconvulsive therapy. In the older adults, the motto of pharmacotherapy treatment is start low and go slow. Older adults typically require lower antidepressant dosage to reach effective blood levels (13). However, even with adequate treatment, less than 50% of older patients respond adequately to first line anti-depressants (18). Also, older adults have a higher rate of relapse (19). Therefore, continued treatment and ongoing evaluation of symptoms is highly important in older adults. Since the older adults are at higher risk with co-morbid illness, have less response to treatment, and higher rates of relapse, it is vital that the focus of health care providers be multimodal. This chapter highlights exercise as an optimal augmentation strategy for depression in the older adults. The ability of exercise to improve depressive symptoms, reduce disability, allow for developmental tasks, and increase social interaction leads to improved life satisfaction.

PHYSICAL EXERCISE

As discussed earlier, the key developmental task in later adulthood is integrating one's life story into an acceptable narrative. Mood stability is important to accurate and positive evaluation of one's life story. Regular physical activity through later adulthood improves independence of activities of daily living, general health, and mood, in turn increasing autonomy, improving self-efficacy, and sense of control over one's life and secondarily life satisfaction and well-being. Exercise may help to set the stage for a more positive evaluation of one's life both present and past.

In order to promote exercise as an intervention for depression, it is important to understand the factors that affect participation in exercise. Determinates of participation in exercise include age, gender, type of activity, accessibility of facilities, and exercise self-efficacy (20). Older women are less likely to exercise than older men. Older adults of lower socioeconomic status (SES) and education have lower exercise self-efficacy and expectations than those with middle SES and education. Better perceived health, lower degree of functional impairment, and delayed onset of chronic disease appears to influence attitudes toward exercise and thereby likelihood to participate in regular exercise (21). Evidence demonstrates that exercise improves these factors and may create a positive feedback loop in which those who exercise are more likely to continue to exercise. Those with social support for exercise are more likely to engage and continue participation. The modifiable variables to increasing participation in exercise include: type of exercise, access to exercise facilities, exercise self-efficacy, outcome expectations, and social support.

Research over the past 30 years has led to the emerging idea that exercise is a key component in attaining life satisfaction in later life. Myriad hypotheses have been proposed as to the nature of this relationship and numerous factors have been found that significantly influence the correlation of exercise and life satisfaction in older adults. Physical activity influences biological, psychological, and social factors that influence life satisfaction. The relationships between physical activity and life satisfaction are complicated. Physical activity improves mood, general health, functionality, and social relationships. Simultaneously, these factors influence likelihood to participate in physical activity. The challenge to utilize these relationships in order to develop interventions to improve life satisfaction is great, however, understanding of the relationships and how to implement that information into practice exists.

BIOLOGICAL FACTORS

The physiological benefits to physical activity have been well documented. Prevention of chronic diseases, improvement in chronic diseases, and maintenance and improvement of function can be attributed to regular physical activity.

Adults age 45 and older who participate in at least 30 minutes of moderate physical activity on five or more days a week or at least 20 minutes of vigorous physical activity on three or more days a week had significantly fewer mentally and physically unhealthy days per month than those engaged in less physical activity according to data collected from the 2001 Behavioral Risk Factor Surveillance System survey (22).

In regard to prevention, leisure time activity is more important for protecting against heart disease in men over 65 than in younger men (23). Data from AHRQ publication, Prevention of Chronic Diseases, demonstrates that regular exercise is effective in the prevention of colon cancer, diabetes, hypertension, and obesity. Regular physical activity reduces risk of falls and injury in older adults. Exercise interventions reduce morbidity of active chronic diseases such as hypertension, depression and arthritis. Individuals involved in regular physical activity have greater survival rates and maintain functionality and independence at greater rates into older age than sedentary adults (3). Prevention of chronic illness and management of existing chronic illnesses through regular physical activity significantly impacts rates of depression in older adults as discussed earlier in the chapter. When to initiate exercise for improvement of life satisfaction becomes of concern when utilizing exercise in a treatment plan.

A cohort of 1,861 Jerusalem residents born in 1920-1921 was surveyed at ages 70, 78, and 85 years (24). The study found that adults who participated in 4 or more hours of physical activity a week, vigorous sports twice a week, or physical activity for at least one hour daily had significantly greater survival rates through age 88 years, maintained greater functionality and independence in performing activities of daily living, were less lonely, and viewed themselves as healthier than adults engaging less than four hours of physical activity weekly. There was a sustained protective effect of physical activity against functional decline. These associations were significant after adjusting for differences in sex, baseline function, and common chronic diseases. Of note, physical activity, even if initiated in later life, has significant association with survival and maintenance of function. Another study showed that among older white women the most recent physical activity levels were more important predictors of longevity than past levels (25). It appears that remaining or starting to be physically active into late adulthood increases likelihood of living longer and staying functionally independent. The idea that it is never too late to begin, instills new hope into what it means to age.

Physical activity is a broad concept and incorporates many different activities of various intensity, duration and frequency. The type of exercise individuals are capable of is determined in part by levels of ability, physical fitness and health co-morbidities. A variety of activities have been found to significantly improve health, functionality, mood, and life

Interplay between mood and physical activity and their effect ... 279

satisfaction. Guidelines for adults age 65 years and older recommend 30 minutes of moderately intense aerobic exercise five days a week. This activity can be accumulated through the day in 10 minute sessions (26). Moderate amount of activity is defined as at least 30 minutes of brisk walking for five or more days of the week, and provides substantial health benefits. To prevent falls, older people need to participate in exercises that promote strength and endurance at least two days a week. Exercises to enhance and maintain flexibility are also recommended (3). Regular activity appears to be more effective than less frequent strenuous activity to improve health and function in older adults (3). Recommended exercises for those with mobility problems include swimming, water exercises, and stretching. Focused strength training and games to help improve function in activities of daily living as well as gentle yoga and tai chi are recommended to improve and maintain functionality (3). Putting these guidelines into practice is difficult in light of the many factors involved in adherence to interventions and barriers to activity that older adults face. Similar to the life satisfaction set point, there is evidence for a physical exercise set point. Studies demonstrate that older adults are likely to have a fairly stable physical activity pattern over middle years (6). Programs that target and attempt to change this set point are essential if we are to have an impact on increasing physical activity and indirectly life satisfaction in older age.

EVIDENCE-BASED EXERCISE PROGRAMS

Numerous exercise treatment programs have been developed in response to the need to translate the research on exercise into a treatment intervention. The Seattle Protocol for Activity in older adults is a nine-session, home-based program that has demonstrated significant success in implementing exercise behaviors and subsequently improving life satisfaction in older adults in a randomized control trial (27). The intervention included instruction in warm-up/cool-down, progressive resistance training with elastic tubing, balance and flexibility training, and recommendation for aerobic training such as walking 30 minutes daily. Classes emphasized safety, making exercise enjoyable, long-term benefits of exercise and benefit to improving independence of activities of daily living. Instruction regarding scheduling challenges and overcoming physical limitations was also included. The program had a lower rate of attrition over 18 months as compared to other community-based programs. Participants in the Seattle protocol program exercised more often, had better general health, greater sense of self control and a higher quality of life after 3 months and maintained improvements at 18 months when compared with those enrolled in health promotion classes or receiving routine healthcare alone. The unique feature of this protocol is that it is a home-based physical activity program. The groups most at risk for not meeting recommended guidelines for leisure-time physical activity (greater than or equal to 1000 kcal/week) were older women, individuals with a lower socioeconomic status, and those with physical impairments. These are the groups at increased risk for difficulty with transportation to exercise centers and for which cost of training classes or equipment may be prohibitive. A home-based program could help those least likely to exercise overcome these barriers. Also, the fact that improvement was maintained at over 18 months may be an important clue as to how exercise might play a role in maintenance of remission in depression. The Seattle

Protocol could provide a guide for implementation of programs for the most at risk individuals.

Among other exercise programs targeting older adults, the Silver Yoga program is promising. In a randomized control trial of 139 adults ages 60 or older, participation in Silver Yoga for 70 minutes three times a week for six months significantly improved sleep quality, physical health perception, mental health perception, daytime dysfunction, and depression state at 3 months and 6 months during the program (28). Silver Yoga was developed by Chen for older adults (29). It is a program that incorporates warm-up, static postures, hatha yoga techniques, gentle stretching, progressive muscle relaxation, guided-imagery and abdominal breathing. The program is less strenuous than traditional yoga practices to accommodate for reduced flexibility in older adults. Among the strengths of this study is the focus on improvement in sleep, an important factor in remission of depression. Improvement in physical and mental health perception contributes to positive assessment of one's life and thereby can improve life satisfaction and sense of well-being.

As communities seek to implement exercise programs for senior adults, the cost of equipment, staff, and facilities becomes a concern. As discussed above, transportation for older adults can be a prohibitive factor in exercise participation. Programs that effectively promote lifestyle change, yet limit cost to the community and individuals are needed. In a translational study of the Active for Life (AFL) and Active Living Every Day (ALED) programs, participation in the programs increased moderate to vigorous physical activity, improved satisfaction with body appearance and function, reduced body mass index, decreased depressive symptoms and reduced perceived stress (30). Participants from 12 diverse community sites across the US were chosen for the participation in the study. For the AFL program, 2503 individuals with an average age of 65.8 years participated and in the ALED program, 3388 individuals with an average age of 70.6 years participated. The programs incorporated social cognitive theory into a lifestyle behavior change program. The ALED program provided group-based instruction targeting lifestyle behavior change to increase participation in exercise over 20 weeks. In the AFL program, one face-to-face meeting with subsequent telephone counseling calls was provided. The focus of the curriculum was setting expectations for regular exercise, formulation of plans and goals with consideration of interests, addressing perceived barriers and benefits to exercise and safety. This study provides a framework for development of programs that can be replicated at a wide variety of settings for a diverse range of older adults. The program required little travel for participants and staff, little investment in equipment and facilities, and limited staff, but resulted in big dividends for healthier, happier participants, and lower healthcare costs for communities.

SOCIAL ASPECTS

Exercise groups and partners can provide encouragement and incentive to regularly engage in physical activity. Barriers to activity in older adults include transportation problems and safety concerns. Exercise groups can help individuals overcome these barriers (3). Role models with similar characteristic to older adults can influence individuals to improve adherence to exercise program (20). Verbal encouragement becomes more important in later

Interplay between mood and physical activity and their effect ...

life for adults to engage in physical activity. Normalizing expectations for physical symptoms during initiation of exercise may increase continuation of exercise. For example, muscle aches, breathlessness, and fatigue may lead to negative evaluation of one's ability to achieve exercise goals. However, challenging this belief and reevaluating expectations of symptoms may lead to more positive evaluation of ability and progress toward the exercise goal. Older adults may find it difficult to find role models of similar age and ability in which to inspire them to exercise. Exercise groups such as running groups, classes, hiking clubs, and senior centers bring together peers with similar goals. Exercise groups also are an opportunity for older adult to interact with those with differing ages and abilities. They may establish relationships within these groups that will help them complete the developmental task of mentoring the younger generation in the "generativity versusstagnation" stage of Erikson's developmental model (16).

The social aspects of exercise also influence the psychological factors involved in exercise. In a study of 309 German adults age 65 years or older, those with support for exercise from friends, acquaintances, and neighbors engaged in more frequent exercise (31). Those with greater self-efficacy engaged in more frequent exercise as well. There existed a synergistic relationship between self-efficacy and social support. Individuals with high levels of either self-efficacy or social support for exercise with low levels of the other factor did not exercise as frequently as those with moderate level of both characteristics. Exercise interventions that target social and psychological aspects simultaneously are more likely to be effective for older adults.

PSYCHOLOGICAL FACTORS

As adults move into the later years of their lives, psychological needs are met less from external resources than from internal resources, such as memories and accomplishments. It is imperative to take into account the developmental stage of the participant to appreciate his or her psychological needs. Whether an exercise intervention is successful is determined by its effectiveness in addressing the psychological needs of the participant. This point is illustrated by a study of centenarians. In analysis of the Georgia Centenarian Study by Oklahoma State University researcher Alex J Bishop, MD, factors associated with happiness were explored. Satisfaction with life in the past was directly associated with current happiness (32). Perceived health, economic status, and social provisions, particularly social support were not significant predictors of happiness in centenarians as they are in younger adults. This appears to be consistent with the task of forming an acceptable life narrative during Erikson's stage of Ego Integrity in late adulthood (15). Notably, most centenarians have successfully delayed impairment and disease until late in life. The maintenance of function and relatively good health of those that live for a century may allow those individuals to more positively assess their past life and current well-being. One may draw the conclusion that happiness and satisfaction with life in late adulthood is associated with a relatively healthy, active life in which one is able to achieve goals and have life experiences on which one can reflect and use to produce an acceptable life narrative.

Dutch anthropologist Arnold van Gennep examined the life cycle from a societal perspective and wrote about rites of passage to assist individuals' transition from one phase of life to the next (33). Much anxiety is involved in the transition from childhood to adolescence and adolescence to adulthood. Similarly, the transition from middle adulthood to late adulthood provokes profound anxiety. Daniel Levinson in his book "The season of a woman's life", hypothesized that "rituals provide a collective vehicle for gaining personal control over anxieties that such transitions generate" (34). Psychiatric pathology, preexisting but in remission, may become exacerbated in these transitions. As is often seen in psychiatric offices and psychiatric hospitals, individuals struggling with the anxiety and role confusion inherent in the transition through phases of the life cycle become distraught, hopeless, and sadly, at times end their lives prematurely. As society evolves and changes, these rites of passage are often themselves in flux or eroded. There is a need to maintain old rites or develop meaningful new rites that individuals may utilize during transition. Exercise groups, amateur running groups, water aerobics groups, hiking clubs and the like, can provide social structure and mentorship opportunities in late adulthood. The multi-generational aspects of these groups, as well as the various levels of physical ability, provide opportunities for older adults in the dominant phase to fulfill the developmental task of mentoring those in the initiation phase. These groups also provide those in old ageopportunity to integrate their life narrative by sharing wisdom through coaching others, utilizing wisdom in their own exercise routine, and testing physical limitations. Exercise becomes the stage on which role fulfillment can be enacted. Individuals who partake in exercise groups are afforded the opportunities to both participate in rites of passage into a new life phase and fulfill their role in that new life phase, and thus are more satisfied with their lives.

TREATMENT PLAN

Mental health is essential to achieving life satisfaction through the life span. As discussed previously depression is a common disorder that significantly impacts older adults. Much evidence exists demonstrating the efficacy of exercise to improve depression. Thirty minutes of moderate to vigorous exercise on all or most days per week has antidepressant effect. It has been shown to effectively improve mild to moderate clinical depression symptoms in adults and particularly aerobic exercise improves symptoms in a dose-response relationship. There is some evidence that aerobic exercise alone can effectively improve depressive symptoms (35). A meta-analysis of 11 randomized, controlled trials supports the use of exercise as an effective intervention for clinical depression (36,37).

The intensity of the exercise intervention is associated with improved mood. In a randomized control trial, progressive resistance training over 10 weeks for older adults with depression and dysthymia significantly improved depression as measured by the Beck Depression Inventory and Hamilton Rating Scale for Depression (38). In a subsequent study, of older adults age 60 or older with depression Singh found that higher intensity progressive resistance training reduced Hamilton Rating Scale for Depression scores more than twice as much as low-intensity resistance training or standard care by a general practitioner alone (49). Exercise as an adjunct to pharmacological treatment for depression may contribute to sustained, long-term recovery (40). Older adults who participated in regular weight lifting over 20 weeks had significantly lower Beck Depression Inventory scores than controls and sustained improved depression scores over 26 months (41).This finding is extraordinary in that it demonstrates a long-term effect on mood symptoms from a time-limited program of vigorous regular exercise.

The treatment plan must be tailored to the individual's severity of depression. Exercise as a treatment or augmentation strategy to pharmacological and psychotherapeutic treatments for mild to moderate depression is more effective than standard treatment alone. However, it must be noted that more severe depression in older adults responds more quickly to medication management (42). Barriers to exercise in severely depressed adults due to mood symptoms such as low energy and motivation and poor sleep may be too great for the individual to overcome to achieve the intensity and frequency threshold needed for a significant effect on mood. Therefore, medication and psychotherapy interventions should always be considered for inclusion into a treatment plan for individuals suffering from severe depression.

Major barriers to achieving adequate participation in exercise are psychological in nature. Attitudes toward exercise have particular importance in predicting involvement in exercise for older adults who face physical disability, chronic illnesses, and misconceptions about ageing and perceived physical ability. According to writing by Bandura, behavior change and maintenance of that change are influenced by self-efficacy and outcome expectations (43). According to Self-Efficacy theory, the strength of the individual's belief in their ability to perform a task predicts the likelihood of the individual to initiate and continue the activity. Outcome expectations are the expected outcomes from a behavior. A number of studies show that use of cognitive-behavioral approaches for implementing lifestyle change are more effective than health education, exercise prescriptions, or instruction alone (27,29,30). Small, achievable goals are highly effective to increase confidence and adherence to exercise programs in the early stage of participation in older adults. Tailored exercise interventions targeting functionality, mood, chronic diseases, and individualized goal-setting are particularly effective to improve participation in exercise (20). These findings point to the effectiveness of modifying beliefs in regard to outcomes expectations and self-efficacy to achieve recommended levels of exercise in older adults. Interventions targeting specific self-esteem toward one's body, health, and specific behaviors may play important roles in self-efficacy and outcome expectations (21). The literature points to self-efficacy, self-esteem and self-sufficiency as key psychological constructs that simultaneously contribute to involvement in exercise and improve with involvement in exercise. These characteristics are also vital to maintaining mood and satisfaction over the life span (44).

EXERCISE + MENTAL HEALTH = LIFE SATISFACTION IN OLDER ADULTS

The concept of quality of life encompasses both life satisfaction and a sense of well-being. There is a great degree of subjectivity involved in an individual's assessment of well-being and satisfaction. In middle to later adulthood, life satisfaction is most strongly influenced by degree of physical disability, depressive mood, and social support (45). Perceived health by older adults influences life satisfaction at rates approaching that of medically defined health (45). Regular exercise participation can improve perception of health and function (28, 29, 30). Prevention and slowing of disability progression is possible with regular exercise. The

Compression of Morbidity concept becomes important when considering life satisfaction in older adults. It suggests that time spent functioning at a high level with limited morbidity burden can be maximized, if disease onset can be delayed and functionality can be maintained. Satisfaction with life may be improved in later years if time spent being sick and disabled can be compressed into a shorter period. The concept has been demonstrated at the Stanford Arthritis Center during a longitudinal study of 537 members of a running club age 50 years and older (46). As compared with age-match controls, members of the running club maintained significantly lower disability levels at eight year follow-up. The ages at which differences were greatest were age 75-79 years. A 20% reduction in musculoskeletal pain and 25% reduction in total medical costs were also observed in the running group. Even after controlling for chronic disease, arthritis, body mass, and smoking, results were still significant. Other forms of selection bias including genetic characteristics, validity of self-report, and rates of development of osteoarthritis were accounted for with the intention-to-treat study design. This study provides strong evidence that vigorous exercise into later life can slow the progression of physical disability and pain without deleterious effects on health. As discussed previously, exercise is effective at improving mood and maintaining mental health through improved self-efficacy and self-esteem. The engagement in physical activity provides a stage on which older adults can participate with others to form supportive social networks, increase and maintain their functionality and independence, improve their sense of satisfaction, and measure success.

FUTURE DIRECTIONS

In light of extensive evidence that regular physical activity significantly improves life satisfaction, morbidity, mortality, and mood in older adults and furthermore has been shown to have a more significant impact in older adults than younger adults, public policies and healthcare organizations would benefit from implementation of programs to increase activity in the older population.Healthcare costs, both directly from utilization of care, and indirectly from lost productivity, would decrease with improvement in adherence to recommended exercise guidelines. The growing rate of inactivity is estimated to cost the U.S. healthcare system $76 billion in year 2000 dollars (47). The challenge is in the translation of the research into practice.

On a community level, developing public policy that emphasizes access to recreational facilities for older adults could increase exercise participation in populations most likely to be sedentary. The US government is a large payer of medical costs for older adults at this time, and costs will continue to grow for older adults as the population ages.

Investment in increasing access to safe parks, pools, and evidence-based exercise programs may decrease costs, and secondarily generate service sector jobs and revenue from more active, productive citizens. On an organization level, several well studied exercise programs have been discussed that could serve as models for communities. The Seattle Protocol, Silver Yoga, Active for Life, and Active Living Every Day programs have incorporated key elements from various studies to target improved compliance, overall health and function as well as mental health in older adults (27,29,30).

On an individual level, incorporating assessments of physical activity into clinical encounters could potentially promote exercise in older adults. According to data from the AHRQ, only half of all adults were asked about physical activity by their healthcare providers and older patients were asked less often than younger patients (3). This is counterintuitive once it is understood that older adults are more sensitive to physical activity as an intervention and are responsive to positive verbal support for exercise.

CONCLUSION

Life satisfaction in later adulthood is a multifaceted concept intricately related to mood and physical activity. Incorporating exercise into the treatment and prevention of late life depression addresses a complex problem in several ways including physical health benefits, social interaction, improvement in mental health, and providing opportunities for mentorship. This approach from a biological, psychological, and social model aims to foster successful aging with improved life satisfaction. With this knowledge, older adults can make changes to live vibrantly in the future.

> Satisfaction lies in the effort, not in the attainment,
> full effort is full victory
> Mahatma Ghandi (1869-1948)

REFERENCES

[1] Diener E, Oishi S, Lucas RE. Subjective well-being: the science of happiness and life satisfaction. In: Snyder CR, Lopez SJ, eds. Oxford handbook of positive psychology, 2nd ed. New York: Oxford University Press, 2009:187-94.

[2] Deeg DJH. Health and quality of life. In: Mollenkopf H, Walker A, eds. Quality of life in old age. International and multidisciplinary perspectives. Heidelberg: Springer, 2007:195-213.

[3] Physical activity and older Americans: Benefits and strategies. Rockville, MD: Agency Healthcare Research Quality, 2002.

[4] Health care spending increases for middle-age Americans. Rockville, MD: Agency Healthcare Research Quality, Rockville, MD. 2009.

[5] Conway P, Goodrich K, Machlin S, Sasse B, Cohen J. Patient-centered care categorization of US health care expenditures. Health Serv Res 2011;46:479-90.

[6] King DE, Mainous AG, Carnemolla M, Everett CJ. Adherence to healthy lifestyle habits in US adults. Am J Med 2009;122(6):528-34.

[7] McGinnis JM, Foege WH. Actual causes of death in the United States. JAMA 1993;270(180);207-12.

[8] American Association for Geriatric Psychiatry. Geriatrics and mental health. The facts. Bethesda, MD: AAGP, 2004.

[9] Katon W, Von Korff M, Lin E, Bush T, Ormel J. Adequacy and duration of antidepressant treatment in primary care. Med Care 1992;30(1):67-76.

[10] Conwell Y. Suicide in later life: A review and recommendation for prevention. J Am Assoc Suicidology 2001;31:32-47.

[11] Koenig HE. Differences between depressed heart failure and pulmonary disease patients. Am J Geriat Psychiatry 2006;14:210-8.

[12] Cole MG, Gendukuri N. Risk factors for depression among elderly community subjects: a systematic review and meta-analysis. Am J Psychiatry 2003;160:1147-56.

[13] Manepalli J, Thaipisuttikul P, Yarnal R. Identifying and treating depression across the life span. Curr Psychiatry 2011;6(10):20-4.

[14] Ortega Y Gasset J. Man and crisis. New York: WW Norton, 1962.

[15] Erikson EH. Childhood and society, 2nd ed. New York: WW Norton, 1964.

[16] Glass TA, De Leon CF, Bassuk SS, Berkman LF. Social disengagement and depressive symptoms in late life: longitudinal findings. J Aging Health 2006;18:604-28.

[17] James BD, Boyle PA, Buchman AS, Bennett, DA. Relation of late-life social activity with incident disability amount community-dwelling older adults. J Gerontol 2011;66A:467-73.

[18] Lenze EJ, Sheffrin M. Driscoll HC, et al. Incomplete response in late-life depression: getting to remission. Diologues Clin Neurosci 2008; 10(4):419-30.

[19] Mueller TI, Kohn R, Leventhal BA, Leon AC, Solomon D, Coryell W, et al. The course of depression in elderly patients. Am J Geriatr Psychiatry 2005;3:22-9.

[20] Lee LL, Arthur A, Avis M. Using self-efficacy theory to develop interventions that help older people overcome psychological barriers to physical activity: A discussion paper. Int J Nurs Stud 2008;45(11):1690-9.

[21] Clark DO. Age, socioeconomic status and exercise self-efficacy. Gerontologist 1996;36(2):157-64.

[22] Brown DW, Balluz LS, et al. Associations between recommended levels of physical activity and health-related quality of life: Findings from the 2001 Behavioral Risk Factor Surveillance System (BRFSS) survey. Prev Med 2003;37:520-8.

[23] Talbot LA, Morrell CH, Metter J, et al. Camparison of cardiorespiratory fitness versus leisure time physical activity as predictors of coronary events in men aged =65 Years and >65 Years. Am J Cardiology 2002;89:1187-92.

[24] Stressman, J, et al. Physical activity, function, and longevity among the very old. Arch Intern Med 2009;169(16):1476-83.

[25] Gregg EW, Cauley JA, Stone K, et al. Study of osteoporotic fractures research group. Relationship of physical activity in relation to mortality among older women. JAMA 2003;289(18):2379-86.

[26] Nelson ME, Rejeski WJ, Blair SN, Duncan PW, Judge JO, King AC, et al. Physical activity and public health in older adults: recommendation from the American College of Sports Medicine and the American Heart Association. Med Sci Sports Exerc 2007;39:1435-45.

[27] Teri L, McCurry SM, Logsdom RG, et al. A randomized controlled clinical trial of the Seattle Protocol for Activity in Older Adults. J Am Geriatr Soc 2011;59:1188-96.

[28] Chen KM, Chen MH, Chao HC et al. Sleep quality, depression state, and health status of older adults after silver yoga exercises: Cluster randomized trial. Int J Nurs Stud 2009;46:154-63.

[29] Chen KM, Tseng WS, Ting LF, Huang GF. Development and evaluation of a yoga exercise programme for older adults. J Adv Nurs 2007; 57(4):432-41.

[30] Wilcox S, Dowda M, Leviton LG, et. al. Active for life: Final results from the translation of two physical activity programs. Am J Prev Med 2008; 35(4);340-51.

[31] Warner LM, et al. Synergistic effect of social support and self-efficacy on physical exercise in older adults. J Aging Phys Activity 2011;19:249-61.

[32] Bishop AJ, et al. Predicting happiness among centenarians. Gerontology 2010;56:88-92.

[33] van Gennep A. The rites of passage. Chicago, IL: University Chicago Press, 1960.

[34] Levinson DJ, Levinson JD. The seasons of a woman's life. New York: Alfred A Knopf, 1996.

[35] Dunn AL, Triveda MH, Kampert JB, et al. Exercise treatment for depression: efficacy and dose response. Am J Prev Med 2005;28(1):1-8.

[36] Stahopoulou G, Powers, MB, Berry AC, et al. Exercise interventions for mental health: a quantitative and qualitative review. Clin Psychol Pract 2006;13(2)179-93.

[37] Sidhu KS, Vandana P, Balon R. Exercise prescription: A practical, effective therapy for depression. Curr Psychiatry 2009;8(6):39-51.

[38] Singh NA, Clements KM, Fiatarone MA. A randomized control trial of progressive resistance training in depressed elders. J Gerontol A BiolSci Med Sci 1997;52(1):M27-35.

[39] Singh NA, Stavrinos TM, Scarbeck Y, et al. A randomized control trial of high versus low intensity weight training versus general practioner care for clinical depression in older adults. J Gerontol A BiolSci Med Sci 2005;60(6):768-76.

Interplay between mood and physical activity and their effect ... 287

[40] Carta MG, Hardoy MC, Pilu A, et al. Improving physical quality of life with group physical activity in the adjunctive treatment of major depressive disorder. Clin Pract Epidemiol Ment Health 2008;4:1.

[41] Singh NA, Clements KM, Singh MA. The efficacy of exercise as a long-term antidepressant in elderly subjects: a randomized, control trial. J Gerontol A BiolSci Med Sci 2001;56(8):M497-504.

[42] Blumentahl JA, Babyak MA, Doraiswamy PM, et al. Exercise and pharmacotherapy in the treatment of major depressive disorder. Psychosom Med 2007;69(7):587-96.

[43] Bandura A. Self-efficacy mechanism in psychological activation and health-promoting beahaviour. In: Madden J, ed. Neurobiology of learning, emotion and affect. New York: Raven, 1991:229-70.

[44] Plante TG, Rodin J. Physical fitness and enhanced psychological health. Curr Psychol Res Rev 1990;9:3-24.

[45] Enkvist A, Ekström H, Elmståhl S. What factors affect life satisfaction (LS) among the oldest-old? Arch Gerontol Geriatr 2011 May 07 [Epub ahead of print].

[46] Fries JF. Physical activity. The compression of morbidity, and the health of the elderly. J R Soc Med 1996;89:64-8.

[47] Pratt M, Macera CA, Wang G. Higher direct medical costs associated with physical inactivity. Phys Sports Med 2000;28(10):63-70.

Submitted: October 16, 2011. *Revised:* November 25, 2011. *Accepted:*December 05, 2011.

In: Alternative Medicine Research Yearbook 2012
Editors: Søren Ventegodt and Joav Merrick

ISBN: 978-1-62808-080-3
© 2013 Nova Science Publishers, Inc.

Chapter 30

QUALITY OF LIFE IN AN EVOLUTIONARY PERSPECTIVE

Bjørn Grinde[*]
Division of Mental Health,
Norwegian Institute of Public Health, Nydalen, Oslo, Norway

ABSTRACT

The main purpose of nervous systems is to direct an animal to behave in a way conductive to survival and procreation. As a rule of thumb that implies either instigation of approach (in the case of opportunities) or avoidance (in the case danger). Three brain modules are essential for this purpose: one for avoidance and two for approach (seeking and consuming). While behavior originally was based on reflexes, in humans these modules operate by the more flexible system of positive and negative affect (good and bad feelings). The human capacity for happiness, in the form of positive feelings, is presumably due to this whim of evolution – i.e., the need for more flexibility in behavioral response. An array of sub-modules has evolved to care for various pursuits, but recent studies suggest that they converge on shared neural circuits designed to generate positive and negative effect. The evolutionary perspective offers both a deeper understanding of what happiness is about, and a framework for improving well-being and mental health.

Keywords: Evolution, quality of life, mental health, brain modules, rewards, punishment

INTRODUCTION

Several lines of scientific inquiry have recently approached the question of happiness: In the social sciences the subject is typically referred to as positive psychology, and measured by questionnaires probing the level of subjective well-being (1,2). In evolutionary biology the

---

[*] Correspondence: Bjørn Grinde, Division of Mental Health, Norwegian Institute of Public Health, PO Box 4404 Nydalen, NO-0403 Oslo, Norway. E-mail: bjgr@fhi.no.

term Darwinian happiness has been used in an attempt to understand why evolution endowed the human species with the capacity to have either pleasant or unpleasant experiences (3,4). Neuroscientists try to locate and understand the neural networks involved (5-7). This chapter draws on all these lines of investigation to generate a novel model for happiness. The model has practical ramifications, not only for the question of improving well-being, but for mental health in general.

Mental health and happiness are closely related issues, as there are two main quandaries associated with a non-optimal functioning of the brain: One, patients are unhappy, i.e., their quality of life suffers; and two, the patients do not function in society, which indirectly may, or may not, cause distress.

These two aspects do not necessarily go together. People with Down syndrome, for example, tend to be happy as long as they are cared for (8); while a depressed person can be deeply unhappy, but still function satisfactory. However, the quality of life is presumably reduced in most individuals with problems related to the mind.

Mental diseases have become the main burden of health in industrialized societies; in terms of the quality of life of citizens, and by disrupting the economy as a major cause of sick leaves and disability. According to estimates, 30–50% of the population suffers from a diagnosable mental disease at some point in life (9,10). The more common problems, such as anxiety disorders, depression and chronic pain, can be understood as malfunctioning of nerve circuits involved in creating negative feelings (11). Even a subclinical level of malfunctioning would be expected to reduce happiness, thus the diagnosable diseases may be the tip of the iceberg as to mental agony and suboptimal quality of life due to excess activity in these circuits.

Preventing or alleviating mental disorders is a first step toward improving well-being in society. The second step would be to create an environment where people thrive beyond what would be expected of an average healthy mind.

THE EVOLUTIONARY PERSPECTIVE

There has been a growing interest in applying the evolutionary perspective to problems of general health (12), as well as to the issue of psychiatric diseases (13) and well-being (4,14). In this perspective, a variety of medical and mental problems are related to an environment at odds with the inherent characteristics of our species. Although all aspects of health may gain from this type of evolutionary analysis, many of the more novel, and applicable, ideas concern mental health.

Evolution selects for survival and procreation – not happiness. Yet there are reasons to assume that the natural state of a healthy mind, in the absence of internal imbalance, external threats, or other stressors, is to be in a good mood. The term default contentment has been coined to reflect this point of view (4). The main argument in favor is that it is in the interest of our genes to rest within an individual with a positive frame of mind – a negative attitude will tend to diminish the effort required for survival and procreation. In further support of the default contentment assumption, there is considerable data suggesting that people are inclined to be overly optimistic – the point is reflected in the tendency to gamble (15). Moreover, when asked about subjective well-being, people claim, on the average, to be on the happy side of neutral (1,2).

Adverse events, such as hunger and fear, may cause negative feelings that temporarily reverse the positive state, but the brain should return to contentment once the particular experience is ended. When discontent is maintained in the absence of adverse events, it is presumably due to unwarranted activity in modules designed to initiate negative states of mind. Hyperactivity in these modules also explains mental ailments such as anxiety and depression. Understanding the nature of these modules may help us improve the mental condition.

BRAIN MODULES

An advanced nervous system is required in order to experience positive or negative feelings; i.e., brains such as those found in mammals.

The mammalian brain has been shaped by evolution to take care of a long list of functions; thus a useful approach to understand the brain is to consider it as divided into various modules – somewhat like a Swiss army knife. Each module deals with a particular need that arouse during our evolutionary history, such as directing movement of a finger, induce hunger in order to initiate food intake, or bring about compassion as a way of establishing relations with fellow humans. Like the various tools of the knife, they can be engaged when required; but while the knife have a dozen or so option, the brain may be divided into perhaps thousands of modules; the number depending on to what extent they are lumped together or split into separate modules.

The brain modules are not easily defined in terms of physical parts of the brain, and are consequently best described in terms of their function. A single module may involve both the conscious and the subconscious brain; and within the conscious part, it may engage both cognitive and affective processes.

In humans, evolution has introduced an overarching unit, roughly speaking the cerebral cortex, which gives us a particularly advanced intellect, as well as the attributes referred to as self-awareness and free will. The various modules involved in conscious thoughts and affects presumably meet in the cortex. Our powerful intellect offers an opportunity to influence both conscious and subconscious affective neurobiology, and thus to some extent control how we feel. Thus, in theory we have the opportunity to manipulate the mind, and consequently the level of happiness, but in practice most people are swayed by environmental stimuli, and by incentives coming from the subconscious parts of the brain.

REWARDS AND PUNISHMENT

Biologically speaking the body is a wrapping designed by the genes with the intent of perpetuating the genes. The brain is part of this wrapping and serves the purpose of orchestrating behavior.

The main objective of primitive nervous systems, such as those found in worms, is to direct the organisms either toward a certain objective, e.g., finding food; or to cause aversion,

292   *Bjørn Grinde*

e.g., avoiding a predator. Thus the first nervous systems, which originated some 600 million years ago, evolved to care for these two primary functions. The corresponding, overarching brain modules – attraction and aversion – are still a key part of the mammalian brain. An important element of brain function is to guide the individual either toward or away from something. In other words, as a gross approximation, the brain is there to direct attention and actions either toward or away from particular situations or opportunities.

In invertebrates, such as worms, the reaction to environmental stimuli involves reflexes or instincts. In order to obtain a more flexible response to various challenges, evolution gradually improved the computational power of the nervous system. Feelings evolved as a means to assess the benefits of various options. Inmammals a positive feeling spurs the animal to move forward, while a negative feeling implies something to be avoided, or a bodily need that should be taken care of. The strength of the feeling indicates the importance of the suggested action. These two main categories of feelings are often referred to as brain rewards and punishment. In biology, rewards may be defined as brain activity that elicits approach and consummatory behavior, while punishments can be defined as activity that elicits avoidance or restoration of bodily homeostasis (16).

The reward module is best understood as two distinct modules, referred to as seeking (some scientists call it wanting) and liking (5,17). Going back to the early nervous systems, they presumably reflect two independent functions: The animals were rewarded first for seeking relevant items in the environment, e.g., food, and subsequently for consuming the items. The two reward functions have distinct neurobiology, yet may, for simplification, in the present context be combined in a single reward module.

The scientific enquiry into the neurobiology behind the modules that are involved in generating feelings, sensations and mood is referred to as affective neuroscience (5).

The neurobiology of reward and punishmentis partly understood (6,7,18). Briefly, certain subcortical parts of the brain serve as a kind of "motor" for positive and negative feeling. The hotspots known to cause activation, in the form of enhanced feelings upon relevant stimulation (either electrodes or local injection of neurotransmitter modulators), are found only in subcortical structures such as the nucleus accumbens and the ventral pallidum. Dopaminergic nerve cells in these regions (and the amygdala) are central in connection with seeking; the opioid system (of much the same brain areas) is involved in wanting. Partly overlapping regions are important for punishing feelings. The cortex apparently serves more like a "dashboard", in the meaning of having a level of conscious control overthe feelings generated in the subcortical brain. The more important cortical regions include the orbitofrontal, lateral prefrontal, insular and anterior cingulate parts.

MOOD MODULES

The brain modules involved in generating positive and negative feelings may be referred to as mood modules. As a first approximation, happiness can be construed as a question of maximizing the net output of mood modules; i.e., stimulating reward modules, while avoiding activity in the punishment module. This way of looking at happiness requires, however, an elaboration.

Quality of life in an evolutionary perspective 293

Most people do not experience life as a stream of either good or bad events, but rather as a relatively steady state of mood interrupted by certain episodes causing a particular surge of pleasure or pain. That does not mean that the modules involved in generating mood are inactive most of the time. It seems more appropriate to envision a tonus of mood caused by the balance of activity between positive and negative modules. This tonus is presumably what some scientists refer to as a set point of happiness (15). Particular events may move you up or down relative to this baseline, but the baseline itself is a consequence of innate factors and previous experiences. While it is easy to find a stimulus that sends your happiness temporarily beyond the baseline; it is more difficult, but not impossible, to boost the baseline itself.

Although the combined activity of the mood modules defines the level of happiness, other parts of the brain, which handle sensory input or cognitive activity, may have considerable impact. A range of modules can affect the tonus of happiness by having neurological connections with the mood modules. Moreover, the cognitive part of the brain determines how the situation is felt – the "flavor" of the reward or punishment. A good meal, for example, offers a rather different experience from the joy of an aesthetic object; yet the pleasure itself may in both cases be cared for by partly the same neurological structures; i.e., the reward module.

The original function of the mood modules can be described as telling the animal whether it is on the right or wrong track toward survival and procreation. In human there is a considerable element of cognitive assessment that influences what is construed as beneficial or detrimental. Collecting butterflies may not improve your chance of survival, but it is possible to prime your brain to accept that acquiring a rare butterfly is the most important thing to do. The human mind is obviously open for this sort of learning and molding.

The mood modules may be activated directly from a sensory experience, such as tasting sweet food or burning a finger; or cognitive modulation may intervene in the process to the effect of either subduing or enhancing the rewarding or punishing feelings. In other words, we may tune in toward pleasure or pain, or try to ignore either. It is possible to activate both at the same time; for example, if you happen to hurt your finger while you are in love. Moreover, one particular sub-module may in certain situations activate reward while causing a punishing feeling at other times – depending on the context.

Fear is an illustrative example. Normally fear is an unpleasant feeling because it is meant to keep you away from dangerous situations. If your eyes catch a stick resembling a snake lying on the ground, you react without thinking. The startle is unpleasant. When upon closer examination you realize that it is only a stick, you relax, which is a pleasant feeling. In other situations the fear may have a positive connotation. A climber appreciates the adrenalin kick of challenging a dangerous mountain. However, if he slips and starts falling, the feeling suddenly becomes disagreeable. The connection between fear and the reward circuitry is explained in biological terms by the evolutionary advantages of occasionally facing treacherous situations. In connection with hunting, for example, one ought to take on a dangerous beast for the purpose of securing food.

Another example concerns grief. Normally this is a negative experience. It is evoked by events that are unfortunate for the genes, such as the loss of a partner or failure to complete a task. The brain reacts by marking the occurrence as something you should try to avoid. On the other hand, the reaction of grief serves a purpose. The mental engagement may help you move on with your life. Moreover, the sorrow is visible in your face, a point that generally means it helps to communicate your feeling to others. In this case the communication may illicit support from friends and thus improve your chance of survival.

The observation that grief may actually improve your fitness implies that, in the appropriate context, you are best served by engaging this emotion; and in order to instigate grief, the emotion presumably connects with the reward module. Consequently, sorrow sometimes feels good. The theory may help explain why people flock to movies that make them cry. When the circumstances indicate that your own situation is not jeopardized, the reward part of grief may overwhelm the negative aspects. In fact, it has been shown that grief may activate either the reward or the punishing module (19).

The point of these examples is to illustrate that it is not obvious whether various situations should make your mood better or worse. The context, the particulars of the situation, and not the least your cognitive assessment, may move the experience toward being either pleasant or unpleasant.

A considerable diversity of external and internal stimuli can impact on the mood modules. Happiness is then a question of moving the balance in a positive direction.

HEDONIA AND EUDAIMONIA

Considering happiness to be a question of stimulating the reward module of the brain is easily confused with the philosophical tradition referred to as hedonism. Hedonia tends to suggest gluttony related to the more typical bodily pleasures; while the alternative concept, eudaimonia, is associated with more positive values, such as socializing and finding a meaning in life.

There is no sign of an alternative neurobiology for eudaimonia. A more parsimonious model is therefore that eudaimonia reflects activity that converges on the same neural networks (the mood modules) as do bodily pleasures. The observation that people suffering from anhedonia have reduced ability to experience all sorts of happiness or contentment, further supports the contention that hedonia and eudaimonia are based on the same neurobiology (7).

The above reasoning does not necessarily imply that the dichotomy is unwarranted, the sources and nature of eudaimonia may differ appreciably from typical hedonic sensations.

One of the foremost items related to eudaimonia is having a "meaningful life". It seems rational for evolution to attach positive feelings to utility, which implies that we are rewarded for doing something considered constructive. Thus "meaning" is presumably a feature installed to avoid having our ancestors turn into "cave potatoes". Similar reasoning may apply to other values typically incorporated in eudaimonia, such as spiritual associations, being virtuous, and showing compassion. Evolutionary speaking, the ultimate objective should be survival and procreation, but all sorts of more proximate purposes may activate reward modules. In other words, the positive affect labeled as eudaimonia may simply reflect a subset of the vast array of stimuli that connect to a share reward motor.

The pleasures typically associated with eudaimonia are either more lasting, less likely to cause harm by misuse, or considered virtuous and beneficial to society. Thus the preference for eudaimonic values may reflect an attempt to coach people toward choosing particular types of rewards. The preferred list would include those more likely to ensure optimal long-

Quality of life in an evolutionary perspective 295

term happiness, and those favored due to social or political priorities. Moreover, the default contentment described above does not require any form of stimuli. Consequently it cannot be misused and would therefore fall in the category of eudaimonic happiness. Yet, it seems likely that the default contentment simply reflects that the mood modules are designed to operate with a net positive value as long as the negative modules are not specifically activated. That is, in a person with proper mental health, whose basal needs are cared for, the setpoint of happiness is positive.

EXERCISING THE BRAIN

It is common knowledge that the size and strength of muscles will develop upon exercise. It may be less obvious that a range of other bodily functions, including the various modules of the brain, also tend to expand (functionally if not anatomically) upon use. The point is easily demonstrated in animals, where it is possible to apply experimentally controlled stimuli and subsequently remove the brain for detailed anatomical analyses. If, for example, the fear module is stimulated excessively, the underlying neurological and endocrine tissues will be enlarged. It seems reasonable to assume that by exercising a brain module, i.e., activating it regularly, it will not only expand, but also tend to have a greater impact on consciousness. For example, by regularly stimulating the fear function, one is more likely to suffer from unwarranted or excessive activity of this module; i.e., more likely to develop anxiety related problems.

A main issue, as to quality of life, may be that modules involved in negative feelings are "exercised" to the extent that they become troublesome. In other words, environmental factors in modern societies may activate modules responsible for negative feelings, and thus cause the underlying nerve circuitry to expand. The modules consequently have a greater impact on conscious experiences than what would be typical for a Stone Age setting.

It should be mentioned that, in the case of humans, cognition allows for "containment" of expanded modules. Anxiety can, for example, be subdued with the help of cognitive therapy. The therapy presumably works not by changing the fear module itself, but by expanding neurological circuits in the brain whose function it is to turn off the fear module. In other words, the therapy may be viewed as exercising this "off-switch".

It is also possible to exercise the modules of the brain associated with rewards. In this case, the daily mood tonus would be expected to improve. Meditation appears to be relevant "brain exercise" in this respect. Certain forms of meditation, such as that based on the Tibetan Buddhist tradition, have been investigated to some detail. This practice has been claimed to be capable of installing in the brain a sufficiently strong reward circuitry to allow for a positive sentiment regardless of the external situation (20). The claim is partly substantiated by measuring activity in brain centers associated with rewards in Buddhist monks during meditation (21).

Engaging in any sort of positive feelings – including those evoked by music and aesthetics – is relevant training of the reward module according to the present model. The typical target of Tibetan Buddhists is, however, of particular interest: They often focus their meditation on compassion. Both pair-bonding and social relations most likely became important during the last 5-7 million years of human evolution; a presumed consequence is that feelings associated with agreeable relationships – including love, compassion and camaraderie – induce powerful brain rewards (22). Moreover, besides being an excellent strategy for personal happiness, expanding the compassion module carries obvious benefits for society.

CAUSES OF REDUCED HAPPINESS

According to the present model, the main threat to quality of life stems from the activation of modules that instigate negative sensations. In their absence, the default state of contentment should secure a good mood. It is therefore useful to take a closer look at the key modules that contribute to an unpleasant frame of mind. By understanding what causes surplus activity in these modules, it may be possible to suggest remedies.

Pain is the classical example. Close to a third of the adult population of Norway suffers from chronic (and presumably inappropriate) pain (23). The pain is often associated with muscle and skeletal problems. One presumed cause, is a lack of physical activity, typically combined with unnatural strain on certain parts of the body, as when sitting all day in front of a computer. Another cause is a misguided immune system, in the form of an easily triggered inflammatory reaction. It is possible to alleviate pain by either cognitive or pharmacological intervention, but preventive measures would be a preferred strategy. Diverse physical activity throughout life is a possible option.

Anxiety may be viewed as a consequence of excessive, or unnatural, activity of the fear function. I have previously described a possible scenario for why anxiety has become such a common problem in Western societies (24). Briefly, infants do not understand that a locked door implies safety, as they rely on parental help to avoid any sort of danger, whether in the form of burglars or wild beasts. Parental proximity is therefore the key to avoid stimulating fear. The present way of handling infants typically involves reduced parental proximity; e.g., strollers instead of carrying, less skin-to-skin contact, and less co-sleeping. The problem may be partly preventable by behavioral changes.

Depression is associated with hyperactivity in a "low mood" module. Patients suffering from anxiety are often at risk for depression as well. It has been estimated that roughly a third of the population over a lifespan suffer from anxiety and/or depression (9,10).

While fear has an obvious biological function, it is less clear why we need a module for low mood. One presumed function is to secure social relations. In the Stone Age a lack of a strong social network, in the form of a tribe, would be a serious threat to survival. The low mood, as exemplified with loneliness, induces negative feelings in order to teach the individual to seek fellowship with others. In other words, the low mood suggests that your social relations are not satisfactory.

The same module may be active when you are unsuccessful in a task, such as missing the game in a hunt or getting lost in the forest. Today, flunking an exam or losing a competition are probably more likely scenarios. Again the feeling induced ought to be unpleasant in order to teach the individual to try to avoid ending up in this situation the next time. The high prevalence of depression may reflect that modern societies are troubled by a suboptimal social environment and by too much pressure on achievement. Altering these conditions may alleviate the problem.

MENTAL HEALTH

Hyperactivity in these three modules – i.e., pain, fear and low mood – is probably the more common cause of reduced happiness in Western societies. In more overt cases, the problem is diagnosed as a mental disorder, while most people may experience a suboptimal quality of life due to more limited, but still inappropriate, activity in these modules. The point should not be to obliterate all activity, only what is excessive or non-functional – pain, for example, is often important for survival. In other words, the main challenge in connection with mental health can be viewed as moving the mind up on the continuous scale (from negative to positive) of mood module activity; without jeopardizing health.

At the face of it, the three negative sub-modules appear to induce completely different types of feelings and experiences. The present model, however, suggest that they all converge on a shared module that generate the tonus of unpleasantness, i.e., the punishment module. Similarly, the various pleasures converge on the reward module (the two reward modules, seeking and liking, if one prefers).

Various evidence supports this notion. Recent neurological research indicates that social situations that are considered either positive or negative activate much the same nerve circuitry as do stimuli such as respectively sweet taste or physical pain (6,7,25-27). The present model is based on an extrapolation of these findings to all sorts of situations that carry an element of positive or negative effect. Jealousy, for example, may touch on the module devoted to punishment; while achievements activate rewards.

The above assumption also fits with current ideas as to how evolution operates. As pointed out above, early nervous systems had limited functions beyond simply directing behavior toward or away from stimuli. The "reflex modules"in charge are present in most invertebrate animals. It is interesting to note thatthe aversion-instigation reflexes use the same neurotransmitters (dopamine, serotonin and opioids) that serve in the mammalian mood modules (5,28,29).

Evolution generally builds on existing structures by expanding on them. Thus it is to be expected that the underlying dichotomy is still present in humans, and that features of the neurobiology is retained, although in a much more advanced and intricate form. In the human brain the functions have expanded to include a range of feelings, as well as all sorts of cognitive ramifications.

It is to be expected that the modules converging on punishment are common causes of complaint. For one, people are unlikely to object if modules offering positive feelings should be hyperactive. Then again, this is less likely to happen. The negative modules are typically involved in some sort of defense; i.e., they are there to avoid dangers and adverse situations. Defense functions are, in general, designed for a low threshold of activation; as it is more important to react with fear once too often, than not to react in times of real danger.

It is better to jump at the sight of a stick resembling a snake, than not to respond when approaching a real snake. The ease of activation implies that these functions are more likely to be "exercised" and thus end up dominating the mind.

The Concept of Discords

Ailments that appear to be more common now than during the Stone Age are typically referred to as diseases of civilization. Some of them are primarily a question of having more people live to a higher age, such as dementia and certain types of cancer. A range of conditions, however, are likely to be a consequence of suboptimal aspects of the present environment – for example, nearsightedness, lung cancer and diabetes. The more common types of mental diseases, including anxiety and depression, probably belong to this latter category.

If one could delineate the actual aspects of the environment that are suboptimal, one would have a strategy for prevention. An illustrative example is to reduce the habit of smoking in order to prevent lung cancer.

According to the present model, the clue to finding preventive measures, in the case of mental problems such as anxiety and depression, rests with finding the factors that contribute to elevated activity. In short, what is causing excessive exercise of the fear and low mood brain modules?

The evolutionary approach is suitable for suggesting candidate factors, but traditional psychological and epidemiological research is required to estimate their actual impact.

As in the case of any animal, humans are adapted to live under certain conditions. In the literature of evolutionary psychology these conditions are commonly referred to as the Environment of Evolutionary Adaptation (EEA); or in more colloquial terms, the Stone Age (30). Differences between present living and life in the EEA are referred to as mismatches. Mismatches may be purely beneficial, such as sleeping on a mattress instead of on the ground or being cured from an infection by the use of antibiotics; but some mismatches have detrimental effects. The latter may be referred to as discords (4,22). Discords are, per definition, responsible for the diseases of civilization (i.e., those that are not consequences of an increased age).

Although any part of the body may suffer from discords, as exemplified with lung cancer, the brain is probably particularly vulnerable. For one, it is a highly complex organ and thus easily thrown out of "balance"; two, it is designed to develop in interaction with the environment, thus when the environment differs from what the genes "expect", the brain is likely to be affected; and three, it is the most important organ of your body in regards to quality of life.

Infancy is a particularly important period. It is during the first years of life that the brain goes through its most dramatic transformation, thus discords affecting infants are more likely to leave lasting "scars" in the brain. It is possible to overcome these scars, but dealing with mental problems tends to be more difficult than curing somatic diseases. Consequently, preventive measures meant to reduce mental agony should focus on how we care for infants.

Conclusion

The present model of happiness incorporates current biological knowledge, including the neurobiology of the human brain, how the evolutionary process works, and the comparative study of animals. The value of the model depends to a considerable extent on a correct interpretation of words such as brain module, mood and happiness.

Chronic pain, anxiety and depression are arguably the most common causes of reduced quality of life. The evolutionary approach offers both an explanation for the current predicament, and possible preventive measures. Happiness depends on tuning down negative modules and tuning up positive modules; where avoiding excessive activity of the negative circuits during childhood and adolescence may be the more important issue. The predictions made as to how one can improve happiness, i.e., avoiding unnecessary stimulation of modules involved in punishment, and exercising modules involved in rewards, can be tested.

It is possible to improve happiness by engaging the reward module, but it appears to be more important to avoid letting the modules impacting on punishment dominate. Indulging in hedonic pleasures is likely to cause health problems later in life; for example in the form of alcoholism, diabetes and obesity.To the extent that the default setting of the brain is one of good mood, it is more important that this sentiment is retained. The foremost advice as to happiness is consequently to avoid enhanced activity in negative circuits.

The model may appear to be somewhat technical, and it does not consider issues typically brought up in connection with happiness studies, such as job related matter, social network, and a meaningful life. These elements are of obvious importance, but their role, according to the present understanding of happiness, is played out by their impact on the mood modules. The model does not refute the relevance of these aspects of life, but suggest an explanation for why they matter.

One suggested rule of thumb is to adjust the conditions of life in accordance with the environment of evolutionary adaptation – i.e., to avoid discords. It is possible to exercise the rewarding sensations, but it should be emphasized that in order to be a viable strategy, the impact of engaging in reward stimuli should be calculated over a lifetime. Moreover, the pursuit of happiness should preferably not reduce the prospect of happiness for future generations.

REFERENCES

[1] Diener E, Oishi S, Lucas RE. Personality, culture, and subjective well-being: emotional and cognitive evaluations of life. Ann Rev Psychol 2003;54:403-25.
[2] Seligman ME, Steen TA, Park N, Peterson C. Positive psychology progress: empirical validation of interventions. Am Psychol 2005;60:410-21.
[3] Grinde B. Happiness in the prespective of evolutionary pshcyhology. J Happiness Stud 2002;3:331-54.
[4] Grinde B. Darwinian happiness. Evolution as a guide for living and understanding human behavior. Princeston, NJ: Darwin Press, 2002.
[5] Panksepp J. Affective neuroscience. Oxford: Oxford Univ Press, 1998.
[6] Leknes S, Tracey I. A common neurobiology for pain and pleasure. Nat Rev Neurosci 2008;9:314-320.
[7] Kringelbach ML, Berridge KC. Towards a functional neuroanatomy of pleasure and happiness. Trends Cogn Sci 2009;13:479-87.
[8] Robinson RJ. Learning about happiness from persons with Down syndrome: feeling the sense of joy and contentment. Am J Mental Retard 2000;105:372-6.
[9] Murray C, Lopez A. The global burden of disease: a comprehensive assessment of mortality and disability from diseases, injuries and risk factors in 1990 and projected to 2020. Harvard: Harvard Univ Press, 1996.

300   *Bjørn Grinde*

[10] Moffitt T, Caspi A, Taylor A, Kokaua J, Milne BJ, Polanczyk G, Poulton R. How common are common mental disorders? Evidence that lifetime rates are doubled by prospective versus retrospective ascertainment. Psychol Med 2010;39:899-909.

[11] Grinde B. Can the concept of discords help us find the causes of mental diseases? Med Hypothesis 2009;73:106-9.

[12] Nesse RM, Williams GC. Why we get sick: the new science of Darwinian medicine. New York: Vintage Books, 1996.

[13] Stevens A, Price J. Evolutionary psychiatry: a new beginning. London: Routledge, 2000.

[14] Grinde B. Darwinian happiness: can the evolutionary perspective on well-being help us improve society? World Futures – J Gen Evol 2004;60:317-29.

[15] Lykken D. Happiness. The nature and nurture of joy and contentment. New York: St. Martin's Griffin, 2000.

[16] Watson KK, Platt ML. Neuroethology of reward and decision making. Phil Trans Royal Soc London B 2008;363:3825-35.

[17] Berridge KC. Pleasures of the brain. Brain Cognition 2003;52:106-28.

[18] Smith KS, Mahler SV, Pecina S, Berridge KC. Hedonic hotspots: generating sesnory pleasure in the brain. In: Kringelbach ML, Berridge KC. Pleasures of the brain. Oxford: Oxford Univ Press, 2010:27-49.

[19] O'Connor MF, Wellisch DK, Stanton AL, Eisenberger NI, Irwin MR, Lieberman MD. Craving love? Enduring grief activates brain's reward center. Neuroimage 2008;42:969-72.

[20] Ricard M. Happiness. A guide to developing life's most important skill. Boston: Atlantic Books, 2007.

[21] Wallace AB. Contemplative science. Where Buddhism and neuroscience converge. New York: Columbia Univ Press, 2007.

[22] Grinde B. An evolutionary perspective on the importance of social relations for quality of life. TheScientificWorldJournal 2009;9:588-605.

[23] Rustøen T, Wahl AK, Hanestad BR, Lerdal A, Paul S, Miaskowski C. Prevalence and characteristics of chronic pain in the general Norwegian population. Eur J Pain 2004;8:555-65.

[24] Grinde B. An approach to the prevention of anxiety-related disorders based on evolutionary medicine. Prev Med 2005;40:904-9.

[25] Eisenberger NI, Lieberman MD, Williams KD Does rejection hurt? An fMRI study of social exclusion. Science 2003;302:290-2.

[26] Moll J, Krueger F, Zahn R, Pardini M, Oliveira-Souza RD, Grafman J. Human fronto-mesolimbic networks guide decisions about charitable donation. Proc Nat Acad Sci USA 2006;103:15623-8.

[27] Takahashi H, Kato M, Matsuura M, Mobbs D, Suhara T, Okubo Y. When your gain is my pain and your pain is my gain: Neural correlates of envy and schadenfreude. Science 2009;323:937-9.

[28] Chase DL, Koelle MR. Biogenic amine neurotransmitters in C. elegans. WormBook 2007;Feb 20:1-15.

[29] Nieto-Fernandez F, Andrieux S, Idrees S, Bagnall C, Pryor SC, Sood R. The effect of opioids and their antagonists on the nocifensive response of Caenorhabditis elegans to noxious thermal stimuli. Invertebrate Neurosci 2009;9:195-200.

[30] Eaton SB, Strassman BI, Nesse RM, Neel JV,Ewald PW, Williams GC, Weder AB, Eaton SB, Lindeberg S, Konner MJ, Mysterud I, Cordain L. Evolutionary health promotion. Prev Med 2002;34:109-18.

Submitted: October 16, 2011. *Revised:* December 03, 2011. *Accepted:* December 07, 2011.

In: Alternative Medicine Research Yearbook 2012
Editors: Søren Ventegodt and Joav Merrick

ISBN: 978-1-62808-080-3
© 2013 Nova Science Publishers, Inc.

Chapter 31

ADOLESCENT LIFE SATISFACTION AND WELL-BEING

Danilo Garcia[1,2]* *and Trevor Archer*[3]

[1]Institute of Neuroscience and Physiology, The Sahlgrenska Academy, University of Gothenburg, Gothenburg, Sweden
[2]Center for Ethics, Law, and Mental Health (CELAM), University of Gothenburg, Gothenburg, Sweden
[3]Department of Psychology, University of Gothenburg, Sweden

ABSTRACT

The aim of the present study was to investigate differences in life satisfaction (LS) and psychological well-being (PWB) among adolescents (N = 141). The relationship between PWB' self-acceptance sub-scale and LS was also investigated. The affective temperaments (AFTs) model was the framework for the research. The AFTs were developed through self-reported affect, generating four temperaments: self-actualizing, high affective, low affective, and self-destructive. Self-destructives reported lower LS and PWB than the other three temperaments. Moreover, PWB, in particular the subscale of self-acceptance, was related to LS for all temperaments. The role of positive emotions and self-acceptance among youth is discussed. The AFTs model is suggested to offer something unique by taking into account the interaction of positive and negative effect.

Keywords: Adolescence, life satisfaction, well-being, mental health

INTRODUCTION

Positive (PA) and negative affect (NA) are indicators or markers of well-being (1). However, according to some researchers PA and NA are two distinctive factors that also reflect stable emotional-temperamental dispositions or signal sensitivity systems (2,3). For instance, Larsen and Ketelaar (4) found that individuals who experience high levels of PA attend and react

---

* Correspondence: Danilo Garcia, CELAM, University of Gothenburg, Wallingsatan 8, SE 431 41 Mölndal, Sweden. E-mail: danilo.garcia@euromail.se.

more intensely to positive stimuli than individuals with low levels of PA. In contrast, individuals with high levels of NA attend and react more intensely to negative stimuli than individuals with low levels of NA. Yet most of the studies use PA and NA to define an emotional state rather than a 'trait-like' temperament. This difference, however, may be addressed by referring to the lack of coherence in the literature—namely; the different measures used in the assessment of affects (see (5) for a large compilation of studies). Moreover, as one of the most used instruments to measure affect, the Positive Affect and Negative Affect Schedule (PANAS by Watson, Clark, & Tellegen) (6), was developed on the idea that PA and NA represent two orthogonal dimensions rather than two ends of one dimension. Consequentially, while some PANAS items (e.g., 'interested') may not be common in other scales, other items (e.g., 'happy') are not included in the PANAS. Additionally, other findings suggest that PANAS items reflect engagement with a stimulus (7). Indeed, PA and NA, as measured by the PANAS show strong stability over time and are probably genetically predisposed in the individual (8,9). In the present study, PA and NA are referred to not only as temperamental dispositions but also as complementary to extraversion and neuroticism. These assumptions are based on the suggestions mentioned above and on research that shows that PA and NA (as measured by the PANAS) involve more mood and social traits than extraversion and neuroticism (10).

In this line of thinking, Garcia and colleagues (11-13) have examined adolescents' judgements of life satisfaction (LS), Psychological Well-Being (PWB) and apprehension for events. As a backdrop for their research, Garcia and his colleagues used the Affective Temperaments model (AFT) originally developed by Norlander, Bood and Archer (14). The model takes into account all characteristics of PA and NA earlier stated and is based on self-reported affects measured by the PANAS. The four temperaments are: self-actualizing (high PA, low NA); high affective (high PA, high NA); low affective (low PA, low NA); and self-destructive (low PA, high NA). Compared to self-destructive, all temperaments report higher levels of LS, PWB and recall more positive than negative life events (11,12). Moreover, while LS is predicted by life events among low PA temperaments (11), PWB predicts LS regardless of temperament (12). More important, although the temperaments differed in several PWB constructs; when Garcia and Siddiqui (12) tested each of the PWB constructs in the prediction of LS among temperaments, self-acceptance emerged as the most important construct for all four temperaments. In a related study, Garcia and colleagues (13) presented adolescents with a short story with different valenced words highlighted in bold type (negative, positive, and neutral). While high affectives and self-actualizers' reaction to negative words predicted the number of positive words in memory, low affectives' reaction to negative words predicted the memory of neutral words. In contrast, self-destructive were unable to self-regulate their reaction of negative words. Hence, all temperaments, with the exception of self-destructives, seem to have the ability to self-regulate their reaction to negative words by better remembering words that were congruent to their own temperament.

Garcia and colleagues (11-13) concluded that there may be two ways of maintaining well-being that are related to the interacting influence of the two signal-sensitivity systems (i.e., PA and NA) and that accepting the self seems important if the adolescent is going to feel satisfied with life. In this context, the researchers related their findings to Fredrickson's (15) suggestions about how positive emotions may also broaden people's mindsets and build enduring personal psychological resources. The effect of broadened thinking may increase the odds of discovering positive meaning in life events (15,16), in turn, enhancing PWB.

Fredrickson (15) goes even further suggesting that high PA balance high negative emotions, thus explaining why high affective adolescents experience high LS and report high PWB despite their experience of high NA. Nevertheless, in Garcia and Siddiqui's studies (11,12) also low affective adolescents (low PA and low NA) reported higher LS and PWB than self-destructive adolescents. In this regard, the researchers noted that Higgins (17) has suggested that it is important to distinguish between strategies used in order to move forward desired end-states (happy) or away from undesired end states (unhappy). Indeed, their findings suggest that self-actualizing and high affective adolescents regulated their reaction to negative words in a story by remembering more of the positive words in the same story. In contrast, low affective adolescents regulated their reaction to negative words by remembering more neutral words (13). In other words, self-actualizing and high affective adolescents approached happiness, while low affective adolescents avoided unhappiness. Hence, the AFT model might offer something unique over and above the single dimensional framework--specifically, with respect to the high and low affective individuals (see figure 1 for a summary of Garcia's findings).

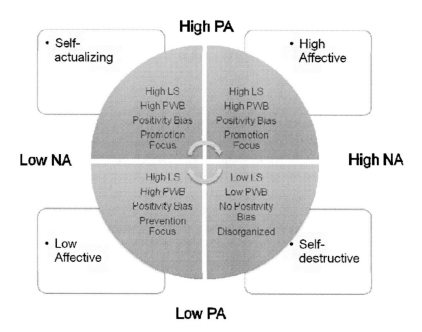

Figure 1. Garcia's findings (11-13) in regard to AFT and different measures of well-being (adapted from a seminar with permission from Professor C Robert Cloninger).

The present study aims to replicate Garcia and Siddiqui's studies (11,12) by investigating if the AFTs differ in their levels of LS and PWB. The role of PWB and self-acceptance in the prediction of satisfaction with life is also examined. Having a sample of adolescents may be important, because in this period of life different events and transitions may influence well-being (18).

In addition, temperament is described is relatively stable in adults, however adolescents' temperament might be less stable due the fact of their neurological development (19). Before trying to disentangle the interesting question of the predictive nature of distinctive measures

Subjective well-being and psychological well-being

In the field of positive psychology, well-being research complements measures of physical (e.g. health) and material (e.g. income) well-being with assessments of optimal psychological functioning and experience (20). Two points of views have been distinctive across studies. One is the hedonic point of view (21), which focuses in people's own judgements and experiences of pleasure versus displeasure. The assessment of this hedonic experience involves individuals' own judgements about life satisfaction, the frequency of positive affect and the infrequency of negative affect (22). The three constructs are summarized as Subjective Well-Being or happiness (SWB) (1). According to Martin and Huebner (23), the multidimensional model of SWB (LS, PA, and NA) is valid for adolescents as well. Thus, a happy adolescent can be assumed to be satisfied with life and to experience more positive than negative affect. LS refers to a comparison process, in which individuals assess the quality of their lives on the basis of their own self-imposed standard (24, 25). The affective part of SWB is computed by subtracting the number of positive emotions from the number of negative emotions that an individual experiences—that is, the affect balance (26).

The current assessment of the affective component can be criticized because it fails to take account of positive and negative aspects of experience independently: an individual experiencing high positive and negative affectivity may end up with the same score as a person who experiences low positive and low negative affectivity (26).

The other point of view is the eudaimonic (27), which sees well-being as a product of "the striving for perfection that represents the realization of one's true potential" (28), hence SWB is a result of full engagement and optimal performance in existential challenges of life (29). In this framework, Ryff (30) proposed six constructs as defining positive psychological functioning: 1) self-acceptance, 2) positive relations with others, 3) autonomy, 4) environmental mastery, 5) purpose in life and 6) personal growth. Ryff (30) compared PWB between young (18-29 years old), midlife (30-64 years old) and old aged (65 years old or more) adults and found different aspects of PWB increasing or decreasing, while other not changing at all. Environmental mastery and autonomy increased with age (especially from young to midlife adults), purpose in life and personal growth decreased (especially from midlife to old aged adults) and no differences where found for self-acceptance and positive relations with others. Although the PWB constructs are not only suggested to promote SWB but also as a measure of well-being, recent research has linked PA as a predictor of PWB. Urry and colleagues (31), for example, tested if eudaimonic behavior (engaging with goal-directed stimuli) contributed to well-being by investigating correlations between individual differences in baseline prefrontal activation and PWB. The results validated the hypothesis and affect, especially approach-related PA (e.g., "interested," "strong"), emerged as an important factor in the prediction of PWB.

The aim of the present study is to replicate Garcia and Colleagues' findings by exploring differences between AFTs with respect to LS and PWB. Furthermore, the present study also investigates the relationship between PWB (specifically the self-acceptance sub-scale) and LS among temperaments. Self-actualizing adolescents might obviously be considered as the

Adolescent life satisfaction and well-being 305

happy ones. On the other hand high affective adolescents' experience of high PA is suggested to not only attenuate their experience of high NA, but also to broaden their thought repertoire, in turn, increasing their PWB. Nonetheless, low affective adolescents' ability to neutralize their reaction to negative stimuli promotes self-regulation and the avoidance of unhappiness. Hence, as in Garcia and Siddiqui's studies (11,12) self-actualizing, high affective and low affective adolescents are expected to show higher LS and PWB than the self-destructive ones. Moreover, PWB and self-acceptance are expected to predict LS for all temperaments.

METHODS

Pupils at a high school in the county of Blekinge, Sweden, participated in the study. The whole population (N = 150) was contacted. A total of 141 pupils (80 girls) with an age mean of 16.89 (SD = .97) agreed to participate. The adolescents had consent from their teachers to participate. All parents were informed of the present and other studies being conducted among adolescents at the school. The nature of the studies was explained (e.g., instruments, confidentiality) and questions addressed at the same meeting. Pupils were told that their involvement was voluntary, confidential and that the studies were about how high school pupils think about their lives. All participants were presented with a battery of instruments including the affect, LS and PWB measure. Participants' PA and NA scores were divided (in high and low) using the following cut-off points recommended in Garcia and colleagues' studies: low PA = 34 or less; high PA = 35 or above; low NA = 22 or less; and high NA = 23 or above.

Instruments

Positive Affect and Negative Affect Schedule (PANAS) (6). The PANAS asks participants to rate to what extent they generally have experienced 20 different feelings or emotions (10 PA and 10 NA) for the last weeks, using a 5-point Likert scale (1 = *very slightly*, 5 = *extremely*). The 10-item PA scale includes adjectives such as strong, proud, and interested (Cronbach's α = .84). The 10-item NA scale includes adjectives such as afraid, ashamed, and nervous (Cronbach's α = .81).

Satisfaction with Life Scale (SWLS) (24). The SWLS asks participants to indicate grade of agreement to 5 items (e.g., "I am satisfied with my life") using a 7-point Likert scale (1 = *strongly disagree*, 7 = *strongly agree*). The LS score was established by summarizing the 5 statements for each participant (Cronbach's α = .83).

Ryff's Short Measurement of Psychological Well-Being (32). The instrument consists of 18 items, three for each construct of PWB. The participants are asked to indicate grade of agreement to three statements for each of the six scales in a 6-point Likert scale (1 = *strongly disagree*, 6 = *strongly agree*).

The three items of the self-acceptance subscale (e.g., "I like most aspects of my personality" Cronbach's α = .76) were summarized to form a separate variable. The total PWB score was computed by simply summarizing all the 18 items (Cronbach's α = .75).

RESULTS

A temperaments x gender between-subjects ANOVA was conducted in order to test differences in LS and PWB. The main effect of gender was not significant for either LS ($F(1,133)$ = 1.42, p = .24) or PWB ($F(1,133)$ = 2.39, p = .12). The main effect of AFTs was significant for both dependent variables: LS ($F(3,133)$ = 11.12, $p <$ .001) and PWB ($F(3,133)$ = 10.07, $p <$.001). A Bonferroni correction to the alpha level showed that, as predicted, self-actualizing ($p <$ .001 for LS; $p <$ .001 for PWB), high affective ($p <$ .001 for LS; p = .001 for PWB) and low affective adolescents ($p <$ .001 for LS; p = .01 for PWB) reported higher LS and PWB than self-destructive adolescents.

The interaction of AFT and gender was not significant for either LS ($F(3,133)$ = .38, p = .77) or PWB ($F(3,133)$ = .70, p = .55), hence the effect of AFTs on LS and PWB was consistent across gender. See Table 1 for mean scores in LS and PWB.

PWB and self-acceptance as a predictor of LS

Four multiple regression analyses (MRAs) were conducted using the whole PWB scale as the independent variable and LS as the dependent variable, one for each temperament. PWB emerged as a significant predictor of LS for each temperament (see table 2).

Nevertheless, self-acceptance was expected to be the main variable related to LS among AFTs (see table 1 for mean scores).

Four MRAs were conducted using self-acceptance as the independent variable and LS as the dependent variable, one for each temperament. Self-acceptance was significantly related to LS for all temperaments. See table 3 for details.

Table 1. Mean Scores in LS, PWB and Self-Acceptance among AFTs

	Self-actualizing n = 40	High affective n = 29	Low affective n = 32	Self-destructive n = 40
Life Satisfaction	26.82±5.30	25.19±5.34	25.05±4.90	19.92±6.40
Psychological Well-Being	82.87±9.08	80.77±9.47	78.82±6.74	71.45±7.33
Self-acceptance	14.24±2.60	14.24±2.83	13.29±2.72	10.93±3.47

Note: Values represent mean scores ± SD.

Table 2. PWB as Predictor of LS among AFTs

	Beta	Adjusted R^2	F
Self-actualizing	.66 ***	.42	F (1,38) = 29.58 ***
High affective	.63 **	.38	F (1,27) = 18.13 ***
Low affective	.52 **	.25	F (1,30) = 11.26 **
Self-destructive	.61 ***	.36	F (1,38) = 22.70 ***

Note: ns = nonsignificant, **p = 0.01, ***$p <$ 0.001.

Adolescent life satisfaction and well-being

Table 3. Self-Acceptance as Predictor of LS among AFTs

	Beta	Adjusted R^2	F
Self-actualizing	.70 ***	.48	$F_{(1,38)} = 37.00$ ***
High affective	.46 **	.18	$F_{(1,27)} = 7.05$ **
Low affective	.42 **	.15	$F_{(1,30)} = 6.25$ **
Self-destructive	.75 ***	.55	$F_{(1,38)} = 49.51$ ***

Note: *ns* = nonsignificant, **$p = 0.01$, ***$p < 0.001$.

DISCUSSION

The aim of the present study was to explore differences between AFTs with respect to LS and PWB. The present study also investigated the relationship between PWB and LS among temperaments. Specifically, the PWB sub-scale of self acceptance was expected to be important in the prediction of LS among temperaments. As in Garcia and Siddiqui's studies (11,12) self-actualizing, high affective, and low affective adolescents showed higher LS and PWB compared to the self-destructive ones. Moreover, PWB and self-acceptance predicted LS for all temperaments.

Although high and low affectives did report higher LS and PWB than self-destructive adolescents, it is important to point out the role of positive emotions in the process of human adaptation. The broaden and build theory (15) posits that the experience of positive emotions is suggested to broad thoughts and behaviors and facilitates more adaptive responses to environments, enhancing well-being (15). Tugade and Fredrickson (33), for example, found that individuals with high affectivity (high PA and high NA) returned faster to their normal cardiovascular activation following a stressful task. Moreover, the absence of PA is a better predictor of mortality and morbidity than the presence of NA (34). Thus, as suggested high affective adolescents' high PA probably neutralizes the effects of their experience of high NA. From this point of view it might be better to be a high affective than a low affective adolescent. For instance, positive emotions, in contrast to negative emotions, are related to adaptive coping, which in turn is related with student engagement among young adolescents (35). In agreement with Larson (36) "a central question of youth development is how to get adolescents' fires lit, how to have them develop the complex of dispositions and skills needed to take charge of their lives." Thus, the promotion of positive emotions should be in focus. It is plausible to suggest that a first step in this direction might be through self-acceptance. Indeed, in concordance to Garcia and Siddiqui's (12) findings, self-acceptance seems to be a predictor of adolescents' LS. That is, if an adolescent is going to be able to successfully adapt, feel good, and resolve problems in life, the adolescent has to accept all different parts of her personality. In Garcia and Siddiqui's study (12) low affectives did not show lower self-acceptance than the high affective adolescents, while showing higher self-acceptance than the self-destructive ones. Perhaps is their ability to accept the self without judgment what makes them to see their life as satisfying.

If it is so, fostering self-acceptance among youth might be crucial for their well-being. According to Magen (37), social skill interventions in the school should include commitment beyond the self. Magen (37) suggested that peer counseling influences adolescents to give and receive help. This mutual interpersonal experience strengthens self-acceptance and fosters their capacity to experience moments of happiness and identity formation (37). The benefits from such interventions are greater "self-esteem, sense of purpose and worth, feeling of accomplishment and mastery, and satisfying interaction with other humans beings" (37).

Limitations

The present study was based on self-reports, the sample was relatively small and cross-sectional. Thus, the generalization value is limited. Although the instruments used to measure LS, PA, and NA (SWLS and PANAS) showed high reliability, appropriate measures for those constructs have been developed and validated for use with adolescents (e.g., Students' Life Satisfaction Scale by Huebner (38) and the PANAS-C by Laurent et al (39)). Nevertheless, evidence of the reliability and validity of the SWLS and the PANAS in adolescents can be found elsewhere (SWLS: (40); PANAS: (41) and (42)).

Suggestions for further investigation

The present study was an important replication of Garcia and colleagues' studies. The AFTs are probably useful in the study and prediction of positive health and indicators of well-being. Nevertheless, to the best of my knowledge no study has investigated if the AFTs actually have different personalities. This is important, since personality appears to be the major determinant of well-being (5) since it is related to reactivity to emotional stimuli, individual differences in intensity to responses to emotional events, and to the duration of emotional reactions (43). If the interacting influence of the two signal-sensitivity systems (i.e., PA and NA) helps maintain well-being, then the AFTs should differ in personality in addition to well-being. In this regard, adolescents that experience high PA could be addressed as extroverts, while high NA adolescents as neurotics. Nevertheless, the AFTs are based in the notion of PA and NA as interacting dispositions, thus high affective adolescents are probably high in both traits. In contrast, low affective might report being low in both Neuroticism and Extraversion. In other words, low affectives might report high LS despite not being extroverts, while high affectives might report high LS despite high neuroticism. If these difference are consistent across samples, the AFT framework can then be suggested as reliable when predicting well-being and useful when interventions seek to increase adolescents satisfaction with their life and PWB. Furthermore, as stated in the introduction temperament is relatively stable in adults, while it might be less stable during adolescence due to neurological development (19). Thus, in order to use PA and NA as trait measures among adolescents, future studies should address the test-retest reliability of the AFT model.

Moreover, although appealing to the senses, dichotomizing (e.g., dividing affect in high and low) has been recently criticized by researchers (44). Thus, the AFTs model should be critically investigated in order to fully assess its usefulness in empirical studies. It is plausible to suggest that the data could be analyzed using a 2 X 2 design (high-low affectivity X positive-negative affectivity). This type of analysis might investigate more directly the interaction of the two signal-sensitivity systems. Finally, although beyond the scope of the present chapter, it is important to address the theoretical question of referring to the AFTs as a model. After all, to the best of my knowledge, the AFTs have not been defined as a model in any study. However, in the present chapter the AFTs are used as a model or representation of the affective system defined as two separate interactive temperamental dispositions. In this line of thinking, individuals can experience affect as described by Norlander and colleagues (14); especially when affect is measured by the PANAS. In other words, individuals probably experience affect in different ways: some are high in both PA and NA while others are low in both; yet, others experience a combination of high and low in the two dimensions. According to Apostel (45) and others (46-48), a scientific model represents phenomena (in this case the affective temperamental system) in a logical but simplified way. Based on the nature and rationale behind the affective temperamental system presented in the introduction, it is reasonable to suggest Norlander's original work as a model of the temperamental affective system.

CONCLUSION

The present study's findings add to the research on adolescents' LS (49-60). More important, the findings add some shades of grey to the belief that the pursuit of a happy life has to be equal to high levels of intensive pleasure. For instance, among adults, individuals who report high levels of SWB seldom experience intense PA (only 2.6% of the time); instead they feel contented or mildly happy very frequently (61, 62). Furthermore, adolescents have a tendency to act in ways that are not congruent to their own self-conceptions (63). False self behavior leads to negative emotional outcomes, if the adolescents engage in such action because they devalue their "true self" (i.e., low self-acceptance). However, if they engage in false self behavior to please others or just for experimentation, such actions do not lead to negative emotions (63). Internalizing external influence from peers leads to self-alienation, in turn, leading to depression, lower levels of hope and SWB (64). Hence, one of the best advices a parent or a teacher can give to adolescents might be that the best shot to a happy life is to stay true to their own nature and to accept all parts of themselves.

"A man cannot be comfortable without his own approval"

Mark Twain

ACKNOWLEDGMENTS

The development of this article was facilitated thanks to the Stiftelse Kempe-Carlgrenska Fonden. We want to thank Patricia Rosenberg and the participants for their help facilitating the study. Appreciation is also directed to reviewers who helped improve the manuscript. Last but not least, we convey our gratitude to Anver Siddiqui, Anders Biel, and Carl Martin Allwood at the University of Gothenburg for their support and encouraging words.

310   *Danilo Garcia and Trevor Archer*

REFERENCES

[1] Diener E. Subjective well-being. Psych Bull 1984;95:542-75.

[2] Watson D, Clark LA. The PANAS-X: Manual for the positive and negative affect schedule—expanded form. Boise, IA: University Iowa Press, 1994.

[3] Tellegen A. Folk concepts and psychological concepts of personality and personality disorder. Psychol Inq 1993;4:122-30.

[4] Larsen RJ, Ketelaar T. Personality and susceptibility to positive and negative emotional states. J Pers Soc Psychol 1991;61:132-40.

[5] Lyubomirsky S, King L, Diener E. The benefits of frequent positive affect: Does happiness lead to success? Psychol Bull 2005;6:803-55.

[6] Watson D, Clark LA, Tellegen A. Development and validation of brief measures of positive and negative affect: The PANAS scale. J Pers Soc Psychol 1988;54:1063-70.

[7] Schimmack U. Methodological issues in the assessment of the affective component of subjective well-being. In: Ong AD, Van Dulmen MHM, eds. Oxford handbook of methods in positive psychology. New York: Oxford University Press, 2007:96-110.

[8] Fujita F, Diener E. Life satisfaction set point: Stability and change. J Pers Soc Psychol 2005;88:158-64.

[9] Lykken D, Tellegen A. Happiness is a stochastic phenomenon. Psychol Sci 1996;7:186-9.

[10] Gunderson JG, Triebwasser J, Phillips KA, Sullivan CN. Personality and vulnerability to affective disorders. In: Cloninger CR, ed. Personality and psychopathology. New York: American Psychiatric Publishing, 1999:3-32.

[11] Garcia D, Siddiqui A. Adolescents' affective temperaments: Life satisfaction, interpretation and memory of events. J Pos Psychol 2009;4: 155-67. DOI: 10.1080/17439760802399349.

[12] Garcia D, Siddiqui A. Adolescents' psychological well-being and memory for life events: Influences on life satisfaction with respect to temperamental dispositions. J Happ Stud 2009;10:387-503. DOI: 10.1007/s10902-008-9096-3.

[13] Garcia D, Rosenberg P, Erlandsson A, Siddiqui A. On lions and adolescents: Affective Temperaments and the influence of negative stimuli on memory. J Happ Stud 2010;11:477-95. DOI: 10.1007/s10902-009-9153-6.

[14] Norlander T, Bood S-Å, Archer T. Performance during stress: Affective personality age, and regularity of physical exercise. Soc Behav Pers 2002;30:495-508.

[15] Fredrickson BL. The broaden-and-build theory of positive emotions. In: Csikszentmihalyi M, Csikszentmihalyi IS, eds. A life worth living: Contributions to positive psychology. New York: Oxford University Press, 2006:85-103.

[16] Fredrickson BL, Branigan C. Positive emotions broaden the scope of attention and thought-action repertoires. Cogn Emot 2005;19:313-32.

[17] Higgins ET. Beyond pleasure and pain. Am Psychol 1997;52:1280-1300.

[18] González M, Casas F, Coenders G. A complexity approach to psychological well-being in adolescence: Major strengths and methodological issues. Soc Indic Res 2007;80:267-95.

[19] Windleand M, Windle RC. Adolescent temperament and lifetime psychiatric and substance abuse disorders assessed in young adulthood. Pers Ind Diff 2006;41:15-25.

[20] Ryan RM, Deci EL. On happiness and human potentials: A review of research on hedonic and eudaimonic well-being. Ann Rev Psychol 2001;52:141-66.

[21] Kahneman D, Diener E, Schwarz N, eds. Well-being: The foundations of hedonic psychology. New York: Russell Sage (1999:213-29.

[22] Pavot W. The assessment of subjective well-being: Successes and shortfalls. In: Eid M, Larsen RJ, eds. The science of subjective well-being. New York: Guilford, 2008:124-67.

[23] Martin KM, Huebner ES. Peer victimization and prosocial experiences and emotional well-being of middle school students. Psychol Sch 2007;44: 199-208.

[24] Pavot W, Diener E. Review of the satisfaction with life scale. Psychol Ass 1993;2:164-72.

[25] Proctor CL, Linley PA, Maltby J. Youth life satisfaction: A review of the literature. J Happ Stud 2009;10:583-630.

[26] Schimmack U, Diener E. Affect intensity: Separating intensity and frequency in repeatedly measured affect. J Pers Soc Psychol 1997;73:1313-30.

[27] Waterman AS. Two conceptions of happiness: Contrasts of personal expressiveness (eudaimonia) and hedonic enjoyment. J Pers Soc Psychol 1993;64:678-91.

[28] Ryff CD. Psychological well-being in adult life. Curr Dir Psychol Sci 1995;4:99-104.

[29] Ryff CD, Keyes CLM, Shmotkin D. Optimizing well-being: The empirical encounter of two traditions. J Pers Soc Psychol 2002;82:1007-22.

[30] Ryff CD. Happiness is everything, or is it? Explorations on the meaning of psychological well-being. J Pers Soc Psychol 1989;57:1069-81.

[31] Urry HL, Nitschke JB, Dolski I, Jackson DC, Dalton KM, Mueller CJ, et al. Making life worth living: Neural correlates of well-being. Psychol Sci 2004;15:367-72.

[32] Clarke PJ, Marshall VM, Ryff CD, Wheaton B. Measuring psychological well-being in the Canadian study of health and aging. Int Psychogeriatr 2001;13:79-90.

[33] Tugade MM, Fredrickson BL. Resilient individuals use positive emotions to bounce back from negative emotional arousal. J Pers Soc Psychol 2004;86:320-33.

[34] Cloninger CR. Fostering spirituality and well-being in clinical practice. Psychol Ann 2006;36:1-6.

[35] Reschly AM, Huebner ES, Appleton JJ, Antaramian S. Engagement as flourishing: The contribution of positive emotions and coping to adolescents' engagement at school with learning. Psychol Sch 2008;45:419-31.

[36] Larson RW. Toward a psychology of positive youth development. Am Psychol 2000;55:170-81.

[37] Magen Z. Exploring adolescent happiness. Commitment, purpose and fulfillment. London: Sage, 1998.

[38] Huebner ES. Initial development of the student's life satisfaction scale. Sch Psychol Int 1991;12:231-40.

[39] Laurent J, Catanzaro SJ, Joiner TE, Rudolph KD, Potter KI, Lambert S, et al. A measure of positive and negative affect for children: Scale development and preliminary validation. Psychol Ass 1999;11: 326-38.

[40] Proctor CL, Linley PA, Maltby J. Youth life satisfaction measures: A review. J Pos Psychol 2009;5: 128-44.

[41] Huebner ES, Dew T. Preliminary validation of the positive and negative affect schedule with adolescents. J Psychoeduc Ass 1995;13:286-93.

[42] McCullough G, Huebner ES, Laughlin JM. Life events, self-concept, and adolescents' positive subjective well-being. Psychol Sch 2000;37:281-90.

[43] Kim-Prieto C, Diener E, Tamir M, Scollon C, Diener M. Integrating the diverse definitions of happiness: A time-sequential framework of subjective well-being. J Happ Stud 2005;6:261-300.

[44] Keren G, Schul Y. Two is not always better than one. A critical evaluation of two-system theories. Perspect Psychol Sci 2009;4:533-50.

[45] Apostel L. Towards the formal study of models in the non-formal sciences. Synth 1960;12:125-61.

[46] Atkinson RC. The use of models in experimental psychology. Synth 1960;12:162-71.

[47] Chakravartty A. Informational versus functional theories of scientific representation. Synth 2010;172:197-213.

[48] Toon A. The ontology of theoretical modelling: models as make-believe. Synth 2010;172:301-15.

[49] Rothbart MK, Jones LB. Temperament, self-regulation, and education. Sch Psychol Rev 1998;27: 479-91.

[50] Fogle LM, Huebner ES, Laughlin JE. The relationship between temperament and life satisfaction in early adolescence: Cognitive and behavioral mediation models. J Happ Stud 2002;3:373-92.

[51] Funk BAIII, Huebner ES, Valois RF. Reliability and validity of a brief life satisfaction scale with a high school sample. J Happ Stud 2006;7:41-54.

[52] Garcia D. Two Models of Personality and Well-Being among Adolescents. Pers Ind Diff 2011;50,1208-1212. DOI: 10.1016/j.paid.2011.02.009.

[53] Garcia D, Rosenberg P, Siddiqui A. Tomorrow I Could Be in Trouble...But The Sun Will Come Out Next Year: The Effect of Temporal Distance on Adolescents' Judgments of Life Satisfaction. J Adolesc 2011;34,751-757. DOI: 10.1016/j.adolescence.2010.08.006.

[54] Garcia D, Kerekes N, Andersson-Arntén A-C, Archer T. Temperament, Character, and Adolescents' Depressive Symptoms: Focusing on Affect. Depress Res Treat 2012. DOI:10.1155/2012/925372.

[55] Garcia D, Moradi S. Adolescents' Temperament and Character: A Longitudinal Study on Happiness. J Happ Stud 2011. DOI: 10.1007/s10902-011-9300-8.
[56] Garcia D. The Affective Temperaments: Differences between Adolescents in the Big Five Model and Cloninger's Psychobiological Model of Personality. J Happ Stud 2011. DOI: 10.1007/s10902-011 -9303-5.
[57] Garcia D, Moradi, S. The Affective Temperaments and Well-Being: Swedish and Iranian Adolescents' Life Satisfaction and Psychological Well-Being. J Happ Stud 2012. DOI: 10.1007/s10902-012-9349-z.
[58] Garcia D, Kerekes N, Archer T. A Will and a Proper Way Leading to Happiness: Self-Directedness Mediates the Effect of Persistence on Positive Affectivity. Pers Ind Diff 2012 DOI: 10.1016/j.paid.2012.07.025.
[59] Garcia D, Sikström S. Quantifying the Semantic Representations in Adolescents' Memories of Positive and Negative Life Events. J Happ Stud 2012.
[60] Garcia D, Archer T, Moradi S, Andersson-Arntén A-C. Exercise Frequency, High Activation Positive Affectivity, and Psychological Well-Being: Beyond Age, Gender, and Occupation. *Psych 2012;*3:328-336.
DOI: 10.4236/psych.2012.32040.
[61] Diener E, Diener C. Most people are happy. Psychol Sci 1996;7:181-5.
[62] Diener E, Seligman MEP. Very happy people. Psychol Sci 2002;13:81-4.
[63] Harter S, Marold DB, Whitesell NR, Cobbs G. A model of the effects of perceived parent and peer support on adolescent false self behavior. Chi Dev 1996;67:360-74.
[64] Wood AM, Linley PA, Maltby J, Baliousis M, Joseph S. The authentic personality: A theoretical and empirical conceptualization and the development of the authentic scale. J Couns Psychol 2008;55: 385-99.

Submitted: September 05, 2011. *Revised:* November 15, 2011. *Accepted:* December 01, 2011.

In: Alternative Medicine Research Yearbook 2012
Editors: Søren Ventegodt and Joav Merrick

ISBN: 978-1-62808-080-3
© 2013 Nova Science Publishers, Inc.

Chapter 32

THE FAMILY ENVIRONMENT IN ADOLESCENCE AS A PREDICTOR OF LIFE SATISFACTION

Liisa Martikainen, PhD *

Unit of Sign Language Interpereting, HUMAK (Humanistinen
Ammattikorkeakoulu), University of Applied Sciences, Helsinki, Finland

ABSTRACT

This study investigates the relationship between family environment-related factors in adolescence and the level of life satisfaction in adulthood. The data were gathered from a representative sample of a Finnish age cohort (born 1968) at two time periods (1984; N=396, and 2001; N=192) via a questionnaire. The research subjects consisted of two subgroups of young adults representing single women living in cities (N=25) and single men living in the countryside (N=36). These groups had previously been found to have the lowest levels of life satisfaction among five distinct groups of Finnish young adults. The statistical methods used were correlation analysis, t-testing and ANOVA. The results showed that for women the most important factor predicting the level of life satisfaction in adulthood was the quality of the mother-daughter –relationship in adolescence. For men the most important factor underlying poor adult life satisfaction was the low occupational status of the fathers; this in turn was related to subjects' poor school achievement and unhealthy living habits at age 15-16 years. The results highlight the importance of a life-span perspective in life satisfaction research.

Keywords: Adolescence, family, life satisfaction

---

* Correspondence: Liisa Martikainen, Unit of Sign Language Interpereting, HUMAK (Humanistinen Ammattikorkeakoulu), University of Applied Sciences, Kansanopistotie 32, 70800 Kuopio, Finland. E-mail: liisa.martikainen@humak.fi.

INTRODUCTION

In recent years, a good many studies have been conducted on life satisfaction and happiness within the fields of psychology, sociology and economic (1). In the main current of life-satisfaction research, satisfaction has usually been studied in relation to subjects' recent life situation. It is quite difficult to find longitudinal studies investigating factors from earlier life phases (such as childhood or adolescence) that might predict life satisfaction in adults (2,3). Thus, the aim of this study was to investigate the relationship between family environment - related factors in adolescence and life satisfaction in adulthood.

Even though this kind of longitudinal research has been very rare in life satisfaction research, there is some evidence from well-being research, that early relationships with one's parents predict mid- to late-life well-being (2,4-6). In theoretical terms, An and Cooney's study (4) is based on Erikson's theory of psychological development, which postulates progression through eight stages in the course of one's life-span (7). These stages represent unique psychosocial developmental challenges, and they must be appropriately resolved so that optimal development can be achieved at the stage in question and in the stages that follow. According to Erikson this applies to early childhood relationships in particular: resolutions of initial developmental crises surrounding trust are central to development across one's life-span (7).

The research of Kafetsios and Sideris (6) was based on the attachment theory put forward by Bowlby, which contends that differences in infant-parent relationships are likely to be similar to individual differences in romantic relationships, and that relationship quality in early life affects social and emotional development in later life-stages (8,9). In similar way to Erikson, Bowlby emphasizes the significance of trust and security in early relationships as predictors of healthy emotional development in later life; from this point of view the quality of early relationships would also underpin adult-life well-being (4,6).

Within psychological and sociological research in general, factors related to the home environment and to family relationships in childhood and adolescence have been seen as important in directing the whole of one's life-span. For example, it has been found that the quality of the parent-child relationship in childhood and adolescence correlates with the quality of romantic relationships in adulthood (10-12). It has also been shown that the parents' socioeconomic status strongly predicts the educational choices and occupational status of the child later in adolescence and in adulthood (13,14). Correspondingly, among adults, marital status and the quality of one's intimate relationships are related to life satisfaction (15-17); so too is occupational status (15,18,19). All things considered, it can be argued that both psychological and sociological factors should be taken into account when investigating the predictors of life satisfaction in longitudinal research.

The findings mentioned above seem to point in the same overall direction, but there remains a need to find out how, and to what extent, the quality of family the environment and of the parent-child relationship in childhood and adolescence predicts the level of life satisfaction in adulthood. The present study seeks to shed some further light on the matter.

In previous research concerning the life satisfaction of Finnish young adults, it was found that the study subjects (N=192) could be divided into five groups -which differed in both - their levels of life satisfaction and the factors underlying it (17). The groups identified were named according to their typical members as i) Settled women living in peaceful areas (these

The family environment in adolescence as a predictor of life satisfaction   315

having the highest level of life satisfaction), ii) Managerial men living in urban areas, iii) Managerial women living in the Helsinki conurbation, iv) Single men living in the countryside and v) Dissatisfied (single) women living in cities (the most dissatisfied group). The groups varied in the importance they attached to marital partnership, friends, health and hobbies as mediators of their level of life satisfaction (17).

The two most dissatisfied groups consisted mostly of young adults who were either single or divorced; in this they differed from the other three groups, whose members were mostly married or living in stable relationships (17).

Nevertheless, the group of single women was not identical with the group of single men in the factors related to their (low) level of life satisfaction. As the most important factors positively relating to life satisfaction, these women emphasized working conditions, health and friends. As a negative factor influencing their life satisfaction the members of this group mentioned the lack of a relationship they could commit themselves to. By contrast for single men, the most important factors positively influencing life satisfaction were work conditions and intimate relationships. Material factors such as a lack of money and problematic living habits were seen as important factors decreasing their level of life satisfaction. In addition, the environmental surroundings of these groups differed. Most of these single men lived in the countryside whereas the single women lived mostly in the cities (17).

The research subjects of the present study consisted of the members of these two subgroups of "most dissatisfied young adults". These two groups were chosen because it has been found that a low level of life satisfaction is in many cases related to deficient life control and –to a low level of perceived health (20-22). One can say with some confidence that the problems related to a low level of life satisfaction are in many cases quite serious, threatening the entire well-being of the individual; hence there is ample reason to attempt to solve them.

The results of the previous research showed that the groups of men differed markedly from the groups of women in their values, and in the daily activities of adult life that underpinned their life satisfaction (17). For this reason the main comparison in the present study were between the dissatisfied group of women and the other groups of women, and between the dissatisfied group of men and the other group of men. However, the dissatisfied men's and women's groups were also compared (see below).

Research questions

In order to explore factors related to the adolescent family environments that might predict the level of life satisfaction in adulthood, the following research questions were specified, focusing particularly on the two groups of "dissatisfied" Finnish young adults mentioned above:

> In what ways does the adolescent family environment of the group of single men living in the countryside differ from the family environment of the other group of men? In what ways are these family-related factors connected to life satisfaction in adulthood?
>
> In what ways does the family adolescent environment of the group of single women living in cities differ from the family environments of the other groups of women? In what ways are these family-related factors connected to life satisfaction in adulthood?

316
Liisa Martikainen

Are the factors related to adolescent family environment that predict life satisfaction in adulthood different between male and female participants? If so, in what way do these groups differ from each other?

METHODS

The data for the present study was taken from questionnaire data obtained from a representative sample of Finnish subjects born in 1968. The questionnaires were administered at two time periods: 1984 (N=396) and 2001 (N=192). In 1984 the data were gathered as part of research project concerning healthy and unhealthy living habits among Finnish adolescents' (23). The 2001 data collection was carried out by the present author as part of a research project concerning the construction of life satisfaction among Finnish young adults (17). During the first data-gathering period the subjects were aged 15-16 years; during the second period they were aged 32-33 years.

The main focus of the present study was on the two subgroups of young adults representing single women living in cities (N=25) and single men living in the countryside (N=36). These two groups were the most dissatisfied out of the five distinct groups of Finnish young adults previously identified (i.e. groups differing both – in their levels of life satisfaction and the factors affecting their life satisfaction).

In the present study the level of life satisfaction in adulthood was measured by the Likert scaled question: "Are you satisfied with the quality of your life these days?" The response categories were very unsatisfied=1, fairly unsatisfied=2, fairly satisfied=3 and very satisfied=4 (19).

The occupational status of one's parents was measured by two open ended questions asked in 1984. The questions took the form "What is the occupational status of your father?" and "What is the occupational status of your mother?" For the purposes of the present study, the answers given to the former question were coded on a 3-point scale: 1= lower occupational status (including mostly blue and pink-collar workers such as waiters and cleaners), 2 = middle occupational status (including mostly white collar workers such as nurses and technicians), and 3 = higher occupational status (including mostly white-collar professionals such as managers and physicians). The answers given to the latter question were coded on a 4-point scale. The additional category was that of "housewife". The subjects' occupational status was coded on the basis of the question: "What is your present occupational status?" with the answers being coded on a 4-point scale (1 = unemployed, 2= lower occupational status, 3 = middle occupational status and 4 = higher occupational status). The socioeconomic status of the family (family SES) was defined using both the father's and mother's occupational status as criteria. The variable for the family was expressed on a 7-point scale (24).

Data on school success (grade point averages) were collected from school archives (recorded when subjects were aged 15 years).The educational aims of the participants were collected in the earlier questionnaire on the basis of the question: "What kind of educational aims do you have for the future?". The response categories were primary school only=1, vocational school=2, college education=3 and university education=4. This was also the way is which way the answers were coded.

The family environment in adolescence as a predictor of life satisfaction   317

The respondents' living habits were measured by two questions concerning personal smoking and drinking. The individuals who did not drink or smoke at all were categorized as having healthy living habits (code=1); those, who either smoked or drank were categorized as an intermediate group (code=2), and those who both drank and smoked were categorized as having unhealthy living habits (code=3). The respondents' living habits were measured at both time periods, i.e. in 1984 and again in 2001.

The variable called maturity of thinking (MOT) was summarized on the basis of four questions asked in 1984: "What would you do, if 1) you were in danger of witnessing a physical fight? 2) someone ridiculed you? 3) you were rejected by the friend? and 4) you failed at school?" The MOT index was coded on 3-point scale on the basis of the appositeness and originality of the answers given to those four questions (25).

The variable called quality of the mother-daughter/son –relationship was summarized on the basis of eight 5-point scaled dimensions, also collected in 1984. The question was formulated as "How would you describe the relationship between you and your mother as regards these dimensions?":

cold – warm;
tense – relaxed;
quarrelsome – peaceful;
insecure – secure;
secretive – open;
judgmental – understanding;
restricted – supporting;
subordinate – equal.

The variable called quality of the father-daughter/son –relationship was formulated and collected in a similar way. The statistical analyses used in this study were: correlation analysis, t-testing and ANOVA.

RESULTS

The results showed that the most significant variable differentiating the family environments of single, less well educated men living in the countryside and managerial men living in urban areas was the father's occupational status, $t(61)=2.21$, $p<.031$. The fathers of the managerial men had an occupational status that was significantly higher ($M = 2.00$, $SD = .83$) than that of the fathers of the other men in the other group ($M = 1.57$, $SD = .73$). The occupational status of the father was in turn strongly correlated to the occupational status of the mother, $r =. 227$, $p<.000$ and thus there was some difference also in the family SES, $t(59) = 1.94$, $p<.057$ of these groups. The occupational status of the father also correlated with the son's school success, educational aims, maturity of thinking and living habits and with the likelihood of their son witnessing a fighting situation when they were aged 15-16 (Table 1).

The lower the occupational status of the father, the lower the school success, the educational aims and the maturity of thinking of the son and the higher the risk of witnessing a fighting situation. One third (31 %) of the members of the group of less well educated men also reported personal experiences of verbal and physical violence within the childhood family or peer group, while only one tenth (11 %) of the managerial men reported such events.

Table 1. Correlations of the variables connected to the male participants life situation (ages 15-16) with the father's occupational status (N=75; Pearson's R)

Variables	r	p
Educational aims	.224**	.008
School success	.408***	.000
Living habits	.194*	.021
Witnessing a fight	.248**	.003
Maturity of thinking	.401***	.000

***p<.001, **p<.01, *p<.05.

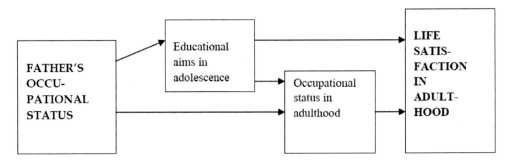

Figure 1. Relationship between the father's occupational status during the subjects' adolescence and the life satisfaction of the subjects in adulthood.

An examination of the relationship between life satisfaction in adulthood and the adolescent family-related variables mentioned above indicates that the educational aims at age 15-16 correlated with life satisfaction at age 32-33, r =.228, p<.049. The educational aims in adolescence also correlated with the occupational status in adulthood, r = .376, p<.000, which in turn was related to life satisfaction in adulthood, r = .430, p<.000. The occupational status of the father and subject's own occupational status also correlated, r = . 233, p<.005. All these relationships can also be seen in figure 1.

On the other hand the most significant variable differentiating the family environments of the three groups of women, i.e. single women living in cities (N=23), managerial women living in the Helsinki conurbation (N=14), and settled women living in peaceful areas (N=49), was the quality of the mother-daughter–relationship during adolescence, F(2, 83) = 3.95, p<.023. The single women living in cities were particularly likely to have described their mothers as being judgmental and their relationship as insecure (see table 2). Every second member of this group (53 %) had also reported their family as hardly ever spending weekends together, while only one third (29 %) of the settled women and two fifths (43 %) of the managerial women had reported such a pattern of family life. When the relationship between life satisfaction in adulthood and above family-related factors in adolescence was analysed, some important indirect relationships were found. The quality of the mother-daughter – relationship at age 15-16 correlated with the women's marital status at age 32-33, r =.155,

The family environment in adolescence as a predictor of life satisfaction   319

p<.036, which in turn strongly correlated with life satisfaction in adulthood, r =.358, p<.000. Marital status was also a factor that differentiated the most dissatisfied group of women from the other groups of women: the dissatisfied women were more likely than the other to be unmarried or divorced, F(2,85)=214.49, p<.000.

Table 2. Dimensions in the mother-daughter –relationship differentiating the three groups of women (ANOVA)

Dimension of mother-daughter relationship	Single women (N=23)		Managerial women (N=14)		Settled women (N=49)		F	p
	M-------------SD		M-------------SD		M -------------SD			
Judgmental-understanding	3.35	1.11	4.29	.825	3.94	.944	4.645**	.012
Secure-insecure	3.91	1.20	4.63	.633	4.33	.922	2.684*	.074

**p<.05,*p<.1.

The quality of the mother-daughter –relationship was also related to experiences of violence in adulthood relationships, r =.212, p<.004, which in turn were related to adult life satisfaction, r =.159, p<.029. The single/divorced women's group had experienced violence in their adulthood relationships more often than the other women, F(2,85)=5.10, p<.008.

Finally, when a comparison was made of factors related to the adolescent family environment in terms of predicting the adult life satisfaction of male and female participants clear differences emerged. For example, whereas the most important factor differentiating the groups of men with different levels of adult life satisfaction was the occupational status of the father, that same factor did not distinguish at all between the groups of women F(2,85)=0.85, p<.831, ns. Conversely, whereas the most important factor differentiating the groups of women with different levels of adult life satisfaction was the quality of the mother-daughter relationship, the mother-son (or the father-son) relationship did not differentiate between the groups of men, t (62)=0.04, p<.965, ns.

DISCUSSION

The results of this study indicate that the roots of life satisfaction in adulthood go back to the family environment in adolescence. The study also suggests that both psychological and sociological aspects should be taken into account in longitudinal life-satisfaction research.

The psychological factors found in this study are in the line with other research results indicating that the quality of intimate relationships in childhood and adolescence is a predictor of the quality of adult intimate relationships (10,12,26) and of adult experiences of loneliness (10). According to the results of the present study, these factors also predict adult life satisfaction (2).

The sociological factors found in this study are also in line with the results of earlier studies indicating that the social class or occupational status of one's parents strongly predicts one's own social class in later life (13,14,24). Nevertheless, the present study goes beyond most earlier studies in finding a connection between the parents' occupational status and the life satisfaction of the offspring in later life.

The results of this study also indicate that life-satisfaction research could benefit from a gender-sensitive approach. As has been shown previously, the factors underlying an individual's life satisfaction are dependent on his/her values (27). Some explanations for this phenomenon can be found from the (persistent) differences that exist in the values of men and women. It has been shown that men usually place a greater emphasis on traditional work-related values such as pay and career development, while women usually place a greater emphasis on social-related values such as altruistic rewards, or taking care of family relationships (17,28).

From the results of this study it could be suggested that abilities that enable women to establish successful intimate relationships, or men to gain a successful working career in later life are important in the construction of adult life satisfaction.

The results do not, of course, tell us anything about the stability of the values identified, or whether these will be in gender-differentiated in generations to come. In the future new values may emerge, leading to the formation of new subgroups, which will have to be investigated without reliance on previous findings.

While it can be claimed that the present study offers some new insights into the construction of life satisfaction in adulthood, much remains to be discovered concerning the variations in personal and societal level factors that can affect the level of life satisfaction over ones' life span. Moreover, there are a number of limitations in the present study that one would seek to correct in future research. For example, broader and more representative samples would be beneficial, since the research sample is relatively small. All in all, it is clear that the relationship between the factors related to early life phases and adult-life satisfaction is a complicated one; hence it is definitely in need of more thorough investigation with a more sophisticated methodology.

REFERENCES

[1] Veenhoven R. World database of happiness, Erasmus University Rotterdam. Accessed 2011 Sep 15. URL: http://worlddatabaseofhappiness.eur.nl

[2] Flouri E. Subjective well-being in midlife: The role of involvement of and closeness to parents in childhood. J Happ Stud 2004;5:335-58.

[3] Diener E, Suh E, Lucas R, Smith H. Subjective well-being: Three decades of progress. Psych Bull 1999;125: 276-302.

[4] An J, Cooney T. Psychological well-being in mid to late life: The role of generativity development and parent-child relationships across lifespan. Int J Behav Dev 2006;30:410-21.

[5] Franz C, McClelland D, Weinberger J. Childhood antecedents of conventional social accomplishment in midlife adults: A 36-year prospective study. J Pers Soc Psychol 1991;60:586-95.

[6] Kafetsios K, Sideridis G. Attachment, social support and well-being in young and older adults. J Health Psychol 2006;11:863-75.

[7] Erikson E. Childhood and society. New York: WW Norton, 1963.

[8] Bowlby J. Attachment and loss. Vol 1: Attachment. New York: Basic Books, 1969.

[9] Bowlby, J. The making and breaking of affectional bonds. Br J Psychiatry 1977;130:201-10.

[10] [10] Hazan C, Shaver P. Romantic love conceptualized as an attachment process. J Pers Soc Psychol 1987;52:511-24.

[11] Race K, Mulkeen P. Relationships with parents and peers: A longitudinal study of adolescent intimacy. J Adolesc Res 1995;10:338-57.

[12] Waters S, Treboux D, Crowell J, Albersheim L. Attachment security in infancy and early adulthood: A twenty-year longitudinal study. Child Dev 2000;71:684-9.

The family environment in adolescence as a predictor of life satisfaction   321

[13] Dubow E, Huesman L, Boxer P, Pulkkinen L, Kokko K. Middle childhood and adolescent contextual and personal predictors of adult educational and occupational outcomes: A mediational model in two countries. Dev Psychol 2006;42:937-49.

[14] Stipek D, Ryan R. Economically disadvantaged preschoolers: Ready to learn but further to go. Dev Psych 1997;33:711-23.

[15] Delhey J. Life satisfaction in an enlarged Europe. Luxembourg: Office Official Publications European Communities, 2004.

[16] Gunderlach P, Kreiner S. Happiness and life satisfaction in advanced European countries. Cross Cult Res 2004;38:359-86.

[17] Martikainen, L. The many faces of life satisfaction among Finnish young adults. J Happ Studies 2009;10:721-37.

[18] Blanchflower DG, Oswald A.J. Well-being over time in Britain and the USA. J Pub Econ 2004;88:1359-86.

[19] Veenhoven, R. Developments in satisfaction-research. Soc Indic Res 1996;37:1-46.

[20] Koivumaa-Honkanen, H. Life satisfaction as a health predictor. Kuopion yliopiston julkaisuja D. Lääketiede 1998;143:1235-303.

[21] Suominen S. Perceived health and life control. Helsinki: Stakes Research Reports 26, 1993.

[22] Söderqvist S, Backman G. Life control and perceived health. Åbo: Åbo Academy, 1988.

[23] von Wright MR, Makkonen M, Markkanen T. Healthy and unhealthy living habits among 15-16 year-old Finnish adolescents. Helsinki: National Board Health, Reports 2, 1986.

[24] Pulkkinen L, Ohranen M, Tolvanen A. Personality antecedents of career orientation and stability among women compared to men. J Voc Behav 1999;54:37-58.

[25] Rauste von Wright M. Maturity of thinking of 15-year-old girls and boys as assessed from the reasons given for answers to questions about their beliefs. Scand J Psych 1983;24:67-74.

[26] Cassidy J. Adult romantic attachments: A developmental perspective on individual differences. Rev Gen Psych 2000;4:111-31.

[27] Oishi S, Diener E, Suh E, Lucas R. Value as a moderator in subjective well-being. J Pers 1999;67:157-82.

[28] Dæhlen M. Job values, gender and profession: a comparative study of the transition from school to work. J Educ Work 2007;20:107-21.

Submitted: October 05, 2011. *Revised:* November 25, 2011. *Accepted:* December 05, 2011.

In: Alternative Medicine Research Yearbook 2012
Editors: Søren Ventegodt and Joav Merrick

ISBN: 978-1-62808-080-3
© 2013 Nova Science Publishers, Inc.

Chapter 33

HOW PEOPLE ASSESS PRESENT AND FUTURE QUALITY OF LIFE IN THE ELDERLY FROM HEALTH STATUS INFORMATION

Maria Teresa Muñoz Sastre and Etienne Mullet[*]
Mirail University, Toulouse and Institute of Advanced Studies, Paris, France

ABSTRACT

We explored the way people judge the quality of life of elderly persons who are in bad health, and the way people anticipate their future quality of life if their health would come to deteriorate. One hundred participants aged 18 to 80 years were presented with vignettes that described elderly people's health status, and they were instructed to judge quality of life in each case. Five attributes were selected for describing the elderly persons' health state: intellectual functioning, presence of anxiety or depression, level of pain or discomfort, ability at conducting daily activities, and mobility. When assessing overall quality of life of elderly persons from these external indices or when anticipating one's future level of quality of life, participants used the information from all the indices, and cognitively integrated it in an additive fashion. Psychological aspects impacted more on quality of life judgments than physical aspects. The mere presence of only one kind of trouble was responsible for a drop in quality of life judgment, a drop that was higher than what the additive-type model predicts. Finally, the way people judge others' quality of life does not differ from the way people anticipate their future quality of life.

Keywords: Quality of life, health, aging, future

INTRODUCTION

Suppose you visit your elderly parents who are in a nursing home. During the visit, you meet various persons whom your parents know and whose health condition is not optimal. Some of

---

[*] Correspondence: Etienne Mullet, Institute of Advanced Studies, Paris, France. E-mail: etienne.mullet@ wanadoo.fr.

them can no longer walk. Others seem slightly demented. Still others seem to express psychiatric troubles. Even without being aware of it, you form a judgment about how miserable these persons maybe, and perhaps about how miserable you would personally be if you were in such situations. The present study was aimed at exploring the way (a) people judge the quality of life of elderly persons who are in bad health, and (b) people anticipate their future quality of life if their health would come to deteriorate.

The way people assess others' quality of life or happiness from external indices has not been much examined. This is unfortunate, because individuals in their role as spouses, parents, friends, or children are often affected by the degree of happiness of others. Affectionate sons or daughters wonder all the time about how happy their elderly parents are. They cannot settle for vague answers to the question "How are you?" Based on various observations of their loved ones, they will get their own idea of their elderly parents' degree of quality of life and will compare it to what they are told. Sons and daughters who believe that the only things necessary to the well-being of their elderly parents are a good place to live, some visits, and some gifts for special occasions will have to face a number of unexpected situations.

Muñoz Sastre (1) examined the way French people judge the well-being of others from five external indices: (a) health (good *vs.* bad), (b) harmony with spouse (good *vs.* bad), (c) harmony with children (good *vs.* bad), (d) friends (has friends *vs.* does not have friends), (e) work (has a satisfying job *vs.* has a poor job), and (f) leisure activities (has pleasant leisure activities *vs.* does not have any leisure activities). She created vignettes describing the current situation of a middle-aged person as a function of these indices, and instructed participants from various age groups to judge this person's probable level of well-being. She showed that (a) three indices had more impact on well-being judgments than others: health status, harmony with spouse, and harmony with children, (b) health status had more impact among middle-aged participants than among younger or older participants, (c) friends had more impact among younger participants than among other participants, and (d) the cognitive rule used for integrating the information conveyed by the six indices was an additive-type rule; that is, each index independently contributed to the overall assessment.

Using the same methodological framework, Macri and Mullet (2) examined the way Greek young people anticipate their future life satisfaction level as a function of three indices: personal employment, spouse employment, and family size. The cognitive rule that best accounted for anticipated life satisfaction judgments was an additive-type rule that may be expressed as: Anticipated Satisfaction = Proximity to optimal personal employment level + Proximity to optimal spouse's employment level + Proximity to optimal family size. This rule was valid as long as acceptable personal (for males) or personal and spouse's (for females) employment levels were considered. When non-acceptable employment levels were considered (e.g., unemployment), satisfaction with life was judged much lower than what could be expected from the model. In other words, the cognitive rule that was applied for assessing future life satisfaction was an additive-type rule with thresholds. This same rule was shown to be operative among young and adult French people (3) and among young French people of Maghrebi origin (4). In other words, this rule has cross-cultural validity.

Theuns, Hofmans and Verresen (5) examined the way in which young students anticipate their future well-being in adulthood from information about (a) material well-being, health status, and quality of family relationships (Study 1), (b) safety, productivity and love (Study 2), and (c) emotional well-being, place in community, and acquaintance intimacy (Study 3).

They showed that, in each case, the cognitive rule used by the students was of an additive-type. In addition, they found that in some cases, there were small deviations from strict additivity: When one level of one factor was low (e.g., bad health status), the impact of this factor was higher; an effect that is highly reminiscent of what had been shown by Bouazzaoui and Mullet (3,4). Theuns et al (6) examined the way in which young students anticipate their future happiness regarding social life in adulthood from information about relations with romantic partner, relations with friends and relations with parents. They found the same kind of additive-type rule, although some deviations from parallelism were present. The relations with partner factor was the most important factor for judging happiness, and when its level was low (e.g., bad relationships), its impact was slightly stronger than when it was high.

The present study

In the present study, we used the same methodology as the one that has been applied in previous studies (1-6). Vignettes were composed that described elderly people's health status and participants were instructed to judge quality of life in each case. Five attributes were selected for describing the elderly persons' health state: (a) intellectual functioning, (b) presence of anxiety or depression, (c) level of pain or discomfort, (d) ability at conducting daily activities (e.g., washing oneself), and (d) mobility.

These aspects were the ones that are constitutive of the EuroQol, a self-reporting measure of health-related quality of life that has been used in a variety of settings and with persons who differed greatly in terms of their health characteristics (7-11)

Our research questions were about the relative importance attributed to the five aspects, and about the nature of the cognitive rule used by the participants for integrating the information. From the five aspects that are listed above, which ones are deemed as truly important at the time of judging or at the time of anticipating quality of life? Are these aspects cognitively combined in an additive way as in the study by Muñoz Sastre (1) or are these aspects combined in such a way that experiencing only one kind of trouble would be enough to consider that quality of life must be low as in the study by Macri and Mullet (2)? Our research questions were also about the possible differences in cognitive processes at work when judging others' quality of life from external indices, and when anticipating one's own quality of life from these same indices.

How to diagnose judgment rules?

Anderson (12) has offered a number of graphical (and statistical) techniques for analyzing judgment rules. These techniques are generally used to characterize the main aspects of the information integration process in a simple fashion. Suppose that the elderly persons' descriptions comprise only three aspects -- patient's intellectual functioning, anxiety or depression, and pain or discomfort, and that these aspects are combined in an orthogonal design, resulting in several concrete descriptions as in the studies reported above (1-6). Suppose that participants judge the overall quality of life that is associated with each description on a continuous scale ranging from "the poorest one" to "the best one".

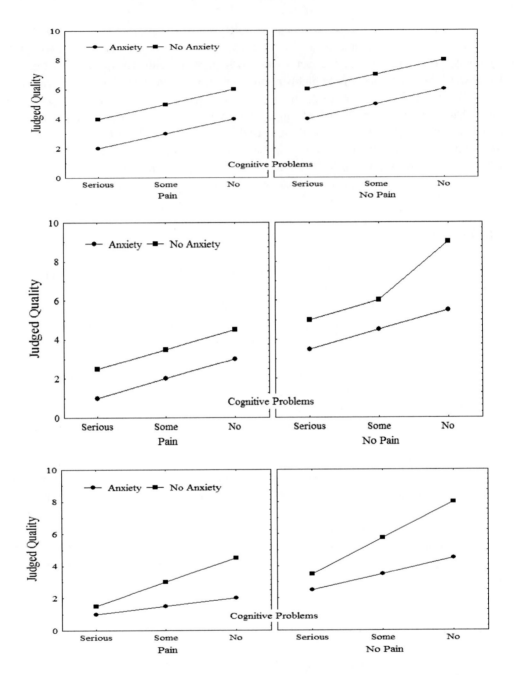

Figure 1. Theoretical predictions from three different models of judgment. The three levels of intellectual functioning used in the descriptions are on the x-axis (from the worst to the best), each curve corresponds to one level of anxiety and each panel corresponds to one level of pain and discomfort. Quality of life judgments are on the y-axis. Top panels show the pattern of results that would be expected from the application of an additive-type information integration rule. Center panels show the pattern of results that would be expected if the basic model was additive, and if, in addition, a single trouble was responsible for a specific drop in quality of life. Bottom panels show the pattern of results that would be expected from the application of a fully interactive information integration rule.

Figure 1 shows the pattern of results that would correspond to the application of a strict additive-type rule. The three levels of intellectual functioning used in the descriptions are on the x-axis (from the worst to the best), each curve corresponds to one level of anxiety and each panel corresponds to one level of pain and discomfort. Quality of life judgments are on the y-axis. Curves are ascending and clearly separated: The better the level of functioning and the better the patients' mood, the higher is the overall level of quality of life. In the right panel, curves are more elevated than they are in the left panel: The lesser the patient's pain, the higher is the overall level of quality of life. More importantly for our purposes, curves are parallel. This parallelism attests to the additive character of the combination rule. In this example, each factor independently adds its effect to the effect of the other factors. As indicated earlier, such a pattern of parallelism has been already observed in studies examining the way people assess the well being or happiness of others (1,13,14). It has also been found in a study on the way physicians and nurses assess patients' level of discomfort from behavioral cues (15).

The pattern of responses that is shown in the top panels is not the only one that could be observed. Participants may not apply a strict additive-type combination rule but instead judge as if the presence of only one trouble would be enough for causing a dramatic disruption in quality of life. The pattern of judgments that would correspond to the application of such a rule is shown in the center panels. As indicated earlier, an interactive pattern of this kind has been observed in studies about anticipated life satisfaction (2-4). Finally, the judgment rule may be a fully interactive one, in which the impact of each factor would depend on the level of the other factors. The pattern of judgments that would correspond to the application of such a rule is shown in the bottom panels. A similar pattern has, for instance, been observed in a study examining people's disutilities for the adverse outcomes of cardiopulmonary resuscitation (16,17).

METHODS

Participants were unpaid volunteers recruited while walking in the streets of Toulouse, a city in the south of France, by Master students trained in the kind of methodology used by Muñoz Sastre (1). The sample consisted of 100 adults (66% females and 33% males). Of those who were asked to participate, 53% accepted; that is, 189 persons in total were solicited to participate). Their ages ranged from 18 to 80 years. Mean age was 35.41 (SD = 16.38). All declared that they were in good health.

Material

The material was composed of 72 vignettes. Each vignette presented the health condition of a person, a question (e.g., What is the current level of quality of life of this person?), and an eleven-point response scale, which anchors were "the poorest state possible" on the left side [0], and "the best state possible" on the right side [10]. The persons' health conditions were described using five factors: (a) mobility (serious difficulties in walking and moving in general versus no special difficulties), (b) daily activities (serious problems in achieving daily life activities such as washing oneself, dressing oneself, and cooking; some problems for achieving these activities or no problems), (c) pain and discomfort (enduring pain and discomfort versus no pain), (d) anxiety and depression (anxious and depressed versus no psychological problems of this kind), and (e) intellectual functioning (seriously impaired; some problems, or no problems).

There were two versions. In one version, the person was somebody else, and the participants' task was to assess this person's quality of life. An example of a vignette used in this version was the following: "Mrs. Lopez currently faces serious troubles in walking, and, more generally, in moving herself around her home. She also faces serious troubles regarding daily activities such as washing herself, dressing, and cooking. She, however, does not experience pain or discomfort of any kind. She does not find herself anxious or depressed. Intellectually speaking, she does not have any problems."

In a second version, participants were instructed to imagine that they were the person described in the vignette. An example of a vignette used in this alternative version is the following: "Suppose that you are now an elderly person. You don't face any trouble in walking or moving yourself in around your home. Furthermore, you do not have any troubles in daily activities such as washing yourself, dressing, or cooking. You, however, experience chronic pain, and much discomfort. You feel yourself very anxious and very depressed. Intellectually speaking you begin to experience some cognitive troubles".

Procedure

The experiment took place in two phases in a single session, in accordance with the standard procedure for applying this methodology (12). The first was the phase of familiarization. The scoring system was explained, 36 vignettes were presented in random order, and the participants were asked to rate each level of quality of life on the response scale. They were given the opportunity to change their ratings, to go back to previous scenarios, and to compare their ratings as often as they wanted. The experimenter answered their questions about the meaning of each outcome, as well as about the experimental procedures, but refrained from making any value judgment.

The second phase was the true experimental phase. It took place in the same fashion as the familiarization phase, except that the participants were presented the whole set of vignettes and they were no longer allowed to look back or to make changes in their ratings. Only the data from this phase were subjected to statistical analyses. Between each phase, the participants were given a rest period. The sessions lasted 30-45 minutes.

RESULTS

An ANOVA was performed on the raw data, with a design of Condition (Other versus Self) x Intellectual functioning x Anxiety x Pain x Daily activities x Mobility, 3 x 2 x 2 x 3 x 2. Owing to the great number of comparisons, the significance threshold was set at .001. The results of these analyses are shown in Table 1. As there were neither main effects for

How people assess present and future quality of life ...   329

participants' age, gender or educational level, nor any interaction of these variables with the intra-subject factors, they were not introduced in the final analysis.

Condition had no significant effect, but the five intra-subject factors were significant. Table 2 shows the mean quality of life assessments that were associated with each level of each factor.

Table 1. Results of the ANOVA conducted on the raw data. All non-reported, higher order interactions are non-significant

Factors	Effect		Error		F	p	η^2_p
	df	MS	df	MS			
Condition (C)	1	14.87	93	39.94	0.37	ns	.01
Intellectual Functioning (I)	2	2 761.16	186	14.06	196.32	.001	.68
Anxiety Depression (A)	1	4 969.36	93	18.94	262.32	.001	.74
Pain Discomfort (P)	1	2 993.42	93	9.59	312.26	.001	.77
Daily Activity (D)	2	914.01	186	3.24	282.07	.001	.75
Mobility (M)	1	2 667.50	93	15.26	174.77	.001	.65
C x I	2	20.90	186	14.06	1.49	ns	.02
C x A	1	5.34	93	18.94	0.28	ns	.00
I x A	2	41.40	186	2.17	19.11	.001	.17
C x P	1	5.61	93	9.59	0.59	ns	.01
I x P	2	53.78	186	1.73	31.07	.001	.25
A x P	1	22.68	93	2.94	7.73	ns	.08
C x D	2	8.28	186	3.24	2.56	ns	.03
I x D	4	14.31	372	1.23	11.62	.001	.11
A x D	2	7.62	186	1.31	5.81	ns	.06
P x D	2	25.96	186	2.62	9.90	.001	.10
C x M	1	4.22	93	15.26	0.28	ns	.00
I x M	2	16.94	186	2.24	7.56	.001	.08
A x M	1	13.11	93	2.40	5.46	ns	.06
P x M	1	7.74	93	1.91	4.05	ns	.04
D x M	2	13.27	186	1.88	7.07	ns	.07
C x I x A	2	10.98	186	2.17	5.07	ns	.05
C x I x P	2	0.49	186	1.73	0.28	ns	.00
C x A x P	1	0.12	93	2.94	0.04	ns	.00
I x A x P	2	29.85	186	1.46	20.47	.001	.18
C x I x D	4	3.38	372	1.23	2.74	ns	.03
C x A x D	2	4.43	186	1.31	3.38	ns	.04
I x A x D	4	6.50	372	1.24	5.24	.001	.06
C x P x D	2	6.44	186	2.62	2.46	ns	.03
I x P x D	4	6.77	372	1.60	4.23	ns	.04
A x P x D	2	25.37	186	1.51	16.82	.001	.15
C x I x M	2	2.08	186	2.24	0.93	ns	.01
C x A x M	1	0.99	93	2.40	0.41	ns	.00
I x A x M	2	9.11	186	1.59	5.72	ns	.06
C x P x M	1	0.10	93	1.91	0.05	ns	.00
I x P x M	2	3.67	186	1.56	2.35	ns	.02
A x P x M	1	13.76	93	1.56	8.81	ns	.08
C x D x M	2	0.93	186	1.88	0.50	ns	.01
I x D x M	4	2.44	372	1.03	2.37	ns	.02
A x D x M	2	1.23	186	1.16	1.05	ns	.01
P x D x M	2	15.92	186	2.25	7.07	ns	.07

Table 2. Mean level of quality of life associated with each level of the five within-subject factors

Factor	Lowest Level	Intermediate Level	Highest Level	Absolute Difference (Impact)
Intellectual Functionning	3.82	4.63	6.00	2.18
Anxiety and Depression	3.96		5.67	1.71
Pain and Discomfort	4.15		5.48	1.33
Mobility	4.19		5.44	1.25
Daily Activities	4.26	4.69	5.50	1.24
Total				7.80

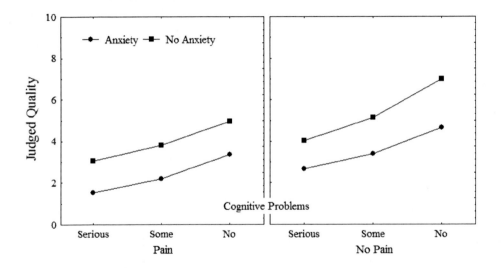

Figure 2. Observed pattern of responses in the case of the Intellectual functioning x Anxiety x Pain interaction.

Between the lowest level and the highest levels of the intellectual functioning and anxiety-depression factors, the difference in quality of life is higher than 1.50 (on a 0-10 scale), whereas between the lowest level and the highest levels of the mobility and daily activities factors, the difference in quality of life is lower than 1.50.

Several two-way and three-way interactions were significant. Figure 2 shows the Intellectual functioning x Anxiety x Pain three-way interaction. Overall, the two sets of curves are parallel, as in the top panels of figure 1, except for one point, the one that corresponds to the combination of good functioning, no anxiety and no pain. As in the center panel of figure 1, this point was higher than expected. The pattern of results that correspond to the other three-way interactions was highly similar to the one shown in figure 2. In each case, deviation from parallelism was observed regarding only one point, the one that corresponds to the complete absence of trouble.

CONCLUSION

Several main findings have emerged from the present study. Firstly, when assessing overall quality of life of elderly persons from external indices, or when anticipating one's future level of quality of life, people use information from all of the indices. This finding was consistent with previous findings (1,6). Secondly, the way people cognitively combine the information from the external indices is basically of an additive-type one; that is, all pieces of information independently impact on the quality of life judgment. As a result, a low level of one factor can be offset by a high level of another factor. This finding was also consistent with previous results (1,5,6,13,14), and it was consistent with the idea that the score structure of the EuroQol is basically an additive one.

Thirdly, psychological aspects (intellectual functioning and anxiety-depression) impact more on quality of life judgments than physical aspects (mobility and daily activities). In other words, quality of life was more associated with psychological intactness than with physical capabilities. This makes perfect sense. In cases of absence of mobility and in cases of other physical troubles, people can still have a meaningful life because somebody else can help compensate for these difficulties. In cases of psychological dysfunctions, drugs can be of some help but it is the meaning of life that begins to be altered. As a result, if some compensation between aspects of quality of life can occur, not all aspects of life can be equally compensated. Compensating for deterioration in psychological aspects will be more difficult than compensating for deterioration in physical aspects.

Fourthly, the mere presence of only one kind of trouble was responsible for a drop in quality of life judgment, a drop that was higher than what the additive-type model predicts. In other words, as soon as one trouble is experienced, a drop is expected in quality of life, and this drop is larger than the one that this trouble would produce if it occurred in association with other troubles. This phenomenon is relatively easy to understand and does not constitute a strong argument against basic additivity. This drop means that there is some kind of bonus in quality of life that is associated, in people's mind, with the absence of any trouble. This finding was consistent with previous findings by Macri and Mullet (2). In that study, for example, when the husband was durably unemployed, life satisfaction was judged to be low even if the spouse's employment level was acceptable and the family size was the expected one (5).

Fifthly, and finally, the way people judge others' quality of life does not differ from the way people anticipate their future quality of life from the same kind of indices. In other words, people have a general cognitive rule for assessing quality of life from external indices, and they apply it in all situations.

REFERENCES

[1] Muñoz Sastre MT. Lay conceptions of well-being and rules used to judge well-being in young adults, middle-aged and elderly people. Soc Indic Res 1999;47:203-31.

[2] Macri D, Mullet E. Employment and family as determinants of anticipated life satisfaction among young Greek adults. Comun Work Fam 2003;6:197-215.

[3] Bouazzaoui B, Mullet E. Workload, family responsibilities, and anticipated life satisfaction: Contrasting young adults' and elderly people's viewpoints J Happiness Stud 2002;3:129-152.

332   *Maria Teresa Muñoz Sastre and Etienne Mullet*

[4] Bouazzaoui B, Mullet E. Employment and family as determinants of anticipated life satisfaction: Contrasting European and Maghrebi people's viewpoints. J Happiness Stud 2005;6:161-185.

[5] Theuns P, Hofmans J, Verresen N. A functional measurement inquiry on the contribution of different life domains to overall subjective well-being. Teor Mod 2007;12:181-9.

[6] Theuns P, Verresen N, Mairesse O, Goossens R, Michiels L, Peeters E, Wastiau M. An experimental approach to the joint effects of relations with partner, friends and parents on happiness. Psicológica Int J Method Exp Psychol 2010;31:629-45.

[7] de Rivas B, Permanyer-Miralda G, Brotons C, Aznar I, Sobreviela E. Health-related quality of life in unselected outpatients with heart failure across Spain in two different health care levels. Magnitude and determinants of impairment: The INCA study. Qual Life Res 2008;18:1229-38.

[8] Xie F, Li S-C, Goeree R, Tarride J-E, O'Reilly D, Lo N-N, Yeo S-J, Yang K-Y, Thumboo J. Validation of Chinese Western Ontario and McMaster Universities Osteoarthritis Index (WOMAC) in patients scheduled for total knee replacement. Qual Life Res 2008;17:595-601.

[9] Serrano-Aguilar P, Munoz-Navarro SR, Ramallo-Farina Y, Trujillo-Martin MM. Obesity and health related quality of life in the general adult population of the Canary Islands. Qual Life Res 2009;18: 171-7.

[10] Suhonen R, Virtanen H, Heikkinen K, Johansson K, Kaljonen A, Leppanen T, Salantera S, Leino-Kilpi H. Health-related quality of life of day-case surgery patients: a pre/posttest survey using the EuroQoL-5D. Qual Life Res 2008;17:169-77.

[11] Versteeg H, Pedersen SS, Erdman RAM, van Nierop JWI, de Jaegere P, van Domburg RT. Negative and positive affect are independently associated with patient-reported health status following percutaneous coronary intervention. Qual Life Res 2009;18:953-60.

[12] Anderson NH. Unified social cognition. New York: Psychology Press 2008.

[13] Singh R, Sidana UR, Saluja SK. Integration theory applied to judgments of personal happiness by children. J Soc Psychol 1978;105:27-31.

[14] Singh R, Sidana UR, Srivastava P. Averaging processes in children's judgment of happiness. J Soc Psychol 1978;104:123-32.

[15] Igier V, Mullet E, Sorum PC. How nursing personnel judge patient's pain. Eur J Pain 2007;11:542-50.

[16] Gamelin A, Muñoz Sastre MT, Sorum PC, Mullet E. Eliciting utilities using functional methodology: People's disutilities for the adverse outcomes of cardiopulmonary resuscitation. Qual Life Res 2006;15:429-39.

[17] Sorum PC, Munoz Sastre MT, Mullet E, Gamelin A. Eliciting patient disutilities for the adverse outcomes of cardiopulmonary resuscitation. Resuscitation 2001;48:265-73.

Submitted: October 15, 2011. *Revised:* December 01, 2011. *Accepted:* December 07, 2011.

In: Alternative Medicine Research Yearbook 2012
Editors: Søren Ventegodt and Joav Merrick

ISBN: 978-1-62808-080-3
© 2013 Nova Science Publishers, Inc.

Chapter 34

CONDITIONS FOR THE DISSATISFYING EFFECT OF REFERENCE GROUP INCOME

Chau-Kiu Cheung [*]
Department of Applied Social Studies,
College of Liberal Arts and Social Sciences,
City University of Hong Kong, Hong Kong, PRC

ABSTRACT

Research has found a weak effect of the income of a supposed reference group on one's life satisfaction and assumed that social comparison theory explains the effect. This assumption is in need of further empirical examination. Specifically, the examination needs to identify the reference group with which one makes income comparisons. Based on this reference group, an elaboration of social comparison theory suggests two conditions for the impact of social comparison. Condition 1 suggests that reference group income is more dissatisfying when the reference group is larger. Condition 2 expects that income disparity is less dissatisfying when more of the reference group has comparable incomes. The test of the conditions in this study employs survey data obtained from 2,079 Hong Kong Chinese adults. Results manifested the two conditions based on personal income. In contrast, the main effect of reference group income on life satisfaction was too weak to be significant. Hence, the dissatisfying effect of reference group income is conditional on reference group size and the non-comparability of reference group income within the group.

Keywords: Life satisfaction, quality of life, income, economics

---

[*] Correspondence: Associate professor, Chau-Kiu Cheung, Department of Applied Social Studies, College of Liberal Arts and Social Sciences, City University of Hong Kong, Hong Kong, PRC. E-mail: ssjacky@cityu.edu.hk.

Introduction

Life satisfaction is an ideal for democracy, meaning that satisfied citizens are more willing to partake in civil activity for the sustenance of democracy (1). Meanwhile, promoting citizens' life satisfaction is at least an implicit promise in democracy. Most modern societies appear to practice or pursue democracy (2). Therefore, promotion of life satisfaction is a concern in most societies, which necessitates related research. In line with the ideal of democracy, the democratic factor of equality is supposedly a contributor to the citizen's life satisfaction (3). The contribution can rest on social comparison theory, such that one is satisfied with life when one finds oneself on par with others, particularly those included in the reference group (4,5). In this connection, personal income and family income are key factors for social comparison. However, the income of the reference group only manifests a very weak effect on one's life satisfaction, even though the effect is statistically significant because of the large sample (4,6). Such an effect is also statistically insignificant sometimes (7,8). This evidence illustrates that merely the income of the reference group is not adequate to reflect the effect of social comparison. That is, the income alone is insufficient to capture social comparison and equality, which are crucial in social comparison theory. Essentially, an elaboration of the theory based on the notion of comparable income is helpful to indicate the impact of income equality on life satisfaction (9). This is the approach adopted in the present study.

The present study is required to elucidate the profound influence of income in the reference group on life satisfaction. It would complement and enrich the majority of research that has not explicitly examined the reference group and social comparison (9). Such research only refers a reference group as other people of the same sex, age, education, time, and place (4,10). It misses the concern of social comparison theory that the reference group is one involved in social comparison (11,12). Essentially, social comparison is the condition for the impact of a reference group. Adhering to social comparison theory, the reference group in this study then explicitly refers to those individuals or families the one compares incomes. This is the self-defined reference group, rather than researcher-imposed group that one is unlikely to have contact, let alone income comparisons (9). The group needs to consist of one's acquaintances, or otherwise, one would have no knowledge about income in the group (13). With respect to social comparison theory, hence, a reference group is one best defined by the individual for comparing incomes (14,15). Comparing incomes with the self-defined income group then identifies a sense of relative deprivation deleterious to life satisfaction (16). Essentially, the self-defined reference group grasps the social comparison that is missing in the externally imposed reference group. That is, one can only compare incomes with acquaintances included in a self-defined reference group and cannot make the comparison with strangers whom one never meets or knows, even though one share the same background with the strangers. As the assumption of social comparison with the externally imposed reference group does not hold, it requires the identification of the self-defined reference group to illustrate the impact due to social comparison. With such identification, the study then elaborates the social comparison effects.

An elaboration of social comparison theory differentiates two comparisons, concerning the range and comparability of the object compared within the reference group (17,18). As regards income, range refers to the ratio of the highest income over the lowest income and comparability refers to the number of people having comparable incomes. The operationalization of comparability is the skew in the distribution of income in the reference group (19,20). This skew indicates the equality of income in the way that many people have relatively low incomes. Accordingly, when the skew is higher, one with low income is more likely to find comparable incomes in others. A paradoxical case is that when the income distribution is more unequal, as measured by the Gini coefficient, people are more likely to find equal incomes within the reference group. The Gini coefficient gauges the concentration of incomes in some group members such that a high score means few members take the large share of incomes and many members have comparably low (21). That is, higher income inequality measured by the Gini coefficient is paradoxically associated with higher income comparability. As social comparison theory expects a positive effect of income comparability on life satisfaction, life satisfaction can be higher in the more unequal income distribution. According to social comparison theory, comparability is favorable to one's life satisfaction because one desires to find others to be similar in order to affirm one's identity (22). This can be an alternative explanation for the positive impact of unequal income distribution in society on life satisfaction (23,24). The explanation is otherwise consistent with the finding of the positive effect of unequal income distribution in a community on the community member's life satisfaction (25).

Pivotal in social comparison theory is social comparison, which presupposes the identification of a reference group for comparison (26). However, social comparison rarely emerges as an explicit concern in research on life satisfaction. Such research often finds that the effect of income relative to that of an assumed reference group is very weak, even though it is occasionally statistically significant (4,6,10). More than examining such an effect, the present study applies social comparison theory to a thorough investigation of the six impacts of income derived from income comparison with a reference group. The impacts are those of:

size of the reference group,
average income of the reference group,
income range of the reference group,
income skew of the reference group,
interaction between reference group size and relative income, and
interaction between reference group income skew and income range or disparity,

The first hypothesis suggests that one who compares incomes with more people or has a larger reference group will have lower life satisfaction. In this connection, reference group size is a relative measure, as a proportion of one's acquaintances. The size is another indicator of social comparison, reflective of the practice of social comparison. Hence, the larger the reference group, the higher the exposure to interpersonal difference will be. Such exposure would create feelings of contrast and envy, which raise aspirations and lower life satisfaction eventually. Regardless of the exact mechanism, social comparison theory expects a negative effect of reference group size on life satisfaction (27).

The second hypothesis suggests that one has lower life satisfaction when the average income of the reference group is higher. This is the usual expectation and finding about the reference group or relative income (4,10). The expectation stems from social comparison theory, which indicates that when the comparison of income is unfavorable, life satisfaction would decline (14).

The third hypothesis expects that one who has a reference group with a larger income range will be less satisfied with life. This is the expectation of social comparison theory, which posits that inequality as reflected by income range erodes life satisfaction (18,20). According to social comparison theory in general, higher range means a greater difficulty to achieve the goal of assimilation in income level (28,29). This difficulty would impede life satisfaction.

The fourth hypothesis asserts that one with a reference group with a larger skew in income will be less satisfied with life. According to social comparison theory, comparison with equals is salutary (13,17). The salutary effect tends to arise from one's desire to find equals, as maintained in the thesis of homophily (30, 31).

The fifth hypothesis envisions that one's life satisfaction is particularly lower when one's reference group is both larger and having higher relative incomes. This hypothesis is the extension of the second hypothesis by adding the consideration of reference group income. Essentially, the hypothesis highlights the importance of social comparison in terms of having a large reference group to realize the negative impact of reference group income. In other words, the interaction between reference group size and reference group income is to register the weighted effect of reference group income. When reference group size represents the commonness of social comparison, it enhances the negative impact of reference group income. The enhancement would illustrate the force of numbers, popularity, or a norm (29,32).

The sixth hypothesis anticipates that one's life satisfaction is particularly higher when one's reference group has higher income skew and range or income disparity. This hypothesis is an elaboration of the third and fourth hypotheses. It suggests that income range in the reference group is less detrimental to life satisfaction when income skew, which reflects equality in the lower income segment, is higher. This tends to happen when income skew, which neutralizes the effect of income inequality, reflected by income range. This interaction effect reflects the positive effect of income inequality in a community or society on life satisfaction, as indicated by the Gini coefficient (23-25). Accordingly, a high level of this income inequality rests on high levels of both income range and income skew. However, income skew is an indicator of income equality, which would tender a positive effect on life satisfaction. More importantly, the high level of income skew reveals that the high level of income range is only incidental. This is the reason for income skew to temper the negative effect of income range. In the view of social comparison theory, when one rarely compares one's income with the highest income, the negative effect of the comparison is unlikely to materialize.

The study examines the above hypotheses for the personal income and family income of employed people and all people as well. This examination is worthwhile because both personal income and family income can be influential on the life satisfaction of employed people and people in general (8,33,34).

Relevance of the study in Hong Kong

Hong Kong is the place for examining the impacts of social comparison on the citizen's life satisfaction. This place is critical for the study because it is both similar with and different from most other modern societies. The similarity would facilitate the application of theory and knowledge usually derived from other, non-Chinese societies to examine and probably enhance their generalization. Nevertheless, the distinctiveness of Hong Kong would render it a sensible and sensitive place to test knowledge arising from non-Chinese societies and identify insights from the amelioration of the knowledge.

Similarly between Hong Kong and the main of modern societies is in economic development, the growth of economic inequality, sociopolitical structure, and immersion in Western culture and the global system (35-38). The similarly also specifically transpires in individualization or the strengthening of individualism, democratization, and reliance on the free market (39,40). Hedonism and the worship of money therefore become normative in Hong Kong (41). Essentially, Hong Kong influences and receives influences internationally, with increasing globalization (42,43). Shear flows of people, commodities, information, and capital just characterize the international nature of Hong Kong (44,45).

Meanwhile, Hong Kong is distinctive in its concentration of Chinese people, dense population, pollution, and social stability, despite the exceptionally high level of income inequality measured by the Gini coefficient (.533) (46,47). As such, physical living conditions in Hong Kong are undesirable (48,49). This may explain the unfavorable health level (50,51). The puzzle is that life satisfaction still maintains a fair level (19,52). Moreover, Hong Kong is not purely Chinese in culture, identity, and local political operation, because it is a special administrative region of China (40,53). It maintains a mental distance with strict security across the border between Hong Kong and Mainland China. Nevertheless, it gradually converges with Mainland China in economic, cultural, and other aspects, making it different from the West (54). These instances of distinctiveness, especially the high level of income inequality measured by the Gini coefficient, makes Hong Kong a suitable place to perform a conservative test of the hypotheses.

In order to examine the hypotheses, a number of background characteristics are required for controlling and adjusting for conditions in Hong Kong. These characteristics include gender, age, education, residency, personal income, family income, poverty, employment, religious faith, marital status, and acquiescence, the latter of which means the tendency of high rating. On the one hand, these characteristics tend to affect life satisfaction (4,10,51,55-57). Particularly, the older person appears to have higher life satisfaction than is the younger one (58,59). Hence, the age of 60 years or above is an indicator to reflect the old age effect. Personal income and family income, notably, are essential determinants of life satisfaction (33). They are particularly crucial as control factors for distilling effects of reference group income (4,10). On the other hand, background characteristics also have potential effects on social comparison and income in the reference group. Notably, the older person tends to show less social comparison than does the younger person (60). In this case, the older person is more likely to compare incomes with the past than with other people. Another reason may be the shrinking reference group of the same age with increasing age (61). Moreover, poverty may provide a reason for the person to have social comparison, because of concern for equity (62). The poorer person is also likely to have a reference group with lower income. Meanwhile, the person who resides in a place longer would have a larger reference group and more opportunities for social comparison (63).

Methods

A telephone survey collected data from 2,079 Hong Kong Chinese adults (aged 18 years and older) in 2009. The survey applied a random sampling procedure to engage respondents. First, the procedure randomly drew telephone numbers from a sampling frame of all residential telephone numbers in Hong Kong. Then, the procedure applied the recent-birthday method to select an adult to respond to the survey, randomly from each of the households contacted using the selected telephone numbers. Accordingly, selecting a household member whose birthday was the latest counted as a random sampling procedure (64). Trained interviewers conducted the telephone survey in the evenings of weekdays to ensure the proper administration of the survey questionnaire and collection of appropriate responses. The survey interview was subject to monitoring to safeguard its quality. Eventually, the response rate was 31.3%, based on the ratio of the number of respondents over the number of people contacted through telephone. This rate was at least favorably comparable to the average response rate (25%) of telephone surveys based on standard practice (65).

The sample had the following major characteristics. There was a fair distribution of respondents of the two sexes, when women represented 58.2% of the sample (see table 1).

The average age was 43.3 years, with a standard deviation of 23.2 years. Duration of residence in Hong Kong, on average, was 36.8 years. The average number of formal education was 10.6 years. A majority (68.4%) of them was not faithful to a religion. Employed adults represented a majority (79.0%), and only 1.3% of the respondents were unemployed. The geometric mean of monthly personal income, which included earnings and allowances from any sources, was US$1,198.3.

Meanwhile, the geometric mean of monthly per capita family income was $2,702.5. Around a fifth (21.4%) of the respondents lived in poverty. In this connection, poverty referred to a condition that reported family spending on food exceeded one third of family income (66). Such a measure of poverty was an alternative to measuring poverty by low personal and family incomes.

Measurement

Life satisfaction was a composite measure of five rating items about current feelings: "In most ways my life is close to my ideal;" "The conditions of my life are excellent;" "I am satisfied with my life;" "So far I have gotten the important things I want in life;" and "If I could live my life over, I would change almost nothing" (67). Each item generated a score ranging from 0 to 100, with 0 for "very little," 25 for "rather little," 50 for "average," 75 for "quite a lot," and 100 for "very much," based on a five-point scale. These items attained a reliability coefficient (α) of .741. The average of item scores gave the composite score.

Reference group size was a relative score representing the percentage of people or families of the respondent's acquaintances with which the respondent regarded as references for comparing incomes. Accordingly, each respondent reported the proportion of acquaintances or acquainted families that the respondent regarded as their references for comparing incomes. One proportion was for comparing personal incomes among acquaintances and another size was for comparing family incomes among acquainted families.

The relative income of the reference group was the ratio of the income of the reference group over the respondent's income. This ratio involved three items, about the highest income, lowest, and average income in the reference group. Three items measured personal incomes in the reference group and another three items measured family incomes in the reference group.

Reference group range was the ratio of the highest income over the lowest income in the reference group. The range generated two scores, one for personal income and another for family income.

Reference group frequency meant the frequency of comparable income within the reference group. A measure of it was the ratio of the gap between the highest and average income in the reference group over the gap between the average and lowest income in the reference group. The higher the ratio, the higher the proportion of the reference group had comparably low incomes. This proportion indicated the frequency of comparable income in the reference group.

Table 1. Means and standard deviations

Variable	Scoring	M	SD
Life satisfaction	0-100	53.1	18.4
Female	0, 100	58.2	49.3
Age	years	43.3	23.2
Age 60+	0, 100	21.8	41.3
Education	years	10.6	4.3
Residency	years	36.8	15.7
Personal income (monthly)	US$	1198.3	2479.7
Family income per capita (monthly)	US$	2702.5	4389.5
Poverty (food expense over one third of family income)	0, 100	21.4	41.0
Nonreligious	0, 100	68.4	46.5
Never married	0, 100	34.0	47.4
Unemployed	0, 100	1.3	11.5
Acquiescence	0-100	45.9	8.7
Personal income disadvantage (based on the same education)	%	48.8	20.4
Comparing family incomes	0-100	11.9	19.7
Comparing personal incomes	0-100	11.4	20.1
Reference group size for family income	%	16.74	37.002
Reference group size for personal income	%	16.10	36.622
Highest family income of the reference group	US$	6501.9	16353.8
Lowest family income of the reference group	US$	1187.0	1577.6
Average family income of the reference group	US$	2564.7	3911.2
Highest personal income of the reference group	US$	4963.2	10265.5
Lowest personal income of the reference group	US$	942.9	1729.2
Average personal income of the reference group	US$	1957.6	3121.0

Essentially, a high ratio reflected that the income distribution in the reference group was unequal, in the sense that most had low incomes and few had high incomes. This inequality, however, indicated that many people had comparable or even equal incomes at the lower end.

340   *Chau-Kiu Cheung*

In all, reference group frequency had two scores, one for personal income and another for family income.

Income disparity was the composite of two measures, reference group range for personal income and income disadvantage. Income disadvantage was the respondent's estimate of the percentage of people having the same education level as the respondent that had higher incomes than the respondent's income. The average of standardized scores of the two measures gave the score of income disparity.

Interactions included that between reference group range for income and that between reference group frequency for income and income disparity. Their scores were the products of standardized scores of constituents, and this scoring minimized the problem of multicollinearity (68).

Acquiescence was the average of all rating items, including those tapping life satisfaction and other aspects included in the questionnaire. It represented the tendency of high rating and served as a control variable in analysis (69). Hence, it would temper confounding due to exaggeration or the method artifact in self-reports.

Analysis

Linear regression analysis estimated the effects of various predictors on life satisfaction with three steps. The first step entered background characteristics into the regression model to tap background influence prior to the consideration of social comparison. The second step added into the model detailed reference group characteristics to examine their main effects. Those reference group characteristics included reference group size, income, range, frequency, and their interactions. The third step of regression analysis then added interaction terms involving reference group characteristics and income disparity. Hence, the analytic steps represented a hierarchical way of examination, involving background, main, and interaction effects progressively. Moreover, the second and third steps involved the social comparison of personal income and family income separately. This was to avoid the problem of mulitcollinearity stemming from correlations between the two sets of income comparison.

RESULTS

Separate analyses of personal income comparison and family income comparison were justified by substantial correlations between the two sets of income comparison (r = .467-.593, see table 2). That is, income comparison with a reference group happened in a parallel manner for personal income and family income. Besides, reference group range and reference group frequency manifested a moderate positive correlation (r = .296 & .278). The correlation indicated that higher income inequality was associated with higher income comparability. That is, when some members in the reference group had very high incomes, more of the members found comparable incomes within the group, as the very high incomes were exceptional. In contrast, average relative income had a negative correlation with income skew in the reference group (r = -.203 & -.177). This reflected the case that income distribution tended to manifest a positive skew such that incomes were more comparable when they were lower. When the average income was higher, the skew would be less positive and hence comparably low incomes would be less likely.

The first step of regression analysis mainly showed the impacts of background or control factors on life satisfaction. Accordingly, life satisfaction was significantly higher in one who was 60 years old or above, had a higher family income per capita, or not remaining single, controlling for other background characteristics and acquiescence (see Table 3). Meanwhile, personal income, poverty, unemployment, education, and other background characteristics did not display significant effects on life satisfaction.

The second step of regression analysis unfolded that reference group size had a significant negative effect on life satisfaction, either based on personal income comparison or family income comparison (β = -.117 & -.123, see Table 3). This finding supports Hypothesis 1, which asserts that more income comparison due to a larger reference group leads to lower life satisfaction.

The second step also showed that average relative income, income range, and income skew in the reference group, either for comparing personal or family incomes, did not spawn significant effects on life satisfaction (see table 3). This null finding lends no support to Hypotheses 2, 3, and 4 concerning the impacts of the details of income comparison. Nevertheless, the effect of average relative personal income of the reference group was negative, albeit weak and insignificant. This finding tends to concur with some existing studies, which employed very large samples to endorse the statistical significance of the weak effect of relative income (4,6,10).

Table 2. Correlations

Correlate	(1)	(2)	(3)	(4)	(5)	(6)	(7)
(1)	1.000						
(2)	.061	1.000					
(3)	-.114**	.041	1.000				
(4)	-.123**	-.203***	.296***	1.000			
(5)	.567***	.085*	-.072*	-.159***	1.000		
(6)	.091*	.467***	-.017	-.034	.147***	1.000	
(7)	-.069	.004	.593***	.202***	-.080*	.019	1.000
(8)	-.109**	-.152**	.182***	.488***	-.154***	-.177***	.278***

Reference group size for personal income.
Average relative personal income of the reference group.
Reference group range for personal income.
Reference group frequency for personal income.
Reference group size for family income.
Average relative family income of the reference group .
Reference group range for family income.
Reference group frequency for family income.
* $p < .05.$ ** $p < .01.$ *** $p < .001.$

The interaction between reference group size for personal income and the highest relative personal income in the reference group revealed a significant negative effect on life satisfaction (β = -.131, see Table 4). The finding is consonant with Hypothesis 5, suggesting the magnifying of the dissatisfying effect of reference group income by social comparison, as represented by reference group size. However, the interaction between reference group size for family income and the highest relative family income in the reference group did not manifest a significant effect (β = -.021, see Table 4). Hence, Hypothesis 5 obtains support based on personal income but not on family income.

The interaction between reference group frequency for personal income and income disparity showed a significant positive effect on life satisfaction (β = .161, see Table 4). That is, life satisfaction would be higher when income disparity occurred in a reference group with a higher frequency of comparable income. In this connection, reference group frequency mitigated the adverse effect of income disparity.

This finding was consistent with Hypothesis 6. However, the similar interaction involving family income did not present a significant effect on life satisfaction. Hence, Hypothesis 6 finds support only in the case of personal income comparison.

Table 3. Standardized regression coefficients for predicting life satisfaction in the first and second steps of the regression model

Predictor	(1)	(2) Personal income	(2) Family income
Female	.069	.077	.084
Age	-.093	-.123	-.127
Age 60+	.135*	.137*	.137*
Education	.004	.016	.012
Residency	.118	.123	.124
Personal income	-.009	-.053	-.100
Family income per capita	.125*	.119	.196*
Poverty	-.034	-.037	-.038
Nonreligious	-.040	-.040	-.030
Never married	-.132*	-.126*	-.122
Unemployed	-.041	-.043	-.049
Acquiescence	.201***	.228***	.223***
Income disadvantage	-.032	-.028	-.037
Reference group size for personal income	-	-.117*	-
Average relative personal income of the reference group	-	-.092	-
Reference group range for personal income	-	.033	-
Reference group frequency for personal income	-	-.016	-
Reference group size for family income	-	-	-.123*
Average relative family income of the reference group	-	-	.062
Reference group range for family income	-	-	.005
Reference group frequency for family income	-	-	.022
R^2	.124	.144	.139

* $p < .05$. ** $p < .01$. *** $p < .001$.

Table 4. Standardized regression coefficients for predicting life satisfaction in the third step of the regression model

Predictor	(3) Personal income	(3) Family income
Reference group frequency for personal income × Income disparity	.160**	-
Reference group size for personal income × Reference group highest relative personal income	-.131*	-
Reference group frequency for family income × Income disparity	-	-.007
Reference group size for family income × Reference group highest relative family income	-	-.021
R^2	.178	.140

Income disparity was the average of reference group range for personal income and personal income disadvantage.
* $p < .05$. ** $p < .01$. *** $p < .001$.

DISCUSSION

Results reveal that the Hong Kong Chinese adult experienced higher life satisfaction when he or she had 1) a smaller reference group for income comparison, 2) both the smaller reference group and lower reference group relative income, or 3) both higher income comparability in the reference group and income disparity. The second condition suggests that the highest reference group relative income is less corrosive to one's life satisfaction when the reference group is smaller. This means that the unfavorable social comparison would be rarer, and its detriment would be slighter. The third condition indicates that income disparity is less harmful to one's life satisfaction when one's reference group has a larger proportion of comparable income. In this connection, income disparity refers to personal income range and the proportion of people of the same education level who have higher personal incomes. Income range means the discrepancy between the highest and lowest income in the reference group. These results are justifiable by social comparison theory, with the notion of comparable income. The theories posit that social comparison is dissatisfying when it involves comparisons with higher income or income discrepancy in the reference group. Hence, the frequency and size of social comparison matter in engendering the dissatisfying effect. Social comparison theory also suggests that whereas income range is dissatisfying, income skew is satisfying. Also consistent with social comparison theory, income range would be less dissatisfying when it is incidental, because the majority in the reference group has comparably low incomes.

Application of social comparison theory enhances the understanding of the impact of reference group income. Consistent with the theories, results show that one's income and reference group income alone do not affect one's life satisfaction. Rather, the impact is contingent on social comparison frequency, reference group size, and income distribution in the reference group. In the absence of social comparison, one's income and income relative to the reference group have only insignificant impacts on one's life satisfaction. Similarly, reference group size and income distribution, in terms of range and skew, are not singularly influential on life satisfaction. Impacts only emanate from interactions among the size, relative income, and income distribution of the reference group. Nevertheless, it is worth noting that the effect of personal income in the reference group size would be statistically significant if the sample size reached 10,000, as shown by weighting the data. This would agree with many existing studies, which have employed very large samples (4,6,10). However, the very weak effects would not be practically meaningful. Instead, effects of interactions among these factors are more noteworthy because they were stronger and statistically significant.

Nevertheless, effects involving the income and relative income are not compellingly strong, even with the moderation of social comparison. This observation echoes views about the insignificance of income for maintaining life satisfaction or subjective well-being in general (12,70). The insignificance may rest on habituation, the diminishing marginal utility of income, and the abundance of alternative resources, which are more salutary than is income. Accordingly, income would have a declining contribution to life satisfaction over time, because of the preference for novelty. In this case, getting a new increase in income may be more satisfying than keeping an income (71). Moreover, the attractiveness of additional income shrinks, as it is not useful for exchanging needed resources and happiness. When people and society are affluent, sufficient in resources, and enjoying fulfilling lives, even the increase in income would not be salutary (3,29,72). Besides, the availability of alternative private and public resources diminishes the need for income to exchange for the resources. This reflects the contribution of decommodification or welfare provision to life satisfaction (1). Nevertheless, the conditions are partly contingent on the affluence of society, which lessens the impact of income on life satisfaction (72,73).

Just as income has at best a conditional effect on life satisfaction through social comparison, income inequality in the reference group or probably in society as well would exert a minimal worsening effect. This is the case in results concerning the insignificant effects of reference group relative income and income disadvantage. According to social comparison theory, income inequality has a negative effect in terms of income range and a positive effect in terms of income skew. Such opposing effects would neutralize any effect from income inequality. Essentially, when income range comes along with income skew, the negative effect of the former would diminish. This is likely to happen when higher income skew implies that upward comparison (i.e., comparing one's income with others' higher incomes) rarely occurs and thus only exerts an insignificant influence. As the co-occurrence of high levels of income range and skew is just the property of income inequality measured by the Gini coefficient, the income inequality is unlikely to weaken life satisfaction. This implication is consistent with the cross-societal finding that income inequality is conducive to life satisfaction (23,24).

Two conditional effects of social comparison were significant for personal income, but not for family income. That is, the effect of relative family income did not vary due to one's reference group size and the frequency or comparability of family income in one's reference group. This finding suggests that the comparison of personal income is more relevant to one's life satisfaction, probably because personal income is more salient and personally important than is family income due to the person's self-centeredness (3). Obviously, personal income is likely a reward to one's effort, ability, and achievement (74,75). In contrast, family income is more likely a result of marriage, family relationships, ethnic backgrounds, and other ascriptive characteristics (76,77). Meanwhile, social comparison is mainly relevant to self-evaluation, and personal achievement is more influential on self-evaluation than are ascriptive factors (78,79). These explain the satisfying effect of personal income comparison rather than of family income comparison. However, family income, rather than personal income, turned out to be a significant contributor to life satisfaction, regardless of income comparison. This finding suggests that resources provided through family income are satisfying (80). It also explains existing evidence that one without personal income can still be satisfied with life (81).

A puzzle in need of explanation and further research is the satisfying effect of income relative to an externally imposed reference group, based on similarity in age, gender, and other background characteristics (4,10). This is a puzzle because of the inability for one to compare incomes directly with such an imaginative reference group. One condition for the influence of the relative income is one's acquaintance with people of the same background. Hence, the imposed reference group is only a proxy of one's reference group and the effect of the former is only an approximation of that of the latter. Another possibility is that the income relative to the imposed reference group simply represents one's extraordinarily high earning capability or overachievement, having nothing to do with income comparison. In this connection, this capability or overachievement is the underlying cause of life satisfaction (80,82). For instance, one's conscientiousness would furnish one's overachievement and eventually life satisfaction (83). Besides, relative income is not influential, ostensibly because it fails to reflect the action of income comparison (9). In this connection, awareness about the income of the reference group does not necessarily entail the comparison of income.

FURTHER RESEARCH

The impact of reference group income on life satisfaction is not yet conclusive because the study only surveyed Hong Kong Chinese adults. Moreover, the study has limitations in the use of cross-sectional design and self-report measures of reference group income. The cross-sectional design at best captures immediate impacts but misses lagged impacts. Nevertheless, the design cannot ensure that the income of the reference group is a causal antecedent to life satisfaction. The uncertainty arises when life satisfaction becomes a stable trait that determines the selection of the reference group. This is possible because life satisfaction can stem from the sable trait of extraversion (84). The self-report measure of reference group income at best reflects effects due to one's experience of social comparison. It may not register the effects of others' income that do not pass through social comparison. A thorough investigation therefore requires further research to extend the sample, design, and measurement. The extension of the sample can involve non-Chinese and various sociocultural settings as well to gauge the generality or specificity of findings drawn from Hong Kong Chinese. In this connection, societal affluence and income inequality are basic factors to examine the contextual moderation of effects of relative income and other social comparison processes. Further research can test the hypothesis that societal affluence tempers the effects of relative income, as well as income (72). Moreover, a panel design is necessary to improve the causal inference and identify lagged effects. It needs to control for prior life satisfaction in order to distill the effect of relative income and other factors emerging later than prior life satisfaction. This need arises because of the possibility of the influences of prior life satisfaction on later life satisfaction and social experiences (85,86). Reference group income based on reports by reference group members is a crucial measure.

Further research is also desirable to elaborate the present findings by elucidating details of social comparison. Such details would explicitly include the frequency and importance of upward and downward comparisons and comparison with comparable income. Examination of details would serve to clarify the moderating effects of reference group size and income comparability. Further research thus expects to find that upward comparison is less dissatisfying when it is rare, and comparison with comparable income is salutary when it is ubiquitous. A promising approach for the elaboration and clarification is the use of qualitative interviews. Such interviews would delve into the details of social comparison and their responses. This approach would offer the merit of illuminating the effects of social comparison and reference group income for selected cases, especially when such effects do not figure in all people.

IMPLICATIONS

Although reference group income displays conditional influences on life satisfaction, the influences are not emphatically strong in a detrimental way. Rather, high relative income in the reference group would be less dissatisfying when the reference group is smaller and its income skew or comparability is higher. The latter suggests that income inequality in the reference group is unlikely to impair one's life satisfaction. This happens when income inequality likely spawns income skew as well, which appears to mitigate the noxious effect of income range. In all, income and its distribution do not strongly affect life satisfaction and do not need to represent indispensable factors for promoting life satisfaction.

In contrast, downplaying the role of social comparison and the reference group would have some contribution to the promotion of life satisfaction. A possible way of such downplaying is the fostering of agreeableness, tolerance, or broadmindedness in the person (78). This is to discourage the calculative, competitive mentality. The approach is likely to hinge on the broadening of the person's exposure and horizons to distract selective attention to a certain group of people (87). Another way of discouraging social comparison is the strengthening of the person's self-confidence (88). In this regard, support for one's autonomy would help in the fostering of self-confidence (89). Such experiences would be vital to sustain one's life satisfaction, particularly when demographic and socioeconomic characteristics just play a minimal role in the sustenance.

REFERENCES

[1] Radcliff B. Politics, market, and life satisfaction: The political economy of human happiness. Am Political Sci Rev 2001;85:938-52.

[2] Inglehart R, Welzel C. Modernization, cultural change, and democracy: The human development sequence. New York: Cambridge University Press, 2005.

[3] Phillips D. Quality of life: Concept, policy and practice. London: Routledge, 2006.

[4] Georgellis Y, Tsitsianis N, Yin TP. Personal values as mitigating factors in the link between income and life satisfaction: Evidence from the European social survey. Soc Indicat Res 2009;91:329-44.

Conditions for the dissatisfying effect of reference group income   347

[5]   Schyns P. Income and satisfaction in Russia. J Happiness Stud 2001;2:173-204.
[6]   Caporale GM, Georgellis Y, Tsitsianis N, Yin YP. Income and happiness across Europe: Do reference values matter? J Econ Psy 2009;30:42-51.
[7]   Drichoutis A, Nayga RM, Lazaridis P. Do reference values matter? Some notes and extensions or income and happiness across Europe J Econ Psy 2010;31:479-86.
[8]   Jorgensen BS, Jamieson RD, Martin JF. Income, sense of community and subjective well-being: Combining economic and psychological variables. J Econ Psychol 2010;31:612-43.
[9]   Clark AE, Frijters P, Shields MA. Relative income happiness and utility: An explanation for the Easterlin paradox and other puzzles. J Econ Lit 2008;46:95-144.
[10] Ferrer-i-Carbonell A. Income and well-being: An empirical analysis of the comparison income effect. J Pub Econ 2005;89:997-1019.
[11] Faunce WA. Work, status, and self esteem: Theory of selective self investment. Lanham, MD: University Press of America, 2003.
[12] Tyler, TR, Boerkmann RJ, Smith HJ, Huo YJ. Social justice in a diverse society. Boulder, CO: Westview, 1997.
[13] Hogg MA. Handbook of social comparison: Theory and research. New York: Kluwer, 2000.
[14] Arthaud-Day ML, Near JP. The wealth of nations and the happiness of nations: Why accounting matters. Soc Indic Res 2005;74:511-48.
[15] Pham-Kanter G. Social comparisons and health: Can having richer friends and neighbors make your sick? Soc Sci Med 2009;69:335-44.
[16] Yngwe, MA, Fritzell J, Lundberg O, Diderichsen F, Surstrom B. Exploring relative deprivation: Is social comparison a mechanism in the relation between income and health? Soc Sci Med 2003;57:1463-71.
[17] Cummins RA, Lau, ALD, Mellor D, Stokes MA, Encouraging governments to enhance the happiness of their nation, step 1: Understand subjective wellbeing. Soc Indic Res 2009;91:23-36.
[18] Parducci A. Happiness, pleasure, and judgment: The contextual theory and its applications, Mahwah, NJ: Erlbaum, 1995.
[19] Cheung CK, Leung KK. Ways by which comparable income affects life satisfaction in Hong Kong. Soc Indic Res 2008;87:169-87.
[20] Hagerty MR. Social comparisons of income in one's community: Evidence from national surveys of income and happiness. J Pers Soc Psychol 2000; 28:764-71.
[21] Milanovic B. A simple way to calculate the Gini coefficient, and some implications. Econ Let 1997;56:45-9.
[22] Buunk BP, Gibbons FX. Health, coping, and well-being: Perspectives from social comparison theory, Mahwah, NJ: Erlbaum, 1997.
[23] Diener E, Suh EM. Culture and subjective well-being. Cambridge, MA: MIT, 2000.
[24] Mookerjee R, Beron K. Gender, religion, and happiness. J Socio-Econ 2004;34:674-85.
[25] Temes N. Income distribution, happiness and satisfaction: A direct test of the interdependent preference model. J Econ Psy 1986;7:425-46.
[26] Diener E, Fujita F. Resources, personal strivings, and subjective well-being: A nomothetic and idiographic approach. J Pers Soc Psycol 1995;68:926-35.
[27] Jasso G. Handbook of sociological theory, New York: Kluwer, 2001.
[28] Diener E. Assessing subjective well-being: Progress and opportunities. Soc Indic Res 1994;31:103-57.
[29] Sirgy MJ, Handbook of quality-of-life research: An ethical marketing perspective. Dordrecht, Netherlands: Kluwer, 2001.
[30] Igaraski T, Kashima Y, Kashima ES, Farsides T, Kim U, Strack F, Werth L, Yuki M, Culture, trust, and social networks. Asian J Soc Psychol 2008;11:88-101.
[31] Kulik L. The impact of spousal variables on life satisfaction of individuals in life adulthood. Int J Comp Soc 2006;67-54-72.
[32] Fiorentine R. Theories of gender stratification. Rationality Soc 1991;5:341-66.
[33] Brockmann H. Why is less money spent on health care for the elderly than for the rest of the population? Health care rationing in German hospitals. Soc Sci Med 2002;55:593-608.
[34] Whelan CT, McGinnity F. Welfare regimes and the experience of unemployment in Europe, Oxford, UK: Oxford, 2000.

[35] Cartier C. Culture and the city: Hong Kong, 1997-2007. China Rev 2008;8:59-83.

[36] Chow NWS. New economy and new social policy in East and Southeast Asian compact, mature economies: The case of Hong Kong. Soc Policy Admin 2003;37:411-22.

[37] Flowerdew J. The discursive construction of an old class city. Discourse Soc 2004;15:579-605.

[38] Zhao X, Zhang L, Sit TOK. Income inequalities under economic restructuring in Hong Kong. Asian Survey 2004;44:442-72.

[39] Chan EHW, Lee GKL. Applicability in Hong Kong of London's experiences on urban redevelopment practices. Property Mgt 2008;26:125-37.

[40] Ku AS. Hegemonic construction, negotiation and displacement: The struggle over right of abode in Hong Kong. Int J Cult Stud 2001;4:259-78.

[41] Guan Y, Bond MH, Huang Z, Zhang Z, Deng H, Hu T, Gao H. Role of personal endorsement of outgroup members' distinctive values and need for cognitive closure in attitude towards the outgroup. Asian J Soc Psychol 2009;12:54-62.

[42] Forrest R, La Grange A, Yip NM. Hong Kong as a global city? Social distance and spatial differentiation. Urban Stud 2004;41:207-27.

[43] Hoover M, Stokes LO. Hong Kong in New York: Global connections, national identity, and film representations. New Polit Sci 2003;25:509-32.

[44] Estes RJ. Development challenges of the New Europe. Soc Indic Res 2004;69:123-66.

[45] Ho SC, Chan CF. In search of a competitive policy in a competitive economy: The case of Hong Kong. J Consumer Aff 2003;37:68-85.

[46] Deutsch FM. How parents influence the life Plans of graduating Chinese university students. J Comp Fam Stud 2004;35:393-424.

[47] La Grange A, Pretorius F. Ontology, policy and the market: Trends to home-ownership in Hong Kong. Urban Stud 2000;37:1561-82.

[48] Tse RYC. Estimating neighborhood effects in house prices: Towards a new hedonic model approach. Urban Stud 2002;39:1165-80.

[49] Yip NM, Forrest R, La Grange A. Cohort, trajectories in Hong Kong's housing system: 1981-2001. Housing Stud 2007;22:121-36.

[50] Lam CLK, Lauder LJ, Lam TP, Gandek B, Population based norming of the Chinese (HK) version of the SF–36 Health Survey. HK Practitioner 1999;21:460-70.

[51] Yamaoka K. Social capital and health and well-being in East Asia: A population-based study. Soc Sci Med 2008;66:883-99.

[52] Sing M. Hong Kong's tortuous, democratization: A comparative analysis, London: Routledge Curzon, 2004.

[53] Huang TYM, Beyond the governance of global city-regions: Discourses and representations of Hong Kong cross-border identities. J Geog Sci 2008;52:1-30.

[54] MacPherson KL, One public, two health systems: Hong Kong and China, integration without convergence. China Rev 2008;8:85-104.

[55] Diez-Nicolas J. Two contradictory hypotheses on globalization: societal convergence or civilization differentiation and clash. Comp Soc 2002;1:465-93.

[56] Frey BS, Stutzer A. Happiness research: State and prospects. Rev Soc Econ 2005;62:207-28.

[57] Groot W, van den Brink HM, van Praag B, The compensating income variation of social capital. Soc Indic Res 2007;82:189-207.

[58] Barrett AE. Social support and life satisfaction among the never married. Res Aging 1999;21:46-72.

[59] Mroczlk DK, Spiro A. Change in life satisfaction during adulthood: Findings from the Veterans Affairs Normative Aging Study. J Pers Soc Psychol 2005;88:189-202.

[60] Redersdorff S, Guimond S. Social comparison and social psychology: Understanding Cognitive, intergroup relations, and culture, Cambridge, UK: Cambridge, 2006.

[61] Kaplan G, Baron-Epel O. What lies behind the subjective evaluation of health status? Soc Sci Med 2003;56: 1669-76.

[62] Zagefka H, Brown R. Social comparison and social psychology: Understanding cognitive, intergroup relations, and culture, Cambridge, UK: Cambridge, 2006.

Conditions for the dissatisfying effect of reference group income

[63] Martinot D, Redersdorff S. Social comparison and social psychology: Understanding cognitive, intergroup relations, and culture, Cambridge, UK: Cambridge, 2006.

[64] Salmon CT, Nichols JS. The next-birthday method of respondent selection. Pub Opin Quart 1983;47:270-6.

[65] Keeter, S, Kennedy C, Dimak M, Best J, Craighill P, Consequences of reducing nonresponse in a national telephone survey. Pub Opin Quart 2006;70:759-79.

[66] Joassart-Marcelli P, Working poverty in Southern California: Towards an operational measure. Soc Sci Res 2005;34:20-43.

[67] Diener E, Emmons RA, Larsen RJ, Griffin S, The satisfaction with life scale. J Pers Assess 1985; 49:71-75.

[68] Cohen J, Cohen P, West SG, Aiken LS. Applied multiple regression/correlation analysis for the behavioral sciences, New York: Wiley, 2003.

[69] Zagorski K. The end of the welfare state? Responses to state retrenchment, London: Routledge, 1999.

[70] Schyns P. Advances in quality of life theory and research, Dordrecht, Netherlands: Kluwer, 2000.

[71] Saris WE. The strength of the causal relationship between living conditions and satisfaction. Soc Meth Res 2001;30:11-34.

[72] Schyns P. Wealth of nations, individual, income and life satisfaction in 42 countries: A multilevel approach. Soc Indic Res 2002;60:5-40.

[73] Lane RE. The market experience. Cambridge, UK: Cambridge, 1991.

[74] Veenhoven R. Return of inequality in modern society? Test by dispersion of life-satisfaction across time and nations. J Happiness Stud 2005;6:457-87.

[75] Motel-Klingebiel A, Gords LR, Betzin J. Welfare states and quality of later life: Distributions and predictors in a comparative perspective. Eur J Aging 2009;6:67-78.

[76] Zhou X, Suhomlinova O. Redistribution under state socialism: A USSR and PRC comparison. Res Soc Stratification Mobility 2001;18:163-204.

[77] Bellair PE, Roscigno VJ. Local labor-market opportunity and adolescent delinquency. Soc Forces 2000;78:1509-38.

[78] Vartanian TP. Adolescent neighborhood effects on labor market and economic outcomes. Soc Serv Rev 1999;73:142-17.

[79] Fujita F. The science of subjective well-being, New York: Guilford, 2008.

[80] Ishida H. Social mobility in contemporary Japan: Educational credentials, class and the labor market in a cross-national perspective, Stanford, CA: Stanford, 1993.

[81] Rettig KD, Leichtentritt RD, Stanton LM. Understanding noncustodial fathers' family and life satisfaction from resource theory perspective. J Fam Issues 1999;20:507-38.

[82] Wong CK, Wong KY, Mok BH. Subjective well-being, societal condition and social policy: The case study of a rich Chinese society. Soc Indic Res 2006;78:405-28.

[83] Hill SE, Buss, DM. The science of subjective well-being, New York: Guilford, 2008.

[84] Prenda KM, Lachman ME. Planning for the future: A life management strategy for increasing control and life satisfaction in adulthood. Psychol Aging 2001;16:206-16.

[85] Schimmack U, Radhakrishnan P, Oishi S, Dzokoto V. Cultural, personality, and subjective well-being: Integrating process models of life satisfaction. J Pers Soc Psychol 2002;82:582-93.

[86] Freitag M. Beyond Tocqueville: The origins of social capital in Switzerland. Eur Soc Rev 2003; 19:217-32.

[87] Thoits PA, Hewitt LN. Volunteer work and well-being. J Health Soc Behav 2001;42:115-31.

[88] Mussweiler T, Ruter K, Epstude K. Social comparison and social psychology: Understanding cognitive, intergroup relations, and culture. Cambridge, UK: Cambridge, 2006.

[89] Leventhal H, Hudson S, Robitaille C. Health, coping, and well-being: Perspectives from social comparison theory. Mahwah, NJ: Erlbaum, 1997.

Submitted: October 16, 2011. *Revised:* December 03, 2011. *Accepted:* December 07, 2011.

In: Alternative Medicine Research Yearbook 2012
Editors: Søren Ventegodt and Joav Merrick

ISBN: 978-1-62808-080-3
© 2013 Nova Science Publishers, Inc.

Chapter 35

SENSE OF COMMUNITY AND INCOME AS INDICATORS OF LIFE SATISFACTION

Evie M Muilenburg-Trevino,* *Megan K Pittman and Mary Guilfoyle Holmes*

Center of Applied Research for Nonprofit Organizations, University of Oklahoma, Tulsa, Schusterman Center, Oklahoma, US

ABSTRACT

A sense of belonging within a community and the ability to meet the most basic human needs such as food, clothing, and shelter impact individuals' sense of life satisfaction. Sense of community is a significant construct in the field of psychology as it is thought to predict individual well-being through a sense of belonging and sense of connectedness. Additionally, previous research indicates that an inverse relationship between poverty and life satisfaction exists. The purpose of this article was to examine the effects of sense of community and income level on life satisfaction. This investigation reports on analysis of variance findings based on data from 217 individuals with Head Start-eligible children. Results indicate a significant main effect for sense of community; in particular, levels of life satisfaction were significantly higher among individuals with a high sense of community compared to those with a low or moderate sense of community. In addition, income was a significant main effect; specifically, life satisfaction was significantly higher among individuals with an income of $31,091 and over compared to those with an income of less than $10,000, an income between $10,001-20,650, and an income between $20,651-31,090. These findings have noteworthy implications. First, fostering communitywide involvement in order to increase members' sense of community may have radiating effects on their overall well-being and sense of life satisfaction. Secondly, economic factors do in fact have an effect on one's overall well-being and life satisfaction, at least for those living in poverty.

Keywords: Life satisfaction, quality of life, well-being, community, income

---

* Correspondence: Evie M. Muilenburg-Trevino, Center of Applied Research for Nonprofit Organizations, University of Oklahoma, Schusterman Center, 4502 E 41st Street, Tulsa, OK 74135-2512 United States. E-mail: emtrevino@ou.edu.

INTRODUCTION

Life satisfaction is an overall evaluation of feelings and attitudes, ranging from negative to positive, about one's life at a particular point in time. Life satisfaction is one of the major indicators of well-being (1), as identified by Diener, along with positive affect and negative affect. Both positive and negative affect refer to the emotional aspect of the construct of well-being, while life satisfaction refers to the cognitive-judgmental aspect. Although researchers typically focus on current circumstances in one's life when measuring life satisfaction, Diener et al included desire to change one's life, satisfaction with the past, satisfaction with the future and significant other's view of one's life in the construct of life satisfaction (2). Research by Seligman and Shueller (3) indicated that pleasure, engagement, and meaning should also be considered as predictors in the conceptualization of subjective well-being and life satisfaction. Shin and Johnson (4) define life satisfaction as a "global assessment of a person's quality of life according to his chosen criteria" (p. 478). Judgments of life satisfaction are based on standards that people individually set for themselves. Typically, individuals compare their individual standards or circumstances to what they believe are appropriate standards or circumstances to evaluate how satisfied they are with their present life. In conjunction, Diener states that it is a hallmark of the subjective well-being area that it centers on the person's own judgments (1), not upon some criterion that is judged to be important by the researcher. According to Davidson and Cotter (5), "people who score high on a subjective well-being scale say they are basically happy, excited, cheerful, and pleased (positive affects); they claim to be relatively free of excessive worry, sadness, anger and guilt (negative affects); and they believe themselves to be competent in handling their lives (perceived efficacy)" (p. 247).

Sense of community and life satisfaction

Sense of community has been an important construct in psychology as it is conceptualized to have an effect on individual well-being. In addition, it stresses the importance of psychological and experiential aspects of individuals in regard to their communities. Since Sarason (6) first introduced the concept of psychological sense of community, McMillan and Chavis (7) have been able to more thoroughly define sense of community as "a feeling that members have a belonging, a feeling that members matter to one another and to the group, and a shared faith that members' needs will be met through their commitment to be together" (p. 9). They base sense of community on the four multidimensional elements of 1) *membership*, which indicates a feeling of belongingness, 2) *influence,* which causes them to believe that they can exert some control over a group and also be influenced by the group, *3) integration and fulfillment of needs,* where the individual believes his or her needs can and are being met through the joint abilities of the group and 4) *shared emotional connection,* deriving from a shared history with the community.

The term community has been distinguished by Gusfield who described community in territorial (neighborhood, town, city, etc.) and relational (volunteer groups, church groups, the workplace, sports etc.) connotations (8). Sense of community takes root in the concept that individuals perceive themselves as part of the "common good" which is available to them

Sense of community and income as indicators of life satisfaction 353

should the need occur. However, while sense of community may be reinforced through actual experiences of social support and strong neighbor-to-neighbor ties, it is not necessarily dependent upon it (9). In addition, those who feel a sense of community tend to take part in local organizations, volunteer, vote, participate in civic duties and be active members in their community (10). Sense of community tends to develop more with age and chances for gathering and associations, presumably favored by working in the community or being an active participant in the community (11), which overall increases subjective well-being and ultimately life satisfaction.

The importance and value of sense of community in everyday life began with Sarason (6), who stressed its significance to the well-being of individuals as well as to society. The intrinsic qualities of sense of community are generally regarded as so imperative to human functioning that their absence can produce feelings of isolation, alienation, loneliness, and depression (6). Without sense of community, a person's psychological health may be affected, causing individuals to possibly lose their sense of well-being or become dissatisfied with life. According to Martini and Sequi (12), sense of community contributes to quality of life, subjectively perceived, and also to individual well-being; it encourages a greater sense of identity and greater self-confidence, facilitating social relations and combating anonymity and loneliness. Subjective well-being is a broad construct that includes people's emotional responses, domain satisfactions (including satisfaction with one's community), and overall opinions of life satisfaction. Because satisfaction with one's community (i.e. sense of community) is a direct predictor of subjective well-being and life satisfaction, it is an important psychological construct. Research by Prezza and Constantini (11) found that sense of community and satisfaction with community services combine into one factor, and self-esteem, perceived social support and life satisfaction merge into another, which correspondingly can be called community and personal well-being. Sense of community produces feelings of worth, membership and emotional connections, which ultimately generates a higher sense of self-esteem. Self-esteem is an indicator of subjective well-being, and as demonstrated by Diener (1), it is the highest predictor of life satisfaction.

Income and life satisfaction

The link between income and life satisfaction has been debated. At the national level, the correlation is quite large, but the relationship is less substantiated at the individual level within nations (13). In part, the correlations may be greater at the national level due to the incidence of higher income countries having other positive characteristics such as health, human rights, modernization and scientific advancement (14). Within nations, the correlation is less marked with the exception of individuals who live in poverty. There is an inverse relationship between poverty and life satisfaction (13), which may be due to the fact that those in poverty are unable to fulfill their basic needs of survival. Once a threshold is established in which basic needs are met, the relationship between income and well-being is less pronounced, thus suggesting the true correlation may be curvilinear in nature.

Veenhoven and Ehrhardt (15) explain this in terms of the livability theory, which states that subjective perceptions of life are based upon objective living conditions. Fundamentally, the better the living condition, the happier individuals will be. Good living conditions are an innate desire of human existence. Livability theory implies that there are universal human needs. In essence, individuals who are able to meet their basic needs will have higher life satisfaction than those living in poorer conditions. This theory supports the idea of curvilinear relationship between income and subjective well-being in that income has a decreasing marginal return (16). While material improvements make a significant difference in the lives of poor people by allowing them to buy essentials such as food and housing, a similar amount of monetary compensation to individuals who are well-off will have less of an effect on their overall satisfaction since their basic needs have already been met (16).

The inability of individuals to provide the most basic of needs such as food, clothing, and shelter likely causes them to experience stress. Thus, stress is closely related to quality of life. Previous studies support the link between stress and low income. Lantz, House, Mero and Williams (17) found that socioeconomic position is related to stress exposure and negative life events, which means that individuals who live in poor economic conditions generally experience more stress. Furthermore, another study indicates that individuals with unmet basic needs exhibited greater stress and a lower sense of well-being (18). As evidence suggests, stress is closely related to poor living conditions, which in turn is directly related to decreased satisfaction with life.

The purpose of the present article was to examine the effects of sense of community and income level on life satisfaction. Because a sense of community has been shown to influence one's overall sense of well-being, it is worthwhile to understand its relationship with life satisfaction. In addition, income level as it relates to poverty also holds significant implications to overall well-being and a sense of life satisfaction.

METHOD

Located in the Midwestern United States, the sample included 217 individuals with Head Start-eligible children. Participants include 88% females with an average age of 32.0 years. Regarding race, participants reported 70.0% Caucasian, 12.0% Hispanic, 11.1% American Indian, and 5.5% African American. Over half (59.4%) of individuals reported married while 17.1% reported single and 12.9% reported divorced. In regard to educational background, 18.6% indicated less than 12th grade, 34.0% indicated Diploma/GED, 27.9% indicated some college, 15.3% indicated college graduate, and 1.9% indicated post-graduate. Finally, income level was reported as follows: less than $10,000 (17.3%), $10,001-20,650 (30.1%), $20,651-31,090 (23.7%), and $31,091 and over (28.9%).

Participants can be described as at-risk for poverty with 72% of individuals having an annual income less than $31,091. In addition, 70% receive Medicaid support, 50% receive food stamps, and 45% receive support from the Women, Infants, and Children (WIC) supplemental nutrition program.

In regard to the number of children in the household, 13% indicated one, 46% indicated two, 23% indicated three, and 18% indicated four or more.

The questionnaire was administered in-person with Head Start family members, as well as at a variety of community events. The questionnaire was furnished in both English and Spanish, but only one Spanish version was returned and not included in subsequent analyses. A total of 257 surveys were returned, 217 of which were usable. The protocol for this study was approved by the university's human subject review board.

Satisfaction with life

The Satisfaction with Life Scale (19) measures global life satisfaction. The 4-item scale is presented in a 7-point Likert type response format ranging from 1-*strongly disagree* to 7-*strongly agree*. Item 5 (If I could live my life over, I would change almost nothing) was not included in the questionnaire. Items were summed to present a composite score with higher scores suggesting higher levels of satisfaction with life. In the current study, the internal consistency reliability was .92 for SWLS scores.

Sense of Community

Sense of community was measured using the eight-item Brief Sense of Community Scale (BSCS) (20). The BSCS was presented in a 7-point Likert-type response format ranging from 1-*strongly disagree* to 7-*strongly agree*. Items were summed to present a composite score with higher scores suggesting higher levels of sense of community. The internal consistency reliability of BSCS scores was .93 in the current study.

Analyses

An Analysis of Variance was computed to examine the impact of sense of community and income on life satisfaction.

Sense of community was grouped into three categories. A composite score that fell within the *strongly disagree* to *slightly disagree* range (overall mean score of 24 or less) was categorized as low, a composite score that fell within the *neither agree nor disagree* range (overall mean score between 25 and 39) was categorized as moderate, and a composite score that fell within the *slightly agree* to *strongly agree* range (overall mean score of 40 or greater) was categorized as high. There were four income categories: less than $10,000, $10,001-20,650, $20,651-31,090, and $31,091 and over. Estimates of effect size were also computed.

RESULTS

Results of the ANOVA indicate a significant main effect for sense of community [F (2, 161) = 18.455; $p <$ .001; η^2 = .187]. The Tukey post hoc comparison indicated that levels of life satisfaction were significantly higher among individuals with a high sense of community (M = 22.22; SD = .64) compared to those with a low sense of community (M = 16.02; SD = 1.22) and a moderate sense of community (M = 17.01; SD = .75).

This indicates that level of life satisfaction increased as level of sense of community increased. See Figure 1 for a graphical representation of mean scores.

Income [F (3, 161) = 5.625; $p =$ .001; η^2 = .095] was also a significant main effect. The Tukey post hoc comparison indicated that life satisfaction was significantly higher among individuals with an income of $31,091 and over (M = 22.33; SD = 1.23) compared to those with an income of less than $10,000 (M = 16.02; SD = 1.14), an income between $10,001-

20,650 (M = 17.02; SD = .85), and an income between $20,651-31,090 (M = 18.28; SD = .93) (see Figure 1). This means that level of satisfaction increased as income increased.

The interaction effect of sense of community and income was non significant [$F(6, 161) = 2.015$; $p = .067$; $\eta^2 = .07$).

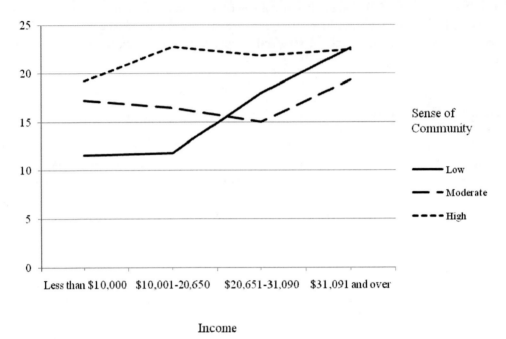

Figure 1. Mean Scores of Sense of Community and Income with Life Satisfaction.

CONCLUSION

The purpose of the present article was to examine the effects of sense of community and income on life satisfaction among a sample of individuals with Head-start eligible children from the Midwestern United States.

Sense of community is a significant construct in the field of psychology as it is thought to predict individual well-being through a sense of belonging and sense of connectedness.

Additionally, previous research indicates that an inverse relationship between poverty and life satisfaction exists (13). Results indicate that higher levels of life satisfaction are observed when a greater sense of community and increased income are present.

Importance of community on life satisfaction

Sense of community is a significant construct in the field of psychology as it is thought to impact individual well being through a sense of belonging and sense of connectedness. The sense of community model, which was developed by McMillan and Chavis (7) is made up of components that include feelings of emotional safety, and a sense of membership and

Sense of community and income as indicators of life satisfaction 357

identification, where one can have some influence over the community while supporting the demands of the community. The shared emotional connection that one feels supports the belief that one will be taken care of by the community.

According to Unger and Wandersman (21), sense of community is implied through neighborly-type behaviors that meet the psychological needs of community members by producing feelings of belonging and connectedness. Members of communities that lack such connections are more likely to have feelings of isolation and loneliness. Sense of community provides the perception that one will have access to the community and its resources if the need should arise, creating a sense of "common good" among its members (9). This study sought to explore the relationships between sense of community and income on life satisfaction. Do these attributes impact perceived happiness in individuals? Previous research has shown a relationship between adults' well being, a construct of life satisfaction and sense of community. The construct of subjective well-being is made up of positive affects (e.g. happiness), negative affects (e.g. worry) and perceived efficacy (e.g. ability to cope). Research by Davidson and Cotter (5) showed that a strong sense of community was significantly related to happiness (positive affect) of the subjective well-being construct, meaning people experience less worry (negative affect). Those that demonstrate positive affect are more likely to be psychologically healthy. Sarason (6) says, "the absence or dilution of the psychological sense of community is the most destructive dynamic in the lives of people in our society" (p. 96). Based on previous research, theoretical literature and the present study, sense of community may be directly associated to one's psychological health and therefore one's life satisfaction.

Importance of income on life satisfaction

The present study indicates that level of life satisfaction increased as income increased. Previous studies have shown that income has a direct effect on well-being while controlling for other variables such as sense of community, civic and political participation and education (22). Those with a lower income are proposed to have a lower level satisfaction. Easterlin (23) proposed that life satisfaction is influenced by the comparison of individual's own incomes with the income of their reference groups. For example, a reference group with a higher income relative to one's own has a downward effect on life satisfaction. In previous studies, the reference group has been defined by Caporale et al. (24) to include whole communities, residents living within the same neighborhood, and individuals who have comparable levels of education, age, etc. A study conducted by Kingdon and Knight (25) measured reference income, calculated as the mean income of one's area of residence (neighborhood, community, etc), showing a positive association with life satisfaction. Therefore, the higher the income in one's community, the higher level of life satisfaction among its residents (25). The present study shows that income is related to psychological variables such as life satisfaction. However, there was no interaction effect between income and sense of community, which suggests their independence. The correlation between income and life satisfaction is a starting point for more studies wishing to look at the potential determinants of individual well-being and life satisfaction.

Implication for practice and future research

Because of its predictive value on life satisfaction and well-being, sense of community is useful as a clinical indicator when assessing vulnerable populations (26) as well as a screening instrument. The present study indicates that sense of community has an effect on life satisfaction. In addition, income is a predictor of life satisfaction. Those living in poverty are typically in frequent contact with social services, which can connect them to community programs and organizations that may foster an overall sense of community and therefore increase life satisfaction.

Limitations

This chapter has some limitations that should be noted. The sample was fairly homogenous, nonrandom, and cross-sectional. Participants were predominantly Caucasian, female, and married. The generalizability of findings should be made with caution given the diversity of groups. In addition, the majority of participants can be described as at-risk for poverty, thus responses may differ from individuals who have greater financial security. Finally, the geographic location may affect study conclusions. Respondents were from the Midwestern United States, thus results here should be compared to those from other regions of the United States.

CONCLUSION

To summarize, the findings of this chapter indicate that sense of community, as we measured it, is significantly related to life satisfaction. In addition, income is significantly related to life satisfaction. Two types of conclusions can be drawn from this study. First, fostering communitywide involvement in order to increase members' sense of community may have radiating effects on their well-being and sense of life satisfaction. Secondly, economic factors do have an effect on one's overall well-being and life satisfaction, at least for those living in poverty.

REFERENCES

[1] Diener E. Subjective well-being. Psychol Bull 1984;95:542-75.
[2] Diener E, Suh EM, Lucas RE, Smith HL. Subjective well-being: Three decades of progress. Psychol Bull 1999;125:276-302.
[3] Schueller SM, Seligman MEP. Pursuit of pleasure, engagement, and meaning: Relationships to subjective and objective measures of well-being. J Positive Psychol 2010;5:253-63.
[4] Shin DC, Johnson DM. Avowed happiness as an overall assessment of the quality of life. Soc Indic Res 1978;5:475-92.
[5] Davidson WB, Cotter PR. The relationship between sense of community and subjective well-being: A first look. Am J Commun Psychol 1991;19:246-53.
[6] Sarason S. The psychological sense of community, Jossey-Bass: San Francisco, 1974.

[7] McMillan D, Chavis, D. Sense of community: A definition and theory. J Commun Psychol 1986; 14:6-23.

[8] Gusfield JR. Community: A critical response, Blackwell: Oxford, 1975.

[9] Pretty GMH, Conroy C, Dugay J, Fowler K, Williams D. Sense of community and its relevance to adolescents of all ages. J Commun Psychol 1996;24:365-79.

[10] Davidson WB, Cotter PR. Psychological sense of community and newspaper readership. Psychol Rep 1997;80:659-65.

[11] Prezza M, Constantini S. Sense of community and life satisfaction: Investigation in three different territorial contexts. J Commun Appl Soc Psychol 1998;8:181-94.

[12] Martini ER, Sequi R. La comunità locale. Roma: Nuova Italia Scientifica,1995.

[13] Diener E, Biswas-Diener R. Will money increase subjective well-being. Soc Indic Res 2002;57:119-69.

[14] Diener E, Diener C. The wealth of nations revisited: Income and quality of life. Soc Indic Res 1995;36:275-86.

[15] Veenhoven E, Ehrhardt J. The cross-national pattern of happiness: Test if of predictions implied in three theories of happiness. Soc Indic Res 1995;34:33-68.

[16] Bernhard C. The relation between life satisfaction and the material situation: A re- evaluation using alternative measures. Soc Indic Res 2010;98:475-99.

[17] Lantz PM, House JS, Mero RP, Williams DR. Stress, life events, and socioeconomic disparities in health: Results from the American's Changing Lives study. J Health Soc Behav 2009;46:274-88.

[18] Ng W, Diener E, Aurora R, Harter J. Affluence, feelings of stress, and well-being. Soc Indic Res 2009;94:257-71.

[19] Diener E, Emmons RA, Larsen RJ, Griffin S. The satisfaction with life scale. J Pers Assess 1985; 49:71-5.

[20] Peterson NA, Speer PW, McMillan DW. Validation of a brief sense of community scale: Confirmation of the principal theory of sense of community. J Commun Psychol 2008;36:61-73.

[21] Unger DG, Wandersman A. The importance of neighbors: The social, cognitive, and affective components of neighboring. Am J Commun Psychol 1985;13:139-69.

[22] Jorgensen BS, Jamieson RD, Martin JF. Income and well-being: Combining economic and psychological approaches. J Econ Psychol 2010;3:612-23.

[23] Easterlin RA. Will raising the incomes of all increase the happiness of all? J Econ Behav Organ 1995;27:35-47.

[24] Caporale GM, Georgellis Y, Tsitsianis N, Yin YP. Income and happiness across Europe: Do reference values matter? J Econ Psychol 2009;30:42-51.

[25] Kingdon GG, Knight J. Community, comparison and subjective well-being in a divided society. J Econ Behav Organ 2007;64:69-90.

[26] Andrèn S, Elmstål S. Family caregivers' subjective experiences of satisfaction in. dementia care: Aspects of burden, subjective health and sense of coherence. Scand J Caring Sci 2005;19:157-68.

Submitted: October 16, 2011. *Revised:* December 03, 2011. *Accepted:* December 07, 2011.

In: Alternative Medicine Research Yearbook 2012
Editors: Søren Ventegodt and Joav Merrick

ISBN: 978-1-62808-080-3
© 2013 Nova Science Publishers, Inc.

Chapter 36

LIFE SATISFACTION IN MACEDONIAN WORK ORGANIZATIONS

*Elisaveta Sardjoska**

Institute of Psychology, Faculty of Philosophy, University St Cyril and Methodius, Skopje, Republic of Macedonia

ABSTRACT

This paper explains the concept and factors of the life satisfaction on an organizational level of analysis and compares the life satisfaction of 514 employees in private and state-owned service and production organizations in the Republic of Macedonia. The three items Life Satisfaction Scale (Tang, Luna-Arocasand Whiteside) scored with five-anchored Lickert's answer scale of contentment was applied. The internal reliability of Life Satisfaction Scale was high (0.826). One-way ANOVA revealed that life satisfaction is significantly higher in private vs. state-owned organizations (F=6.226 sig=0.013), and in private-service vs. other types of organizations (F=3.441 sig 0.017). Life satisfaction is almost significantly higher in service vs. production organizations (F=3.260 sig 0.072).We explain the results with the impact of the social transition lasting for more than two decades in Macedonia over the process of privatization of organizations. Higher life satisfaction in private-service organizations is due to their capability to adapt quickly to changes in business strategy and policy than the other organizations can. Changes refer to new work values, market oriented economy and culture, competition, searching for new markets and resources, globalization of services, production, science, administration and trade. In addition, the new technology creates a great demand for service activities, so service organizations become attractive workplaces with high quality work life, performance, job contentment and life satisfaction of employees. We suggest some intervention programs to the management of other types of Macedonian organizations in order to attain high quality of work life and its positive organizational and individual outcomes in the new societal context of the transition process.

Keywords: Life satisfaction, job satisfaction, quality of life, work organization

---

* Correspondence: Elisaveta Sardjoska, University St Cyril and Methodius, Faculty of Philosophy, Institute for Psychology, Skopje, Republic of Macedonia. E-mail: elisasar2004@yahoo.com; elisaveta@fzf.ukim.edu.mk.

INTRODUCTION

The substantial body on the life satisfaction research points at the societal (macro) and individual (micro) level survey on this phenomenon with insufficient data about the organizational (meso) level of analysis. It seems appropriate to replenish this gap in organizational research with an adequate study of the life satisfaction in work organizations due to the world we live in consisting of different types of organizations. On the one hand, work organizations supply material and service societal demands and provide the economic growth entailing the national affluence, employment, high incomes and beneficiaries for a great number of citizens. On the other hand, employees feel satisfied with their work organizations if they do accomplish work worthy for society and its development.

Radcliff (1) emphasizes social democratic values that a government of the society from any ideological provenientia attaches to, as a base for national level of life satisfaction. Such values including political freedom, access to knowledge, opportunities for individual growth, human rights allow one's own choice of a life-style and career, thus enhancing general level of life satisfaction. Whereas national level of the life satisfaction depends on the democratic political ideology of government parties including the quality and extent of wellbeing provisions theretofore subjective wellbeing is the appraisal of one's own life compared to cultural standards that are established in his/her nation varying from the other nations' standards.

Veenhoven (2) cites social indicators embodied in literacy, education, health-care, eradication of epidemic disease and poverty and elimination of hunger reflecting in the societal level of wellbeing. He mentions mental health and social relationships as subjective wellbeing indicators. In addition, he (3) distinguishes four qualities of life considering life-chances (events) and life- results (outcomes) on the one hand as well as outer and inner qualities on the other hand, among which the satisfaction with a life is a prominent outcome. One outer quality of life (livability of environment) encompassing favorable socio-economic, political, historic and cultural conditions is necessary for a social and subjective wellbeing, the other one reflects one's contribution to the social wellbeing through his/her work, engagement and position in society (utility of life). One inner quality of life refers to the individual capacity, skills and arts-of-living (life-ability of the person), the other one represents the individual feeling about and an appraisal of his/her life (satisfaction with life).

Life satisfaction may be passing or enduring and may relate to a part (domain) of the life or to a life-as a-whole. Only the satisfaction with a life- as- a- whole due to its endurance and integrity refers to the concepts of happiness and subjective wellbeing. The other three types of life satisfaction represent a part satisfaction, pleasure, top (peak) experience, the former being enduring, and the latter ones are passing. Usually, we expect the highest level of satisfaction for the top experience following by that of a pleasure whereas a part satisfaction and satisfaction with a life-as-a whole may vary among high, average or low level of satisfaction. The pleasure is passing enjoyment of sensoric or mental feeling and the top experience is intense positive feeling taking hold of the whole person interim. The part satisfaction is enduring positive feeling about a part (domain) of life like work, career, family, income, partner/spouse, health state. The satisfaction-with-life-as-a-whole incorporates affective and cognitive components designating one's feelings about and appraisal of his/her life respectively. The affective level of life satisfaction is equal to the balance of positive and negative affects one feels during definite time span in his/her life.

The preponderance of pleasures (positive affects) embodies hedonism in one's life constituting a state of happiness. Partisans to the affective theory of a life satisfaction emphasize human nature as a base for need gratification, so frequent attainment of personal important wants and needs makes a person feel satisfied enduringly. The cognitive level of life satisfaction encompasses an appraisal and a comparison of one's life against some social standard. The culture represents a base of the cognitive theory determining standards for the cognitive comparison. We accept a mixed theory about life satisfaction implying a presence of more pleasures and enjoyment in the life than pains (affective level) and a positive appraisal of the life comparing to pertinent social standards (cognitive level). There are also relative, trait and livability theories on life satisfaction. The relative theory considers the life satisfaction dependent on cognitive comparison including judgment of actual against the ideal life circumstances both at individual and societal level. Contrary, the trait theory considers life satisfaction as inherited and immutable personal characteristic accentuating the role personality plays in determination of the life satisfaction level. Personal characteristics may include the assertiveness, psychological resilience, internal control of life, empathy, extroversion, openness to experience. The liability theory emphasizes the impact of objective conditions on the level of happiness and it is close to understanding for the importance of situational factors (life circumstances and life events) in determination of the life satisfaction. We agree that both personality and environmental circumstances are indispensable factors of inner and outer impact on life satisfaction respectively accord to Sousa and Lyubomirsky (4).

Historically in relatively near past, life satisfaction became a topic of interest in the 18th century during the enlightment period emphasizing the value of the life itself contrary to its mission as a service to God or King. In the 19th century, the utilarian creed about the best society taking care for the happiness of a great number was a dominant one. It entails the political parties from different ideology to put the economic growth on the first place of their political agenda in order to eliminate poverty, epidemic diseases, hunger, and illiteracy ensuring a good economic standard in society, happiness and life satisfaction for the most people. The economic growth has shown accelerated growth through 20th century to 1960th when the interest passed from the materialistic to post-materialistic values embodied in the movement for a quality of life. This trend continues in the 21th century with social indicators guiding the social policy of the political governments from different ideology. Quality of life presents a form of mind, everyday human activities, culture of living, style and philosophy of operation offering products, services and processes for need gratification of citizens in any society. Good quality of life and socially responsible society enable wellbeing, life satisfaction, enhanced work motivation and efficacy of its inhabitants guiding to high economic standard and productivity on societal level. Quality of life importantly affects each individual, all social levels, work organizations and institutions, and the development of the community-as a-whole through level of employment, sustainable and competitive economy of any society. Quality of life and its outcomes are even important both for work organizations in developed countries as well as in developing countries. We are especially interested to study life satisfaction of employees in work organizations in one developing country undergoing the process of social transition for the last twenty years.

We can study life satisfaction in the same way people answer when we ask them for an appraisal of the contentment with their life applying bottom-up or top-down approach. The first approach means addition of satisfactions with different domains of life (e.g. family, health-state, children, financial situation, partner/spouse, job, career, income, education level) resulting in a global average measure of life satisfaction. The other approach sets off the quality and quantity of contentment with a life-as-a-whole concluding if he/she is satisfied or dissatisfied with life and/or particular parts of life.

This paper aimed to enrich research on life satisfaction of employees comparing various work organizations on this organizational outcome in the Republic of Macedonia. The paper attempts to explain macroeconomic changes in Macedonian society during the process of transition from socialism into capitalism evoking changes in the structure and functioning of work organizations that in turn affect life satisfaction of employees. Key socio-economic indicators of transition enduring for the last 20 years represent privatization of state-owned organizations, market oriented economy, competition and shareholding, guiding to changes in employee basic assumptions, beliefs, cognitions, attitudes and to new work values represented in protestant work ethics of hard working, self-efficacy, inner locus of control. Following cross-cultural research of transitional economies, it seems that the process of transition is unique and specific for each country although it has been unfolding simultaneously in Eastern Europe, former Soviet Union, China etc. Even if research on characteristics of work organizations in a same country undergoing transitional process pointed at differences in organizational culture and climate, work setting, productivity, quality of work life, employee wellbeing, and contentment with a job and satisfaction with a life due to the varying impact of a social transition.

Diener (5) asserts life satisfaction is a cognitive, judgmental process apart from the other two affective, emotional aspects of subjective wellbeing presenting a positive affect and negative affect respectively. Further, he defined life satisfaction as a global assessment of a person's quality of life according to standards, which each individual sets for him or herself (5). The choice of comparison criteria is internally imposed to individual although they are culturally determined and hence differ from standards other cultures have established. Albeit, according to Drenth and Groenendijk (6) individual social standards express prevailing and generally accepted cultural values of "a contemporary man/woman" – an openness to new ideas, an independence from traditional authorities, a trust in science and medicine, an ambition. Sousa and Lyubomirsky (4) hold life satisfaction is a subjective assessment of the quality of one's life. They defined satisfaction with one's life as a contentment or acceptance of one's life circumstances, or the fulfillment of one's wants and needs for one's life as a whole. They used the concepts of appraisal and contentment with one's life in general to denote cognitive aspect of the life satisfaction prevails against its affective components.

Life satisfaction refers to the degree to which individuals evaluate positively the quality of their life in total according to Radcliff (1). Veenhoven (7) considers life satisfaction as an enduring and integrative contentment with one's life-as-a whole, so it refers to the concepts of happiness and subjective well-being too. We conceive that life satisfaction incorporates affective and cognitive components designating one's feelings about and appraisal of his/her life as a whole respectively.

METHODS

We explored life satisfaction of 514 employees from 25 work organizations including 7 private-service, 4 private-production, 10 state owned-service and 4 state owned-production organizations. High school completed 49 percent, two years college 22 percent and four years college 29 percent of respondents. Men represented 45 percent and women 55 percent of the sample. The respondents were among 19 and 63 years old with an average of 39 years. Their total job experience was between 4 months and 40 years with an average of 16 years.

The three items Life Satisfaction Scale according to Tang, Luna-Arocas and Whiteside (8) scored with five-anchored Lickert's answer scale of contentment (1=very dissatisfied, 2=dissatisfied, 3=neutral, 4=satisfied, 5=very satisfied) was applied. The instruction to fill up life satisfaction scale is How satisfied are you with the following aspects of your life? The items are:

My work/family/personal life in general
My life as a whole these days
My overall life satisfaction

Mean life satisfaction score may range from one (low satisfaction) to five (high satisfaction). The internal reliability of Life Satisfaction Scale is high (0.826) allowing its application albeit it is a short scale.

RESULTS

One-way ANOVA revealed that life satisfaction is significantly higher in private vs. state-owned organizations (F=6.226 sig=0.013) (see table 3), and in private-service vs. other types of organizations (F=3.441 sig 0.017) (see table 1). Life satisfaction is almost significantly higher in service vs. production organizations (F=3.260 sig 0.072) (see table 4).

In addition, multiple comparisons of mean differences (MD) point at almost significantly higher life satisfaction in private-service organizations than it is into state owned-service and state owned-production organizations respectively (MD= .236 sig .072; MD= .2728 sig .066) (see table 2).

Table 1. One-way ANOVA results on employee life satisfaction in Macedonian work organizations

Life satis.	Private service org.	State-owned service org.	Private production org.	State-owned production org.	F	sig
N (514)	(158)	(190)	(50)	(116)		
M 3.6984	3.8734	3.6368	3.6067	3.6006	3.441	.017
SD .8346	.7633	.8481	.8669	.8650		

Elisaveta Sardjoska

Table 2. Multiple comparisons on life satisfaction means among Macedonian work organizations with Scheffe

(I) org.	(J) org.	Mean Difference (I-J)	sig
Private-service (3.8734)	State owned-service (3.6368)	.2366	.072
	Private-production (3.6067)	.2668	.270
	State owned-production (3.6006)	.2728	.066

Table 3. One-way ANOVA results on life satisfaction in Macedonian private and state-owned organizations in general

Life satis.	Private org.	State owned org	F	sig
N (514)	(208)	(306)	6.226	.013
M 3.6984	3.8093	3.6231		
SD .8346	.7955	.8533		

Table 4. One-way ANOVA results on satisfaction in Macedonian service and production organizations in total

Life satis.	Service org.	Production org	F	sig
N (514)	(348)	(166)	3.260	.072
M 3.6984	3.7443	3.6024		
SD .8346	.8181	.8629		

DISCUSSION

Results have shown that private organizations in general are happier and healthier places to work at, due to higher level of a life satisfaction of employees compared with state owned organizations in total. Due to better adjustment of private organizations to the new market and work values imposed with the process of privatization, they succeed to attain good quality of work life that in turn guides to employee job satisfaction and work motivation, efficacy and productivity on individual and organizational level.

The next finding refers to service organizations in general as preferring workplaces against production organizations due to the nature of work into the latter ones characterized with substantive workload, strain, hard regime of work and work conditions.

Private-service organizations in various business areas distinguish among other types of organizations as specially attractive workplaces offering services and jobs based on application of new information technology, projects, team working, transformational leadership, employee autonomy, self-efficacy and flexible role orientations according to Turner, Barling and Zacharatos (9).

Transition economies in general distinguish with insufficient physical, psychic and social well-being of their inhabitants. Mental health and social relationships are significant psychosocial indicators of life satisfaction, happiness and well-being according to Veenhoven

(7). Organizations in developing countries ought to find out purposeful strategies for acceptance of new values of market economy and provision of high quality of work life in a new societal context of work. Quality of life-in-total encompasses quality of work life and quality of private life, and balance between life and work. The life satisfaction, happiness and well-being on subjective and societal level are principal outcomes of quality of life. The life satisfaction brings on a job satisfaction because the satisfaction with life-as-a-whole spills over the work and career. High quality of work life is a prerequisite for a job satisfaction, work motivation, efficacy and effectiveness on individual and organizational level.

This paper has shown that the life satisfaction in Macedonia is significantly higher in private-service organizations due to their capability to adapt quickly to changes in business strategy and policy during transition compared to the other types of organizations (state-owned organizations in general, production organizations in total, state owned-service organizations and state owned-production organizations). Changes refer to new work values, market oriented economy and culture, competition, searching for new markets and resources, globalization of services, production, science, administration and trade. In addition, the new technology creates a great demand for service activities, so service organizations become attractive workplaces with high quality work life that in turn brings on to high performance, job contentment and life satisfaction of employees. The management of the other types of Macedonian organizations ought to implement some intervention programs in order to attain high quality of work life and its positive organizational and individual outcomes. Such interventions and strategies may be flexible work time, financial assistance, employee health-care and well-being programs, work/life balance, services for taking care for individuals depending on employees, paid leave according to Business for Social Responsibility Advisory Services- 2005 (10).

REFERENCES

[1] Radcliff B. Politics, markets, and life satisfaction: The political economy of human happiness. Am Political Sci Rev 2001;95(4):939-52.

[2] Veenhoven R. The study of life satisfaction. In: Saris WE, Veenhoven R, Scherpenzeel AC, Bunting B, eds. A comparative study of satisfaction with life in Europe. Budapest: Eötvös University Press, 1996:11-48.

[3] Veenhoven R. How do we assess how happy we are? Tenets, implications and tenability of three theories. Paper presented at conference on 'New Directions in the Study of Happiness: United States and International Perspectives', University of Notre Dame, USA, 2006 Oct 22-24.

[4] Sousa L, Lyubomirsky S. Life satisfaction. In: Worell J, ed. Encyclopedia of women and gender: Sex similarities, differences, andthe impact of society on gender. San Diego, CA: Academic Press, 2001:667-76).

[5] Diener E, Emmons RA, Larsen RJ, Griffin S. The satisfaction with life scale. J Pers Assess 1985;49(1):71-5.

[6] Drenth JDP, Groenendijk B. Organizational psychology in a cross-cultural perspective. In: Drenth JDP, Thierry H, de Wolff JC, eds. Handbook of work and organizational psychology. East Sussex: Psychology Press, 1998:133-60.

[7] Veenhoven R. Greater happiness for a greater number. Is that possible and desirable? J Happiness Stud 2010;11:605-29.

[8] Tang TLP, Luna-Arocas R, Whiteside HD. Attitudes toward money and demographic variables as related to income and life satisfaction: USA vs. Spain. Proceedings of the 22nd Annual Colloquium of

368   *Elisaveta Sardjoska*

the International association for Research in Economic Psychology: Proceedings of the International Colloquium of Economic Psychology, Valencia, Spain (1997;1:256-66.

[9] Turner N, Barling J, Zachartos A. Positive psychology at work. In: Snyder CR, Lopez SJ, eds. Handbook of positive psychology. New York: Oxford University Press, 2002:715-28.

[10] Business for Social Responsibility Advisory Services, 2005 Executive Summary on Work Life Quality. Accessed 2011 Sep 11. URL:
http://www.bsr.org/CSRResources/IssueBriefDetail.cfm?DocumentID=50965

Submitted: October 16, 2011. *Revised:* December 03, 2011. *Accepted:* December 07, 2011.

In: Alternative Medicine Research Yearbook 2012
Editors: Søren Ventegodt and Joav Merrick

ISBN: 978-1-62808-080-3
© 2013 Nova Science Publishers, Inc.

Chapter 37

THE TRANSITION TO COHABITATION: THE MEDIATING ROLE OF SELF-EFFICACY BETWEEN STRESS MANAGEMENT AND COUPLE SATISFACTION

Antonella Roggero, Maria Fernanda Vacirca, Adele Mauri and Silvia Ciairano*

Department of Psychology, Turin University, Turin, Italy

ABSTRACT

In the present study we focused on self-efficacy for couples: each partner's perception about his/her ability to communicate with, to support, to respect and value his/her partner, to manage conflicts and disagreements, and to avoid the intrusion of third parties. In particular, the study is aimed at investigating: 1) satisfaction, stress and self-efficacy in people who are going to marry; 2) the relationships between self-efficacy and: a) stress, in terms of tension, depression and tiredness, and the physical manifestation of stress; b) couple satisfaction; 3) the mediating role of self-efficacy between stress management and satisfaction. In this study 385 people of both genders participated, with a mean age of 32.6 years (st.dev. 5.5). The participants Were administered a self-reporting questionnaire to evaluate their self-efficacy, stress and satisfaction. This survey was administered on the day they went to the municipality to hand over marriage documents in a big city in the northwest of Italy. Their satisfaction is negatively related with psychological tension ($r=-.11$; $p<.02$) and with depression and tiredness ($r=-.18$; $p<.001$); the participants with high levels of self-efficacy also show higher levels of satisfaction [$F(2,300)=28.55$; $p<.0001$; $\eta2=.16$]. Finally, the negative relationship between stress and satisfaction is fully mediated by self-efficacy: $\beta=-.39$ $p<.0001$; $z=-3.7$ for psychological tension; and $\beta=-.39$, $p<.0001$; $z=-3.5$ for depression. Self-efficacy is an important resource for mastering stress during the transition to cohabitation. In particular it influences the couple's satisfaction both directly and indirectly by buffering the negative role of stress.

Keywords: Life satisfaction, quality of life, marriage, cohabitation

---

* Corresponding author: Antonella Roggero, Department of Psychology, Turin University, Turin, Italy. E-mail: antonella.roggero@unito.it.

INTRODUCTION

In the last few decades, the transitions marking every life's path are becoming increasingly interesting for researchers because of their ecological meaning (1) in fact these transitions always represent experiences of reciprocal adjustment between people and their contexts. An ecological transition takes place every time that the position of the person in his/her context changes: this change implies a change in his/her role, and thus of his/her and others' expectations about behavior and experiences (1). The formation of a stable couple relationship and cohabitation is one of the more relevant transitions for the development of identity and the psychosocial well-being of the person along their life span (2). Today the transition to cohabitation is realized in different forms, from civil to religious marriage to simply living together (3). Such forms of cohabitation are present in every Western country, although they have different proportions because of various cultural factors, such as the prevalence of Catholic beliefs about the family, and political issues such as the legal protection of unmarried couples (4). Italy, the country where we conducted this study, has no legal protection for unmarried cohabiting couples. However, also in Italy, exactly as it is happening at a global level (5), the number of cohabiting couples is increasing while the number of marriages is decreasing (6). Nevertheless, in Italy to marry at the civil and/or religious level is still more common than to cohabit, and unlike the countries of north-western Europe, marriage in Italy has maintained a crucial role in the process of family formation (7). In Italy, from the Church-State agreement of 1929, a Catholic marriage is valid also at the civil level. In fact, cohabitation is often just a pre-marriage stage and the decision to marry is undertaken after the birth of the first child (6). In all these cases the transition to the construction of a stable couple is better articulated and it occupies a longer temporal interval than when people marry before they cohabitate.

Whatever form cohabitation takes, from just living together to marrying, constructing a stable couple is the result of a complex transition and as such it implies elaborating and acting out processes of adjustment that involve the person's activities, roles and relationships (1). These processes of adjustment require the overcoming of different developmental tasks such as the construction of a relationship based on sharing, empathy, reciprocal collaboration and openness. These processes imply relatively high levels of communication, reciprocal and long-term engagement, and sharing of future projects (8). In fact a good and satisfactory couple life guarantees that the partners have support with difficulties as well as pleasant occasions of sharing interests and leisure. A partnership offers the possibility of confiding daily worries within a climate of openness and reciprocal trust, contributing to a decrease in anxiety levels and tension and increases the ability of managing stressful situations (9,10).

In sum, the transition to couple life, which implies projecting and personally engaging in reaching a satisfactory level of cohabitation, is a challenge that requires the person to be able to acknowledge and to successfully use his/her resources. Several studies have already investigated the various social and/or cultural factors that are positively related to couple satisfaction (11-13).

At the individual level some studies investigated the personality characteristics of the partners (14,15); their similarities (16,17); the coping strategies they use (18,19); their relational patterns as support within the couple (20), the quality of communication (21), and the positive and negative dimensions of partner behaviors (22).

Among all of the other personal characteristics, we are particularly interested in the positive relationship between personal self-efficacy in the couple and their satisfaction with living together (10) because self-efficacy can be trained and improved in people differently than other personal characteristics (23). Personal self-efficacy, which expresses the beliefs of individuals to successfully master the course of actions necessary to adequately face situations and to get the expected outcomes is among the best predictors of well-being and psychosocial adjustment (24). In particular, the belief of successfully mastering the various tasks and activities that characterize a romantic relationship was positively associated with the quality of the communication, conflict resolution styles, and the degree of reciprocal support and satisfaction of the partners (25). Caprara and Steca (26) showed in Italian adults from four different age groups that beliefs of personal self-efficacy in couples positively influence the subjective well-being of married men and women. That is, self-efficacy promotes the global experience of "well-being" as it is experienced, evaluated and declared by an individual. Despite the acknowledged role of self-efficacy as a potential protective factor for couples, the underlying processes by which it works have not been investigated yet. For instance, we still do not know whether self-efficacy has a direct effect only on satisfaction and/or if it is able to buffer the unavoidable negative consequences of stressful life events on the couple's satisfaction with their partner.

Among all the other potential risk factors for couple satisfaction, we are interested in the role of stress because it has been recently acknowledged as a relevant risk element for the well-being of couple life (27). Stress can play an important role in understanding the quality and stability of close relationships (28). Also in the case of stress, its possible consequences for each one of the partners or for the couple's life have already been investigated. In particular, we already know that the accumulation of stressful events may deteriorate the quality of the relationship because it implies a reduction of the time the two partners spend together, a decline in the opportunity to share common experiences as well as the general well-being of the couple (29). Stress seems to have a central role in many stages of the couple relationship: from the division of domestic labor to the failure of the relationship (30-32). Kinnunen and Taru (33) found that poor economic circumstances were linked to economic strain, which was related to increased psychological distress, and psychological distress in its turn was negatively reflected in marital adjustment. Recently, the study by Lederman et al (21), which used the dyad instead of the individual as the unit of analysis, showed that a person's relationship stress is more strongly related with their own external stress than with the partner's external stress and that the quality of communication buffers the effect of stress on the couple's relationship. However, as anticipated, what is still lacking is the analysis of the personal characteristics that may buffer the negative consequences of unavoidable stressful life events to the little daily hassles.

It is on the basis of previous findings that we focused our study on the relationships between beliefs of self-efficacy, perceived stress of the partners and their satisfaction with the couple relationship. Furthermore, we concentrated on couples who are in the middle of the transition to cohabitation. Until now the great majority of previous studies investigated *marital satisfaction*, measured by way of different kinds of instruments, in couples who have been already been married for a number of years (34). Scarce attention has been paid to the couples who are making the transition into stable cohabitation. We think that this transition is of particular interest because of its ecological meaning and also because the manner in which the partners face this transition may have dramatic consequences for the couple and future dynamics between the partners. In fact, the perception of couple life by the partners and their expectations towards the new experience may be determinant in defining their attitude and the investment of resources with which the partners face the transition and their new life. Self-efficacy is one of the factors that can have relevant consequences not only for people's behavior but also for their projects and future choices. In fact, people settle their goals, their levels of engagement in reaching these goals, how long they persist in facing difficulties and the amount of recovery after failures on the basis of their self-efficacy. Besides this, people also derive their standards in reaching their goals from their self-efficacy. When people feel high levels of self-efficacy they are also more likely to negotiate and mediate difficulties in a positive way, they have high levels of expectation, they are also able to intensify their efforts if it is functional to their goals, they are also more likely to recover quickly after a failure, and finally to experiment with success by seeking out new experiences (24).

The present study concentrates on couples nearing marriage, independently of whether they will have a religious or a civil marriage, and thus are all involved in a relevant experience of ecological transition. In particular, we consider self-efficacy in terms of the perceived ability of the partners to communicate efficiently, to offer their partner the required support, to value their partner's uniqueness, to handle conflicts and frustration in disagreements and criticism, to maintain the balance between self-fulfillment and respect for the partner, and finally to avoid intrusions by third parties, such as the partners' parents and/or other relatives (25). We also consider the couple's perceived satisfaction and stress because, as previous studies already showed, they may greatly influenced the quality of life and the well-being of both the couple and the individual partners (29).

Starting with the hypotheses that high levels of self-efficacy would reduce the potential negative features of the couple and would potentiate personal satisfaction and well-being, this study is aimed at investigating: 1) satisfaction, stress and self-efficacy in adults who are going to marry; 2) the relationships between self-efficacy and: a) stress, in terms of tension, depression and tiredness, and the physical manifestation of stress (35); b) satisfaction with living as a couple; 3) the mediating role of self-efficacy between stress management and satisfaction.

METHODS

This study concerns 385 people upon the day they went to the municipality to hand over marriage documents in a big city in the northwest of Italy. Fifty-one percent were women (N=194). The great majority (78%) lived in the city, 20% lived near the city, and only 2% resides in another region.

The participants were between 19-55 years (mean age 32.6 years, st.dev. 5.5): 11% is between 19-26 years, 54% is between 27-33 years, 27% is between 34-40 years, and finally 8% is between 41-55 years old. These data are in line with ISTAT (2009-2010). ISTAT is the Italian National Institute for Statistics and it is the main supplier of official statistical information in Italy (www.istat.it). It collects and produces information about socio-demographic, economic and contextual data in Italy. These statistics highlight that people below 35 years show a clear decrease in their propensity to marry. In actuality the mean age at the first marriage is 33 for men and 30 for women.

With respect to their level of education, 15% of the participants attended compulsory primary school, 48% finished high school, 34% completed university, and 3% had some kind of further professional specialization more than a university degree.

We coded professions according to the categories given by ISTAT: 36% of the participants were white-collar workers (N=134), 16% were employed with a technical profession (such as teachers, agents of commerce, and nurses; N=58), 15% had an intellectual or scientific profession with a high specialization (such as university professors, doctors and architects; N=56), 13% (N=49) were artisans or specialized blue-collar workers, 7% (N=27) worked in the commercial sector, 4 % (N= 14) of managers and entrepreneurs. With respect to the categories noted by ISTAT made up of conductors of facilities, semi-qualified blue-collar workers, unqualified workers and people who serve in the army, each one of these categories was present in our sample at 1% for a total of 4%. We also found 2% (N= 7) housewives, 2% (N= 6) unemployed and 1% (N=5) students.

With respect to aspects directly linked to the couple relationship, the participants were engaged for a mean of 54 months (d.s.38). In the further descriptive analyses, the months of engagement were dichotomized using the mean as a cut off: <=54 months of engagement and from 55 months on: 58% of the participants were engaged for 3-54 months and 42% for more than 55 months. From the data by ISTAT the period of engagement until 1964 for a first marriage was shorter (about 3 years) than in later years. From 1993 engagements lasted about 5 years (a length similar to that we found, which was about 4.5 years). Furthermore, the participants were equally divided into people who are already cohabiting (50%) and people who are not (50%). For 96% it is their first marriage. According to ISTAT, in Italy the proportion of premarital cohabitation dramatically increased in the last decades: it was about 10% between 1984-1993, 15% between 1994-1998, 25% from 1999-2003. More recent data are not shown.

Procedure and measures

Considering that marriages in this part of Italy are usually celebrated during spring and summer and that typically people apply for their documents at least three months earlier than the date of their marriage, before planning our study we interviewed the marriage officer in the municipality in order to find out the best three-month periods of the year during which to contact our participants. According to the marriage officer's suggestions we selected the period of the year between mid-January and mid-April.

The participants were contacted directly by researchers specialized in self-reporting questionnaire administration on the day they went to the municipality to hand over their documents for a civil or religious marriage. The partners were offered the self-reporting questionnaire about their current transition to marriage.

The municipal marriage officer made space available for the researchers to distribute and fill in the questionnaire. While no incentives were offered for participation, we registered a few cases of refusal to participate: only five couples (corresponding to 10 people) and one of the two members of a couple refused and the reasons for this refusal were mainly attributed to very practical problems such as time constraints due to employment and/or impending medical appointments. The administration of the entire questionnaire lasted for about 30 minutes.

In the first part, the questionnaire investigated self-efficacy in the context of the couple relationship (36). As Bandura highlighted (37), knowledge of the particular context of activities drives the aspects of personal self-efficacy that are important to measure. Furthermore, the scales of self-efficacy need to be linked and constructed for relevant and specific activities in order to be able to estimate if and why the beliefs of self-efficacy operate in different contexts.

In particular, our study focused on self-efficacy for the couple, i.e. each partner's perception about his/her ability to communicate with, to support, to respect and value their partner, to manage conflicts and disagreements and to avoid the intrusion of third parties. In particular, the scale consists of 13 items investigating some of the most common situations in a couple relationship: finding time to talk about the relationship, discussing worries, expectations, things to do together, to avoid conflicts leading to insults, to respect the opinions of the partner also when different from one's own, to face difficulties together and avoiding reciprocal criticism.

The modalities of responses were from "Not at all ability" (coded as 1), "A little" (2), "Enough" (3), "A lot" (coded as 4). The potential range of the responses varies from 13 to 76 (Alpha = .84). The real range varies from a minimum of 43 and the maximum of 76 (mean 62.7, st.dev. 6.2). In some descriptive analyses, the self-efficacy was trichotomised using the mean plus or minus half of the standard deviation as the cut-offs. That is, participants were considered to have low self-efficacy when they scored less than 57, at an intermediate level of self-efficacy when they scored between 57 and 68, and at a high self-efficacy level when they scored 69 and above.

A subsequent part of the questionnaire was aimed at investigating if and how much the participants perceived the preparation for marriage as a potentially stressful event.

We used the *tolesian scale of stress* (35). This scale considers that the coping strategies used by the person for facing a problematic condition, in terms of both strategies aimed at the safeguarding of one's own identity and strategies aimed at projecting one's own future, are essentially interdependent and reciprocally influencing elements and also that these strategies have an influence on the answer of the person during the stressful situation.

The entire scale consists 15 items with 5 modalities of answers from 1 (Never), 2, 3, 4 to 5 (Very often). The range varies from 15 to 75; Alpha = .93. Parallel to what Tap and Vasconcelos did in order to validate this scale and its sub-components, we used a truncated analysis of principal components (*Varimax method*) that highlighted the presence of three components in agreement with what Tap and Vasconcelos found (35).

In concordance with their method, the first component was called "Psychological tension and depression" (29% of explained variance), the second dimension was called "Tiredness" (20% of explained variance) and the last dimension represents the "Physical manifestation of stress" (13% of explained variance). In table 1 we reported the weight of each item in the three dimensions.

Starting with these analyses, we constructed the scale of " Psychological tension and depression" (8 items, Alpha = .89; mean 19.2, st.dev. 7.4), alla " Tiredness" (5 items, Alpha = .79; mean 12.1, st.dev. 4.4) e alle "Physical manifestation of stress" (2 items, Alpha = .74; mean 5.6, st.dev. 2.2).

For investigating couple satisfaction, we used one item asking the participants to evaluate how much he/she is satisfied on a four-point scale range from "Not at all" (1) to "Very much" (4): mean 3.7, st.dev. .46. We know that there are plenty of different scales evaluating

The transition to cohabitation　　375

different aspects of couple satisfaction (34) but we decided to use the simplest one because we are interested in the very general construct of satisfaction.

Table 1. Components of the stress scale

When I think about or am busy with the wedding preparations, sometimes…	Components (Weight of rotated components)		
	1	2	3
	Psychological tension and depression	Tiredness	Physical manifestation of stress
My heart runs very fast.	.105	.095	.900
I feel upset.	.500	.220	.648
I bite my nails.	.541	-.002	.463
I have the feeling of losing control	.685	.128	.405
I ruminate on the same ideas.	.807	.175	-.011
I don't handle difficulties well.	.816	.190	.077
I am worried.	.815	.256	.207
I feel tense.	.700	.331	.282
I feel pressure.	.573	.344	.314
I am anxious with respect to my future.	.519	.407	.174
I forget appointments, objects, or things to do.	-.004	.711	.014
I have difficulties with time management.	.216	.655	.045
I have little energy.	.226	.786	.090
I feel tired.	.288	.745	.057
I have difficulties in falling asleep or I sleep poorly.	.214	.589	.250
Eigenvalue	6.6	1.7	1.0
Percentage of explained variance	29%	20%	13%

Analytic plan

In describing how much the participants perceive themselves to be efficient in mastering the couple relationship, are satisfied with the relationship and are stressed during the wedding preparation, we used analyses of frequency and χ^2. For investigating the relationships between self-efficacy and stress and couple satisfaction we used correlations, ANOVA, and linear regression. For investigating the possible mediating effect of self-efficacy for the couple relationship we calculated the indirect effect by way of z-test and the Sobel-test (38).

The proposed mediating role of a couple's self-efficacy in the relationship between stress management and couple satisfaction was tested using the criteria described by Baron and Kenny (39) and Holmbeck (40). In order to demonstrate the mediation the following conditions should be met: a) the predictor variable has an effect on the mediator, b) the mediator variables have an effect on the outcome variables when controlling for predictor variables, and c) the effect of the predictor variable on the outcome is significantly less when the mediator is included in the model than when it is not included. Linear regression analyses were used to assess mediation.

Mediation analysis was conducted as follows (41): the direct effect (stress in terms of tiredness and psychological tension and depression → couple satisfaction) was evaluated to verify the influence of the predictor on the outcome variable. If the direct effect was significant, the mediator was included in the analyses.

Theoretically, if the mediation exists, the coefficients of the direct path (stress→ satisfaction), and the paths from the predictor variable to the mediator (stress →self-efficacy), and the mediator to the outcome variables (self-efficacy→ satisfaction), should all be significant and in the directions predicted. A mediation effect is present if, when the mediating paths are included, the overall fit of the model improves and the coefficient from predictor to outcome is lowered. If the direct effects between the predictor and the outcome is no longer statistically significant, the mediation is said to be *full*.

If the significance of the direct paths are lower but still significant, the mediation effect is said to be *partial*. First, the relationship between stress and the self-efficacy was investigated by way of linear regression. Second, we tested the direct effect of stress on couple satisfaction. After having controlled for the significance of those correlations, we assessed the final model (stress and self-efficacy → satisfaction). With regard to model indices of fit, we used an R square change for the linear regression.

RESULTS

The first goal of the study was to analyze the couple's self-efficacy, couple satisfaction, and stress (in terms of tension and depression, tiredness, and physical manifestations of stress) for marriage preparation.

With respect to the couple's self-efficacy, that is each partner's perception about his/her ability to find time to talk about the relationship, share worries, expectations, things to do together, avoid disagreements leading to insults, to respect the opinions of the partner even when they are different from one's own, to face difficulties together and avoiding reciprocal criticism, 66% of the participants were at intermediate levels, while 15% were at low and 19% at high levels. We did not find any gender difference. However, by increasing the age of the participants the proportions in the two extremes were higher: Generally speaking, older participants were more likely than younger ones to perceive low levels of self-efficacy (the proportion is 37% after the age of 40 years; Chi square=15.87; d.f.=6; p=.014).

The great majority (72%) was very much satisfied with his/her relationship (mean = 3.7 and st.dev.=.46) and we did not find any great gender and/or age difference. With respect to stress in general, the mean value is at intermediate levels (range 17-71, mean= 36.7; st.dev.= 11.9. However, women perceived higher stress than their partners [women = 39 vs. men = 34: $F(1, 364) = 18.5$; p=.0001, n^2=.05]. In particular women perceived more stress than men in two out of the three components of stress (Graph 1): psychological tension and depression [$F(1, 372) = 18.6$; p=.0001, n^2=.05], and the physical manifestation of stress [$F(1, 374) = 36.4$; p=.0001, n^2=.09]. Aside from this, people aged 34 to 40 perceived lower stress than all the other participants but especially lower than the youngest [F(3, 344) = 5.2; p=.002, n²=.04].

People aged from 34 to 40 years were less stressed than the other participants with respect to both psychological tension and depression [F(3, 349) = 3.8; p=.011, n²=.03] and the physical manifestation of stress [F(3, 351) = 7.6; p=.0001, n²=.06].

Those who were already living together perceived lower stress than the other participants [already cohabiting = 34 vs. not cohabiting = 39 [F(1, 360) = 13.8; p=.0001, n²=.04]. In particular, those who already cohabit perceived lower levels of stress than the other participants in all three components of stress (Graph 4): psychological tension and depression [F(1, 368) = 13.5; p=.0001, n²=.04], tiredness [F(1, 367) = 9.3; p=.003, n²=.03], and the physical manifestation of stress [F(1, 370) = 6.2; p=.013, n²=.02].

Our second goal was to investigate the relationships between the different aspects considered. The correlational analyses showed that couple satisfaction is negatively related with psychological tension and with depression (r=-.11; p<.05) and tiredness (r=-.18; p<.001). We did not find any correlation to the physical manifestation of stress.

The individual's self-efficacy within the couple relationship is positively correlated to his/her couple satisfaction (r=.40; p<.01) and negatively correlated with psychological tension and depression (r=-.23; p<.01), and with tiredness (r=-.21; p<.01). In particular, the participants with high levels of self-efficacy also showed higher levels of satisfaction [F(2, 300) = 28.5; p<.0001; n²=.16] the mean of satisfaction was 3.33, d.s.=.52 at low self-efficacy; 3.73, d.s.=.44 at intermediate self-efficacy; 3.96, d.s=.18 at high self-efficacy and the post hoc differences among the three groups were all statistically significant.

Finally, we investigated the possible mediation effect of self-efficacy between stress (in terms of its components: psychological tension, depression, and tiredness) and couple satisfaction. In order to do so, we performed some linear regressions in which satisfaction in the relationship in Step 1 was used as the outcome or dependent variable and the components of stress, and in Step 2 self-efficacy in the couple relationship was used as predictors.

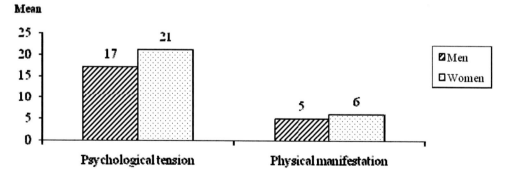

Graph 1. Gender differences with respect to psychological tension and depression and the physical manifestation of stress.

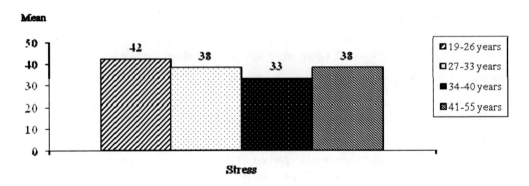

Graph 2. Age differences with respect to stress.

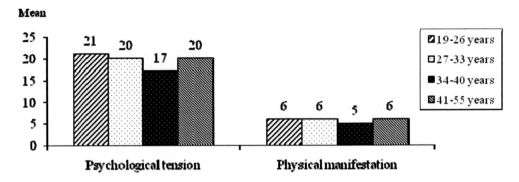

Graph 3. Age differences with respect to psychological tension and depression and the physical manifestation of stress.

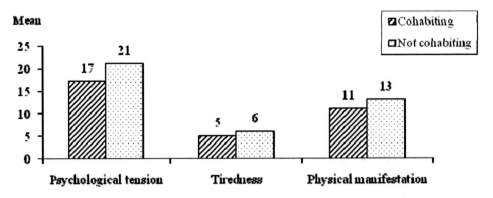

Graph 4. Cohabitation differences with respect to psychological tension and depression and the physical manifestation of stress.

Table 2 shows the results of our main effects model. Results showed that psychological tension and depression were negatively significantly associated with couple satisfaction ($\beta = -.12$, $p = 039$). Likewise our results also showed that couple's self-efficacy was positively significantly associated with satisfaction ($\beta = 0.391$, $p < .0001$).

The transition to cohabitation 379

Table 2. Standardized regression coefficients between psychological tension and depression, self-efficacy, and couple satisfaction

	Couple satisfaction		
	β estimate	SE	P
Psychological tension and depression	-.12	.003	.039
Self-efficacy	.391	.04	.0001

Table 3. Non-standardized regression coefficients of couple satisfaction (outcome), psychological tension and depression, and self-efficacy (predictor)

	Couple satisfaction		
	B	SE	P
Step 1 Psychological tension and depression	-.007	.004	.039
Step 2 Psychological tension and depression	-.002	.003	.55
Self-efficacy	.029	.004	.0001

Psychological tension and depression > Self-efficacy > Couple satisfaction

In order to test if the indirect effect of psychological tension and depression on couple satisfaction via the mediator perception of the couple's self-efficacy was significantly different from zero, first we established that psychological tension and depression were associated with the couple's self-efficacy. As expected, the coefficient between the predictor variable and our mediator was significant (β = -.12, p < .05). The coefficient for the regression association between psychological tension and depression (predictor) on couple satisfaction (outcome) was also significant (β = -.23, p = .0001). We observed a decrease in the coefficient once the mediator perception of the couple's self-efficacy was included in the regression model of their psychological tension and depression (predictor) on satisfaction (outcome) (β = -.032, p > .05).

Finally, the Sobel test for mediation that determines if the coefficient decrease is significant/reliable indicated the mediation model was fully mediated (z =-3.7 p= .0001).

Table 4. Standardized regression coefficients between tiredness, self-efficacy, couple satisfaction

	Couple satisfaction		
	β estimate	SE	P
Tiredness	-.19	.006	.001
Self-efficacy	.394	.04	.0001

Table 4 showed that tiredness was negatively significantly associated with couple satisfaction (β =-.19, p = .001). Likewise our results also showed that the self-efficacy was positively significantly associated with satisfaction (β = 0.394, p <. 0001).

Table 5. Non-standardized regression coefficients of the couple satisfaction (outcome), tiredness and self-efficacy (predictor)

	Couple satisfaction		
	B	SE	P
Step 1			
Tiredness	-.020	.006	.001
Step 2			
Tiredness	-.011	.006	.06
Self-efficacy	.030	.004	.0001

Tiredness > Self-efficacy > Couple satisfaction

In order to test if the indirect effect of tiredness on couple satisfaction via the mediator perception of self-efficacy was significantly different from zero, also in this case we first established that tiredness was associated with self-efficacy. As expected, the coefficient between the predictor variable and our mediator was significant (β = -.21, p < .0001). The coefficient for the regression association between tiredness (predictor) on couple satisfaction (outcome) was also significant (β = -.19, p = .001). We observed a decrease in the coefficient once the mediator perception of self-efficacy was included in the regression model of their tiredness (predictor) on satisfaction (outcome) (β = -.100, p > .05).

Finally, in this case we also found that the negative relationship between tiredness and couple satisfaction was totally mediated by beliefs of self-efficacy (z = -3.5 p = .0001).

DISCUSSION

This study was aimed at investigating the role of self-efficacy, which is a central dimension in individual development and adjustment during an important life transition: the construction of a stable couple. This transition is normatively characterized by strong psychological and emotional involvement because during the process, as in every ecological transition a meaningful resettlement of the relationship between the individual and his/her life contexts, the restructuring of his/her roles, and the redefinition of personal and others' expectations usually takes place (1). In the case of the transition to marriage, all of these things happen during a relatively defined time, where waiting and preparation for the marriage assumes a central dimension. Preparation for marriage may come with the experience of stress and fatigue, which in their turn may affect the condition of well-being and the perception of personal and couple satisfaction. In fact the preparation for marriage is usually characterized by strong projecting and a number of shared choices which concern both the public celebration of the civic or religious marriage and the preparation of the spouses' first home, unless they already cohabit. The spouses are often confronted with relevant expectations and interventions of practical and economic support by their families, who in Italy are generally very involved. The new couple is constructed as such by the way of a process of legitimization and of differentiation by their families (8). Facing all this complexity is likely to affect the relational dynamics and the shared experiences of the partners, the characteristics of the time they spend together and their accommodation of choices and desires, with relevant consequences for the well-being and the perception of couple satisfaction.

Thus, believing themselves to be more or less able to face the couple relationship is likely to be very important during this sensitive time of transition. We also know that self-efficacy affects the skill of mastering and controlling levels of stress and depressive conditions that intense or difficult situations may generate (23). In sum, we thought it would be interesting to investigate the relationship between self-efficacy, transitional stress and couple satisfaction. We turned our attention to a group of participants, the majority of which were young adults but also included older adults, who were comparable in terms of socio-demographic characteristics in their same age group in the national population (6).

We found that both self-efficacy and couple satisfaction were at intermediate-high levels for the majority of the participants and that there were no gender differences. These findings confirm that the people who decide to engage in a stable couple relationship are generally characterized by adequate instruments for bridging this transition and that their choice is driven by a general condition of satisfaction and well-being with their partner. The lack of gender differences with respect to the couple satisfaction was underlined previously in married couples (42).

However we also found that stress due to wedding preparations is at an intermediate-high level. The transition to marriage seems to contain elements that may lead to psychological tension and depression, tiredness and other physical manifestations of stress. In the case of stress, we found gender differences in that women reported higher levels of stress than men at both the general stress dimension and the two components of psychological tension in depression and physical manifestations of stress. On the contrary we did not find gender differences with respect to tiredness. A first interpretation of these findings could be based on the study by Shulz, Cowan, Cowan and Brennan (43). These authors found that the gender differences in tiring aspects of the daily life of a couple are enhanced under stress. Thus, the different perception of men and women of the psychological and physical manifestation of stress could be increased by the stress itself in a vicious circle. Another, not necessarily alternative, interpretation could instead refer to the type and the quantity of duties women and men usually have to face during the wedding preparations and those tasks could be unequally distributed between the two genders. In fact women are probably more likely than men to be busy with several organizational and practical aspects and also to face tensions linked to her own expectations and/or the expectations from her family with respect to the wedding ceremony and the couple's future life. The second interpretation seems indirectly confirmed by another finding and in particular by the fact that the people who were already cohabiting and/or had already have their home ready were also much less stressed than the other participants. Nevertheless, our study does not allow us to claim that previous cohabitation represents some kind of psychological or practical help in facilitating the transition to marriage. It seems likely that both the two previously mentioned aspects are present. In fact, people who already cohabit are more likely to have already been trained to successfully face little daily hassles and lesser or greater problems with their partner. Their transition may be more articulated and takes place during a longer time with respect to those who start cohabiting only after marriage. This articulation and timing may be related to lower levels of stress with respect to people who suddenly change their living condition. However, people who already cohabit and those who already have a home available certainly have fewer practical problems to solve before the wedding date.

Furthermore, we found that the most stressed among our participants were the youngest group aged 19-26 years. The youngest participants reported higher levels of stress than the others considering both the general level of stress and two out of its three components, psychological tension and depression and the physical manifestation of stress. It is possible to also interpret this finding only at a provisional level. In fact we have no information that could help us in attributing age differences to specific factors such as low economic stability and/or high work instability of the youngest group of participants. Previous studies by Ciairano et al (44,45) already showed that job instability may represent a threatening condition especially for some and it may lead to low levels of general life satisfaction. Job instability seems particularly powerful in affecting romantic relationships. However, at least another two alternative interpretations are possible. First, family pressure may be stronger in the cases of the youngest participants, probably because they are likely to be less economically independent from their families than the older participants. Second, and probably also more importantly, the youngest group might not be psychological ready to face the transition to marriage. In certain way their transition appears anticipated with respect to the mean age of marriage in both our group of participants and the Italian national population as a whole. Hendry and Kloep (46) already underlined that to get involved in a transition in advance with respect to same age may have negative effects for the individual adjustment and wellbeing. In particular, making a transition in advance is likely to be related to miss important occasions of self-fulfillment in the career and also to low levels of support in one's own broad social context. All these aspects may affect the way these participants experience their transition.

Another central aim of our study was to investigate the relationships between self-efficacy on the one side, and stress on the other in terms of tension, depression and tiredness, the physical manifestation of stress (35) and couple satisfaction. We showed that couple satisfaction is negatively related with psychological tension and depression and tiredness. This finding is in line with what we already know about the central role of stress in numerous phases of the couple's life. For instance, Bodenmann (29) highlighted that the accumulation of stressful events can deteriorate the quality of the relationship and consequently also the satisfaction perceived by the partners.

We also wanted to know whether or not the belief of being able to successfully master the different situations and experiences a person can encounter in their relationship with the partner may be positively related with couple satisfaction and negatively related with stress. In particular we expected that a person who believes him/herself to be able to manage a couple relationship is also more satisfied with this relationship and perceives lower levels of stress with respect to someone else who does not believe him/herself to be able to face daily tasks and hassles. Our findings seem to confirm our expectations: The participants with high levels of self-efficacy were also more satisfied with their couple relationship and they also felt less tension and depression during the wedding preparations. This finding confirms what other studies have already highlighted in married couples: couple satisfaction is greatly affected by the personal skills of the partners, especially in terms of the communication skills, understanding of the partner, and of facing problems (47,48). It seems plausible to hypothesize that self-efficacy and couple satisfaction are factors that reciprocally influence each other by involving the partners in positive dynamics. In fact both self-efficacy and couple satisfaction may improve reciprocity in the constructive dimensions of the relationship and consequently the perception of well-being in the relationship by each member of the couple. Such aspects may represent relevant protective factors for combating the unavoidable negative sides of relationships, which include conflicts and misunderstandings. When people possesses adequate levels of personal resources, conflicts and misunderstanding may appear less threatening and they are more likely to be faced successfully (49).

Finally, and more specifically, we wanted to know whether or not self-efficacy may mediate or buffer the relationship between perceived stress in wedding preparations and couple satisfaction. As expected, we found that self-efficacy really can fulfill this buffering role. In fact the negative relationship between stress and satisfaction is fully mediated by self-efficacy. That is, the higher the levels of self-efficacy, the lower the negative effects of high levels of psychological tension, depression, and tiredness on perceived satisfaction.

In sum, our study showed that during the transition to cohabitation, as well as in other contexts, self-efficacy may represent a fundamental resource for mastering stress and fatigue. The strong adaptive value of self-efficacy, which translates into social, cognitive, emotional and behavioral skills to successfully face lesser or greater daily challenges and hassles (24) is also confirmed when the transition to couple life is concerned. The increasing number of relationship failures, such as divorces and broken relationships in general, indicates that not all people possess adequate skills for facing this transition and that there are great individual differences in these skills. However, our study showed the important role that self-efficacy, and especially in the dimensions of communication and problem solving within relationships, can contribute towards the stability of the couple and in their stress management.

Self-efficacy has an interesting characteristic from an applied perspective: it can be improved by specific training programs. Thus, we think that our findings fit perfectly with the increasing awareness of the importance of some enrichment programs that have been introduced recently and that are precisely aimed at improving the personal skills of people who are going to marry in order to construct and to maintain a satisfactory marriage and decrease the divorce rate (50). Such enrichment programs are usually aimed at promoting reflection and experiential learning in order to improve and potentiate the couple relationship by enhancing protective factors and limiting the negative consequences of risk factors (51). These programs generally focus on skills and competence. That is to say, they concentrate not on the personality of the partners but rather on something that can be learned, or at least be trained and thus improved, and/or on something than the partners perhaps already have but need to learn how and when to use it in a more appropriate and mindful manner.

Our study certainly has several limits. First, we need to apply a similar study with a longitudinal design in order to investigate whether or not self-efficacy, satisfaction and stress for couple relationships and the relationship patterns between them are stable or change after marriage. Bodenmann and Cina (48) in a 5-year prospective longitudinal study found that the stable and satisfied couples were characterized by a lower level of stress or by more functional skills in facing stress at both the individual and the couple levels. By using a longitudinal design, we may further investigate the role of some socio-demographic or functional factors that can contribute to promoting or preventing the transition to a stable relationship. Second, especially considering that couples unavoidably involve two partners, we need to go beyond the individual level of analyses and toward the dyadic level. In the field of study of interpersonal relationships a few studies have started to focus on the dyad because the interdependence between partners is the basis of their reciprocal influence. With respect to couple relationships, there are a few recent studies such as those by Brock and Lawrence (52) and Ledermann et al (21) that investigated stress in married couples. Today, to use the dyad

384   *Antonella Roggero, Maria Fernanda Vacirca, Adele Mauri et al.*

as the level of analyses also becomes possible because specific models of analyses have recently been introduced. Among others, interdependence among the partners is considered in the *Actor-Partner Interdependence Model* (APIM) by Kashy and Kenny (53). This model integrates a rigorous theoretical approach to the unavoidable interdependence between two people, with appropriate analyses to test these interdependences (54). We plan to continue our research on couple relationships pursuing both the path of the longitudinal design and that of the dyadic level of analysis.

ACKNOWLEDGMENTS

We would like to thank Sezin Koehler for her professional assistance in editing this manuscript.

REFERENCES

[1] Bronfenbrenner U. The ecology of human development: Experiments by nature and design. Cambridge, MA: Harvard University Press, 1979.
[2] French A, Williams K. Depression and the psychological benefits of enteringmarriage. J Health Soc Behav 2007;48(2):149-63.
[3] ISTAT, Annuario statistico italiano 2007. Roma: ISTAT, 2004. Accessed 2011 Oct 01. URL: http://www.istat.it (2007).
[4] Asprea S. [La famiglia di fatto in Italia e in Europa]. Milano: Giuffré, 2003. [Italian]
[5] Mensch BS, Singh S, Casterline JB. Trends in the timing of first marriageamong men and women in the developing world. Populat Council 2005;2: 1–59.
[6] ISTAT Il matrimonio in Italia: anno 2008. Roma: ISTAT, 2010.
[7] Rosina A, Fraboni R. Is marriage losing its centrality in Italy? Demographic Res 2004;11(6):149-72.
[8] Scabini E, Iafrate R. [Psicologia dei legami familiari]. Bologna: Il Mulino, 2003.
[9] Hendrick SS, Hendrick C. Love and satisfaction. In: Sternberg RJ, Hojjat M, eds. Satisfaction in close relationships. New York: Guilford, 1997:56-78.
[10] Tani F, Steca P. [Soddisfazione di coppia e benessere della persona: determinanti personali e relazionali]. Età evolutiva 2007;86:67-76. [Italian]
[11] Bradbury TN, Fincham FD, Beach SRH. Research on the nature and determinants of marital satisfaction: A decade in review. J Marriage Fam 2000;62:964–80.
[12] Van denTroost A, Matthijs K, Vermulst AA, Gerris JRM, Welkenhuysen-Gybels J. Effects of spousal economic and cultural factors on Dutch marital satisfaction. J Fam Econ Issues 2006;27(2):235-62.
[13] Halliday J, Lucas A. Economic factors and relationship quality among young couples: Comparing cohabitation and marriage. J Marriage Fam, 2010;72(5): 1141-54.
[14] Blum JS, Mehrabian A. Personality and Temperament Correlates of Marital Satisfaction. J Personality, 1999, 67(1):93–125.
[15] Bouchard G, Sabourin S, Lussier Y, Wright J, Richer C. Predictive validity of coping strategies on marital satisfaction: Cross-sectional and longitudinal evidence. J Fam Psychol 1998;12(1):112-31.
[16] Burpee LC, Langer EJ. Mindfulness and marital satisfaction. J Adult Dev 2005;12(1):43-51.
[17] Gaunt R. Couple similarity and marital satisfaction: Are similar spouses happier? J Personality 2006;74(5):1401-20.
[18] Bouchard G, Lussier Y, Sabourin S. Personality and marital adjustment: Utility of the five-factor model of personality. J Marriage Fam 1999;61(3);651-60.
[19] Bodenmann G, Shantinath SD. The couples coping enhancement training (CCET): A new approach to prevention of marital distress based upon stress and coping. Fam Relat 2004;53(5):477-84.
[20] Cramer D. Satisfaction with a romantic relationship, depression, support and conflict. Psychol Psychother Theory Res Pract 2004;77:449–61.

[21] Ledermann T, Bodenmann G, Rudaz M, Bradbury T. Stress, Communication, and Marital Quality in Couples. Fam Relations, 2010;59:195–206.

[22] Ducat WH, Zimmer-Gembeck MJ. Romantic Partner Behavioursas Social Context: Measuring Six Dimensions of Relationships. J Relatsh Res 2010; 1:1–16.

[23] Bandura A. Self-efficacy in changing societies. Cambridge: Cambridge University Press, 1995.

[24] Bandura A. Self-efficacy: The exercise of control. New York: Freeman, 1997.

[25] Caprara GV, Regalia C, Scabini E. Autoefficacia familiare. In GV Caprara (Ed). [La valutazione dell'autoefficacia]. Trento: Erickson, 2001:63–86. [Italian]

[26] Caprara GV, Steca P. The contribution of self-regulatory efficacy beliefs in managing affect and family relationships to positive thinking and hedonic balance. J Soc Clin Psychol 2006; 25:601–25.

[27] Van Steenbergen EF, Kluwer ES, Karney BR. Workload and the Trajectory of Marital Satisfaction in Newlyweds: Job Satisfaction, Gender, and Parental Status as Moderators. J Fam Psychol 2011; 9:345–55.

[28] Randall AK, Bodenmann G. The role of stress on close relationships and marital satisfaction. Clinic Psychol Rev 2009; 29:105–15.

[29] Bodenmann G. Dyadic coping and its significance for marital functioning. In: Revenson TA, Kayser K, Bodenmann G. Emerging perspectives on couples' coping with stress. Washington: APA, 2005: 47-62.

[30] Hahlweg K, Markman HJ, Thurmaier F, Engl J, Eckert V. Prevention of maritaldistress: Results of a German prospective longitudinal study. J Fam Psychol 1998; 12:543–56.

[31] Pittman JF, Solheim CA, Blanchard D. Stress as a driver of the allocation of housework. J Marriage Fam 1996; 58(2): 456–68.

[32] Whisman MA, Uebelacker LA. Impairment and distress sassociated with relationship discord in a national sample of married or cohabiting adults. *J Fam Psychol* 2006; *20*:369–77.

[33] Kinnunen U, Taru F. Economic stress and marital adjustment among couples: analyses at the dyadic level. Eur J Soc Psychol 2004; 34(5):519–32.

[34] Graham JM, Diebels KJ, Barnow ZB. The Reliability of Relationship Satisfaction: A Reliability Generalization Meta-Analysis. J Fam Psychol 2011; 25(1):39–48.

[35] Tap P, Vasconcelos ML. Précarité et vulnérabilité psychologique. Fundação Bissaya-Barreto. CEICI (Coimbra), Ramonville Saint-Agne: Editions Erès, 2004.

[36] Caprara GV. [La valutazione dell'autoefficacia]. Trento: Erickson, 2001. [Italian]

[37] Bandura A. [Autoefficacia: Teorie e Applicazioni]. Trento: Erickson, 2000. [Italian]

[38] Sobel ME. Asymptotic confidence intervals for indirect effects in structural equationmodels. In Leinhardt S. Sociological Methodology. Washington DC: Americ Sociol Ass, 1982: 290-312.

[39] Baron RM, Kenny DA. The Moderator-Mediator Variable Distinction in Social Psychological Research: Conceptual, Strategic, and Statistical Considerations. J Pers Soc Psychol 1986; 51(6):1173-82.

[40] Holmbeck GN. Toward terminological, conceptual, and statistical clarity in the study of mediators and moderators: Examples from the child-clinical and pediatric psychology literatures. J Consulting Clinic Psychol 1997; 65:599-610.

[41] Hoyle RH, Smith GT. Formulating clinical research hypotheses as structural equation models: A conceptual overview. J Consulting Clinic Psychol 1994; 62(3):429-40.

[42] Kurdek LA. Gender and Marital Satisfaction Early in Marriage: A Growth Curve Approach. J Marriage Fam 2005; 67:68–84.

[43] Schulz MS, Cowan PA, Cowan CP, Brennan RT. Coming Home Upset: Gender, Marital Satisfaction, and the Daily Spillover of Workday Experience Into Couple Interactions. J Fam Psychol 2004; 18(1): 250–63.

[44] Ciairano S, Callari TC, Rabaglietti E, Roggero A. Precariousness of job, sensc of coherence and life satisfaction in Italianadults. In Psychol Satisf. Hauppauge, NY: Nova Science Publishers (publicationpending).

[45] Ciairano S, Rabaglietti E, Roggero A, Callari TC. Life satisfaction, Sense of Coherence and Job Precariousness in Italian Young Adults. J Adult Dev 2010; 17(3)):177–89.

[46] Hendry LB, Kloep M. [Lo sviluppo nel ciclo di vita]. Bologna: Il Mulino, 2003. [Italian]

[47] Rogge RD, Bradbury T. Predicting marital distress and dissolution: refining the two factor hypothesis. J Fam Psychol 2006; 20(1):156-9.

[48] Bodenmann G, Cina A. Stress and Coping Among Stable-Satisfied, Stable-Distressed and Separated/Divorced Swiss Couples. J Divorce Remarriage 2006; 44(1):71–89.

[49] Acitelli LK, Douvan E, Veroff J. The changing influence of interpersonal perceptions on marital well-being among black and white couples. J Soc Pers Relatsh 1997; 14:291–304.

[50] Van Widenfelt B, Markam HJ. Prevention of relationship problems. In Halford WK, Markam HJ. Clinical handbook of marriage and couples intervention. Chichester, England: Wiley, 1997: 651-78.
[51] Giuliani C, Iafrate C. [L'enrichment familiare]. Roma: Carocci, 2006.[Italian]
[52] Brock RL, Lawrence E. A Longitudinal Investigation of Stress Spillover in Marriage: Does Spousal Support Adequacy Buffer the Effects? J Fam Psychol 2008; 22(1):11–20.
[53] Kashy DA, Kenny DA. The analysis of data from dyads and groups. In Reis HT, Judd CM. Handbook of research methods in social and personality psychology. Cambridge: Cambridge University Press, 1999: 110-36.
[54] Cook WL, Kenny DA. The actor-partner interdependence model: A model of bidirectional effects in developmental studies. Internat J BehavDev 2005; 29:101–9.

Submitted: October 18, 2011. *Revised:* December 06, 2011. *Accepted:* December 18, 2011.

SECTION FOUR – POSITIVE YOUTH DEVELOPMENT

In: Alternative Medicine Research Yearbook 2012
Editors: Søren Ventegodt and Joav Merrick

ISBN: 978-1-62808-080-3
© 2013 Nova Science Publishers, Inc.

Chapter 38

SPIRITUALITY AS A POSITIVE YOUTH DEVELOPMENT CONSTRUCT: A CONCEPTUAL REVIEW

Daniel TL Shek, PhD, FHKPS, BBS, JP[1,2,3,4,5] *

[1]Department of Applied Social Sciences, The Hong Kong Polytechnic University, Hong Kong, PRC
[2]Public Policy Research Institute, The Hong Kong Polytechnic University, Hong Kong, PRC
[3]Department of Social Work, East China Normal University, Shanghai, PRC
[4]Kiang Wu Nursing College of Macau, Macau, PRC
[5]Division of Adolescent Medicine, Department of Pediatrics, Kentucky Children's Hospital, University of Kentucky College of Medicine, Lexington, Kentucky, US

ABSTRACT

The concept of spirituality as a positive youth development construct is reviewed in this paper. Both broad and narrow definitions of spirituality are examined and a working definition of spirituality is proposed. Regarding theories of spirituality, different models pertinent to spiritual development and the relationship between spirituality and positive youth development are highlighted. Different ecological factors, particularly family and peer influences were found to influence spirituality. Research on the influence of spirituality on adolescent developmental outcomes is examined. Finally, ways to promote adolescent spirituality are discussed.

Keywords: Adolescence, positive youth development, spirituality

---

* Correspondence: Professor Daniel TL Shek, PhD, FHKPS, BBS, JP, Chair Professor of Applied Social Sciences, Faculty of Health and Social Sciences, Department of Applied Social Sciences, The Hong Kong Polytechnic University, Room HJ407, Core H, Hunghom, Hong Kong. E-mail: ssdaniel@inet.polyu.edu.hk.

INTRODUCTION

There are research studies showing that spiritual and religious involvement is an important dimension in adolescent development. For example, Gallup and Bezilla reported that 95% of American adolescents believed in God (1). Based on the data collected from "The Project Teen Canada", Bibby found that 75% of the respondents regarded themselves as members of a religion, 60% viewed spirituality as important, and 48% indicated they had spiritual needs (2). In a study based on 112,232 freshmen in 236 colleges and universities in the United States, Astin et al. reported that 77% of the students agreed that they were "spiritual beings" and roughly four-fifth of them indicated that they had interest in spirituality and they believed in the sacredness (3). These findings are consistent with the view of Benson and Roehlkepartain (4) that "most young people view spiritual development as an important part of their lives" (p. 14). King and Boyatzis (5) similarly commented that adolescence "may be a particularly important time period in which to study spiritual and religious development"(p. 2).

Using life meaning as an illustration, adolescents tend to think in abstract terms and explore future possibilities when they are cognitively mature. They commonly ask questions about life, including: What is the meaning of life? What is a meaningful life? Why do we exist? What should we accomplish in life? These questions commonly fall within the large scope of "meaning of life" or "purpose in life", which addresses three inter-related issues which that are the meaning of life (e.g., what life signifies, personal reasons, and importance of existence), meaningfulness of life, (e.g., whether life is worth living or purposeful) and purpose in life (e.g., life goals, life purpose, things to be accomplished, ideals to be attained).

The importance of the meaning of life in adolescent behavior is clearly reflected in human history. For example, in the 1930's, young people supported Hitler in Nazi Germany when they believed that building an ethnically superior Germany was their life mission.

During the Cultural Revolution in Communist China in the 1960's, the Red Guards fiercely fought against "enemies" of the proletarians when they saw that building a Communist utopia was their sacred life goal. In the contemporary world, many young people in Africa participate in military activities to look for changes for their countries.

Unfortunately, despite the importance of spirituality in adolescent development, a review of the literature showed that less than 1% of the literature on children and adolescents had examined issues on spirituality and religiosity (6). As commented by King and Boyatzis (5), "adolescents' spirituality and religion haven been relatively neglected in the developmental sciences" (p. 2).

In addition, there is a huge research gap in the study of spirituality in the clinical literature (7). Against this background, this paper attempts to review the concept of spirituality in adolescence. Besides definitions and theories, antecedents of adolescent spirituality and its effects on developmental outcomes are presented. Finally, ways to promote adolescent spirituality are presented.

DEFINITION OF SPIRITUALITY

Various definitions of spirituality have been put forward by different researchers. Based on qualitative analyses of various definitions of religiousness and conceptions of spirituality, Scott reported (cited by 8, p63) that the conceptions distributed over nine content areas, with no category containing most of the definitions (8). These content areas include: 1) connectedness or relationship; 2) processes contributing to a higher level of connectedness; 3) reactions to sacred or secular things; 4) beliefs or thoughts; 5) traditional institutional structures; 6) pleasurable existence; 7) beliefs in the sacred or higher being; 8) personal transcendence; and 9) existential issues and concerns. Markow and Klenke pointed out there were more than 70 definitions of spirituality at work (9).

Perhaps the first clarification that should be made is the distinction between spirituality and religion. Pargament (10) argued that religion is "the search for significance in ways related to the sacred" whereas spirituality is "the search for the sacred" (pp. 11-12). Worthington, Hook, Davis and McDaniel (11) defined religion as "adherence to a belief system and practices associated with a tradition in which there is agreement about what is believed and practiced" whereas spirituality as "a more general feeling of closeness and connectedness to the sacred. What one views as sacred is often a socially influenced perception of either (a) a divine being or object or (b) sense of ultimate reality or truth" (p. 205). With reference to this conception, while religion is related to institutional beliefs and the sacred, the divine and institutional religion is not necessarily related to the definition of spirituality. According to Worthington et al. (11), there are four types of spirituality, with the first one more related to religion: religious spirituality (closeness and connection to the sacred defined by religion); humanistic spirituality (closeness and connection to mankind); nature spirituality (closeness and connection to nature); cosmos spirituality (closeness and connection to the whole of creation) (11). In the project on the role of spirituality in higher education at the Higher Education Research Institute at the UCLA, Austin and his associates distinguished spiritual attributes and religious attributes. While spiritual attributes includes spiritual quest (answers to life's questions), ecumenical worldview (transcendence of ethnocentrism and egocentrism), ethics of care (compassion), charitable involvement (services to others), and equanimity (inner peace), religious attributes includes religious commitment (degree of identification with the religion), engagement (behavioral aspect of religion), conservatism (identification with orthodox beliefs), skepticism (questions raised on the beliefs), and struggle (unsettlement about religion).

Broad as well as narrow definitions of spirituality exist in the literature. An example of a broad definition was put forward by Myers, Sweeney and Witmer (12) who defined spirituality as "personal and private beliefs that transcend the material aspects of life and give a deep sense of wholeness, connectedness, and openness to the infinite" (p. 265). According to this conception, spirituality includes: a) belief in a power beyond oneself; b) behavior in relation to the infinite such as prayer; c) meaning and purpose of life; d) hope and optimism; e) love and compassion; f) moral and ethical guidelines; g) transcendental experience. Another broad definition can be seen in Lewis who conceived spirituality as the life affirmed in a relationship with God, self, community, and environment which leads to the nurturance and celebration of wholeness (13). Within this context, spiritual needs include meaning, purpose and hope, transcendence circumstances, integrity and worthiness, religious participation, loving and serving others, cultivating thankfulness, forgiving and being forgiven, and preparation for death and dying. On the other hand, there are relatively narrower definitions of spirituality such as focus on existential or transcendental questions, belongingness to involvement of cardinal values underlying every aspect of life, and self-reflective behavior. For example, Worthington et al (11) conceived spirituality as "general feeling of closeness and connectedness to the sacred" (p. 205).

An integration of the literature shows that several elements are commonly employed in the definition of spirituality. These include meaning and purpose of life, meaning of and reactions to limits of life such as death and dying, search for the sacred or infinite, including religiosity, hope and hopelessness, forgiveness, and restoration of health (14). Lau pointed out that three key elements of spirituality had been identified in the literature (15). The first element is horizontal as well as vertical relationships in human existence (16). While horizontal relationships are related to oneself, others and nature, vertical relationship involves a transcendental relationship with a higher being. The second element is beliefs and values which are integral to answers to spiritual questions such as life and death. The third element is the meaning of life. In this review, a broader conception of spirituality (i.e., horizontal and vertical relationships, beliefs, meaning of life) is adopted.

ASSESSMENT OF SPIRITUALITY

Two broad strategies are commonly used to assess the construct of spirituality: quantitative approach and qualitative approach. To maximize the strengths and minimize the limitations of both approaches, researchers commonly use both approaches to assess spirituality. In the quantitative approach, either single items or scales are used to assess spirituality. For example, researchers have used single items to assess a respondent's ranking of the importance of things in life, such as wealth, family, health, friends, social status and peace of mind. Also commonly, researchers use a few items to assess religiosity and religious involvement. Obviously, both single-item measure and multiple-item measures are problematic because their reliability and validity are usually not examined. To overcome such problems, psychological scales have been developed to measure the construct of spirituality. Some examples include the Spiritual Well Being Scale, Purpose in Life Questionnaire, Templer's Death Anxiety Scale, Enright Forgiveness Inventory and Herth Hope Index. Unfortunately, there are few validated measures of spirituality for Chinese adolescents (14,17). Furthermore, few researchers use advanced statistical techniques such as structural equation modeling to assess spirituality.

Qualitative methods (such as open-ended questions, drawing, verbal commentary techniques, and case studies) are also employed to examine spirituality, particularly in the clinical settings. The common features of qualitative research include naturalistic inquiry, inductive analysis, holistic perspective, qualitative data, personal contact and insight, dynamic system, unique case orientation, empathetic neutrality and design flexibility. For example, children have been invited to draw pictures about their attitudes towards death and dying. While qualitative study can capture the perspectives of the informants and is a more naturalistic form of research, it is often criticized as biased and polluted by ideological preoccupations. As such, ways to enhance the credibility of data collection, analyses, and interpretations are important issues to be considered.

THEORIES OF SPIRITUALITY

There are three categories of theories of spirituality. The first category of theories focuses on the nature of spirituality in relation to different aspects of human development. For example, there are theories suggesting that spirituality is part of quality of life. In the model of psychological well-being proposed by Ryff and Singer (18), meaning, purpose, growth, and self-actualization are basic components of well-being, and psychological well-being includes self-acceptance, environmental mastery, positive relations with others, purpose in life, personal growth, and autonomy. In the Wellness Model proposed by Adams, Bezner, Drabbs, Zambarano and Steinhardt, emotional centeredness, intellectual stimulation, physical resilience, psychological optimism, social connectedness, and spiritual life purpose are basic dimensions (19).

The second group of theories concerns the nature of spiritual development. In Erikson's theory of psychosocial development (20), the major task of an adolescent is to develop an identity, with ego identity versus role confusion as the basic psychosocial crisis. In Marcia's framework, crisis and commitment are two basic dimensions of identity, particularly in religious or spiritual identity (21). In the spiritual development model proposed by Fowler (22), there are six stages of faith development, with Stage 3 and Stage 4 most relevant to spiritual development of adolescents. In Stage 3, faith development takes the form of "synthetic-conventional" faith which is characterized by conformity with little reflection on one's religious beliefs. This stage is quite typical in the Chinese culture. In Stage 4, "individuative-reflective" faith is characterized by personal struggle and choice. It is argued that the existence of personal struggle and choice are important elements of mature spirituality.

In the faith development model suggested by Genia (23), five stages were proposed. Following the stages of Egocentric Faith (Stage 1) and Dogmatic Faith (Stage 2), the third stage is Transitional Faith where adolescents can critically examine their spirituality which is prompted by adolescents' gradual maturation in cognitive ability and interpersonal perspective taking. If the transition in Stage 3 is successful, adolescents will progress to Stage 4 (Reconstructed Internalized Faith) and Stage 5 (Transcendent Faith) where transcendent faith is characterized by flexible system of faith, universal principles, and permeable psycho-spiritual boundaries.

The third group of theories is on the relationship between spirituality and positive youth development. In the model proposed by Benson (24), there are 40 developmental assets in adolescent development, where life meaning and positive beliefs are important internal assets that influence adolescent development. Dowling et al. proposed a model in which spirituality was hypothesized to influence thriving with religiosity as a mediating factor (25). In a review of 77 positive youth development programs in the United States, Catalano et al. concluded that positive youth development constructs are intrinsic to the successful programs, with spirituality as one of the constructs identified which is defined as the development of purpose and meaning in life, hope, or beliefs in a higher power (26). There are many recent

394 Daniel TL Shek

publications highlighting the relationship between positive youth development and spirituality (27-29).

ANTECEDENTS OF ADOLESCENT SPIRITUALITY

Benson and Roehlkepartain (4) concluded three processes intrinsic to adolescent spirituality. The first process is awareness or awakening which contributes to the development of spiritual identity, meaning and purpose. The second process is interconnecting or belonging which involves seeking or experiencing relationships with others, including divine beings. The final process is a way of life where a person expresses one's spiritual identity through different activities and relationships. This model further proposed that these three processes shaping adolescent developmental outcomes are related to other dimensions of development which are influenced by context (e.g., family, peers and neighborhood), culture, (e.g., media) and meta-narratives (e.g., stories). Besides ecological models, there are other accounts on the factors influencing adolescent spirituality. For the channeling hypothesis, it is stated that children are "channeled" into different social groups based on the religious expectations of the parents (30). The spiritual modeling perspective based on the social learning premise indicates that adolescents model their religious behavior of their parents (31). The role of significant-others in shaping adolescent spirituality is also highlighted by Fry who explicitly stated that "it is through supportive and sharing relationships within a trusting and accepting atmosphere that the adolescent gains the courage to explore what experiences make sense or providing meaning even in the face of doubts" (p. 98), thus emphasizing the role of intimate relations in the development of adolescent purpose in life (32).

There are research findings showing that family and peers exert influence on the spiritual development in adolescents. In a longitudinal study based on individuals, parents, peers, schools, and community, Regnerus et al. found that while parents and friends strongly influenced religious behavior of adolescents, county level influences were weak (31). In their study of parent and peer relationships and relational spirituality in adolescents and young adults, Desrosiers, Kelley and Miller (33) showed that parents and peers, particularly maternal communication and paternal affection facilitated the development of relational spirituality.

With specific focus on the Chinese culture, Shek (17) reviewed ecological factors that influence the development of meaning in life among Chinese adolescents. Regarding the socio-demographic correlates of meaning in life in Chinese adolescents, it was found that gender, age and economic disadvantage were related to adolescent life meaning, although the effect sizes were small. For example, regarding gender differences, there are research findings showing that male adolescents displayed a higher level of life purpose than did female adolescents, although such gender differences are not consistent across studies (17). Within the family context, two types of family experiences that may shape the meaning of life in adolescentsare dyadic family processes (e.g., parent-child relationship and marital quality of the parents) and systemic family attributes (e.g., family functioning and communication patterns). Shek (17) reported that there were several cross-sectional studies showing that the quality of parenting was positively related to adolescent meaning of life indexed by the Chinese Purpose in Life Questionnaire. Besides, in a series of studies examining the relationship between family processes and adolescent development, positive parenting attributes (such as parental support and involvement) were related to existential well-being in several samples. There are longitudinal research findings showing that parenting characteristics and parent-adolescent conflict were related to adolescent life meaning. Finally, research evidence also supporting supports that family functioning is related to adolescent meaning in life, both concurrently and longitudinally. cross-sectional and over time.

SPIRITUALITY AND ADOLESCENT DEVELOPMENTAL OUTCOMES

Regarding the relationship between spirituality and quality of life, there are four possibilities. First, spirituality is a cause of quality of life. Second, spirituality is a concomitant of quality of life. Third, spirituality is a consequence of quality of life. Finally, the relationship between spirituality and quality of life are is moderated and/or mediated by other factors. While studies have been conducted to examine the first two possibilities, research on the latter two possibilities is almost non-existent (14,17).

There are theoretical accounts suggesting that spirituality is an antecedent of quality of life (i.e., first possibility). In the theory of logotherapy proposed by Victor Frankl (34), it is asserted that when there is existential vacuum (i.e., loss of meaning in life), mental problems come in to fill the vacuum. Frankl's conceptualization about human nature is based on the premise of "will to meaning". When a person fails to find meaning in life and a state of vacuum of perceived meaning in personal existence (i.e., existential vacuum) is present, he or she is confronted by "existential frustration", which is characterized by the feeling of boredom (35). Although the occurrence of existential vacuum does not necessarily lead to noogenic neuroses, it was contended that existential vacuum is an etiological factor of psychopathology. Based on the above reasoning, it could be assumed that purpose in life is causally related to adolescent developmental outcomes. In a review of the relationships among meaning in life and well-being, psychopathology and spirituality, research showeds that people experiencing greater life meaning reported greater well-being, less psychopathology and more positive experience of spirituality (36). Emmons also argued that religion provides goals and value system contributes to life meaning which would eventually shape different aspects of a person's life (37).

In the area of adolescent spirituality, despite their findings that spiritual attributes were related to global and life domains, Sawatzky, Gadermann and Pesut (38) commented that there are few studies on spirituality and quality of life in adolescents and the mechanisms underlying the relationship remains relatively unknown. They remarked that "few studies have examined the relevance of spirituality in adolescents with respect to their quality of life (QOL), despite empirical literature suggesting that religion and spirituality are important to adolescents" (p. 6).

Rew and Wong reviewed the association between religiosity/spirituality and adolescent health attitude and behavior (39). The review showed that although roughly half of the studies indicated that religiosity/spirituality had positive effect on adolescent health attitude and behavior, there were theoretical and methodological limitations of the studies. In a review of research on adolescent religiosity and mental health, Wong, Rew and Slaikeu (40) found that most studies showed a positive relationship between religiosity/spirituality and adolescent mental health. Cotton et al reviewed religiosity/spirituality and health outcomes (41). They differentiated distal domains (service attendance, frequency of prayers and meditation, self-rated religiosity) and proximal domains (meaning and peace, religious coping, church support) and reviewed the related studies on adolescent developmental outcomes. While studies showed negative relationship between religiosity/spirituality and adolescent health risk, positive relationship between religiosity/spirituality and physical/mental health were reported.

Reviews showed that spiritual well-being is was positively related to health outcomes, although there are were possible confounding effects in the reported relationships (42). Regarding the relationship between spirituality and physical health, Powell, Shahabi and Thoresen tested nine hypotheses with reference to mediated models (evaluation of the impact of religion or spirituality on health, regardless of whether or not such a relationship was mediated by established risk/protective factors) and independent models (evaluatinged religion or spirituality as an independent protective factor after controlling other effects) and concluded that church/service attendance protects healthy people against death (43). Meanwhile, the authors also pointed out the need for more methodologically sound studies in the field.

The role of spiritual intervention has also received increasing attention in the literature. On one hand, patients expect helping professionals to address their spiritual needs (42). On the other hand, different professional bodies give more attention to spiritual care. For example, the National Consensus Project for Quality Palliative Care regarded spiritual, religious and existential aspects of care as a domain of quality palliative care requiring spiritual care (Domain 5). In addition, the White House Office of Faith-Based and Community Initiatives was established in the Bush administration. Theoretically, Lent argued that it is important to understand spiritual variables such as meaning in life so that client growth and rehabilitation can be promoted (44).

Under the assumption that spirituality influences health outcomes, spiritual intervention with the aims of treatment or restoration and improvement of quality of life has been developed. In a meta-analysis of 51 samples from 46 studies examining psychotherapies in which religious or spiritual (R/S) beliefs are were incorporated, Worthington et al (11) drew several conclusions. First, compared with patients receiving secular psychotherapies, patients receiving R/S psychotherapies had better improvement in psychological and spiritual outcomes. Second, in contexts where spiritual outcomes are important, psychotherapies with R/S is a treatment of choice. Third, practitioners could consider offering psychotherapies with R/S to highly religious or spiritual patients.

With specific reference to the Chinese culture, there are research findings showing that purpose in life was negatively associated with psychological symptoms, including general psychological problems, trait anxiety, depression and hopelessness. Furthermore, participants with different existential statuses also displayed different levels of psychological symptoms. There are also longitudinal data showing the adverse relationship between purpose in life and psychological symptoms over time. Besides psychiatric symptoms, meaning in life was found to be related to positive mental health measures (14,17). Shek, Siu and Lee (45) also reported that the spirituality subscale score of the Chinese Positive Youth Development Scale was positively associated with other positive youth development constructs, including bonding, resilience, social competence, emotional competence, cognitive competence, behavioral competence, moral competence, self-determination, self-efficacy, beliefs in the future, clear and positive identity, recognition for positive behavior, prosocial involvement, and prosocial norms. These findings are generally consistent with the views of Ryff and Singer (18) that sense of meaning and sense of self-realization are two key components of positive mental health, where meaning in life provides the necessary inner resources to fuel optimal functioning. There are also research findings showing that meaning in life was related to prosocial behavior and antisocial behavior while negatively associated with problem behavior.

Consistent with this notion, there are research findings suggesting that meaning in life is an important factor in helping adolescents to face adversity. Shek (46) showed that adolescents with stronger endorsement of positive Chinese beliefs (or weaker endorsement of negative Chinese beliefs) about adversity generally had better psychological well-being and school adjustment and less problem behavior. Although adolescents' degree of agreement with Chinese cultural beliefs about adversity was generally associated with adolescent adjustment, this relationship was stronger in adolescents with economic disadvantage than in adolescents without economic disadvantage. Nevertheless, while this study is pioneering in Hong Kong, replication of the findings is necessary in view of the worsening of income disparity and inequality in Hong Kong.

PROMOTION OF SPIRITUALITY
IN ADOLESCENTS

Given the importance of spirituality, there are several ways to promote adolescent spirituality. The first strategy is to understand different forms of religions and spirituality via different media, including print and non-print media. Enhanced understanding is important as far as religious and spiritual beliefs are concerned. However, understanding alone is not enough. Active reflection and experience are important processes in the development of spirituality. "Why do we exist? Where are we going? Is there any life after death? What should we do when we are still conscious?" These are important spiritual questions demanding conscious reflection. Besides gaining more experience and having personal reflections, joining religious groups, church activities, and spiritually related gatherings provide a good opportunity to develop spirituality. Bruce and Cockreham proposed different ways of promoting spirituality in adolescent girls via group work approach (47). Besides, as significant-others surrounding adolescents (such as parents, teachers and peers) have an important influence on adolescent spirituality, how to shape adolescent spirituality through such significant personal relationships could be considered.

Finally, curricular-based programs can be utilized to promote spirituality in adolescents. For example, Hui and Ho (48) evaluated a forgiveness training program via quantitative and qualitative methods. Although there was no significant improvement in self-esteem and hope among the participants based on the pretest and posttest scores, participants showed better conception of forgiveness and had a positive attitude to using forgiveness. They concluded that it was "viable to promote forgiveness as a classroom guidance program" (p. 477). In the Project P.A.T.H.S. which attempts to promote holistic development in Chinese adolescents, units on spirituality are included in the Secondary 1 to Secondary 3 curricula (49-51). Finally, in the course entitled "Tomorrow's Leader" developed in The Hong Kong Polytechnic

University, the following elements pertinent to the construct of spirituality are included: definition and basic concepts of spirituality, theories of spirituality, antecedents of spirituality, spirituality and adolescent developmental outcomes, spirituality and leadership, and ways to promote spiritual leadership.

EXISTING RESEARCH GAPS AND FUTURE RESEARCH DIRECTIONS

King and Boyatzis (5) described that adolescence is "an age period of intense ideological hunger, a striving for meaning and purpose, and desire for relationships and connectedness" (p. 2). Given its importance, what are the research directions as far as the study of adolescent spirituality is concerned? Conceptually speaking, although literature shows that ecological factors at the individual, interpersonal and family contexts are related to adolescent spirituality, there are several conceptual gaps. First, although there are views suggesting that spirituality influences adolescent developmental outcomes, how developmental outcomes may influence the development of purpose in life is far from clear (i.e., bi-directional relationships between purpose in life and developmental outcomes). Obviously, accumulation of research findings in this area would help to enrich Frankl's idea on the role of existential vacuum in human behavior.

Second, based on the ecological model, further studies should be conducted to examine how individual factors (e.g., religiosity and values), family factors (e.g., global parenting versus specific parenting practice, behavioral control and psychological control) and social factors (e.g., endorsement of Chinese superstitious beliefs) are related to adolescent spirituality. This research direction is consistent with the argument of Fry (32) that "whether adolescents' life meaning and wisdom will grow and unfold from being relatively straightforward to being mature and complex will depend invariably on the presence or absence of a number of other intervening and moderating influences and contextual factors" (p. 93). It would be theoretically interesting to look at the relationships among life meaning, character building and religiousness, and subjective well-being.

Third, although the present review highlights the importance of family processes in adolescents' purpose in life, further work is needed to examine how specific family processes and related experiences are related to purpose in life among adolescents. For example, it would be interesting to study how purpose in life of the parents is related to that of their adolescent children. It is important to examine the achievement of life meaning through love in close relationships.

Finally, although there are research findings in the area of human development examining the influence of spirituality on developmental outcomes in different stages of life span, Ellison and Lee (52) stated that spiritual struggles, including troubled relationships with God, negative interaction in religious settings and chronic religious doubting were related to psychological distress. The possible "dark side" of adolescent spirituality should be considered.

REFERENCES

[1] Gallup G, Bezilla R. The religious life of young Americans: aA compendium of surveys on the spiritual beliefs and practices of teenagers and young adults. Princeton, NJ: GH Gallup International Institute, 1992.

[2] Bibby RW. The boomer factor: What Canada's most famous generation is leaving behind. Toronto, ON: Bastian Books, 2006.

[3] Astin AW, Astin HS, Lindholm JA, Bryant A, Szelenyi K, Calderone S. The spiritual life of college students: A a national study of college students' search for meaning and purpose. Los Angeles, CA: Higher Education Research Institute, UCLA, 2005.

[4] Benson PL, Roehlkepartain EC. Spiritual development: a missing priority in youth development. New Dir Youth Dev 2008;118:13–28.

[5] King PE, Boyatzis CJ. (2004) Exploring adolescent spiritual and religious development: current and future theoretical and empirical perspectives. Appl Dev Sci 2004;8(1):2–6.

[6] Benson PL, Roehlkepartain EC, Rude SP. Spiritual development in childhood and adolescence: toward a field of inquiry. Appl Dev Sci 2003;7:205–13.

[7] Wong PTP, Fry PS, eds. The human quest for meaning: A a handbook of psychological research and clinical applications. Erlbaum, Mahwah, NJ: Lawrence Erlbaum, 1998.

[8] Scott AB. Categorizing definitions of religion and spirituality in the psychological literature: a content analytic approach. Unpublished manuscript. Cited in Hill PC, Pargamnet KI, Hood RWJr, McCullough ME, Swyers, JP, et al. Conceptualizing religion and spirituality: points of commonality, points of departure. J Theor Soc Behav 2000;30:51–77.

[9] Markow F, Klenke K. The effects of personal meaning and calling on organizational commitment: An an empirical investigation of spiritual leadership. Int J Organ Anal 2005;13(1):8–27.

[10] Pargament KI. The psychology of religion and spirituality? Yes and no. Int J Psychol Relig 1999; 9:3–16.

[11] Worthington EL, Hook JN, Davis DE, McDaniel MA. Religion and spirituality. J Clin Psychol 2011;67:204–14.

[12] Myers JE, Sweeney TJ, Witmer JM. The wheel of wellness counseling for wellness: a holistic model for treatment planning. J Couns Dev 2000;78:251–66.

[13] Lewis MM. Spirituality, counseling, and elderly: an introduction to the spiritual life review. J Adult Dev 2001;8:231–40.

[14] Shek DTL. The spirituality of Chinese people. In: Bond MJ, ed. Oxford handbook of Chinese psychology. Oxford: Oxford University Press, 2010:343–66.

[15] Lau PSY. Spirituality as a positive youth development construct: conceptual bases and implications for curriculum development. Int J Adolesc Med Health 2006;18(3):363–70.

[16] Carson VB. Spiritual dimensions of nursing practice. Philadelphia, PA: WB Saunders, 1989.

[17] Shek DTL. Life meaning and purpose in life among Chinese adolescents: What can we learn from Chinese studies in Hong Kong? In: Wong PTP, ed. The human quest for meaning: tTheories, research, and applications. London: Routledge, 2012:335-56., in press.

[18] Ryff CD, Singer B. The contours of positive human health. Psychol Inq 1998;9:1–28.

[19] Adams TB, Bezner JR, Drabbs ME, Zambarano RJ, Steinhardt MA. Conceptualization and measurement of the spiritual and psychological dimensions of wellness in a college population. J Am Coll Health 2000;48:165–73.

[20] Erikson EH. Identity, youth, and crisis. New York: Norton, 1968.

[21] Marcia JE. Identity in adolescence. In: Adelson J, ed. Handbook of adolescent psychology. New York: John Wiley, 1980:159–87.

[22] Fowler JW. Stages of faith. New York: Harper Row, 1981.

[23] Genia V. Interreligious encounter group: a psychospiritual experience for faith development. Counsel Val 1990;35:39–51.

[24] Benson PL. All kids are our kids: wWhat communities must do to raise caring and responsible children and adolescents. San Francisco, CA: Jossey-Bass, 1997.

[25] Dowling EM, Gestsdottir S, Anderson PM, von Eye A, Almerigi J, Lerner RM. Structural relations among spirituality, religiosity, and thriving in adolescence. Appl Dev Sci 2004;8:7-16.

[26] Catalano RF, Berglund ML, Ryan JAM, Lonczak HS, Hawkins JD. Positive youth development in the United States: rResearch findings on evaluations of positive youth development programs, 2002. [Cited 2011 Oct 11]. available from Accessed 2011 Oct 11. URL: http://aspe. hhs.gov/hsp/PositiveYouthDev99/

[27] Roehlkepartain EC, King PE, Wagener L, Benson PL, eds. The handbook of spiritual development in childhood and adolescence. Thousand Oaks, CA: Sage, 2006.

[28] Lerner RM, Roeser RW, Phelps E. Positive youth development and spirituality. West Conshohocken, PA: Templeton Press, 2008.

[29] Warren AEA, Lerner RM, Phelps E, eds. Thriving and spirituality among youth: Research research perspectives and future possibilities. New YorkHoboken, NJ: John Wiley & Sons. IncWiley, New York, 201211.

[30] Martin TF, White JM, Perlman D. Religious socialization: a test of the channeling hypothesis of parental influence on adolescent faith maturity. J Adolescent Res 2003;18:169–87.

[31] Regnerus MD, Smith C, Smith B. Social context in the development of adolescent religiosity. Appl Dev Sci 2004;8:27–38.

[32] Fry PS. The development of personal meaning and wisdom in adolescence: a reexamination of moderating and consolidating factors and influences. In: Wong PTP, Fry PS, eds. The human quest for meaning: A a handbook of psychological research and clinical applications. Erlbaum, Mahwah, NJ: Lawrence Erlbaum, 1998:91-110.

[33] Desrosiers A, Kelley BS, Miller L. Parent and peer relationships and relational spirituality in adolescents and young adults. Psychol Relig Spirituality 2011;3(1):39–54.

[34] Frankl VE. Psychotherapy and existentialism: Selected papers on logotherapy. New York: Simons Schuster, 1967.

[35] Crumbaugh JC. Cross validation of purpose in life test based on Frankl's concepts. J Indiv Psychol 1968;24:74–81.

[36] Wong PTP, ed. The human quest for meaning: Theories, research, and applications. London: Routledge, 2012.

[37] Emmons RA. Striving for the sacred: personal goals, life meaning, and religion. J Soc Issues 2005;61(4):731-45.

[38] Sawatzky R, Gadermann A, Pesut B. An investigation of the relationships between spirituality, health status and quality of life in adolescents. Appl Res Qual Life 2009;4:5–22.

[39] Rew L, Wong YL. A systematic review of associations among religiosity/spirituality and adolescent health attitudes and behaviors. J Adolesc Health 2006;38:433–42.

[40] Wong J, Rew L, Slaikeu KD. A systematic review of recent research on adolescent religiosity/spirituality and mental health. Issues Ment Health Nurs 2006;27:161–83.

[41] Cotton S, Zebracki K, Rosenthal SL, Tsevat J, Drotar D. Religiosity/spirituality and adolescent health outcomes: A a review. J Adolesc Health 2006;38:472–80.

[42] Sinclair S, Peperira J, Raffin S. A thematic review of the spirituality literature within palliative care. J Palliat Med 2006;9(2):464–79.

[43] Powell LH, Shahabi L, Thoresen CE. Religion and spirituality: lLinkages to physical health. Am Psychol 2003;58(1):36–52.

[44] Lent RW. (2004) Towards a unifying theoretical and practical perspective on well-being and psychosocial adjustment. J Couns Psychol 2004;51(4): 482–509.

[45] Shek DTL, Siu AMH, Lee TY. The Chinese positive youth development scale: A a validation study. Res Soc Work Pract 2007;17:380–91.

[46] Shek DTL. Chinese cultural beliefs about adversity: its relationship to psychological well-being, school adjustment and problem behavior in Hong Kong adolescents with and without economic disadvantage. Childhood 2004;11(1): 63–80.

[47] Bruce MA, Cockreham D. Enhancing the spiritual development of adolescent girls. Prof Sch Couns 2004;7:334–42.

[48] Hui EKP, Ho DKY. Forgiveness in the context of developmental guidance: implementation and evaluation. Br J Guid Couns 2004;32: 477–92.

[49] Shek DTL, Sun RCF. Effectiveness of the Tier 1 Program of Project P.A.T.H.S.: findings based on three years of program implementation. Scientific World Journal 2010;10:1509–19.

[50] Shek DTL, Ma CMS. Impact of the Project P.A.T.H.S. in the junior secondary school years: individual growth curve analyses. Scientific World Journal 2011;11: 253–66.

[51] Shek DTL, Yu L. Prevention of adolescent problem behavior: longitudinal impact of the Project P.A.T.H.S. in Hong Kong. Scientific World Journal 2011;11:546–67.

[52] Ellison CG, Lee JW. Spiritual struggles and psychological distress: is there a dark side of religion? Soc Indic Res 2010;98:501–17.

Submitted: October 01, 2011. *Revised:* November 15, 2011. *Accepted:* December 01, 2011.

In: Alternative Medicine Research Yearbook 2012
Editors: Søren Ventegodt and Joav Merrick

ISBN: 978-1-62808-080-3
© 2013 Nova Science Publishers, Inc.

Chapter 39

BELIEFS IN THE FUTURE AS A POSITIVE YOUTH DEVELOPMENT CONSTRUCT: A CONCEPTUAL REVIEW

Rachel CF Sun, PhD[*,1] *and Daniel TL Shek, PhD, FHKPS, BBS, JP*[2,3,4,5,6]

[1]Faculty of Education, The University of Hong Kong, Hong Kong, PRC
[2]Department of Applied Social Sciences, The Hong Kong Polytechnic University, Hong Kong, PRC
[3]Public Policy Research Institute, The Hong Kong Polytechnic University, Hong Kong, PRC
[4]Department of Sociology, East China Normal University, Shanghai, PRC
[5]Kiang Wu Nursing College of Macau, Macau, PRC
[6]Division of Adolescent Medicine, Department of Pediatrics, Kentucky Children's Hospital, University of Kentucky College of Medicine, Lexington, Kentucky, US

ABSTRACT

Beliefs in the future is an internalization of hope and optimism about future outcomes. This paper reviews and compares several theories of hope and optimism, and highlights the features constituting beliefs in the future. This paper points out that beliefs in the future includes a series of goal-directed thoughts and motivation, such as setting up valued and attainable goals, planning pathways, and maintaining self-confidence and mastery, so as to keep adolescents engaged in the pursuit of goals. This kind of personal mastery, together with socio-cultural values, family, school and peers are the antecedents leading to beliefs in the future, which is related to adolescents' well-being and positive development. In order to cultivate adolescents' beliefs in the future, enabling their ability to manipulate goal-directed thoughts and motivation, and providing a supportive environment including their family, school, peers and the society, are recommended.

---

[*] Correspondence Assistant Professor Rachel CF Sun, PhD, Faculty of Education, The University of Hong Kong, Pokfulam Road, Hong Kong, PRC. E-mail: rachels@hku.hk.

404   *Rachel CF Sun and Daniel TL Shek*

Keywords: Adolescence, positive youth development, beliefs in the future, hope, optimism

INTRODUCTION

Catalano, Berglund, Ryan, Lonczak, and Hawkins (1) defined "beliefs in the future" as "an internalization of hope and optimism about possible outcomes". That is, beliefs in the future entail the concepts of hope and optimism, and the ability to internalize both in anticipating future outcomes. It plays a vital role in the growth of adolescents who are encountering an increasing number of future life options, such as studies, careers and heterosexual relationships (2)) that needs them to set up personal goals. Research findings showed that adolescents aged between 12 and 19 were able to generate various personal goals relating to school, future trajectory, material, free time, relationship, self, health and body, though there were differences in the goal content and pursuit between younger and older adolescents (3).

It is because the progressive cognitive development enables adolescents to conduct reasoning, test hypotheses, set personal goals and plan more realistically (4,5), which allows them to play an active role in envisaging and manipulating their future possibilities. Moreover, the cognitive advancement allows adolescents to evaluate goal attainment, generate alternative pathways and modify goal planning, that are closely interlinked with their self-efficacy, optimism, resiliency against adversities and persistence (6)

As such, beliefs in the future, as well as hope and optimism, are regarded as important personal strengths in positive psychology (7,8) and positive youth development (1).

In regard of this, this paper reviews and compares several theories of hope and optimism, and highlights the features constituting beliefs in the future. It looks at the antecedents leading to beliefs in the future, and the relationships of hope and optimism to adolescents' well-being and positive development.

As hope and optimism share a common theme of future orientation that keeps one engaged in the pursuit of goals (9,10), this paper translates hope and optimism into a series of goal-directed thoughts and motivation so as to enable adolescents to internalize both in expecting future outcomes. It also discusses several ways to nurture adolescents' beliefs in the future.

DEFINITION OF BELIEFS IN THE FUTURE

Based on the definitions given by Catalano et al. (1) and Sun and Lau (11), hope and optimism constitute "beliefs in the future" that include (i) goal-directed thoughts, such as setting up valued and attainable goals and planning primary and alternative goal-directed pathways; and (ii) goal-directed motivation, such as self-confidence and mastery that are derived from positive appraisal of one's capability and effort.

These thoughts and motivation influence each other reciprocally in the process of goal-pursuit, and would rejuvenate when the goals are successfully attained.

HOPE

There are two lines of research in understanding the definition of hope. One is the emotion-based model which states that hope is "an emotion that occurs when an individual focuses on an important future outcome that allows little personal control, so the person is unable to take much action to realize the outcome" (12, p.348).

In this perspective, hope is conceptualized as an emotion, usually a positive affect that keeps adolescents engaged with the future outcomes, though one may not control the outcome. As such, the future outcome needs to be valuable, so that one can carry positive expectancy despite the likelihood of occurrence is low (13).

Unlike the emotion-based model of hope, the cognitive-motivation-based model argues that adolescents can control future outcomes as hope is "the perceived capability to derive pathways to desired goals, and motivate oneself via agency thinking to use those pathways" (14, p.249).

Hope is perceived as a trait comprising the will and the ways to attain the goals (15). Such a goal-directed hope is acknowledged because one can exercise a certain level of mastery while anticipating future possibilities – "yet hope is not necessarily a bad thing because mental time travel to the future can sometimes affect the present... It can set goals, develop plans, impel action, and thus transform the hypothetical future into reality" (16, p.140).

According to Snyder (14), goals, pathways (planning to meet goals) and agency (goal-directed energy) are the three important cognitive and motivational components in the trilogy concept of hope. These three components are interactional, and adolescents can exercise their personal control in setting goals and manipulating their pathway and agency thinking in the goal-pursuit process.

The role of emotion is not completely denied. In fact, successful goal attainment, as well as positive affect that resulted from successful goal attainment, feedback and energize a series of goal-directed thoughts, motivation and behaviors, and further contribute to forward flow of hope (6).

Goals

There are different types of goals serving different levels of purposes (14). Some goals are positive and approachable, such as those (a) going to be reached for the first time, (b) sustaining of a present goal, and (c) furthering upon which already has been initiated. On the other hand, some goals are negative including those (a) stopping something before it happens, and (b) delaying the unwanted. These goals are purposes to be achieved, which generate a series of actions to attain the goals; if not, they are simply desires. Adolescents need to identify the purpose and value of what they are doing, and to set up realistic goals of which they can achieve and succeed (17). The fact is having valued and attainable goals can keep adolescents engaged and confident in accomplishing these goals (18). Otherwise, adolescents are less motivated in goal pursuit particularly when there is either too low or too high probability of success. In short, it is essential to set up goals that are valued enough to arouse motivation to attain (i.e., agency thinking), as well as realistic enough to elicit concrete planning (i.e., pathway thinking).

Pathway thinking

Pathway thinking is "goal-directed thoughts" referring to adolescents' cognitive ability to plan feasible ways to meet their desired goals, as well as to generate alternative pathways when they encounter obstacles in goal attainment (6,19). It is evolving throughout one's trials and errors, as Snyder noted, "pathway thinking should become increasingly refined and precise as the goal pursuit sequence progresses toward the goal attainment" (14, p.251). Trait was found to make a difference in which high hope people are more quickly to set up and refine their primary routes to reach their goals in an effective manner than low hope people (5). Nevertheless, pathway thinking can be made explicit and translated into a series of goal-setting and goal-planning skills that enable low hope people to make improvement and high hope people to make advancement.

With reference to the advancement in abstract thinking and reasoning (4,5), adolescents are capable of setting up concrete and realistic goals for planning feasible ways of goal attainment. For instance, adolescents can set up achievable short-term goals in which a series of connected short-term goals would become a long-term goal, or set up a long-term goal which can be broken down into several consecutive short-term goals to make goal attainment more realistic. Moreover, they can focus on a single goal, or set up multiple goals that allow flexibility and reservation when the pursuit of a goal failed. Most importantly, they have to be informative of the situation, be evaluative of their ability within the time and resource constraints/available, and be able to prioritize multiple goals in accordance with their values. For such global thinking and reasoning help setting up measurable and manageable goals, that not only enable adolescents to plan feasible pathways and alternatives to attain within one's capability, but also allow them to evaluate successes or failures which become reference points for future modification and progress of their pathway thinking in the process of goal attainment.

Agency thinking

Agency thinking is "goal-directed motivation" referring to adolescents' appraisal of their capability to move along the pathways to achieve their goals, which is associated with one's confidence, mental will power and perseverance in the course of goal attainment (6,19). Agency thinking is similar to self-efficacy that refers to "people's beliefs about their capabilities to produce designated levels of performance that exercise influence over events that affect their lives" (20, p.71). According to Bandura (20), adolescents who had higher appraisal of their capabilities tend to set higher goals and are more committed to plan courses of action to realize those goals. Hence, the central inquiry is how adolescents appraise their capabilities, for such an appraisal would affect their goal-pursuit motivation and behavior. Generally speaking, one way of appraising one's capability to reach a goal is to derive from past experiences – attribution of the causes of successes and failures (21). If adolescents attribute their past successes to their "ability" (an internal and stable factor), it definitely enhances their self-efficacy and confidence in achieving future goals. However, if they attribute their past failures to their ability which is also an uncontrollable factor, they will become frustrated and hopeless when they think it is hard to change the "cause" (i.e., ability) and so as the negative "outcome" (i.e., failure). On the other hand, if adolescents attribute their past successes and failures to causes within internal locus of control such as "effort" (21,22), the sense of mastery would energize them to be more persistent to achieve success or to avoid failure. Moreover, the beliefs that one can succeed (because of one's ability and/or effort) can be self-fulfilling, and further motivate adolescents to exercise control in the goal pursuit process. Therefore, it is important to have an optimal appraisal of one's ability and effort in achieving goals, for such agency thinking is motivational that keeps adolescents cognitively and behaviorally engaged in creating pathways, as well as generating alternatives in times of encountering obstacles.

In sum, according to the cognitive-motivation-based model (14), hope is future-oriented thoughts and motivation, embracing (i) setting up valued and attainable goals, (ii) planning primary and alternative goal-directed pathways, and (iii) having positive appraisal of one's capabilities and effort, that benefit goal-pursuit.

OPTIMISM

Optimism refers to positive expectancy about the future (23). It is a kind of personality that has an obvious benefit in psychological and physical well-being (24). However, unrealistic optimism can be detrimental if people only expect good things to happen and rarely prepare themselves to cope with the situations, or do not make an accurate evaluation of their life and over-anticipate to having a brighter future (25). It reveals that optimism embraces some cognitive components, such as a goal or an expectation that regulate behavior. Optimism can then be learnt (26) while it is dispositional, for enabling goal attainment, positive growth and well-being, and vice-versa.

Based on the conceptual framework of expectancy-valued models of motivation, Carver and Scheier (18) pointed out that optimism embraces (i) valued and attainable goal which keeps adolescents engaged in the process of goal attainment; and (ii) a sense of confidence which encourages adolescents to carry out effortful behaviors, even in the face of adversity. Research findings showed that optimistic expectations for future goal pursuit influenced immediate acts (27), and helped overcoming anticipated obstacles in goal pursuit (28). Hence, this positive expectancy about the future is similar to goal-directed motivation (agency thinking) (14) and self-efficacy (20) discussed in the previous section. However, the difference is positive expectancy alone elicits goal-directed behaviors in the conception of optimism, whereas both pathway thinking and agency thinking are equally important in bringing forth goal-directed behaviors in the conception of hope.

Another difference is optimists engage their effort to reach goals as long as there is positive expectancy for eventual success, whereas self-efficacious people drive towards their goals as long as they believe they can.

Alternatively, Seligman, Reivich, Jaycox, and Gillham (29) adopted an attribution explanatory model to elucidate optimism. Optimistic adolescents explain good events as having permanent and pervasive causes, hence they are confident and will try harder to achieve positive outcomes in the future. In addition, optimistic adolescents make realistic judgment on one's responsibility when things go wrong. Even when they blame themselves for the faults, they will attribute them to temporary, specific and internal causes, such as effort that they can adjust. Again, like the agency thinking of hope, this positive and realistic explanatory style generates self-confidence and a sense of mastery to achieve, to make changes and to overcome challenges in the process of goal attainment.

On the other hand, pessimism, which is at the other end of the pole, is not totally detrimental to goal attainment. Hazlett, Molden, and Sackett (30) found that people who simply look for maintenance, safety and security performed better when they preferred pessimistic forecasts, whereas people who are motivated for attainment, growth and advancement performed better in goal pursuit when they preferred optimistic forecasts of their future.

That means, different types of goals can be achieved, provided that one's motivation orientation (preventive or promotional) and self-regulatory preferences (pessimistic or optimistic) are matched. In positive youth development, thus, it is crucial to encourage adolescents to pursuit growth and advancement and to adopt a positive self-regulation. As such, optimism refers to positive expectancy about the future (23), including setting valued and attainable goals, and developing a sense of confidence that can be generated from positive and realistic attribution of one's experiences.

RELATIONSHIP BETWEEN HOPE AND OPTIMISM

In contemporary research studies, the psychometrically validated Hope Scale (31) and Life Orientation Test (32) are commonly used to measure hope and optimism, respectively among children and adolescents. These two scales were found to have convergent validity, and were highly recommended for research use after comparing with other instruments (33). In addition, there were several empirical findings showing that both hope and optimism are related yet distinct constructs (9,34), predicting life satisfaction (35) and well-being (36). All these lend support to the conceptual understanding that both hope and optimism are closely inter-related concepts of future orientation and positive expectancy (10), and thus hope and optimism are regarded as the components of beliefs in the future that contributes to adolescent development and well-being.

BELIEFS IN THE FUTURE AND ADOLESCENT DEVELOPMENTAL OUTCOMES

Relating beliefs in the future as goal-directed thoughts and motivation, a review showed that adolescents' goal content and pursuit is are connected to their behavior, health and well-being (37). For the goal content, research findings showed that goals related to learning and mastery (38) and intrinsic values of self-acceptance and affiliation (39) had stronger contribution to student well-being.

In the goal-pursuit process, students having lower goal-related self-efficacy, greater goal-attainment difficulty and frustration were found to have poorer well-being (3). In contrast, resilience to challenges, such as using emotional regulation, goal regulation and social support, was contributory to student well-being when encountering adversity in the goal-pursuit process (40).

Moreover, hope is considered as one of the character strengths contributory to life satisfaction among youth (41), predicting self-esteem (42) and positive affect (7), lowering internalizing behavior and moderating the negative effects of life stress on adolescent psychological well-being (7). Furthermore, hope was found to be a strong predictor of academic achievement over years among high school students in Australia (43) and college students in the United States (44). In particular, pathway thinking was found to be a unique predictor of academic achievement, when controlling the effects of intelligence, personality and previous academic achievement among a group of university undergraduate students in the United Kingdom (45). On the other hand, agency thinking was found to be a strong and consistent predictor of life satisfaction across college students and adults in the United States (46).

Similarly, optimism is regarded as a personal strength (8), predicting life satisfaction among Taiwan adolescents (47), and mediating the relationship between meaning in life and psychosocial problems among Hong Kong adolescents (48). Both optimism and hope were found to significantly predict life satisfaction and negatively predict depression among Singaporean adolescents (35), whereas optimism and life satisfaction were found to negatively predict depression among Hungarian adolescents (49). Furthermore, a combination of both optimism and hope, as a goal attitude, was found to be a significant predictor of academic grade among university students in the United States (50).

Research studies comparing students with different levels of hope showed that students having high hope felt more inspired, energized, confident, and challenged by their goals (31), had higher levels of self-worth and lower levels of depression (51,52), and had higher academic achievement (53) when compared with students having low hope. In particular, middle and high school students having high hope were found to have less school maladjustment and emotional distress, higher personal adjustment, life satisfaction and academic achievement, and participate more school extracurricular activities (54), and be less likely to drop out even though they were at risk for dropping out (55). Also, college students with high hope were found to have greater problem-solving abilities and coping than low hope students (56).

In the same vein, when compared with pessimistic students, studies found that optimistic students had lower stress levels and fewer depressive and physical symptoms (57), and were more able to use a variety of problem-solving and emotion-focused strategies to cope with stress (58). It was also found that optimists had more positive evaluation of their past and present and made more realistic anticipation of the future than pessimists (25). Like hope, optimism has positive associations with adolescents' psychological and physical health and adaptive coping (24).

ANTECEDENTS OF BELIEFS IN THE FUTURE IN ADOLESCENTS

A survey of the literature showed that there are various socio-demographic antecedents (e.g., age, gender, ethnicity, socio-economic status, family, peers, school, and social and political environment) and individual's psychological and behavioral problems affecting adolescents' goal content and pursuit (37).

According to the human ecological model (59,60), adolescents' beliefs in the future are products of the environmental influences and their own manipulation of such influences.

As the role of "personal mastery" (14,23,30) was discussed in the earlier parts of the paper, the following environmental factors (i.e., socio-cultural values, ideologies, family, school and peers influences) affecting adolescents' beliefs in the future are discussed.

Socio-cultural values and ideologies

Some researchers highlighted that there are differences in the conceptualization of optimism between the Western and Chinese cultures (e.g.,61). Therefore, when adopting the Western conceptions of hope and optimism to understand Chinese adolescents' beliefs in the future, the influences of Chinese cultural values and social contexts cannot be overlooked. In Chinese culture, high value is placed on academic success as it is associated with prospective studies, rewarding careers and wealth (62).

These messages are transmitted both explicitly and implicitly through mass media, comparison and competition, social communication and expectation. When adolescents internalize these values, they tend to perceive getting academic success and prosperous careers as their learning goals, and thus are intrinsically motivated to study well so as to achieve.

They put in effort to attain their goals, because such a personal control is highly acknowledged in the Chinese proverbs, like "jin ren shi an tian ming" (try our best but leave the fate to heaven) and "cheng shi zai tian, mou shi zai ren" (men can plan but the outcomes are determined by heaven), albeit the ultimate success is determined by fate.

Several beliefs, e.g., "failure is the mother of success" and "there is light at the end of the tunnel" also keep adolescents being optimistic and autonomous in the process of goal attainment, even when encountering difficulties or failures. Therefore, with unique values and ideologies, several studies found that adolescents living in different socio-cultural contexts had different goal orientations (63,64).

Moreover, socio-cultural expectation of gender roles, which is traditionally rooted as well as being reinforced by mass media, also affects adolescents' goal orientation, aspirations and perceived pathways. Research studies showed that there were significant gender differences in adolescents' goals related to future careers, education, family, marriage, leisure activities and properties (65,66,67), and girls tended to report having more obstructed goals, greater goal frustration and lower goal-related self-efficacy than boys (3).

These might be related to the gender stereotypes in careers, such as "men are breadwinners; women are housewives". However, Greene and DeBacker (68) indicated that there has been a change in women's roles, and so does their future orientations that are not restricted to family aspect only, but include both family and career expectations simultaneously.

Family influences

In family, parental support, involvement, nurturance, attainment beliefs and aspirations for the children were revealed to have significant influences on adolescents' goal setting and attainment (37). Fitzsimons and Finkel (69) also added that interpersonal processes played a crucial role in affecting adolescents' goal-setting and pursuit. Taking parenting as an illustration, if parents are demanding but responsive to the growing needs of their children, it will facilitate their children to set achievable goals and find plausible ways to attain. It was evidenced by research findings that perceived parental authoritativeness (demanding but responsive) was related to higher levels of hope over years, whereas perceived parental authoritarianism and permissiveness did not show significant correlations with hope (70). Another longitudinal research study also found that optimism mediated the predictive effects of authoritative parenting on students' self-esteem, depression and school adjustment (71). In short, parental acceptance and support are essential in fostering adolescents' beliefs in their future.

On the other hand, negligence, conflicts, and uncontrollable traumatic events in family (such as being abused) will dampen adolescents' hope and optimism. For instance, research studies showed that Chinese adolescents who had more parent-child conflicts were likely to have feelings of hopelessness (72), whereas Arab adolescents who were physically and psychologically maltreated in family or witnessed violence and aggression between parents reported having hopelessness, low self-esteem, and psychological adjustment problems (73,74).

School influences

Between schools, differences in the environment and educational tracks were found to have different influences on adolescents' goal setting and attainment (37). Within a school, differences in educational and developmental preparation in different grade levels were related to the age differences in goal-setting, in which younger students tended to focus more on school goals whereas older students tended to focus more on future trajectory goals and have higher levels of goal-related self-efficacy (3). In addition, social comparison, which is inevitable under the competitive learning environment and assessment system, can affect students' perceptions of their future. In particular, academic failure would lead to learned hopelessness, particularly among academically low achievers who had already studied hard (75).

Nevertheless, school-based intervention programs, for instance, the Penn Optimism Program (76) and the Penn Resiliency Program (77) were found to be effective in increasing students' levels of hope, optimism and resiliency and reducing their levels of depression and anxiety (78). Other hope-based interventions designed to enhance the goal-directed thinking in children (79), and at the same time in collaboration with parents and teachers (80), were also found to be effective in enhancing children's hope, life satisfaction and self-worth.

Peer influences

Peer support was shown to contribute to adolescents' goal pursuit (82) and hope (83). However, students who did not have adequate peer and family support and positive perceptions about school and oneself were more likely to have hopeless feelings (84). Furthermore, being victimized by peers in school would also lead to social hopelessness and thus suicidal ideation, though family support could act as a buffer (85). It indicated that having adequate social support, ranging from one to multiple networks including family, peers and school, is pertinent for maintaining adolescents' psychological well-being and positive development (1).

CULTIVATING ADOLESCENTS' BELIEFS IN THE FUTURE

There are several ways to foster students' beliefs in the future. First, schools can arrange curricula-based programs (76,77,86,87), since these programs were evidenced to enhance students' hope, optimism and well-being. These programs can focus on strengthening adolescents' competence and resilience, such as setting up valued and attainable goals, planning primary and alternative pathways, and appraising one's capability and effort positively. Moreover, these programs can incorporate some positive cultural values and ideologies to cultivate adolescents' optimistic and hopeful orientation towards the future. At the same time, schools need to develop a goal-directed learning environment and arrange more opportunities both inside and outside the classrooms for students to master the learnt skills and maintain their aspirations. Besides, developmental group work can be carried out to promote students' beliefs in the future, when more intensive intervention is needed. Of course, materials in the curricula-based programs can be used in the group work context. In addition, specialized intervention programs such as adventure-based counseling can be attempted. All these programs require the joint hands between teachers and social workers, and the utilization of peers as a supportive resource.

Second, career education and guidance (88) can be provided primarily by teachers and social workers, with the support of the potential mentors in the community. It not only guides students to link up school learning with one's future career in the society, but also widens their career horizon. It is believed that early career awareness and preparation can stimulate students' future orientation. Also, it can let students to have better self-understanding and self-acceptance, which help tackling gender stereotypes and myths about career choices and pathways.

Third, school teachers and social workers can collaborate with students' parents so as to encourage parental involvement and support in fostering adolescents' beliefs in the future. Parenting skills workshops can be attempted to remind parents to accept and respect their children of who they are and what they could achieve, be responsive to their children's growing needs, and be demanding but avoid setting unrealistic expectations. All in all, adolescents themselves, as well as their family, peers, school and the community can jointly work together to nurture adolescents' beliefs in the future.

CONCLUSION

Promotion of beliefs in the future for positive youth development deserves greater attention since there is growing research evidence demonstrating its positive effects on adolescent well-being. Noting that hope and optimism are the two core components of beliefs in the future, it is necessary to help adolescents to internalize both hope and optimism by facilitating them to manipulate their goal-directed thoughts and motivation, and by providing a supportive environment including their family, school, peers and the community.

REFERENCES

[1] Catalano RF, Berglund ML, Ryan JAM, Lonczak HS, Hawkins JD. Positive youth development in the United States: research findings on evaluations of positive youth development programs 20021988.URL: http://aspe.hhs.gov/hsp/PositiveYouthDev99/

[2] Allen JP, Philliber S, Herrling S, Kupermine Kuperminc GP. Preventing teen pregnancy and academic failure: experimental evaluation of a developmentally based approach. Child Dev 1997;64(4):729-42.

[3] Massey EK, Gebhardt WA, Garnefski N. Self-generated goals and goal process appraisals: relationships with sociodemographic factors and well-being. J Adolescence 2009;32:501-18.

[4] Piaget J. The language and thought of the child. 3rd ed. London: Routledge Kegan-Paul, 1962.

[5] Piaget J. The development of thought: equilibration of cognitive structures. Blackwell: Oxford, 1977.

[6] Snyder CR. Handbook of hope theory, measures, and applications. San Diego, CA: Academic Press, 2000.

[7] Valle MF, Huebner ES, Suldo SM. An analysis of hope as a psychological strength. J School Psychol 2006;44(5):393-406.

[8] Seligman MEP. Positive psychology, positive prevention, and positive therapy. In: Snyder CR, Lopez SJ. Handbook of positive psychology. New York: Oxford University Press, 2002:3-9.

[9] Bryant FB, Cvengros JA. Distinguishing hope and optimism: two sides of a coin, or two separate coins? J Soc Clin Psychol 2004;23(2):273-302.

[10] Snyder CR, Sympson SC, Michael ST, Cheavens J. Optimism and hope constructs: variants on a positive expectancy theme. In: Chang EC. Optimism and pessimism: implications for theory, research, and practice. Washington, DC: American Psychological Association, 2001:101-23.

[11] Sun RCF, Lau PSY. Beliefs in the future as a positive youth development construct: conceptual bases and implications for curriculum development. Int J Adolesc Med Health 2006;18(3):409-16.

[12] Bruininks P, Malle BF. Distinguishing hope from optimism and related affective states. Motiv Emotion 2005;29(4):327-55.

[13] Averill JR, Catlin G, Chon KK. Rules of hope. New York: Springer-Verlag, 1990.

[14] Snyder CR. Hope theory: rainbows in the mind. Psychol Inq 2002;13(4):249-75.

[15] Snyder CR, Irving L, Anderson JR. Hope and health: measuring the will and the ways. In: Snyder CR, Forsyth DR. Handbook of social and clinical psychology: the health perspective. New York, Elmsford: Pergamon, 1991:285-305.

[16] Ross M, Newby-Clark IR. Constructing the past and future. Soc Cognition 1998;16(1):133-50.

[17] Wigfield A, Eccles JS. Expectancy-value theory of achievement motivation. Contemp Psychol 2000;25(1):68-81.

[18] Carver CS, Scheier MF. Optimism, pessimism, and self-regulation. In: Chang EC. Optimism and pessimism: implications for theory, research, and practice. Washington, DC: American Psychological Association, 2001:31-54.

[19] Snyder CR, Rand KL, Sigmon DR. Hope theory: a member of the positive psychology family. In: Snyder CR. Handbook of positive psychology. New York: Oxford University Press, 2002:257-76.

[20] Bandura A. Self-efficacy. In: Ramachaudran VS. Encyclopedia of human behavior Vol. 4. New York: Academic Press, 1994:71-81.

[21] Weiner B. Human motivation. New York: Holt Rinehart Winston, 1980.

[22] Rotter J. Social learning and clinical psychology. Englewood Cliffs, NJ: Prentice-Hall, 1954.

[23] Scheier MF, Carver CS. On the power of positive thinking: the benefits of being optimistic. Curr Dir Psychol Sci 1993;2(1):26-30.

[24] Scheier MF, Carver CS. Effects of optimism on psychological and physical well-being: theoretical overview and empirical update. Cognitive Ther Res 1992;16(2):201-28.

[25] Busseri MA, Choma BL, Sadava SW. "As good as it gets" or "The best is yet to come"? How optimists and pessimists view their past, present, and anticipated future life satisfaction. Pers Indiv Diff 2009;47(4):352-56.

[26] Seligman MEP. Learned optimism: how to change your mind and your life. New York: Vintage, 2006.

[27] Zhang Y, Fishbach A, Dhar R. When thinking beats doing: the role of optimistic expectations in goal-based choice. J Consum Res 2007;34(4):567-78.

[28] Zhang Y, Fishbach A. Counactering obstacles with optimistic predictions. J Exp Psychol Gen 2010;139(1):16-31.

[29] Seligman MEP, Reivich K, Jaycox L, Gillham J. The optimistic child. Boston, MA: Houghton Mifflin, 1995.

[30] Hazlett A, Molden DC, Sackett AM. Hoping for the best or preparing for the worst? Regulatory focus and preferences for optimism and pessimism in predicting personal outcomes. Soc Cognition 2011;29(1):74-96.

[31] Snyder CR, Harris C, Anderson JR, Holleran SA, Irving LM, Sigmon ST, et al. The will and the ways: development and validation of an individual-differences measure of hope. J Pers Soc Psychol 1991;60(4):570-85.

[32] Scheier MF, Carver CS. Optimism, coping, and health: assessment and implications of generalized outcome expectancies. Health Psychol 1985;4(3):219-47.

[33] Steed LG. A psychometric comparison of four measures of hope and optimism. Educ Psychol Meas 2002;62(3):466-82.

[34] Magaletta PR, Oliver JM. The hope construct, will, and ways: their relations with self-efficacy, optimism, and general well-being. J Clin Psychol 1999;55(5):539-51.

[35] Wong SS, Lim T. Hope versus optimism in Singaporean adolescents: contributions to depression and life satisfaction. Pers Indiv Differ 2009;46(5-6):648-52.

[36] Avey JB, Wernsing TS, Mhatre KH. A longitudinal analysis of positive psychological constructs and emotions on stress, anxiety, and well-being. J Leadership Organ Stud 2011;18(2):216-28.

[37] Massey EK, Gebhardt WA, Garnefski N. Adolescent goal content and pursuit: a review of the literature from the past 16 years. Dev Rev 2008;28(4):421-60.

[38] Kaplan A, Maehr ML. Achievement goals and student well-being. Contemp Educ Psychol 1999;24(4):330-58.

[39] Schmuckh P, Kasser T, Ryan RM. Intrinsic and extrinsic goals: their structure and relationship with well-being in German and U.S. college students. Soc Indicators Res 2000; 5059(2):225-41.

[40] Neely ME, Schallert DL, Mohammed SS, Roberts RM, Chen YJ. Self-kindness when facing stress: the role of self-compassion, goal regulation, and support in college students' well-being. Motiv Emotion 2009(1);33:88-97.

[41] Park MN, Peterson C, Seligman MEP. Strengths of character and well-being: a closer look at hope and modesty. J Soc Clin Psychol 2004;23(5):628-3403-19.

[42] Halama P, Dedova M. Meaning in life and hope as predictors of positive mental health: do they explain residual variance not predicted by personality traits? Stud Psychol 2007;49(3):191-200.

Beliefs in the future as a positive youth development construct 415

[43] Ciarrochi J, Heaven PCL, Davies F. The impact of hope, self-esteem, and attributional style on adolescents' school grade and emotional well-being: a longitudinal study. J Res Pers 2007;41(6): 1161-78.

[44] Snyder CR, Shorey HS, Cheavens J, Pulvers KM, Adams III VH, Wiklund C. Hope and academic success in college. J Educ Psychol 2002;94(4):820-6.

[45] Day L, Hanson K, Maltby J, Proctor C, Wood A. Hope uniquely predicts objective academic achievement above intelligence, personality, and previous academic achievement. J Res Pers 2010;44(4):550-3.

[46] Bailey TC, Eng W, Frisch MB, Snyder CR. Hope and optimism as related to life satisfaction. J Posit Psychol 2007;2(3):168-75.

[47] Wu CH, Tsai YM, Chen LH. How do positive views maintain life satisfaction? Soc Indic Res 2009;91(2):269-81.

[48] Ho MYYM, Cheung FM, Cheung SF. The role of meaning in life and optimism in promoting well-being. Pers Indiv Differ 2010;48(5):658-63.

[49] Piko BF, Kovacs E, Fitzpatrick KM. What makes a difference? Understanding understanding the role of protective factors in Hungarian adolescents' depressive symptomatology. Eur Child Adoles Psy 2009;18(10):617-24.

[50] Rand KL. Hope and optimism: latent structures and influences on grade expectancy and academic performance. J Pers 2009;77(1):231-60.

[51] Snyder CR, Hoza B, Pelham WE, Rapoff M, Ware L, Danovsky M, et al. The development and validation of the children's hope scale. J Pediatr Psychol 1997;22(3):399-421.

[52] Snyder CR, Sympson SC, Ybasco FC, Borders TF, Babyak MA, Higgins RL. Development and validation of the State Hope Scale. J Pers Soc Psychol 1996;70(2):321-35.

[53] Snyder CR, Cheavens J, Michael ST. Hoping. In: Snyder CR. Coping: the psychology of what works. New York: Oxford University Press, 1999:205-31.

[54] Gilman R, Dooley J, Florell D. Relative levels of hope and their relationship with academic and psychological indicators among adolescents. J Soc Clin Psychol 2006;25(2):166-78.

[55] Worrell FC, Hale RL. The relationship of hope in the future and perceived school climate to school completion. School Psychol Quart 2001;16(4):370-88.

[56] Chang EC. Hope, problem-solving ability, and coping in a college student population: some implications for theory and practice. J Clin Psychol 1998;54(7):953-62.

[57] O'Brien WJ, VanEgeren L, Mumby PB. Predicting health behaviors using measures of optimism and perceived risk. Health Val 1995;19(1):21-8.

[58] Scheier MF, Weintraub JK, Crarver CS. Coping with stress: divergent strategies of optimists and pessimists. J Pers Soc Psychol 1986;51(6):1257-64.

[59] Bronfenbrenner U. The ecology of human development: experiments by nature and design. Cambridge, MA: Harvard University Press, 1979.

[60] Bronfenbrenner U. Interacting systems in human development. Research paradigms. Present and future. In: Bolger N, Caspi A, Downey G, Moorehouse M. Persons in context: developmental processes. New York: Cambridge University Press, 1988:25-47.

[61] Lai JCL, Yue X. Measuring optimism in Hong Kong and mainland Chinese with the revised life orientation test. Pers Indiv Differ 2000;28(4):781-96.

[62] Yang KS. Chinese personality and its change. In: Bond MH. The psychology of the Chinese people. Hong Kong: Oxford University Press, 1986:106-70.

[63] Nurmi JE, Poole ME, Kalakoski V. Age differences in adolescent future-oriented goals, concerns, and related temporal extension in different sociocultural contexts. J Youth Adolescence 1994;23(4): 471-87.

[64] Seginer R, Halabi-Kheir H. Adolescent passage to adulthood: future orientation in the context of culture, age, and gender. Int J Intercultural Rel 1998;22(3):309-2838.

[65] Francis B. Is the future really female? The impact and implications of gender for 14-16 year olds' career choices J Educ Work 2002;15(1):75-88.

[66] Honora DT. The relationship of gender and achievement to future outlook among African American adolescents. Adolescence 2002;37(146):301-16.

[67] Nurmi JE, Poole ME, Seginer R. Tracks and transitions – a comparison of adolescent future-oriented goals, explorations, and commitments in Australia, Israel and Finland. Int J Psychol 1995;30(3): 355-75.

[68] Greene BA, DeBacker TK. Gender and orientations toward the future: links to motivation. Educ Psychol Rev 2004;16(2):91-120.

[69] Fitzsimons GM, Finkel EJ. Interpersonal influences on self-regulation. Curr Dir Psychol Sci 2010;19(2):101-5.

[70] Heaven P, Ciarrochi J. Parental styles, gender and the development of hope and self-esteem. Eur J Personality 2008;22(8):707-24.

[71] Jackson LM, Pratt MW, Hunsberger B, Pancer SM. Optimism as a mediator of the relation between perceived parental authoritativeness and adjustment among adolescents: finding the sunny side of the street. Soc Dev 2005;14(2):273-304.

[72] Shek DTL. Family functioning and psychological well-being, school adjustment, and problem behavior in Chinese adolescents with and without economic disadvantage. J Genet Psychol 2002;163(4):497-502.

[73] Haj-Yahia MM. The incidence of witnessing interparental violence and some of its psychological consequences among Arab adolescents. Child Abuse Neglect 2001;25(7):885-907.

[74] Haj-Yahia MM, Musleh K, Haj-Yahia YM. The incidence of adolescent maltreatment in Arab society and some of its psychological effects. J Fam Issues 2002;23(8):1032-64.

[75] Au RCP. Academic failure and learned hopelessness in Hong Kong academically low achievers. Bull Hong Kong Psychol Soc 1995;34-35:83-100.

[76] Shatte AJ, Gillham JE, Reivich K. Promoting hope in children and adolescents. In: Gillham JE. The science of optimism and hope. PhiladephiaPhiladelphia: Templeton Foundation Press, 20022000: 215-34.

[77] Gilliam Gillham J, Reivich K. Cultivating optimism in childhood and adolescence. Ann Am Acad Polit S S 2004;591:146-63.

[78] Reivich K, Gillham JE, Chaplin TM, Seligman MEP. From helplessness to optimism: the role of resilience in treating and preventing depression in children and youth. In: Goldstein S, Brooks RB. Handbook of resilience in children and youth. New York: Kluwer, 2005:223-37.

[79] Lopez SJ, Rose S, Robinson C, Marques SC, Pais-Ribeiro JL. Measuring and promoting hope in school children. In: Gilman R, Huebner ES, Furlong MJ. Handbook of positive psychology in the schools. Mahwah, NJ: Lawrence Erlbaum, 2009:37-51.

[80] Marques SC, Lopez SJ, Pais-Ribeiro JL. "Building hope for the future": a program to foster strengths in middle-school students. J Happiness Stud 200911;12(1):139-52.

[81] Miller DN, Gilman R, Martens MP. Wellness promotion in the schools: enhancing students' mental and physical health. Psychol Schools 2008;45(1):5-15.

[82] Wentzel KR. Relations of social goal pursuit to social acceptance, classroom behavior, and perceived social support. J Educ Psychol 1994;86(2):173–82.

[83] Harter S, Whitesell NR. Multiple pathways to self-reported depression and psychological adjustment among adolescents. Dev Psychopathol 1996;8(4):761-77.

[84] Yilmaz V, TürkümTurkum AS. Factors affecting hopelessness levels of Turkish preteenagers attending primary schools: a structural equation model. Soc Behav Personal 2008;36(1):19-26.

[85] Bonanno RA, Hymel S. Beyond the hurt feelings: investigating why some victims of bullying are at greater risk for suicidal ideation. Merrill-Palmer Quart 2010;56(3):420-40.

[86] Shek DTL, Ma CMS. Impact of the Project P.A.T.H.S. on adolescent developmental outcomes in Hong Kong: findings based on seven waves of data. Int J Adolesc Med Health In press.

[87] Shek DTL, Sun RCF. Effectiveness of the Tier 1 Program of Project P.A.T.H.S.: findings based on three years of program implementation. ScientificWorldJournal 2010;10:1509-19.

[88] Gysbers NC. Career guidance and counseling in primary and secondary educational settings. In: Athanasou JA, Van Esbroeck R. International handbook of career guidance. Netherland, Dordrecht: Springer, 2008:249-63.

Submitted: October 01, 2011. *Revised:* November 15, 2011. *Accepted:* December 03, 2011.

In: Alternative Medicine Research Yearbook 2012
Editors: Søren Ventegodt and Joav Merrick

ISBN: 978-1-62808-080-3
© 2013 Nova Science Publishers, Inc.

Chapter 40

COGNITIVE COMPETENCE AS A POSITIVE YOUTH DEVELOPMENT CONSTRUCT: A CONCEPTUAL REVIEW

Rachel CF Sun, PhD*
and Eadaoin KP Hui, PhD, CPsychol BPS, Reg Psy HKPS
Faculty of Education, University of Hong Kong, Hong Kong, PRC

ABSTRACT

This paper focuses on discussing critical thinking and creative thinking as the core cognitive competence. It reviews and compares several theories of thinking, highlights the features of critical thinking and creative thinking, and delineates their inter-relationships. It discusses cognitive competence as a positive youth development construct by linking its relationships with adolescent development and its contributions to adolescents' learning and well-being. Critical thinking and creative thinking are translated into self-regulated cognitive skills for adolescents to master and capitalize on, so as to facilitate knowledge construction, task completion, problem-solving and decision-making. Ways of fostering these thinking skills, cognitive competence and ultimately positive youth development are discussed.

Keywords: Adolescence, positive youth development, cognitive competence, critical thinking, creative thinking

INTRODUCTION

According to Piaget (1,2), cognitive competence constitutes the cyclical processes of assimilation and accommodation, which indicates that people can manipulate their personal experiences as well as organize and adapt their thoughts to guide their behavior. Similarly,

---

* Correspondence: Assistant Professor Rachel CF Sun, PhD, Faculty of Education, The University of Hong Kong, Pokfulam Road, Hong Kong, PRC. E-mail: rachels@hku.hk.

Fry (3) pointed out that cognitive competence comprises three interwoven and interdependent components: cognitive structures, cognitive processes and overt behaviors. Among them, "cognitive processes", such as metacognition, cognitive styles of self-regulation, and cognitive skills of thinking, reasoning, analyzing problems and information processing, can affect one's "behaviors" like task performance, problem-solving and decision-making, as well as "cognitive structures", such as self-schemas and goal orientation. It further points out that people can make a difference in their cognitive development and capability by manipulating their mental processes and cognitive styles via using appropriate thinking skills. It is also argued that cognitive competence is more than an ability to manipulate and strategize information, but an ability to internalize, self-regulate and transfer these cognitive skills to construct knowledge and make sense of the surroundings (4,5).

In the literature, there are various types of thinking, for instance, logical thinking and reasoning (1,2), legislative, executive, and judicial thinking styles (6), synthetic, analytic and practical intellectual skills (7), divergent thinking and evaluative thinking (8-10), and lateral thinking and vertical thinking (11). There are also important features of adolescent thinking, for instance, being able to think abstractly, test hypotheses, conduct reasoning, and make causal inferences (1,2). All these are used to facilitate knowledge construction, task completion, problem-solving and decision-making, but their application commonly requires critical thinking and creative thinking. Indeed, numerous studies have demonstrated that adolescents who were equipped with critical thinking and creative thinking had better academic performance (12,13), health (14,15), cognitive development (16), psychosocial development (17) and identity development (18), and were less likely to engage in unhealthy or problem behavior (19,20). Therefore, both critical thinking and creative thinking are regarded as generic transferable life skills for adolescents (11,21-23), who have to deal with various developmental stresses and challenges, such as puberty changes, adjustments in social roles and expectations, school transition, examination, pursuit of further studies, preparing for or entering the labor market, expansion of social circles, and development of romantic relationship. Nonetheless, there are also situations that adolescents still engage in problem behaviors even though they understand the pros and cons, or make numerous imaginative solutions of which none of them are realistic to solve the problems. Therefore, it is of paramount importance to guide adolescents to master the thinking skills well in order to foster learning (24,25), leadership (26-28), and positive youth development (29,30).

In regard of this, the present paper focuses on discussing critical thinking and creative thinking as the core cognitive competence. It reviews and compares several theories of thinking, highlights the features of critical thinking and creative thinking, and delineates their inter-relationships. It discusses cognitive competence as a positive youth development construct by linking its relationships with adolescent development and its contributions to adolescents' learning, well-being and positive development. It shows how critical thinking and creative thinking can be translated into self-regulated cognitive skills for adolescents to master and capitalize on to achieve better task performance, generate precise solutions to problems and make right decisions. It is believed that these thinking skills not only facilitate life-long learning and holistic development among youngsters, but also prepare youngsters to be the future masters of the society who are able to solve social problems and contribute to global development.

DEFINITION OF COGNITIVE COMPETENCE

There are broad definitions of cognitive competence (1-5), as well as narrow definitions (29). Building on the definition given by Sun and Hui (29), the present paper refers critical thinking and creative thinking as the core cognitive competence, though it is noted that cognitive competence includes, but is not limited to these two thinking. Critical thinking refers to reasoning and making inferences, and creative thinking means stretching one's spectacles, evaluating multiple ideas and alternatives, and generating novel and practical ideas. The definitions of critical thinking and creative thinking, and the specific cognitive skills involved are reviewed in the followings.

CRITICAL THINKING

According to Paul (31), "critical thinking is the intellectually disciplined process of actively and skillfully conceptualizing, applying, analyzing, synthesizing, and/or evaluating information gathered from, or generated by, observation, experience, reflection, or communication, as a guide to belief and action" (p.22). Moreover, "critical thinking refers to the use of cognitive skills or strategies that increase the probability of a desirable outcome. Critical thinking is purposeful, reasoned, and goal-directed. It is the kind of thinking involved in solving problems, formulating inferences, calculating likelihoods, and making decisions" (p.70) (32). Therefore, critical thinking is a process that activates certain cognitive skills so as to make the best judgments regarding on what to believe and what to do (33).

"Reason" and "inference" are the two main cognitive skills in critical thinking (34), that are used when making judgments or decisions, accepting beliefs, and developing ideas and alternatives. It is important to make good and objective reasons for one's beliefs, by recognizing one's subjective point of view, gathering multiple and diverse points of view, coordinating various views (including those for and against the concerned issues), for generating sufficient reasons and reliable evidence before making a judgment (34,35). Since there are no explicit guidelines for judging what sufficient and reliable reasons are, it may run the risk of developing under- or over-critical judgments. Therefore, rational thinking is needed (35). Lipman (36) further elaborated that when engaging in critical thinking, one should make reference to reliable, strong, and relevant criteria, such as norms, shared values, laws, rules, definitions, facts, and values, and pay attention to the situational factors, such as special circumstances and limitations, and variations in culture, context, time, and people. One should also be reflective and self-correcting so as to question one's own thoughts, identify the errors in one's own thinking, and then make reasonable corrections. In other words, critical thinking means one needs to be critical to the concerned issues as well as one's thinking, so that one can proceed to make inference and deduction from the information collected for doing a rational evaluation and making a reasonable decision (34). Paul (31) added that critical thinkers like to reason about their reasoning and make inferences and conceptualization with rational justification. Their habitual inspection of the thinking is, in fact, "an action of ongoing creation" contributing to their cognitive and intellectual advancement. In sum, critical thinking includes the skills of reasoning and making inferences, and it is both evaluative and productive (37) that encompasses the ideas of rationality and creativity, respectively (38,39).

CREATIVE THINKING

Creative thinking refers to thinking that is novel, and that produces ideas that are of value (40). According to Sternberg (6,7), creative thinking is autonomous and people can choose to capitalize on certain "thinking styles" and "intellectual skills" to maximize their creativity (41,42). Among the thirteen thinking styles, research findings showed that five of them, including legislative, judicial, hierarchical, global and liberal (i.e., Type I intellectual styles) are related to creative thinking (43,44). Adolescents choose to regulate their thinking processes and behaviors accordingly can thus learn to master creative thinking. Therefore, it is preferable that, adolescents, when performing a task, can evaluate the task (judicial thinking style) and choose to develop their own ideas, rules, and procedures (legislative thinking style), instead of simply following rules and instructions (executive thinking style). When doing multiple tasks, adolescents can rank things in priority and distribute attention to the tasks in accordance with the value of the tasks (hierarchical thinking style). Besides drilling the details of a task (local thinking style), adolescents can also look at the overall picture of the task (global thinking style). Moreover, adolescents can be proactive in choosing works involving novelty and ambiguity (liberal thinking style). All these are in parallel with the synthetic, analytic and practical intellectual skills for solving problems (7), in which creative people would interpret problems in a new way and avoid being bounded by conventional thinking (synthetic skills), identify the most valuable and novel idea (analytic skills), and make out ways to demonstrate the values of that idea (practical skills). In short, creative thinking refers to the cognitive skills of stretching one's spectacles, generating and evaluating multiple ideas and alternatives, and generating novel and practical ideas. Similarly, creative thinking (the components of judicial thinking style and analytic skills) entails critical thinking, because adolescents have to be skeptical enough to criticize their own ideas so as to initiate positive changes in their thinking. It is believed that after continuously practicing these thinking styles and skills, adolescents would learn to welcome changes and innovations, to think globally and progressively rather than conservatively, and become habitual in generating novel and realistic ideas that help task completion, problem-solving and decision-making.

RELATIONSHIP BETWEEN CREATIVE THINKING AND CRITICAL THINKING

Conceptually, creative thinking and critical thinking are not dichotomous and conflicting (7,31,45). Both of them operate together productively to leading to creative and effective problem-solving, just as "divergent thinking" and "evaluative thinking" do (8-10,44,46). Adolescents are activating creative thinking when they use divergent thinking to generate numerous and diverse solutions to a problem, in which they redefine problems in novel ways that other people usually do not see (originality), select relevant information to conceptualize a problem (flexibility), draw an analogy between the old problem and the new interpretation, and combine the information in a novel way (fluency) (47,48). To find out the most sensible novel solution, adolescents also activate evaluative and critical thinking to perform valuation. Likewise, creative thinking and critical thinking are comparable to de Bono's conceptions of "lateral thinking" and "vertical thinking" (11,49), in which the former requires people to see things from multiple perspectives and arrive at the solutions from new angles, whereas the later requires people to see things sequentially and conventionally and generate solutions from a deeper investigation. He highlighted that both thinking are equally important in generating novel and practical ideas for problem-solving, because solutions generated by lateral thinking solely are not realistic enough for tackling problems, whereas solutions generated by vertical thinking lack novelty for energizing progressive advancement though the problem is practically solved. Some empirical studies also revealed that both creative thinking and critical thinking (or divergent thinking and evaluative thinking, or lateral thinking and vertical thinking) are complementary with each other in effective problem-solving and decision-making (50,51).

Research findings also showed that both critical thinking and creative thinking are closely related to each other to facilitate learning and knowledge construction (52). In learning, simply recalling the facts and information are usually being accused of a straight-forward surface approach. However, it is argued that recalling is a step to build up a solid foundation of knowledge, so that one can further execute the higher-order cognitive processes of critical thinking and creative thinking to understand the meanings of the information and to apply the learnt knowledge to daily life situations (53). To further constructing one's own knowledge and meaningful learning, more sophisticated critical thinking skills are indispensable for analyzing (such as differentiating, organizing and attributing) and evaluating (e.g. checking and critiquing) multiple information, followed by using creative thinking to create (such as generating, planning and producing) knowledge with originality and novelty. Paul (31) stressed that "the creative dimension of thinking is best fostered by joining with the critical dimension" (p.21).

It demonstrates that there is a close linkage between critical thinking and creative thinking in problem-solving and learning, and therefore acquiring and mastering of these thinking skills are of paramount importance. Adolescents should be encouraged to utilize these thinking skills effectively, not simply to get problems solved and to know more, but to achieve effective problem-solving and meaningful knowledge construction.

ANTECEDENTS OF COGNITIVE COMPETENCE

There are various factors, such as heredity, environmental stimuli, socioeconomic status, culture, and maturation, contributing to adolescents' cognitive competence (54). Among them, the role of cognitive development and maturation is indispensable. According to Piaget (1,2), one's cognitive competence become sophisticated throughout four developmental stages according to one's age. Children aged between 7 and 11 years are at the concrete operational stage. Their logical reasoning is developed which allows them to mentally arrange and compare things. Critical thinking starts to blossom as their thinking becomes decentered and less egocentric, which allows them to consider others' perspectives and clarify one's thoughts (1,55). These logical and critical thinking become advanced when they reach the formal operational stage (age 12 or above) because they are able to think systematically, manipulate mental objects, test hypotheses and draw conclusions based on reasoning. It reveals that developmental age and maturation are related to the development of cognitive competence, and at the same time, adolescents' cognitive competence is changing progressively via their active manipulation of the mental processes.

Meaningful social interaction is another factor helping adolescents excel cognitively. Vygotsky (4,5) believed that through conversation, collaboration, modeling, guidance and encouragement, adolescents learn better ways of thinking, reasoning and solving problems from more competent peers and adults, when compared with performing the task alone. Creative imagination and thinking also become more sophisticated during adolescence, when youngsters actively use private speech to conceptualize their own ways of problem-solving from those learnt from social models (56). Empirical findings also showed that students were cognitively advanced when they could internalize, self-regulate and transfer these cognitive skills, so as to complete the tasks independently without the help of the others (52).

Socio-cultural contexts and settings, e.g., family, classroom, school and educational system, also account for cognitive competence among adolescents. Thus, another critical antecedent of cognitive competence is whether there is "mediated learning experience" that provides the opportunities for adolescents (i) to learn the thinking skills, and (ii) to become aware of these thinking skills and processes that help them to excel in task performance, and also become more self-regulatory and self-efficacious in transferring the skills to wider contexts. There are many research findings demonstrated that structured programs, activities, scaffolding instructions and guidance, and social interactions are effective in helping children and adolescents to equip and transfer these thinking skills. For instance, the Philosophy for Children Program in training critical thinking (21), the Purdue Creative Thinking Program in training divergent thinking (20,23); and the de Bono Cognitive Research Trust Program for Creative Thinking (CoRT Program) in training lateral thinking and vertical thinking (11) which could facilitate the fluency, flexibility and originality of thinking (50,51). Mushrooming evidences also showed the potential of incorporating creative thinking in classroom teaching for mainstream students (24,25) and outside classroom context among gifted students (26,27) for them to transfer the skills to independent learning and problem-solving.

COGNITIVE COMPETENCE AND ADOLESCENT DEVELOPMENTAL OUTCOMES

With reference to the holistic development of adolescents, there are interconnections and reciprocal influences among cognitive, moral, behavioral, emotional, social, physical, aesthetical and spiritual domains. Hence, cognitive competence is vital in contributing to adolescent development in specific domains as well as their holistic well-being. In education, critical thinking was revealed to play a crucial role in students' self-regulatory learning by influencing their mastery of learning goals and deep information processing (57). Some studies also found that critical thinking significantly predicted students' academic performance (12,13). Apart from the positive effects on intellectual development, health education research studies showed that strengthening adolescents' critical thinking skills was one of the important components that enabled students' autonomy in identifying their health needs and making healthy choices (14), developing healthy body image and preventing disordered eating patterns (19). Critical thinking was also found to help adolescents to be more pragmatic about media messages and thus less likely to internalize some distorted messages regarding beauty standard (15), and had lower intention of substance use in the future (20).

In addition, compared with those having lower levels of creative thinking, adolescents having higher levels of creative thinking were found to have higher levels of internal control and self-acceptance (58), lower levels of depression and more likely to adopt a positive attributional style (59). A series of research studies, which were mainly conducted with Chinese university students by Zhang and her colleagues also demonstrated that creativity-generating styles (i.e., Type I intellectual style) were positively related to academic achievement (60-62), self-esteem (63) and emotion management(64), and contributory to cognitive development (16), psychosocial development (17,65) and identity development (18). The long-term positive effects of creative thinking was also demonstrated, as an 18-year longitudinal research study found that creative thinking and creative performance, rather than school grade at adolescence were better predictors of life accomplishment in adulthood (66).

All these show that critical thinking and creative thinking are the developmental assets and strengths. Adolescents who are equipped with these thinking skills tend to have better learning, well-being and positive development. In regard of these beneficial effects on adolescent development, promotion of cognitive competence in education (67,68) and developmental programs aiming at preventing youth problems and promoting healthy growth (29,69) has have been advocated over recent decades.

Taking Hong Kong as an example, nurturing students' independent and critical thinking and creativity is clearly spelt out in the objectives of the senior secondary education and higher education (70), for such thinking skills are believed to be indispensable generic skills helping students to learn how to learn, and so as to become independent life-long learners.

In addition, cognitive competence is regarded as one of the core psychosocial competencies facilitating adolescent holistic development in a curricula-based positive youth development program adopted by numerous secondary schools in Hong Kong since 2005 (30).

FOSTERING COGNITIVE COMPETENCE IN ADOLESCENTS

To foster cognitive competence among adolescents, one of the ways is to introduce creative thinking and critical thinking skills and provide social opportunities for adolescents to master these skills. The central issues are to let students to understand "What are these practical skills?', "How can they be carried out?", and "Why do I use these skills?", so as to help them to internalize, self-regulate and transfer the learnt skills. It can be done explicitly or implicitly, both inside and outside schools, in the following three ways.

DIRECT TEACHING (BOLT-ON APPROACH)

Thinking skills can be taught explicitly to students in context-free situation. For instance, the Instrumental Enrichment aims at developing students' generic thinking skills that enable their ability to solve problems and transfer their problem-solving skills to a wider context (71). As aforementioned, there are many programs targeting at training students' critical and creative thinking skills, e.g., Philosophy for Children Program (21), the Purdue Creative Thinking Program (22,23) and the CoRT Program (11). In addition, thinking skills can also be directly introduced in developmental programs, like leadership training (26,27) and positive youth development program (29,30,72), in which students' cognitive competence are fostered and sharpened leading to the forward flow of positive developmental attributes, and vice versa. In such kind of direct teaching, teachers play a crucial role in a series of structural "mediated learning experiences" to guide students to master the skills in defining problems, developing plans and strategies, and transferring the classroom learning to other life aspects. As there is a spiral of learning to think and thinking to learn, arranging more opportunities for students to practice, reflect and evaluate the skills is necessary for them to assimilate, accommodate, internalize, advance and transfer the thinking strategies and processes.

EMBEDDED APPROACH

Embedded approach means that thinking skills are taught and practiced within a subject in school formal curriculum, e.g., in Social Studies (73), Liberal Studies (70) and Sciences (24,25). This approach allows students to apply critical and creative thinking skills in a meaningful subject context, and at the same time, to develop a deep understanding of the subject matters through utilizing the skills. "Inquiry teaching" (74,75) can be adopted, in which students are enabled to evaluate existing information and proceed to construct new knowledge of that subject. In the learning process, reasoning skills are emphasized and students are guided to form hypotheses, test hypotheses, make predictions, select cases, distinguish consider alternative hypotheses, examine misconceptions in their current reasoning, ask questions and challenge authorities. Moreover, probing questions and dialoging can stimulate and challenge students' thoughts, sharpen their skills and motivation to reason, to make inferences, and even to generate creative and valuable ideas.

At the same time, "problem-based learning" can be incorporated. The problems need to be novel, ambiguous or challenging, so as to generate cognitive conflicts and stimulate higher-order thinking (1). In other words, the problems need to be structured with reference to the students' prior knowledge in that subject areas and existing levels of thinking skills, with the purpose to progress students' generic skills of critical thinking and creative thinking in analyzing and solving the problems. Collins and Stevens (74) noted that, "by turning learning into problem solving, by carefully selecting cases that optimize the abilities the teacher is trying to teach, by making students grapple with counterexamples and entrapments, teachers challenge the students more than by any other teaching method. The students come out of the experience are able to attack novel problems by applying these strategies themselves" (p.229). Therefore, the students can become more skillful, esteemed and motivated to master the thinking skills inside and outside their school learning.

INFUSION APPROACH

Infusion means having the subject matters and thinking skills learnt together across curriculum. There is no specific lessons design to teach thinking skills, but teachers plan and deliver lessons with an emphasis on thinking, and to let students developing the feelings of competence and autonomy via self-regulation that encourages them to transfer the mastered skills across different subject areas and life situations. The overarching goal is to let student master these generic and transferable skills, take the responsibility in self-regulatory learning, and become a person with independent thinking. An example is the project of Activating Children's Thinking Skills (52) for primary school children in Northern Ireland, in which metacognitive skills of critical thinking, creative thinking, searching for meaning, problem-solving and decision-making are infused across curriculum, demonstrated with significant effects on students' cognitive advancement as well as social and behavioral improvement. However, the infusion approach cannot succeed without structured pedagogy, for instance, engaging students in open-ended activities, collaborative activities, classroom dialogue, and joint meaning making (76) are some strategies of social construction of learning (4,5).

To help students to transfer thinking skills to other tasks, teachers can also give examples or ask students to generate examples, so as to guide them of how these forms of reasoning, inference-making and idea-generating can be applied inside the subject areas as well as outside. Paul and his colleagues (77,78) have given detailed suggestions of how critical thinking and creative thinking can be incorporated into teaching and curriculum.

CONCLUSION

In this paper, cognitive competence is defined as critical thinking and creative thinking skills which facilitate effective problem-solving, decision-making and learning for positive youth development. However, there are several conceptual and research gaps that need to be filled. First, as the narrow definition was adopted, further review is needed to elucidate the broad conception of cognitive competence. Second, although the literature showed that both critical thinking and creative thinking are inter-related thinking skills, more empirical research on their relationships is needed. Third, there were studies showing that critical thinking and creative thinking are beneficial to adolescents' cognitive advancement, psychosocial well-being, life-long learning and accomplishment. However, most of these were separate studies. Further research is needed to demonstrate their unique effects as well as their interactive effects on adolescents' problem-solving, decision-making, learning and development. Lastly, while three ways are discussed to promote adolescents' cognitive competence, it is necessary to have more vigorous research studies to evaluate and compare the effectiveness of these approaches across age groups and cultural settings. It is hoped that tailor-made curriculum or programs can be offered to cater to the unique characteristics and needs of adolescents for their cognitive advancement and positive development.

REFERENCES

[1] Piaget J. The language and thought of the child, 3rd ed. London: Routledge Kegan-Paul, 1962.

[2] Piaget J. The development of thought: equilibration of cognitive structures. Oxford: Blackwell, 1977.

[3] Fry PS. Fostering children's cognitive competence through mediated learning experiences: frontiers and futures. Springfield, IL: CC Thomas, 1991.

[4] Vygotsky LS. Thought and language. Cambridge, MA: MIT Press, 1962.

[5] Vygotsky LS. Mind in society: the development of higher psychological process. Cambridge, MA: Harvard University Press, 1978.

[6] Sternberg RJ. Mental self-government: a theory of intellectual styles and their development. Hum Dev 1988;31:197-224.

[7] Sternberg RJ. The nature of creativity. Creativity Res J 2006;18(1): 87-98.

[8] Baer J. Evaluative thinking, creativity, and task specificity: separating wheat from chaff is not the same as findings needles in haystacks. In: Runco MA, eds. Critical creative processes. Cresskill, NJNew Jersey: Hampton Press, 2003:129-51.

[9] Runco MA. Idea evaluation, divergent thinking, and creativity. In: Runco MA. Critical creative processes. Cresskill, NJ: Hampton Press, 2003:69-94.

[10] Runco MA. Creativity: theories and themes: research, development, and practice. Burlington, MA: Elsevier Academic Press, 2007.

[11] De Bono E. The direct teaching of thinking in education and the CoRT method. In: Maclure S, Davies P. Learning to think: thinking to learn. Oxford: Pergamon, 1991:1-14.

[12] Lun VMC, Fischer R, Ward C. Exploring cultural differences in critical thinking: is it about my thinking style or language I speak? Learn Individ Differ 2010;20(6):604-16.

[13] Phan HP. Unifying different theories of learning: theoretical framework and empirical evidence. Educ Psychol UK 2008;28(3):325-40.

[14] Rindner EC. Using freirean empowerment for health education with adolescents in primary, secondary, and tertiary psychiatric settings. J Child Adol Psychiat Nur 2004;17(2):78-84.

[15] Irving LM, DuPen J, Berel S. A media literacy program for high school females. Eat Disord: J Treat Prev 1998;6(2):119-3231.

[16] Zhang LF. Thinking styles and cognitive development. J Genet Psychol 2002;163(2):179-95.

[17] Zhang LF. Further investigating thinking styles and psychosocial development in the Chinese higher education context. Learn Indivd Differ 2010(6);20:593-603.

[18] Zhang LF. Thinking styles and identity development among Chinese university students. Am J Psychol 2008;121(2):255-71.

[19] Kater KJ, Rohwer J, Levine MP. An elementary school project for developing healthy body image and reducing risk factors for unhealthy and disordered eating. Eat Disord: J Treat Prev 2000;8(1):3-16.

[20] Scull TM, Kupersmidt JB, Parker AE, Elmore KC, Benson JW. Adolescents' media-related cognitions and substance use in the context of parental and peer influences. J Youth Adolescence 2010;39(9):981-98.

[21] Lipman M. Thinking skills fostered by philosophy for children. In: Segal JW, Chipman SF, Glaser R. Thinking and learning skill Vol. 1: relating instruction to research. Hillsdale, NJ: Lawrence Erlbaum, 1985:83-108.

[22] Feldhusen JF, Treffinger DJ, Bahlke SJ. Developing creative thinking: the purdue creative creativity program. J Creative Behav 1970; 4(2):85-906:114-35.

[23] Speedie SM, Treffinger DJ, Feldhusen JF. Evaluation of components of the purdue creative thinking program: a longitudinal study. Psychol Rep 1971;29(2):395-8.

[24] Cheng VMY. Teaching creative thinking in regular science lessons: potentials and obstacles of three different approaches in an Asian context. Asia Pac Forum on Sci Learn Teach 2010;11(1):1-21.

[25] Cheng VMY. Infusing creativity into Eastern classrooms: evaluation from student perspectives. Think Skills Creativity 2011;6(1):67-87.

[26] Chan DW. Developing the creative leadership training program for gifted and talented students in Hong Kong. Roeper Rev 2000;22(2):94-7.

Cognitive competence as a positive youth development construct   427

[27] Chan DW, Cheung PC, Chan ASK, Leung WWM, Leung KW. Evaluating the Chinese University summer gifted program for junior secondary school students in Hong Kong. J Secondary Gifted Educ 2000;11(3):136-43.

[28] Gardner H. Leading Minds: an anatomy of leadership. New York: Basic Books, 1995.

[29] Sun RCF, Hui EKP. Cognitive competence as a positive youth development construct: conceptual bases and implications for curriculum development. Int J Adolesc Med Health 2006;18(3):401-8.

[30] Shek DTL, Sun RCF. Development, implementation and evaluation of a holistic positive youth development program: project P.A.T.H.S. in Hong Kong. Int J Disabil Hum De 2009;8(2):107-17.

[31] Paul RW. The logic of creative and critical thinking. Am Behav Sci 1993;37(1):21-39.

[32] Halpern DF.Teaching for critical thinking: helping college students develop the skills and dispositions of a critical thinker. New Dir Teach Learn 1999;80:69-74.

[33] Flage DE. The art of questioning: an introduction to critical thinking. NJ: Pearson, 2004.

[34] Ennis RH. Critical thinking. Upper Saddle River, NJ: Prentice Hall, 1996.

[35] Moshman D. Adolescent psychological development: rationality, morality, and identity. Mahwah, NJ: Lawrence Erlbaum, 1999.

[36] Lipman M. Thinking in education. 2nd ed. Cambridge: Cambridge University Press, 2003.

[37] Norris SP, Ennis RH. The practitioners guide to teaching thinking series: evaluating critical thinking. Pacific Grove, CA: Critical Thinking Press Software, 1989.

[38] Brookfield S. Developing critical thinkers. San Francisco, CA: Jossey-Bass, 1987.

[39] Meyers C. Teaching students to think critically: a guide for faculty in all disciplines. San Francisco, CA: Jossey-Bass, 1986.

[40] Sternberg RJ, Lubart TI. Defying the crowd: cultivating creativity in a culture of conformity. New York: Free Press, 1995.

[41] Sternberg RJ, Lubart TI. An investment theory of creativity and its development. Hum Dev 1991;34(1):1-32.

[42] Sternberg RJ, Lubart TI. Creativity: its nature and assessment. School Psychol Int 1992;13(3):243-53.

[43] Zhang LF, Sternberg RJ. A threefold model of intellectual styles. Educ Psychol Rev 2005;17(1):1-53.

[44] Zhu C, Zhang LF. Thinking styles and conceptions of creativity among university students. Educ Psychol 2011;31(3):361-75.

[45] Runco MA, Chand I. Cognition and creativity. Educ Psychol Rev 1995(3);7:243-67.

[46] Runco MA. Divergent thinking and creative performance in gifted and nongifted children. Educ Psychol Meas 1986;46(2):375-84.

[47] Guilford JP. Creativity. Am Psychol 1950;5(9):444-54.

[48] Guilford JP. Creativity, intelligence and their educational implications. San Diego, CA: EDITS, 1968.

[49] Dingli S. Thinking outside the box: Edward de Bono's lateral thinking. In: Rickards T, Runco MA, Moger S. The Routledge companion to creativity. New York, NY: Routledge, 2009:338-50.

[50] Edwards J. Research work on the CoRT Method. In: Maclure S, Davies P. Learning to think: thinking to learn. Oxford: Pergamon, 1991:19-30.

[51] Ritchie SM, Edwards J. Creative thinking instruction for Aboriginal children. Learn Instr 1996;6(1):59-7975.

[52] Dewey J, Bento J. Activating children's thinking skills (ACTS): the effects of an infusion approach to teaching thinking in primary schools. Brit J Educ Psychol 2009;79(2):329-51.

[53] Anderson LW, Krathwohl DR. A taxonomy for learning, teaching and assessing: a revision of Bloom's Taxonomy of educational objectives. New York: Longman, 2001.

[54] Feuerstein R, Rand Y, Hoffman MB, Miller R. Instrumental enrichment. Baltimore, MD: University Park Press, 1980.

[55] Tudge JRH, Winterhoff PA. Vygotsky, Piaget, and Bandura: perspectives on the relations between the social world and cognitive development. Hum Dev 1993(2);36:61-81.

[56] Smolucha FC. A reconstruction of Vygotsky's theory of creativity. Creativity Res J 1992;5(1):49-67.

[57] Phan HP. Relations between goals, self-efficacy, critical thinking and deep processing strategies: a path analysis. Educ Psychol UK 2009;29(7):777-99.

[58] Pufai-Struzik I. Self-acceptance and behaviour control in creatively gifted young people. High Abil Stud 1998;9(2):197-205.

[59] DeMoss K, Milich R, DeMers S. Gender, creativity, depression, and attributional style in adolescents with high academic ability. J Abnorm Child Psych 1993;21(4):455-67.

[60] Bernardo ABI, Zhang LF, Callueng CM. Thinking styles and academic achievement among Filipino students. J Genet Psychol 2002;163(2):149-63.

[61] Zhang LF, Sternberg RJ. Thinking styles, abilities, and academic achievement among Hong Kong university students. Educ Res J 1998(1);13:41-62.

[62] Grigorenko EL, Sternberg RJ. Styles of thinking, abilities, and academic performance. Except Children 1997;63(3):295-312.

[63] Zhang LF, Postiglion GA. Thinking styles, self-esteem, and socio-economic status. Pers Indiv Differ 2001;31(8):1333-46.

[64] Zhang LF. Thinking styles and emotions. J Psychol 2008;142(5):497-515.

[65] Zhang LF. Anxiety and thinking styles. Pers Indiv Differ 2009;47(4):347-51.

[66] Milgram RM, Hong E. Creative thinking and creative performance in adolescents as predictors of creative attainments in adults: a follow-up study after 18 years. Roeper Rev 1993;15(3):135-9.

[67] Glevey KE. Promoting thinking skills in education. Lond Rev Educ 2006;4(3):291-302.

[68] Pithers RT, Soden R. Critical thinking in education: a review. Educ Res 20012000;42(3):237-49.

[69] Scales P. Developing capable young people: an alternative strategy for prevention programs. J Early Adolescence 1990;10(4):420-38.

[70] Education Commission. Reform proposal for the education reform in Hong Kong. Hong Kong: Education Bureau, The Government of the Hong Kong Special Administrative Region 2000. URL: http://www. e-c.edu.hk/eng/reform/annex/Edu-reform-eng.pdf.

[71] Feuerstein R, Jensen MR, Hoffman MB, Rand Y. Instrumental enrichment, an intervention program for structural cognitive modifiability: theory and practice. In: Segal JW, Chipman SF, Glaser R. Thinking and Learning Skills Vol. 1: relating instruction to research. Hillsdale, NJ: Lawrence Erlbaum Associates, 1985:43-82.

[72] Catalano RF, Berglund ML, Ryan JAM, Lonczak HS, Hawkins JD. Positive youth development in the United States: research findings on evaluations of positive youth development programs 20021988. URL: http://aspe.hhs.gov/hsp/PositiveYouthDev99/

[73] Johnson A. How to use thinking skills to differentiate curricula for gifted and highly creative students. Gifted Child Today 2001;24(4):58-63.

[74] Collins A, Stevens AL. A cognitive theory of inquiry teaching. In: Goodyear P. Teaching knowledge and intelligent tutoring. Norwood, NJ: Ablex, 1991:203-30.

[75] Kind PM, Kind V. Creativity in science education: perspectives and challenges for developing school science. Stud Sci Educ 2007;43(1):1-37.

[76] McGuinness C. Teaching thinking: theory and practice. Brit J Educ Psychol 2005;20:107-26.

[77] Paul RW, Binker AJA, Martin D, Vetrano C, Kreklau H. Critical thinking handbook: 6th-9th grade for remodeling lesson plans in Language Arts, Social Studies and Sciences. Santa Rosa, CA: Foundation for Critical Thinking, 1995.

[78] Paul RW, Martin D, Adamson K. Critical thinking handbook: high school, a guide for redesigning instruction. Santa Rosa, CA: Foundation for Critical Thinking, 1995.

Submitted: October 01, 2011. *Revised:* November 15, 2011. *Accepted:* December 03, 2011.

In: Alternative Medicine Research Yearbook 2012
Editors: Søren Ventegodt and Joav Merrick

ISBN: 978-1-62808-080-3
© 2013 Nova Science Publishers, Inc.

Chapter 41

EMOTIONAL COMPETENCE AS A POSITIVE YOUTH DEVELOPMENT CONSTRUCT: A CONCEPTUAL REVIEW

Patrick SY Lau, PhD*
and Florence KY Wu, BA, MA

Department of Educational Psychology, The Chinese University of Hong Kong,
Hong Kong, PRC

ABSTRACT

The concept of emotional competence as a positive youth development construct is reviewed in this paper. Differences between emotional intelligence and emotional competence are discussed and an operational definition is adopted. Assessment methods of emotional competence with an emphasis on its quantitative nature are introduced. In the discussion of theories of emotional competence, the functionalist and developmental perspectives and the relationships with positive youth development are highlighted. Possible antecedents, especially the influence of early child-caregiver, and expected outcomes of emotional competence are examined. Practical ways to promote emotional competence among adolescents, particularly the role of parents and teachers, and the future direction of research are also discussed.

Keywords: Adolescence, positive youth development, emotional competence

INTRODUCTION

Cognitive intelligence has received much attention as the single most important predictor of human performance (1). However, the notion of emotional competence is gaining more attention and has been signified as a strong predictor of life success (2). Emotional

---

* Correspondence: Patrick SY Lau, PhD, Department of Educational Psychology, The Chinese University of Hong Kong, Hong Kong, PRC. E-mail: patricklau@cuhk.edu.hk.

competence (EC) can be understood as a group of generic skills that can be applied to many types of emotion-related skills (3). The ability to identify and discriminate emotions is especially important in youth development (4) and may be influenced by a person's initial orientation to his/her emotion-related problems. When an individual has an ineffective orientation, he/she will try to avoid thoughts and feelings related to the problem (5). In such a case, he/she may fail to identify emotions, and thus be less able to resolve emotional problems in constructive ways and less likely to accept his/her own feelings.

Although references on developing competence related to emotions have been found in both UK and US government reports, the research field is not yet very developed (2). In the United Kingdom, emphasis on the "well-being" of children has been amplified. The government has set various goals for the educational settings to develop government-approved materials in developing emotional competence in Britain's youth. Government-determined national targets give rise to the need for young people to excel in social and emotional skills. In the United States, the government is equally focused on child well-being, with its "No Child Left Behind" legislation representing a commitment to ensure that all children are provided with effective learning and the opportunity to achieve through development of emotional skills.

The debate in the literature over the terms, "Emotional Intelligence (EI)" or Emotional Competence remains active. Some researchers even deliberately avoid the use of the term, "emotional intelligence" as the distinction between EC and EI is still not clear (4). Lau (6) articulated the difference between emotional intelligence and emotional competence in his review. The review places the emphasis of EI primarily on in-born ability while the proponents of EC emphasize the skills acquired through cultural and contextual interferences as one develops. In this paper, we take Saarni's (7) "Emotional competence" as the more general and neutral term. We agree with Saarni that the regulation and stabilization of emotions may not assemble general intelligence that is inherited or in-born. Emotional competence can be nurtured and developed as a person grows.

DEFINITION OF EMOTIONAL COMPETENCE

In the 1920s and 1930s, many psychologists explored emotional intelligence in the arena of "social intelligence" as a single concept (8). Goleman (9) furthered his research in emotional competencies in relation to two key domain facets: ability and target. Salovey and Mayer (10) first used the term "emotional intelligence" and stated it in four domains: knowing one's emotions, knowing others' emotions, handling one's emotions and handling others' emotions. Recently, psychologists have been paying attention to the complexity of the construct and describing it in terms of multiple capabilities and competencies (11,12). The multiplicity and integration of the concepts provide a more comprehensive framework for investigating the emotional competence. Emotional competence is understood as the capabilities that are used as predictors of performance and effectiveness in management and leadership (13). Boyatzis et al. (13) offer a descriptive definition of emotional competence that "a person demonstrates the competencies that constitute self-awareness, self-management, social awareness, and social skills at appropriate times and ways in sufficient frequency to be effective in the situation" (p.3).

Emotional intelligence is a "convenient phrase" that focuses on human talent (13). However, EI has been challenged for having too broad a definition of all positive personality traits that result in positive outcomes. The famous model proposed by Goleman (8,9) does not mention the ways to distinguish the level of a person's EI. Zeidner et al. (14) state that the definition of EI may be mixed with social intelligence (SI) as both constructs measure the individual differences relative to how much an individual exhibits traits. In their review, Zeidner et al. (14) point out that EI is mostly defined as a stable quality of the individual. However, most of the adaptive responses to different emotional circumstances are dynamic and situation dependent. In this sense, using the causal model among the constructs of EI is meaningless. Hence, it would be better to define EI as a set of supporting adaptations of emotional skills, which the proponents of EC emphasize, that would form the causal, positive outcomes (15).

Carroll (16) comments that the EI construct lacks the comprehensive models established for conventional mental abilities and Zeidner et al. (14) echo that it is difficult to differentiate EI from multiple constructs due to the difficulty in conceptualization. The developmental psychologists find that the term "intelligence" focuses more on the "mental ability" (17) and characteristics of the person (18) without the notion of contextual influences on the individual. Most recently, there has developed a separate strand of research, focusing on the conceptions, awareness, understanding, and applications of the emotions in social interactions (3). EI can thus be viewed as a snapshot of emotional competencies and the term "emotional competence" is adopted in a more neutral way (7). The word, "competence" signifies the generalization of the most emotive situations (14). As such, we agree with Ciarrochi and Scott (4) that emotional competence includes the ability to identify emotions and an individual difference in how effectively people deal with emotions and emotionally charged problems.

The ideations between the constructs of EC and EI are substantially overlapping yet conceptually different. The trait EI, one of the two predominant perspectives in conceptualizing EI, sees EI as a kind of competence that indicates "one's ability to succeed in coping with environment demands and pressures" (11, p.14). Trait EI shares some commonalities with EC, in that it conceptualizes "intelligence" as "competences" and qualities of individuals to aid them to utilize the competence in real-life situations (19). The major differentiation between EC and EI is the conceptualization of learning the emotions. The essence of EI is more on an individual's traits and personality in response to the emotion displayed. Yet the proponents of EC are prone to the strand of developmental approach. The competence is gained through development of skills acquired by context- and cultural-related experiences with others. Children can learn specific emotional behaviors for their culture as a result of social interaction. Emotional competence is transactional within self and between self and others, yet EI is less transactional as the model is centered within the individual (20). Saarni (21) furthers this distinction in her recent review, stating that there are three significant conceptual differences between EI and EC, which are (1) EC is seen as a set of developed skills; (2) individuals that are emotionally competent are reacting to the emotion-eliciting environments with skills whereas emotionally intelligent individuals are responding with traits residing within those individuals; (3) the contribution of personal integrity to mature, emotionally competent functioning. Therefore, we take EC as the discussion focus as we believe that the focus of growth should be on how much the individuals apply their potential and skills in life contexts, rather than emphasizing internal ability in dealing with emotion-laden situations.

Furthermore, the word "competence" could also be referred to a person's mastery of some skills in the traditional western psychology (22). Based on this tradition, Saarni (7) proposed eight skills as the components of emotional competence to handle emotion-eliciting social transactions. In brief, these eight skills include: (1) being aware of one's own emotions; (2) discerning and understanding others' emotions; (3) using the vocabulary of emotion and expression; (4) having the capacity for empathic involvement; (5) differentiating internal, subjective emotional experience from external, emotional expression; (6) coping adaptively with aversive emotions and distressing circumstances; (7) being aware of emotional communication within relationships; and (8) possessing the capacity for emotional self-efficacy. Lau (6) classified these eight skills into two broad domains: skills (1) and (2) form the perceptual domain and the others form the behavioral domain. Integrating the key concepts of emotional competence in the literature, Lau (6) then summarized three major components of emotional competence as its operational definition. These three components include the skills for identifying personal feelings and those of others; the skills for communicating emotions with others; and the skills for coping with negative emotions and set-backs. In this review, this operational definition of emotional competence is adopted.

THEORIES OF EMOTIONAL COMPETENCE

Theories of the emotional competence construct are crucial to understanding the application of skills of the individuals to the emotion-laden environments (23). There are two dimensions to infer the theories of emotional competence; (1) the construct related to the socialization in respect of functionalist and developmental perspectives; and (2) the relationship between the construct and positive youth development.

Lazarus (24) and Campos et al. (25) first proposed to view competences related to emotions from a functionalist point of view and Saarni (21,23) advanced this perspective from both the functionalist and developmental angles. In the functionalist perspective, the purpose of responding the stimulations of significant events or situations is stressed. The emotional competence can be developed in response to the dynamic interactions with significant others in the environment. An individual gains the interpretation of different emotions by the environmental and interpersonal stimuli as he or she moves through different developmental stages. In line with the functionalist perspective, Saarni (23) discussed EC under the assumption that emotional development would be affected by the interactions among human beings and with the "ethno-psychological ecology", that is, the culture and social world. The skills in managing and regulating emotions can be acquired through learning and the interpretation of the emotion-eliciting environment with the emphasis on the interpersonal and social interactions within it. Although the competence can be gained developmentally, Saarni (18,21,23) remarks that the acquisition of emotional competence would not be sequential. Each skill "reciprocally influences the differentiation of the other skills" in human development (23, p.30).

The second dimension in understanding the theories of the construct is in relation to positive youth development. The perception of the problems generated in the emotion-laden contexts exerts influences on adolescents' emotional well-being. Concerning the well-being of the adolescents, emotional problems were found to be one of the key competence variables in a large cross-sectional study by Ciarrochi et al. (26). Ineffective orientation to emotion-related problems is related to the difficulty in indentifying the emotions. The individuals would then turn to destructive forms of emotional management, such as alcohol abuse (27). Ciarrochi and Scott (4) administered a longitudinal study to investigate causal relations and the link between emotional competence and well-being. They found that people with effective problem orientation were less likely to experience depression, anxiety, and stress and were more likely to experience positive moods. Catalano et al. (28) state that the enhancement of competence can help prevent other negative outcomes and is indicative of positive youth development.

In her review of the influence of the emotional competence in teaching and learning, Garner (3) articulated the theories derived from psychology and education that affect the development of emotional competence in adolescents. The theories denote the relationship between the positive and stable emotions and academic performance in schools. As shown in past studies, Garner (3) agreed that adolescents with better managed emotions would perform, both academically and socially, better in schools.

Under the influence of globalization, adolescents are exposed to divergence of their own culture and other cultures. As school-aged children and adolescents are experiencing the trials of understanding emotions and emotional changes (3), the intention of increasing the awareness of the consideration of the cultural norms and the social partners, or "audience" as Saarni (7) claims, becomes the priority. Gross and Levenson (29) echo this priority with reference to the emotional display rule that would help adolescents to identify the socially and culturally unaccepted emotions. The knowledge of the cultural rule is transmitted by the emotion-eliciting situations in the adolescents' culture. As the learning process of emotions is procedural (21), rehearsals of responding to the social contexts would contribute to one's emotional competence.

ASSESSMENT OF EMOTIONAL COMPETENCE

There is a considerable number of assessment tools for EI developed for measuring emotion-related competencies. The measurements originally developed for EI have been commonly used in studying EC, reflecting that these measurements are compatible for assessing EC. Although there are two approaches for assessing EC, namely quantitative and qualitative methods, the methods generally used are quantitative in nature.

A number of assessment instruments were developed in the past decades and have provided valuable information on social-emotional behaviors in young children (30). Nevertheless, there are two concerns in using the assessment instruments of EC. The first is that there are few measures available to assess the EC of adolescents (31). Consistent findings appear in different reviews (30,32) that few measures are found to be relevant to assess the EC of pre-school and young children. The second concern is the speculation regarding the psychometric properties of the related instruments or inventories (2,33). Although Bar-On Emotional Quotient Inventory (Bar-On EQ-i) (11) is a popular and commonly used assessment instrument for measuring EC, its validity is frequently challenged and criticized (34).

In addition, self-perception reports are commonly used to report the scale of emotion competence. Some researchers may challenge the format of the measurement. Austin, Saklofske, Huang, and McKenny (35) doubt the consistency of the factor structure of the Schutte Self Report Inventory (SSRI) (33) although the internal reliability for overall construct of the scale is good. Most of the measurements of the emotional competence share the basis of self-report measures (1). It is possible that respondents may inflate their ratings as a result of social desirability (36). The intention to assess the respondent's tendency of unconscious self-deception should be emphasized in these self-report measures. As such, further development on the consistency of the self-perception reports should be considered.

Despite the inadequate psychometric properties of the Bar-On EQ-i, Saarni (23) commented that this inventory came closest to the construct of EC in providing "a combined social-emotional and personality attribute assessment of children's self-reported emotion-related functioning" (p. 18). In order to supplement the quantitative data obtained by using Bar-On EQ-i in assessing EC, Saarni (23) proposed a series of qualitative methods, such as interviewing the subjects about their emotional experiences, asking the parents and teachers of the subjects to systematically rate and describe the subjects' emotions, observing them directly in emotion-eliciting situations. Thus, combining both quantitative and qualitative methods may be of greater value and should be considered in assessing EC.

POSSIBLE ANTECEDENTS OF EMOTIONAL COMPETENCE

The social environment influences the emotional development of the individual. Using attachment theory, Harris (37) and Colle and Del Giudice (38) agree that attachment status and early child-caregiver relationships contribute to children's understanding of emotions and affect children's emotional functioning at all levels (39). The different attachment patterns of the individuals might have impact on the development of emotional competence from infancy to adulthood. The secure milieu provided by the caregivers, with their openness of expressivity and co-regulation efforts, enhances the internalization of effective emotion regulation of children. Hence, children grow in a more stable emotional state and with higher tendency to engage in active problem solving and coping. In contrast, if the children's emotions are not attended with support and care, hyperactivating and deactivating styles of coping strategies will be developed (38). Hyperactivating children would regulate emotions ineffectively and feel helpless as they fear losing the attention and care of the caregivers. This may hamper the empathic connection with others and the children may have difficulty in acquiring the social skills and emotional communicative strategies for friendship development (23). Children with deactivating style will avoid expressing their emotions, especially negative emotions, and eventually become less aware of their own feelings and emotions (38). This kind of suppression lasts into adulthood. In the attachment interview of Roisman, Tsai and Chiang (40), an increase of electrodermal response, interpreted as high arousal of suppressed emotions, was found in adult participants who lived in a rare care-giving milieu.

Scharfe (41) suggests that the maternal expressivity influences children's capacity of expressing emotions. The role of secure caregivers (usually maternal care) and the sense of security are highlighted in the research conducted by Colle and Del Giudice (38). Secure children were found to be more capable of regulating their emotions and maintaining organized behaviors during the times of emotional arousals and were showing higher tolerance to frustrations than those children of dismissed and disorganized attachment style. It seems that the sense of security facilitates children to come up with reflective and effective coping strategies that may benefit in managing the negative emotions in social contexts when they grow older (38). The related literature emphasizes the maternal role in influencing the development of the emotional competence of children.

In line with the recent investigations and findings on the genetic factors contributing to the development of EI, Cassidy (42) suggests that children's temperament, which is found to be genetically inherited, would influence the development and regulation of emotions. The mental status and ability of the individuals exert influence over the understanding emotions too. McAlpine et al. (43) indicate in their research that individuals with mental disabilities, like attention-deficit hyperactivity disorder (ADHD) or learning difficulties are less proficient in identifying and understanding emotions.

EMOTIONAL COMPETENCE AND ADOLESCENT DEVELOPMENTAL OUTCOMES

There is a large number of empirical studies on the expected developmental outcomes of emotional competence among adolescents (e.g. 7,44,45) with special references on the three intriguing consequences: skills in managing one's emotions, a sense of subjective well-being, and adaptive resilience (18).

Colle and Del Guidice (38) point out that the development of emotional competence reaches its critical phase in middle childhood, which would be the time for children to gain understanding of complex emotions and employ emotion regulation strategies. In middle childhood, children start to experience the complexity of the human world and learn how to cope with these situations. Regulating and controlling oneself becomes an essential ability in the context of social life for children at this crucial stage. By adolescence, young people start to become aware of the variations in emotion-evocative situations and try to respond to these changing contexts with proper expressions. Adolescents learn how to develop socially desirable coping strategies with increased maturity and broad exposure of social interactions. Sufficient provision of training on emotional competence to cope effectively with stressful life events is indispensable and beneficial for adolescents during this turbulent life stage.

Although their well-being has been found to decrease in early to middle adolescence and reach its lowest point at age 16 years (46), emotional competence is generally hypothesized to be a good predictor of one's sense of subjective well-being (19). There is an assumption that emotional competent individuals will have richer sense of subjective well-being. Zeidner and Shemesh (19) summarize four reasons for this assumption. First, emotionally competent individuals are more aware of their emotions and more able to regulate them, which will contribute to experience higher levels of well-being. Second, the individuals with emotional competence are assumed to have richer social connections and are able to demonstrate better coping strategies. Third, with more accurate interpretation of the information yielded by the emotions and the environment, individuals with emotional competence can sustain a better sense of well-being. Fourth, provided that those with emotional competence would have the propensity to experience more positive effects, individuals are more prone to a richer sense of subjective well-being.

Having an opportunity to be educated and being young are contributors to subjective well-being (47). In the educational settings, school success and academic achievement are crucial to adolescent development. Parker et al (48) reviewed the association between emotional competence and academic achievement of adolescents and conducted a research investigating the relationship between the two. Emotional competence was found to be a significant predictor of academic success for students of all grades without any gender differences (2,48). The result is consistent with other studies (49,50) stating that students with better academic achievements have better management of emotional dimensions including interpersonal, intrapersonal, adaptability and stress management. However, the directionality works both ways: students with better emotional competence may perform better academically.

Given that the traditional constructs of intelligence do not predict life success (51, the importance of prediction by emotional competence is demonstrated. In predicting life success or life satisfaction of school children and adolescents, adolescents who are more emotionally competent are found less aggressive (52) and less likely to have had unauthorized absence from school (53). There is also evidence that EC moderates the link between stress and mental health, hopelessness and suicidal ideation (54). The term, resilience, denotes the "defensive connotations" and assumes that the danger or distress must be overcome by personal qualities (55). Saarni (18) explains these personal qualities as individuals behave with emotional competence—using effective coping strategies and regulating the stressor-eliciting emotions. In their research, Murphy and Moriarty (56) found that if children could behave emotional-competently when they were exposed to stressors that were within their coping capacity, they were more likely to develop new coping strategies and thus the ability to overcome future stressors would be increased. In other words, adaptive resilience could be a consequence of the development of emotional competence.

PROMOTIONS OF EMOTIONAL COMPETENCE AMONG ADOLESCENTS

In promoting emotional competence among adolescents, three practical methods are introduced in this review: 1) provision of the platform for discussing emotions; 2) modeling from significant others and the role of family and 3) scaffolding provided by school-based interventions.

Clore et al (57) suggest that most emotion processes operate without consciousness. With the provision of a platform for the discussion about emotions, adolescents can gain knowledge in expressing emotions appropriately. The platform is well-situated in familial and school settings. If we take the hypothesis of emotional competence as being related to the development of actual skills and the construct is more prone to the individual's perceptions, emotional competence can be taught within social contexts such as family and school settings. While the competence of emotion is the accumulation and understanding of life experiences within the environment (2,58), the acquisition of EC should involve the teaching of social skills and emotion knowledge (59). In the process of teaching, the social information processing model is usually adopted to teach children and adolescents the interpersonal cognition (the interpretation of the social interactions among peers) and intrapersonal cognition (the application of actual social skills through the conceptions of their emotions) (60). Therefore, integrating these concepts and the model in the school curriculum assists the promotion of emotional competence in adolescents. A simple yet logical assumption follows: if emotional skills are taught through a curricular approach in schools, the emotional competence of adolescents will be increased.

In order to assist adolescents to enhance the sensitivity of the learning of emotions, parents can perform as role models to articulate the learning experiences in these situations in their daily life contexts. Saarni (23) emphasizes that the emotion socialization processes of the families of origin are crucial to children's development. If the child is living under a secure and supportive family, the child may experience diverse emotions in a safe and predictable place (61), enabling the child to learn effective coping strategies and be more pro-social. Moreover, emotional management of children is facilitated by a parent who "sympathetically hears what the child has to say, provides reasoned alternatives" (23, p.28). The supportive parent would act as a good emotion coach to help the child regulate emotional challenges and arousal. In Chinese societies, however, children are socialized and taught to control and suppress emotions within the family (6,62). Lau (6) emphasizes that his traditional and patriarchal familial teaching may inhibit the expression of emotions of Chinese children. The difficulty in modulating the emotions leads the Chinese to display more emotional problems when compared with their western counterparts. In addition, the patriarchal culture of Chinese families also affects girls' expressivity of emotions. Girls are perceived as more verbally and facially expressive than boys. However, bing influenced by the traditional teaching, Chinese girls are more passive and less willing to exhibit their emotions to others. Lau (6), therefore, suggests that the gender differences should be taken consideration when designing curricula for youth development.

The importance of promoting emotional education is questioned in the educational settings and the response of the educators to the importance of emotional education is mixed. Some claim that emotional education is 'the missing piece" (63) yet some teachers may view it with skepticism as they believe that academic achievement is more important. However, as indicated by substantial literature, there is a direct link between the emotional status of the students and their performance in tests and examinations: increased anxiety and stress equates with poorer performance in these areas. Emotional stability indicates the wide array of expected and favorable outcomes. Emotional competence is seen as the knowledge about ourselves and others. It is also of the prime indicator of academic success (64) and this helps to have the capacity to solve problems adaptively, which is the crucial foundation for academic learning. Emotional competence of adolescents could be promoted by school-based intervention programs. The education can be carried out in diverse formats, such as classroom instruction, extra-curricular activities, or curricular-based programs. The emotional education programs aim at promoting skills "to listen or focus, to feel committed and responsible for work, to rein impulses, and to cope with upsetting events" (11, p.222). This scaffolding provided by school-based programs becomes an important factor for developing students' emotional competence.

CONCLUDING THOUGHTS WITH FUTURE RESEARCH DIRECTIONS

In reviewing the literature, there are constant, overlapping ideations and ambiguity of conceptual formulations of the constructs, EI and EC. Many researchers have addressed the issue and attempted to differentiate these two; yet overlaps still exist. Therefore, conceptual clarification of the two constructs should be emphasized. The validity of the two constructs is challenged and criticized as discussed in the preceding text. Additional studies are needed to validate the uniqueness of both EI and EC.

Much of the research output is investigated in a cross-sectional nature (2,3,58); more longitudinal investigations are expected to inquire into the influences of emotional competence at different time points and stages of life. Different methodological techniques should be adopted in the future investigations on emotional competence. In addition to the traditional and static investigation methods by the quantitative approach, multiple modes of portrayal of emotions and other qualitative methods, such as interviews and observations can be adopted, as emotions are dynamic and fluid in nature.

The influence of school and family is highlighted in the review, yet the role of personnel, like the influence of teachers and parents, needs further exploration. Researchers are showing interest in inquiring into the teachers' or parents' understanding of the students' emotions in relation to adolescents' development of emotional competence in the socialization of emotions (3,65). However, the idea of teachers and parents as agents of emotion socialization has received limited research attention. The work in this arena is still in its infancy and requires further investigation.

REFERENCES

[1] Wang N, Young T, Wilhite SC, Marczyk G. Assessing students' emotional competence in higher education: development and validation of the Widener Emotional Learning Scale. J Psychoeduc Assess 2011;29(1):47-62.

[2] Qualter P, Gardner KJ, Whiteley HE. Emotional intelligence: review of research and educational implications. Pas Care Educ 2007;25(1): 11-20.

[3] Garner PW. Emotional competence and its influences on teaching and learning. Educ Psychol Rev 2010;22:
297-321.

[4] Ciarrochi J, Scott G. The link between emotional competence and well-being: A longitudinal study. Br J Guid Couns 2006;34(2):231-43.

[5] Frauenknecht M, Black DR. Social Problem-Solving Inventory of Adolescents (SPSI-A): development and preliminary psychometric evaluation. J Pers Assess 1995;64:533-9.

[6] Lau PSY. Emotional competence as a positive youth development construct: conceptual bases and implications for curriculum development. Int J Adolesc Med Health 2006;18(3):355-62.

[7] Saarni C. The development of Emotional Competence. New York: Guilford Press, 1999.

[8] Goleman D. Emotional Intelligence. New York: Bantam, 1995.

[9] Goleman D. An EI-based theory of performance. In Cherniss C, Goleman D. The emotionally intelligent workplace: how to select for, measure, and improve Emotional Intelligence in individuals, groups, and organizations. San Francisco: Jossey-Bass, 2001:27-44.

[10] Salovey P, Mayer JD. Emotional intelligence. Imagin Cog Pers 1990;9:185-211.

[11] Bar-On R. The Emotional Intelligence Inventory (EQ-i): technical manual., Toronto, Canada: Multi-Health Systems, 1999.

[12] Goleman D. Working with Emotional Intelligence., New York: Bantam, 1998.

Emotional competence as a positive youth development construct 439

[13] Boyatzis RE, Goleman D, Rhee K. Clustering competence in emotional intelligence: insights from the Emotional Competence Inventory (ECI). In Bar-On R, Parker JDA. Handbook of Emotional Intelligence., San Francisco: Jossey-Bass, 1999:2-35.

[14] Zeidner M, Roberts RD, Matthews G. Can emotional intelligence be schooled? A critical review. Educ Psychol 2002;37(4):215-31.

[15] Zeidner M. Intelligence and conation: current perspectives and directions for future research. In Messick S, Collis J. Intelligence and personality: bridging the gap in theory and measurement. Mahwah, NJ: Lawrence Erlbaum, 2001:195-213.

[16] Carroll JB. Human cognitive abilities: a survey of factor-analytic studies. New York: Cambridge University Press, 1993.

[17] Wong SS, Ang RP. Emotional competencies and maladjustment in Singaporean adolescents. Pers Indiv Differ 2007;43:2193-2204.

[18] Saarni C. Emotional competence: a developmental perspective. In Bar-On R, Parker JDA. Handbook of Emotional Intelligence., San Francisco: Jossey-Bass, 2000:68-91.

[19] Zeidner M, Olinick-Shemesh D. Emotional intelligence and subjective well-being revisited. Pers Indiv Differ 2010;48:431-5.

[20] Halberstadt A, Denham S, Dunsmore J. Affective social competence. Soc Dev 2001;10:79-119.

[21] Saarni C. Emotional competence and effective negotiation: the integration of emotion understanding, regulation, and communication. In Aquilar F, Galluccio M. Psychology and political strategies for peace negotiation. NY: Springer Science+Businesss Media, 2011:55-74.

[22] White RW. Motivation reconsidered: the concept of competence. Psychol Rev 1959;66:297-333.

[23] Saarni C. The development of emotional competence: pathways for helping children to become emotionally intelligent. In: Bar-On R, Maree JG, Elias MJ. Educating people to be emotionally intelligent., Westport, CT: Praeger, 2007:15-35.

[24] Lazarus RS. Emotion and adaptation. New York: Oxford University Press, 1991.

[25] Campos J, Mumme D, Kermoian R, Campos R. A functionalist perspective on the nature of emotion. In: Fox N, ed. The development of emotion regulation. Monogr Soc Res Child Dev 1994;59:284-303.

[26] Ciarrochi J, Scott G, Deane FP, Heaven PCL. Relations between social and emotional competence and mental health: a construct validation study. Pers Indiv Differ 2003;35:1947-63.

[27] Taylor GJ. Recent developments in alexithymia theory and research. Can J Psychiat 2000;45:134-42.

[28] Catalano RF, Berglund ML, Ryan JAM, Lonczak HS, Hawkins JD. Positive youth development in the United States: research findings on evaluations of positive youth development programs. Ann Am Acad Polit Soc Sci 2004;591:98-124.

[29] Gross JJ, Levenson RW. Hiding feelings: the acute effects of suppressing negative and positive emotion. J Abnorm Psychol 1997;106:95-103.

[30] McCabe PC, Altamura M. Empirically valid strategies to improve social and emotional competence of preschool children. Psychol Sch 2011;48(5):513-40.

[31] Merrell KW. Behavioral, social, and emotional assessment of children and adolescents. Mahwah, NJ: Lawrence Erlbaum, 2003.

[32] Stewart-Brown S, Edmunds L. Assessing emotional intelligence in children: a review of existing measures of emotional and social competence. In: Bar-On R, Maree JG, Elias MJ, eds. Educating people to be emotionally intelligent. Westport, CT: Praeger, 2007:241-257.

[33] Schutte NS, Malouff JM, Hall LE, Haggerty DJ, Cooper JT, Golden CJ, Dornheim L. Development and validation of a measure of Emotional Intelligence. Pers Indiv Differ 1998; 25:167-77.

[34] Matthews G, Zeidner M, Roberts RD. Emotional Intelligence: science and myth. Cambridge, MA: MIT Press, 2002.

[35] Austin EJ, Saklofske DH, Huang SHS, McKenny D. Measurement of trait emotional intelligence: testing and cross-validating a modified version of Schutte et al.'s (1998) measure. Pers Indiv Differ 2004;36:555-62.

[36] Ellington JE, Sackett PR, Hough LM. Social desirability corrections in personality measurement: issues of applicant comparison and construct validity. J Appl Psychol 1999;84:155-66.

[37] Harris PL. Individual differences in understanding emotion: the role of attachment status and psychological discourse. Attach Hum Dev 1999;1: 307-24.

[38] Colle L, Del Giudice M. Patterns of attachment and emotional competence in middle childhood. Soc Dev 2011;20(1):51-72.

[39] Cassidy J, Shaver PR. Handbook of attachment: theory, research and clinical applications. 2nd ed. New York: Guilford, 2008.

[40] Roisman GI, Tsai JL, Chiang KS. The emotional integration of childhood experience: psychological, facial expressive and self-reported emotional response during the adult attachment interview. Dev Psychol 2004;40:776-89.

[41] Scharfe E. Development of emotional expression, understanding and regulation in infants and young children. In: Bar-On R, Parker JDA, eds. Handbook of emotional intelligence. San Francisco, CA: Jossey-Bass, 2000:244-62.

[42] Cassidy J. Emotion regulation: influences on attachment relationships. The development of emotion regulation: Biological and behavioural considerations. Monogr Soc Res Child Dev 1994;59(2-3): 228-49.

[43] McAlpine C, Singh NN, Kendall KA, Ellis CR. Recognition of facial expressions of emotion by persons with mental retardation. Behav Mod 1992;16:543-58.

[44] Parke RD, Cassidy J, Burks V, Carson J, Boyum L. Familial contribution to peer competence among children: the role of interactive affective processes. In Parke R, G Ladd. Family-peer relationships: modes of linkage. Hillsdale, NJ: Erlbaum, 1992:107-34.

[45] Thompson RA. Emotional regulation and emotional development. Educ Psychol Rev 1991;3:269-307.

[46] Csikszentmihalyi M, Hunter J. Happiness in everyday life: the uses of experience sampling. J Happiness Stud 2003;4:185-99.

[47] Wilson W. Correlates of avowed happiness. Psychol Bull 1967;67:294-306.

[48] Parker JDA, Creque RE Sr, Barnhart DL, Harris JI, Majeski SA, Wood LM, et al. Academic achievement in high school: does emotional intelligence matter? Pers Indiv Differ 2003;37:1321-30.

[49] Petrides KV, Fredrickson N, Furnham A. The role of trait emotional intelligence in academic performance and deviant behaviour at school. Pers Indiv Differ 2004;36:277-329.

[50] Trinidad DR, Johnson CA. The association between emotional intelligence and early adolescent tobacco and alcohol use. Pers Indiv Differ 2002;32:95-105.

[51] Reiff HB, Hatzes NM, Bramel MH, Gibbon T. The relation of LD and Gender with emotional intelligence in college students. J Learn Disabil 2001;34:66-78.

[52] Rubin MM. Emotional intelligence and its role in mitigating aggression: a correlational study of the relationship between emotional intelligence and aggression in urban adolescents. Dissertation. Pennsylvania: Immaculata College, 1999.

[53] Qualter P, Whiteley HE, Hutchinson JM, Pope DJ. Supporting the development of emotional intelligence competencies to ease the transition from primary to high school. Educ Psychol Practice 2007;23:79-95.

[54] Ciarrochi J, Deane FP, Anderson S. Emotional intelligence moderates the relationship between stress and mental health. Pers Indiv Differ 2002;32:197-209.

[55] Damon W. What is positive youth development? Ann Am Acad Polit Soc Sci 2004;591:13-23.

[56] Murphy L, Moriarty A. Vulnerability, coping, and growth. New Haven, CT: Yale University Press, 1976.

[57] Clore G, Storbeck J, Robinson M, Centerbar D. Seven sins in the study of unconscious affect. In Barret LF, Niedenthal P, Winkielman P. Emotion and consciousness. New York: Guilford, 2005:384-408.

[58] Zeidner M, Matthews G, Roberts RD, Maccann C. Development of emotional intelligence: towards a multi-level investment model. Hum Dev 2003;46:69-96.

[59] Weare K. Developing the emotionally literate school. UK: Paul Chapman Publishing, 2004.

[60] Crick NR, Dodge KA. A review and reformulation of social informational processing mechanisms in children's social adjustment. Psychol Bull 1994;115:74-101.

[61] Valiente C, Eisenberg N, Fabes R, Shepard S, Cumberland A, Lysoya S. Prediction of children's empathy-related responding from their effortful control and parents' expressivity. Dev Psychol 2004;40:911-26.

Emotional competence as a positive youth development construct

[62] Shek DTL, Chan LK. Hong Kong Chinese parents' perceptions of the ideal child. J Psychol 1999;33(3):291-302.

[63] Elias MJ, Zins JE, Weissberg RP, Frey KS, Greenberg MT, Haynes NM, Kessler R, Schwab-Stone ME, Shriver TP. Promoting social and emotional learning: guidelines for educators. Alexandria, VA: Association for Supervision and Curriculum Development, 1997.

[64] Zeidner M. Hebrew adaptation of the OCEANIC. Haifa: Center for Interdisciplinary Research on Emotions Press, Univ Haifa, 2002.

[65] Calkins SD, Hill A. Caregiver influences on emerging emotion regulation: biological and environmental transactions in early development. In Gross JJ. Handbook of emotion regulation. New York: Guilford, 2007:229-48.

Submitted: October 03, 2011. *Revised:* November 16, 2011. *Accepted:* December 04, 2011.

In: Alternative Medicine Research Yearbook 2012
Editors: Søren Ventegodt and Joav Merrick

ISBN: 978-1-62808-080-3
© 2013 Nova Science Publishers, Inc.

Chapter 42

SELF-EFFICACY AS A POSITIVE YOUTH DEVELOPMENT CONSTRUCT: A CONCEPTUAL REVIEW

Sandra KM Tsang*, PhD, FHKPS, CPsych, RSW, RCP (HKPS)[1], Eadaoin KP Hui, PhD, FHKPS, CPsychol (BPS)[2] and Bella CM Law, BSocSc[1]

[1]Department of Social Work and Social Administration, The University of Hong Kong, Hong Kong, PRC
[2]Faculty of Education, The University of Hong Kong, Hong Kong, PRC

ABSTRACT

Self-efficacy denotes people's beliefs about their ability to perform in different situations. It functions as a multi-level and multi-faceted set of beliefs that influence how people feel, think, motivate themselves and behave during various tasks. Self-efficacy beliefs are informed by enactive attainment, vicarious experience, imaginal experiences, and social persuasion as well as physical and emotional states. These beliefs are mediated by cognitive, motivational, affective and selection processes to generate actual performance. Self-efficacy development is closely intertwined with a person's experiences, competencies and developmental tasks in different domains at different stages in life. This paper reviews the literature to outline the definition and theoretical conceptualizations of the construct originally devised by Bandura that have flourished since the 1990s. Drawing from the studies of the construct to assess self-efficacy, and to inform positive youth development, the paper will present the determinants of the development of self-efficacy beliefs and identify the connection between self-efficacy and adolescent developmental outcomes. The paper will conclude with strategies to enhance youth self-efficacy and proposals for future research directions.

Keywords: Adolescence, positive youth development, self-efficacy

---

* Correspondence: Sandra KM Tsang, PhD, Reg ClinPsy and FHKPS, CPsy (BPS), BSS, RSW, Head, Department of Social Work and Social Administration, The University of Hong Kong, Hong Kong, PRC. E-mail: sandratsang@hku.hk.

INTRODUCTION

Since the 1970s, the Social Cognitive Theory proposed by Bandura (1-3) has been one of the most influential theories used to guide the understanding of human behavior and the motivational determinants of such behavior. The theory advocates a theme of "Triadic reciprocity" which asserts that a person's behavior is constantly under the reciprocal influence of the environment and personal cognitions. When applied in the context of adolescent development, such as academic performance, this theory suggests that an adolescent's academic performance (behavior) is influenced by how this adolescent's beliefs (cognitions) are affected by the support provided by his or her significant others, including parents, teachers and peers (the environment). Bandura argues that self-efficacy is the most pivotal factor affecting a person's cognition, and his assertion has popularized self-efficacy studies since the 1990s.

The following sections aim to present findings and observations from a review of the literature on the definition, assessment, theoretical conceptualizations, adolescent development outcomes and promotion strategies of self-efficacy, with specific reference to positive youth development. Identified research gaps and suggestions for future research will also be presented.

DEFINITION OF SELF-EFFICACY

Self-efficacy refers to one's beliefs in one's capability to organize and execute the courses of action required to achieve given results (4). In the 1994 Encyclopedia of human behavior (5), Bandura emphasized that "Self-efficacy beliefs determine how people feel, think, motivate themselves and behave" (p.71). The concept has been used in research in two different ways: as "task self-efficacy" denoting the perceived ability to perform a particular behavior, and as "coping self-efficacy" denoting the perceived ability to prevent, control, or cope with potential difficulties that might be encountered when engaged in a particular performance (6,7). In the context of seeking evidence-informed ways to promote positive youth development, these two perspectives are both very useful because adolescents enjoy optimal physical growth and energy and are open to the formulation of their self-identity (8). They actively address the potentials and possibilities as well as the challenges and crises of their adolescent developmental stage (9). Their beliefs in their self-efficacy for different tasks and the cumulative effects of such beliefs will significantly influence their immediate and long term development

Self-efficacy is experimentally validated through substantial causality-testing research projects involving "different modes of efficacy induction, diverse populations, using both inter-individual and intra-individual verification, in all sorts of domains of functioning, and with micro level and macro level relations" (Bandura, 1997, as cited in p.18 (10)). Results suggest that self-efficacy functions as a multi-level and multi-faceted set of beliefs, each differing in level, strength and generativity (11). That means, aside from a general perception of self-efficacy, there can be very specific beliefs in self-efficacy regarding different domains of oneself (e.g. physical strength in soccer, or the stamina to prepare for a difficult mathematics test). Self-efficacy beliefs also vary in level, strength and generativity across different domains.

Using language self-efficacy for an illustration, the self-efficacy level refers to variations of self-efficacy beliefs across the mastery of a first and second language; the strength of perceived self-efficacy is indicated by the degree of certainty in using the language in social or formal occasions; while generativity refers to the transfer of self-efficacy beliefs across different language assignments (e.g. written or oral presentations). Each belief and its impact are sensitive to variations in situation, context and task, and they orchestrate and steer a person's course of actions (performance) that generate outcomes in the form of positive or negative physical, social and self-evaluation effects (4).

ASSESSMENT OF SELF-EFFICACY

Self-efficacy assessment is needed for understanding the nature and strength of beliefs that influence performance. Quantitative and qualitative assessment measures and strategies have been devised to assess general self-efficacy, as well as sources and processes of self-efficacy. Self-efficacy is best assessed within the consideration of contextual factors in order to discern whether it plays a mediating, moderating or other role in a behavioral performance. In the case of secondary school students' development, contextual factors like gender, ethnicity, academic ability, and academic domain should be priority concerns.

Usher and Pajares (12) described and critically reviewed both quantitative and qualitative means to assess sources of self-efficacy in school. They found that scales using Likert-type items have been created to assess sources like mastery experience, vicarious experience, social persuasions, and physiological state. These sources have varied psychometric properties when tested with construct or explanatory factor-analysis, or construct validity and internal reliability. However, they also found that the reliability measures on vicarious experiences have consistently been notably low, and more studies are needed to strengthen such measures.

Usher and Pajares (12) also identified some qualitative methods that can be used to assess self-efficacy and sources of self-efficacy under different personal, social, situational and temporal conditions. Methods include grounded theory, ethnography, classroom observations, case studies, interviews, self-reports on recalled reasons for self-efficacy judgments, and self-assigned weights of self-efficacy regarding academic performance. It was found that the semi-structured interview is most useful for capturing both the objective and subjective aspects of self-efficacy beliefs, and the nature and processes of the influence of these beliefs on performance.

Qualitative methods are particularly useful for studying cases where individuals still harbor disabling self-doubts even though they have been recognized to have more than adequate competence in performing the task in question. Thus it is important to synthesize the assessment of such sources with an assessment of psychological processes like motivation, emotion management, strategies in task selection, and problem-solving resourcefulness.

In view of the fact that self-efficacy is complex and context-specific, there is a need for researchers to develop thorough measures that effectively assess the multidimensionality of the hypothesized sources and processes of self-efficacy, together with the strengths and dynamic interactions of these sources and processes. O'Sullivan and Strauser(13) once stated that "It should be noted that for almost any behavior that can be imagined an efficacy scale has been developed" (p.257) (e.g. Diabetes Management Efficacy Scale, Science-teacher Efficacy Scale; Internet Use Efficacy Scale, etc.).

While it appears that great advancement has been achieved in the assessment of self-efficacy, it has to be noted that generating some very task-specific assessment measures in the changing world where young people learn and live can be a time consuming and even endless pursuit. It seems that while striking the right balance between generality and specificity, future research should still try to find the core elements of self-efficacy beliefs that are sensitive to intervention and that can be reliably and validly measured and compared for changes.

In Hong Kong, attempts to develop a self-efficacy scale for Chinese junior secondary school students have been made (14), and the psychometric properties of that scale are satisfactory. The scale consists of 7 items including statements like "When I face life difficulties, I feel helpless" that are to be answered in a 6 point Likert format. It is still a rather general self-efficacy scale for youths, but it is a big step forward in devising ways to measure culture-specific self-efficacy in young people in China. This is important as China is having an increasing influence on the world both in terms of the size of its population and its resource potentials. There is also evidence showing that because Chinese parents and children still value academic achievement as the most important facilitator for upward social mobility, they assert so much concern on academic performance that often high academic achievers still suffer from low academic self-efficacy (15-17).

All these things suggest that for Chinese, in addition to a general self-efficacy scale, other scales focusing on more specific domains like academic, social, sports, moral, information technology management and social services, also need to be developed in order to fully address the different aspects of youth talents and performance, and to yield information on possible means of intervention.

THEORIES ON SELF-EFFICACY

Research-informed theoretical formulations of self-efficacy drew from learning, cognitive, and social cognitive theories, and were able to shed light on the nature, sources, and psychological processes involved in the formation of self-efficacy beliefs. Learning theories attempting to explain the emergence of behavior first focused on conditioning, and then on the consequences of behavior. Cognitive theories of learning introduced cognition into the behavior generation process, and emphasized the consideration of gains or losses resulting from performing the said behavior as significant deciding factors. According to Klassen and Usher (18), "Bandura's Social Cognition Theory marks human functioning as the product of a dynamic interplay of personal, behavioral and environmental influences. These factors exert their influence through a process of reciprocal determinism, by which (a) personal factors in the form of cognition, affect, and biological events, (b) behavior, and (c) environmental influences interact" (p.3).

Research along this line shows that people's self-efficacy beliefs about their capabilities and about the outcomes of their efforts are particularly predictive of actual behavior, like academic performance and even vocational choices. Self-efficacy is also "associated with key motivational constructs like causal attributions, self-concept, optimism, achievement goal orientation, academic help-seeking, anxiety, and value" (p.751) (12), and is thus the most important construct of the Social Cognitive Theory. The theory asserts that self-efficacy beliefs work through the four major psychological processes listed below to produce actual performance:

- *Cognitive processes:* These include self-appraisal of capabilities, skills and resources; goal selection; construction of success and failure scenarios in the goal accomplishment processes; generation and selection of problem-solving options; and sustaining the necessary attention and functioning for task completion.
- *Motivational processes:* Self-efficacy beliefs affect one's self-regulation of motivation. Three cognitive motivators, namely "attribution", "value of expected outcomes" and "clarity and value of goals" have been identified as being influenced by self-efficacy beliefs.
- *Affective processes:* A person's self-perception of coping abilities affects the person's arousal threshold and their tolerance of emotional threats like anxiety and depression (11). Even the process and outcome of threat management can be affected by procedures like guiding imagery to adjust anxiety symptoms when encountering stressors (19).
- *Selection processes:* Decisions on choice of residence, career, family set up, and even use of time can directly influence a person's functioning. In order to attain the outcomes they are interested in, people with high self-efficacy are more proactive in selecting and creating a physical and social environment that matches their perceived capabilities and resources. Their chances of successful goal attainment and personal development are also maximized in the process.

According to Bandura (4) and Maddux and Gosselin (7), self-efficacy beliefs formed through the above processes are not static. They are constantly informed, energized or depleted through at least five identifiable primary sources that are affected by a person's interpretations of former and current experiences:

- *Mastery experiences:* Cognitive processes working on the previous experience of mastery or success in an actual task performance will raise self-efficacy. Successful perseverance through some hardship in the task completion process can even reinforce the durability of self-efficacy. That explains why the adventure-based type of experiential training is both welcomed by young people and found to have a positive impact on their growth and development.
- *Vicarious experience:* Observation of successful task performance by social models (like parents and teachers), and by those whose capabilities are similar to oneself (like peers for young people), generates a strong sense of self-efficacy. Effective mastery and coping models, such as parents, teachers or peers who cope competently with challenges, can demonstrate and stimulate the learning of skills and strategies (20). These models can also promote the readiness of young people to put ideas into action, thus creating more chances for success that will further enhance self-efficacy.

- *Social persuasion:* Convincing verbal persuasion given by significant others, like parents and teachers (21-22), can enhance a young person's self-efficacy, provided that the youth really possesses the capabilities in question. Failure to complete a task that was based on false expectations can do more to damage self-efficacy beliefs than to build them up. Successful social persuasion should include manipulation of all variables in the triadic reciprocity process: expansion of the behavior repertoire through skills training, and environmental control to facilitate successful performance, as well as convincing persuasion of the desirability of the outcome. In recent years, there has been an emerging trend to introduce mature and successful adults from the community to serve as mentors for young people in order to expand the social capital of young people beyond family and school boundaries. The role modeling and guidance of these mentors should provide useful self-efficacy sources for young people.

- *Physiological and affective states*: Actual and perceived physiological and emotional conditions work directly through the affective processes described in the above section to influence a person's self-efficacy beliefs. These physiological and emotional conditions include physical and mental readiness for action, vulnerability to fatigue and susceptibility to a decision to continue or give up. These states also influence the person's subscription to different ways of interpreting and handling all this information. These are particularly important for young people because young people possess important developmental resources like physical energy and emotional accessibility and can benefit greatly if such sources are optimized in time.

- *Imaginal experiences:* Imaginal rehearsal of successful or unsuccessful performance, be it deliberate or while ruminating, can improve coping strategy and enhance self-efficacy (7). Examples include imagination-based interventions such as systematic desensitization and covert modeling(23). In promoting youth self-efficacy, the use of experiential exercises and role playing in skills practice has been found to be helpful in expanding youth experience and preparation (24).

Careful understanding and manipulation of the above psychological processes and sources that influence the formation and functioning of self-efficacy beliefs should create promising avenues for the promotion of self-efficacy. In the context of positive youth development, Usher and Pajares (12) critically reviewed the literature on the sources of self-efficacy in school and proposed directions for research and enhancement strategies.

Suggestions include (a) paying attention to both a quantitative and a qualitative assessment of self-efficacy in order to fine tune the theory and the conceptualization of the nature and the function of its sources and processes; (b) making self-efficacy considerations more context, task, age, gender, academic domain, academic level, and culture sensitive, while also examining their generalizability; (c) utilizing the relationship between the sources of self-efficacy to introduce even more creative enhancement strategies; and (d) identifying if there are other sources of self-efficacy in addition to the four proposed by Bandura.

Specifically, Usher and Pajares identified an invitational approach (25) that suggests that the beliefs people develop about themselves and about others jointly form the perceptual lenses through which people view the world and appreciate new experiences. The messages (or invitations) that people receive and send are pivotal in creating self-efficacy beliefs.

Bandura also stated that the interplay amongst the self-efficacy sources can be additive, relative, multiplicative or configurative.

While Bandura nearly exclusively emphasizes the causal importance of self-efficacy beliefs in influencing final behavior, there is also increasing evidence drawing due attention to the importance of outcome expectancies in producing behavior. Some of the recent applications on young people include expectancy studies on indulgent behavior, like gambling, smoking (26) and cyber-addiction (27). There should also be more discussion on how to manage possible mismatches between self-efficacy and the knowledge and skills necessary for task performance, and how to help youths with low competence and inadequate work attitudes but high self-efficacy build up functional competence and attitude. More studies are still needed to establish the specific role of each self-efficacy source and process, and the role they play in informing and enhancing actual performance.

In recent years, self-efficacy studies have been giving more attention to the environmental variable, and to discussing individual versus collective self-efficacy. In a context like secondary schools where adolescents are constantly in close interaction with their peers and teachers, research should go beyond individual efficacy studies and examine the collective efficacy of the whole class; subgroups in the class; teachers and students as subgroups in a school; or one school versus others in open competitions with other schools (18).

As adolescents are still mainly under the influence of families and schools in their development, attempts to theorize and enhance adolescent development and performance should also give more attention to the efficacy beliefs of parents and teachers. The quality of the role performance of parents and teachers should be examined together with the impact of such on the development of young people's study habits, values and attitudes, health and social habits, as well as how they can avoid at risk behavior.

SELF-EFFICACY AND ADOLESCENT DEVELOPMENTAL OUTCOMES

Pajares (28) reviewed over 20 years of self-efficacy research and identified two main lines of study: (a) connecting self-efficacy beliefs with college major and vocational choices and (b) surveying the connections amongst self-efficacy, other psychological constructs, and academic performance. There are numerous research studies showing that self-efficacy beliefs help determine both task performance (whether people choose to attempt certain tasks, how they attempt the tasks) as well as coping (how people tackle challenges arising from trying to complete the task, and the degree of anxiety and frustration they experience in the process). In the case of adolescents, Pajares and Urdan (29) showed that self-efficacy predicts academic areas and levels, while Brown and Lend (30) identified that self-efficacy predicts students' college major and career choices. In their 2008 review of the literature since 1977 on the sources of self-efficacy in school, Usher and Pajares (12) observed that self-efficacy is "associated with key motivational constructs such as causal attributions, self-concept, optimism, achievement goal orientation, academic help-seeking, anxiety, and value" (p.751). Self-efficacy is also connected to self-regulated learning, including students' decision to stay in school (31), and academic procrastination (32).

Aside from academic performance and study style, self-efficacy also has an impact on adolescents' performance in extra-curricular activities like soccer (19). A review of two school intervention projects aiming to promote students' self-efficacy and school mental health in Germany found that individualized task demands and specific teacher feedback enhances student self-efficacy, while social self-efficacy is fostered through a positive class climate with mutual support amongst students, and when teachers are sensitive to the individual needs of the students (24). The students who finished the projects reported improved motivational orientations, coping with stress, and conflict solving. Cicognani (33) studied 342 adolescents and found coping resources like self-efficacy helped them survive minor stressors and fostered psychological well-being and social support.

In recent years, research into the role of self-efficacy in the regulation of involvement in peer aggression and defending the victim (34), or in indulgent behavior like smoking (35), drinking (36), drug addiction (37) and internet usage (38) has also produced very promising results.

PROMOTION OF SELF-EFFICACY
IN ADOLESCENTS

There is plenty of research evidence indicating that timely and strategic cultivation of positive self-efficacy in early adolescence is important and possible. In 1998, Richard Catalano and his colleagues in the University of Washington reviewed 25 effective "Positive Youth Development Programs in the United States" and found that each of these programs included a component to promote self-efficacy (39). Popular themes included the enhancement of skills, responsibility, supportive relationships and belonging. There is also an increased indication that the promotion strategies have to be age, gender, task and culture specific to show the best results, and using self-efficacy evaluation measures tailored for the task to be mastered will also show the clearest intervention effect (18). These findings have informed teaching in Hong Kong and research demonstrating their usefulness is just beginning to build up. Some of the strategies found useful for Chinese school children were competitions in vicarious learning for writing tasks (40), and delivering individual and formative evaluative feedback to foster self-efficacy in English vocabulary acquisition (41).

Aside from work done with individual adolescents, increasing attention is being paid to cultivate collective self-efficacy (18). A whole class in a secondary school, or a group in a team project, or even a whole school, can also be used as a collective unit, depending whether it is a class, group or school-based task. Inclusion of the belief in efficacy, be it the team leader, a fellow student, or the responsible teacher or trainer, is also found to be useful in appreciating the full sources and dynamics of self-efficacy.

Since most children stay at home and then go to primary and secondary school for education before they enter tertiary education, parents and teachers should be important contextual agents to be included in studies of social cognitive theory. Surprisingly, a review of 244 articles on self-efficacy from the period 2000-2009 found that some 40% studied teachers while only 2% studied parents (18). Fan and Williams (21) found that parental advising on study in English, and family rules for watching television were positively linked to students' engagement and intrinsic motivation towards both English and Mathematics. As

Self-efficacy as a positive youth development construct

most Chinese parents put a very high priority on supporting their children to achieve academically, and as home-school cooperation has been found to provide useful support for adolescent development (22), it is important that self-efficacy studies draw adequately from these two important contextual agents.

RESEARCH GAPS AND FUTURE RESEARCH DIRECTIONS

Considering the current literature, and the review of self-efficacy studies from 1977 up to 2007 by Usher and Pajares (12) (Usher and Pajares used sources, antecedents, self-efficacy and development in various combination as search items), as well as the review by Klassen and Usher on 244 articles from 65 journals of self-efficacy studies (18), the following is recommended for future self-efficacy research, especially where adolescent positive development is concerned:

- *Refine the measurement of the self-efficacy sources:* Each of the four named self-efficacy sources differs in nature and they vary according to the task and the context in question, so that there should be source and task-specific assessments to detect any changes with adequate sensitivity.
- *Foster new methods of inquiry:* Aside from purely quantitative measures, qualitative and mixed method assessment should also be used. In addition to self-administered questionnaires, interviews, and self-reported recall tasks, innovative research design should also be developed to capture the full interplay amongst the person, their behavior, and the environment in human functioning.
- *Consider new elements and paths in social cognition theory:* This might include new sources of self-efficacy like the invitational approach (25), optimism and positive psychology, as well as the role of outcome expectancy (42). There should be more investigation into the transformative experience in the formation of self-efficacy. Exploration into the neurobiological basis of self-efficacy, in adolescence and across the human life-span, should also be another productive agenda.
- *Attend to collective efficacy*: Klassen and Usher(18) found that during the period 2000-2009, education-related studies on collective efficacy were few and focused on teachers rather than students. It is high time such collective beliefs were better understood, and that individual and collective efficacies were put into proper perspective.
- *Attend to gender, age and cultural variations*: According to a ten-year review (18), over 60% of the 244 articles reviewed were on N. America, with only 20% on Asia. With the growing impact of globalization, and communication without-borders on the internet, more attention should be paid to different forms of culture when trying to understand the nature and dynamics of self-efficacy. Aside from describing the effects of gender, age and cultural differences on self-efficacy, it is also important to find out the causes for such differences. As an example, the roles of an individual's gender orientation and personal style, as well as the role of the home, culture, school, and the mass media should all be clearly discerned to sharpen the effectiveness of interventions. With a growing number of children with special educational needs,

REFERENCES

[1] Bandura A. Self-efficacy: toward a unifying theory of behavioral change. Psychol Rev 1977; 84:191-215.
[2] Bandura A. Social foundations of thought and action. New York: Prentice-Hall, 1986.
[3] Bandura A. Social cognitive theory: an agentic perspective. Annu Rev Psychol 2001;52:1-26.
[4] Bandura A. Self-efficacy: the exercise of control. New York: WH Freeman, 1997.
[5] Bandura A. Self-efficacy. In: Ramchaudran VS. Encyclopedia of human behavior Vol. 4. New York: Academic Press, 1994:71-81.
[6] Kirsch I. Self-efficacy and outcome expectancy. In: Maddux JE. Self-efficacy, adaptation, and adjustment: theory, research and application. New York: Plenum, 1995:331-45.
[7] Maddux JE, Gosselin JT. Self-efficacy. In: Leary MR, Tangney JP. Handbook of self and identity. New York: Guilford Press, 2003:218-37.
[8] Tsang SKM, Yip FYY. Positive identity as a positive youth development construct: conceptual bases and implications for curriculum development. In: Shek DTL, Ma HK, Merrick J. Positive youth development: development of a pioneering program in a Chinese context. Tel Aviv: Freund Publishing House, 2007:227-35.
[9] Erikson EH. Identity, youth, and crisis 1st Ed. New York: Norton, 1968.
[10] Bandura A. Self-efficacy: the foundation of agency. In: Walter JP, Alexander G. Control of human behavior, mental processes, and consciousness: essays in honor of the 60th birthday of August flammer. NJ, Mahwah: Lawrence Erlbaum, 2000:17-34.
[11] Ehrenberg MF, Cox DN, Koopman RF. The relationship between self-efficacy and depression in adolescents. Adolesc 1991;26(102):361-74.
[12] Usher EL, Pajares F. Sources of self-efficacy in school: critical review of the literature and future directions. Rev Educ Res 2008;78(4):751-96.
[13] O'Sullivan D, Strauser DR. Operationalizing self-efficacy, related social cognitive variables, and moderating effects: implications for rehabilitation research and practice. Rehabil Couns Bull 2009;52(4):251-8.
[14] Shek DTL, Siu AMH, Lee TY, Cheng H, Tsang SKM, Lui J, et al. Development and validation of a positive youth development scale in Hong Kong. Int J Adoles Med Health 2006;18(3):547-58.
[15] Organization for Economic Co-operation and Development. Learning for tomorrow's world: first result from PISA 2003. France: Organization for Economic Co-operation and Development, 2004.
[16] Rao N, Moely BE, Sachs J. Motivation beliefs, study strategies, and mathematics attainment in high- and low-achieving Chinese secondary school students. Contemp Educ Psychol 2000;25:287-316.
[17] Shek DTL, Chan LK. Hong Kong Chinese parents' perceptions of the ideal child. J Psychol 1999;133(3):291-302.
[18] Klassen RM, Usher EL. Self-efficacy in educational settings: recent research and emerging directions. In: Karabenick S, Urdan TC. Advances in motivation and achievement Vol. 16A: the decade ahead: theoretical perspectives on motivation and achievement. UK, Bingley: Emerald Books, 2010:1-33.
[19] Munroe-Chandler K, Hall C, Fishburne G. Playing with confidence: the relationship between imagery use and self-confidence and self-efficacy in youth soccer players. J Sports Sci 2008;26(14):1539-40.
[20] Schunk DH, Zimmerman BJ. Influencing children's self-efficacy and self-regulation of reading and writing through modeling. Read Writ Q 2007;23:7-25.
[21] Fan W, Williams CM. The effects of parental involvement on students' academic self-efficacy, engagement and intrinsic motivation. Educ Psychol 2010;30(1):53-74.
[22] Tsang SKM, Leung C. Positive psychology and enhancement of home-school support for students with dyslexia: evaluative study. Int J Learn 2006;12(6):245-54.

Self-efficacy as a positive youth development construct   453

[23] Williams SL. Self-efficacy, anxiety, and phobic disorders. In: Maddux JE. Self-efficacy, adaptation, and adjustment: theory, research and application. New York: Plenum, 1995:69-107.

[24] Jerusalem M, Hessling JK. Mental health promotion in schools by strengthening self-efficacy. Health Educ 2009;109(4):329-41.

[25] Purkey S. What students say to themselves: internal dialogue and school success. CA, Thousand Oaks: Corwin, 2000.

[26] Bektas M, Ozturk C, Armstrong M. An approach to children's smoking behaviors using social cognitive learning theory. Asian Pac J Cancer Prev 2010;11:1143-9.

[27] Lin MP, Ko HC, Wu JYW. The role of positive/negative outcome expectancy and refusal self-efficacy of internet use on internet addiction among college students in Taiwan. Cyber Psychol Behav 2008;11(4):451-7.

[28] Pajares F. Self-efficacy beliefs in academic setting. Rev Educ Res 1996;66:543-78.

[29] Pajares F, Urdan T. Adolescence and education Vol. 5. Self-efficacy beliefs of adolescents. CT, Greenwich: Information Age, 2006.

[30] Brown SD, Lent RW. Preparing adolescent to make career decisions: a social cognitive perspective. In: Pajares F, Urdan T. Adolescence and education Vol. 5 Self-efficacy beliefs of adolescents. CT, Greenwich: Information Age, 2006:201-33.

[31] Caprara GV, Fida R, Vecchoine M, Del Bove G, Vecchio GM, Barbaranelli C, et al. Longitudinal analysis of the role of perceived self-efficacy for self-regulated learning in academic continuance and achievement. J Educ Psychol 2008;100:525-34.

[32] Klassen RM, Krawchuk LL, Rajani S. Academic procrastination of undergraduates: low self-efficacy to self-regulate predicts high levels of procrastination. Contemp Educ Psychol 2008;33:915-31.

[33] Cicognani E. Coping strategies with minor stressors in adolescence: relationships with social support, self-efficacy, and psychological well-being. J Appl Soc Psychol 2011;41(3):559-78.

[34] Barchia K, Bussey K. Predictors of student defenders of peer aggression victims: empathy and social cognitive factors. Int J Behav Dev 2011;35(3):1-9.

[35] Veselska Z, Geckova AM, Reijneveld SA, Dijk JP. Self-efficacy, affectivity and smoking behavior in adolescence. Eur Addict Res 2011;17(4):55-64.

[36] Connor JP, George SM, Gullo MJ, Kelly AB, Young RM. Cognition and behavior: a prospective study of alcohol expectancies and self-efficacy as predictors of young adolescent alcohol misuse. Alcohol Alcohol 2011;46(2):161-9.

[37] Hyde J, Hankins M, Deale A, Marteau TM. Interventions to increase self-efficacy in the context of addiction behavior: a systematic literature review. J Health Psychol 2008;13(5):607-23.

[38] Tsai MJ, Tsai CC. Junior high school students' internet usage and self-efficacy: a re-examination of the gender gap. Comput Educ 2010;54:1182-92.

[39] Catalano R F, Berglund M L, Ryan JAM, Lonczak HS, Hawkins JD. Positive youth development in the United States: research findings on evaluations of positive youth development programs. Prev Treat, 2002;5(15):111. Accessed 2004 Dec 15. URL: http://www.jounrals.aps.org/prevention/volume5/pre0050015a.htm

[40] Chan JCY, Lam SF. Effects of competition on students' self-efficacy in vicarious learning. Br J Educ Psychol 2008;78:95-108.

[41] Chan JCY, Lam SF. Effects of different evaluative feedback on students' self-efficacy in learning. Instr Sci 2010;38(1):37-58.

[42] Williams DM. Outcome expectancy and self-efficacy: theoretical implications of an unresolved contradiction. Pers Soc Psychol Rev 2010;14(4):417-25.

Submitted: October 05, 2011. *Revised:* November 17, 2011. *Accepted:* December 04, 2011.

In: Alternative Medicine Research Yearbook 2012
Editors: Søren Ventegodt and Joav Merrick

ISBN: 978-1-62808-080-3
© 2013 Nova Science Publishers, Inc.

Chapter 43

SELF-DETERMINATION AS A PSYCHOLOGICAL AND POSITIVE YOUTH DEVELOPMENT CONSTRUCT

Eadaoin KP Hui, PhD, FHKPS, CPsychol (BPS)[*,1]
and Sandra KM Tsang, PhD, FHKPS, CPsych, RSW, RCP (HKPS)[2]

[1]Faculty of Education, The University of Hong Kong, Hong Kong, PRC
[2]Department of Social Work and Social Administration, The University of Hong Kong, Hong Kong, PRC

ABSTRACT

This paper presents a review of self-determination as a positive youth development construct. The definition and conceptualization of the concept are examined from the perspective of self-determination theory and the functional theory of self-determination. Theories of self-determination from the perspective of motivation and skills enhancement are examined. Factors contributing to self-determination, such as autonomy-supportive teaching and parenting style, culture, efficacy of intervention programmes and the educational benefits of self-determination for students are discussed. Strategies to promote self-determination in an educational context and implications for further research and practice are discussed.

Keywords: Self-determination, autonomy, positive youth development, adolescence

INTRODUCTION

Adolescence is a critical phase of life during which young people face physical, psychological, intellectual and emotional concerns and challenges, search for self-identity, explore new roles, and deal with transition to secondary schools and later from school to work

---

[*] Correspondence: Associate professor Eadaoin KP Hui, PhD, Head of Division of Learning Development and Diversity, Faculty of Education, University of Hong Kong, Room 414, Runme Shaw Building, Hong Kong, PRC. E-mail: eadaoin@hku.hk.

and adulthood. Individuation and separation are processes that adolescents have to go through.

Achieving independence and autonomy, setting personal goals and making plans, and acquiring values and ethics are developmental tasks that all adolescents have to realize. Being self-determined is a developmental task that all young people have to confront and is pertinent to their whole-person development.

DEFINITION OF SELF-DETERMINATION

Self-determination, as a psychological construct, refers to volitional actions taken by people based on their own will, and self-determined behaviour comes from intentional, conscious choice and decision (1). The conceptualization and definition of self-determination varies according to its theoretical orientations. The self-determination theory (SDT) proposed by Deci and Ryan (2), for example, focuses on the motivational aspect of self-determination and the role of self-determined motivation and autonomy on students' learning and education (3). Self-determination is defined as "the capacity to choose and to have those choices....be the determinations of one's action" (p.38) (4).

In the field of special education with youth and adults with disabilities, researchers focus more on the development of cognitive, social and behavioural components which are essential dispositional characteristics for self-determined behaviour. Wehmeyer (5), for example, refers self-determined behaviour as "volitional actions that enable one to act as the primary causal agent in one's life and to maintain or improve one's quality of life" (p.117). Self-determination is defined as skills, knowledge, beliefs which facilitate goal-directed, self-regulated and autonomous behaviour(6).

In the context of positive youth development, self-determination is defined as "the ability to think for oneself and to take action consistent with that thought" (p.105) (7). Self-determination of young people is fostered through positive youth development programmes which target at promoting autonomy, independent thinking, self-advocacy, empowerment of young people, and their ability to live according to values and standards. Such conceptualization is in line with the emergence of positive psychology which emphasizes fostering of human strengths (8).

In short, people who are self-determined are self-initiated, self-directed, and make things happen in their lives. Self-determination is about the competence of young people in engaging in volitional behaviour, and their autonomy in making choices and decisions, which are nurtured in supportive social environments.

SELF-DETERMINATION FROM THE HUMAN MOTIVATION PERSPECTIVE

Theoretical framework of SDT

SDT is based upon the assumption that human persons are active and growth-oriented agents, inclined to organize and initiate their actions with reference to their values and interests, with the tendency to integrate social norms and practices, intrinsically motivated to pursue personal goals, and striving to master the environments. The development of these tendencies and qualities are dependent upon the kind of support they receive from the socializing environments, which may promote or undermine their intrinsic motivation and internalization (2,9).

SDT postulates that the satisfaction of the three basic psychological needs, namely, competence, relatedness and autonomy, is pertinent for the optimal development and functioning of human persons. Competence refers to having the feeling of being capable to meet the demands of environments and face daily challenges. Such need can be fulfilled by the experiences of enacting and achieving desired goals and having effective outcomes. Autonomy is about being volitional and self-endorsing in one's behaviour and having the control to make choices from one's own will. The need for autonomy differs from being independent, selfish, and having freedom of choices (2,10). The essential elements which facilitate autonomy include self-awareness of one's motives, emotions and external demands, having active involvement, and having the chances for self-direction and choice making. Satisfaction of the need for autonomy at home and in a school environment is likely to facilitate the development of intrinsic motivation and internalization (2). In addition, both the needs for competence and autonomy are necessary and essential for the maintaining of intrinsic motivation (11). Relatedness is about the need to achieve a sense of closeness, connectedness and belongingness with others. The satisfaction of the need for relatedness will provide emotional security for further exploration. Feelings of closeness to the significant others such as parents and teachers will facilitate the process of internalization of values, social norms and practice. Hence, socio-emotional relatedness is pertinent to internalization and the subsequent motivation and self-regulation to engage in tasks demanded by others (2,11).

SELF-DETERMINATION AND EDUCATIONAL OUTCOMES

Research studies have provided evidence that support for students' psychological needs for autonomy, competence and relatedness facilitates autonomous self-regulated learning, academic performance and well-being (11). High levels of autonomy, relatedness and competence are associated with more satisfying learning experiences (3). Academic achievement is strongly associated with autonomous motivation (12).

Young people who are regulated by autonomous and intrinsic motivation experience more positive educational outcomes at schools. For example, students who were autonomously motivated had higher academic achievement, self-esteem, perceived competence, personal control and creativity (13), and showed a more adaptive learning attitude, and academic success (14).

Students taught by autonomy-supportive teachers were found to have increased intrinsic motivation, higher competence and self-esteem, more interest for lessons, greater creativity, flexibility in thinking and conceptual understanding, and more active involvement in information processing than were their counterparts whose teachers were controlling (13,15,16).

Autonomous motivation was also found to be associated with psychological well-being (17). Research studies have shown that autonomously motivated students reported more positive affect and emotions, having more enjoyment of academic work, experiencing greater life and school satisfaction, and having lower ill-being such as depression (11,12).

In addition, higher autonomy in schools is associated with lower dropout rates, lower level of anxiety, more positive coping strategies (18). Students whose environments are supportive of their needs have a greater tendency to engage in learning which promotes hope (19).

FACTORS CONTRIBUTING TO THE DEVELOPMENT OF SELF-DETERMINATION

Parenting styles

According to SDT, the social contexts that are responsive and supportive can facilitate young people to engage in self-initiated, self-regulated and volitional behaviour (2). Parents in the context of family play a very important role in the cultivation of self-determination. First, parents who meet their children's needs for autonomy contribute to their self-regulation and motivation. Research studies have provided evidence that parents who are autonomously supportive provide their children with choices and options, allow them to explore and enact according to their own interests and values (20,21). By showing genuine interest to their children's needs and being empathic to their views and perspectives (22), parents help their children to develop themselves as active and volitional agents. Research by Soenens and Vansteenkiste (9) has shown that parental autonomy support contributed significantly to self-determination in the domain of school and peer relationship. On the other hand, a controlling parental style which focuses on outcome rather than process and on controlling techniques tend to undermine children's intrinsic motivation and internalization (23,24). Second, the provision of structure by parents, such as giving clear expectation about behaviour, promotes children's competence, understanding of ways to attain success, and perceived personal control (24). Third, parental involvement facilitates children's motivation to achieve, internalization of values, and students' academic self-regulation (24,25). A caring and supportive home environment also satisfies children's needs for relatedness. In short, parental autonomy support, structure and involvement are pertinent to fostering autonomous self-regulation in children.

Teacher autonomy-supportive style

SDT suggests that teacher autonomy support and structure are pertinent to help students to attain optimal learning. Autonomy support and structure, though different, are student-focused and positively related. Teachers who provide students with structure and guidelines tend to have a more autonomy-supportive style (26). Research studies have found positive relationships between teacher autonomy support and students' scholastic self-determination, school engagement and school adjustment (9). Autonomy-supportive teachers, similar to autonomy-supportive parents, contribute to students' self-determination through offering choices, providing rationale for choices, empathizing with students' perspectives, and minimizing the use of controlling language in the classroom environments (26). Autonomy-supportive teachers also identify, cultivate, and develop students' inner motivational resources (27). These practices provide students with the opportunity to pursue personal goals and interest and to satisfy their needs for autonomy and competence.

In addition, an autonomy-supportive learning environment contributes to the enhancement of students' perceived competence, interest and enjoyment(28). Students with a low autonomy level benefit particularly in an autonomy-supportive environment, where they learn to be more autonomous and self-regulated, leading to improvement in learning performance.

Culture and self-determination

SDT posits that the needs for competence, autonomy and relatedness are innate, universal and compatible. Hence, fulfilment of these needs contributes to the optimal functioning of all individuals across cultures and societies (29). SDT acknowledges that people are influenced by their culture in assigning meaning and interpretation to their autonomous experience as positive or negative, to be supported or to be prevented (3). Individuals' expressions of their needs for competence, autonomy and relatedness may differ within cultures that hold different values. Yet, they reckon that the benefits of self-determination and the negative consequences of being non-autonomous are across culture. Cross-cultural psychologists, however, argue that the constructs of self-determination and autonomy are influenced by western cultural values. For example, autonomy is considered as a value upheld in individualist societies(30), reflecting an independent view of self (31). Hence, the need for autonomy is in conflict with the need for relatedness and interdependent relationships cherished in collectivistic societies (32, 33). However, other researchers argue that autonomy from the SDT perspective is about being volitional in one's act, which is different from asserting independence from significant others and having freedom of choices. In a collectivist culture, the need for autonomy can be met through internalization of the demands of others and self-endorsement of the choices (10). A recent research by Hui, Sun, Chow and Chu (34) has demonstrated that these three psychological needs are pertinent to academic motivation in the East as well as in the West. Competence was found to be the most significant predictor of academic motivation among Chinese students. Following competence, relatedness with parents was salient in predicting academic motivation. Autonomy had a strong positive association with relatedness, revealing that the higher autonomous support the students perceived from their parents, the greater the connection they felt with their parents. Another study with Chinese students from the People's Republic of China also illustrated the benefits of autonomous academic motivation to adaptive learning attitudes, academic success and well-being (14).

SELF-DETERMINATION FROM THE PERSPECTIVE OF SKILLS ENHANCEMENT

Theoretical framework and approaches

According to the functional theory of self-determination, people act as causal agents who make things happen. Actions that are self-determined are related to the function they serve. The essential characteristics of self-determined actions include that the person acts autonomously and in a self-realizing manner, the behaviour is self-regulated, and the act is a self-initiated response to events in a psychologically empowered manner (35). As the functional theory of self-determination adopts a person-environment interaction framework in its conceptualization, the development of self-determination is influenced by both individual dispositional characteristics as well as environmental experiences. The ecological model of self-determination, on the other hand, considers attaining personal control over one's life as the ultimate goal of self-determination (36). According to this model, the skills, knowledge and beliefs which a person holds interact with the environment to facilitate the attainment of goals and desirable outcomes.

Promoting self-determination has been a major concern for youth with disabilities. Research studies have suggested that youth with disabilities lack skills, knowledge and beliefs which are important for their self-determination (37). Further, students with disabilities are less self-determined than their peers without disabilities. Hence, fostering self-determination has been a major issue in the field of special education, and has become best practice in secondary education and transition service (38).

In recent years, the emergence of positive psychology has had considerable impact on the field of positive youth development. Grounded in developmental theories such as Erikson's identity development theory and Bowlby's attachment theory, the positive youth development approach emphasizes identifying young peoples' strengths and competencies. The approaches are grounded in humanistic psychology which emphasizes individuals' potentials and capabilities. It can be seen that the assumptions of humanistic theories are very similar to those that self-determination is based on, for example, emphasizing individuals' subjective awareness of themselves and others, individuals having choice and capability for self-actualization (4). Self-determination is one of the fifteen psychological constructs to be taught as skill development for youth with or without disabilities in Positive Youth Development Programmes and Project P.A.T.H.S in Hong Kong Schools (7).

Factors contributing to self-determination of students with disabilities

The development of self-determination, according to functional theory, is influenced by an individual's capacity, that is, the personal characteristics and the environmental factors and instructional experiences. Regarding personal characteristics, intelligence was found to have a positive relationship with self-determination, in which individuals high in IQ scores have higher self-determination scores (39).

Research examining the effect of gender on self-determination has been limited and has produced mixed findings. Gender was not found to be significant in the study by Wehmeyer and Gardner (40). Other studies however found gender to assert effect on self-determination (Nota et al 2007 and Shogren et al 2007 cited in (41)). External factors, such as choice opportunity rather than intelligence, were found to be the primary predictor of self-determination among people with intellectual disabilities (40). The living and working environments contribute to self-determination, with people in community-based settings having greater autonomy and more choice opportunities, whereas people from restrictive settings were lower in self-determination (42). A recent research by Lee, Wehmeyer, Palmer, Williams-Diehl, Davies, et al (41) found that instructional, knowledge and dispositional factors were stronger predictors of students' self-determination than personal factors such as age, gender and intelligence level. Self-efficacy and outcome expectancy, student-directed transition planning instruction, and students' pre-intervention transition planning knowledge were strong predictors of students' determination.

Environmental factors which contribute to self-determination include provision of self-determined role models, self-determination skill instruction and support, opportunities for choice to make decision, positive communication patterns within the school institutions and personal relationships, and provision of student support by teachers and peers (43). In addition, developing supportive relationships with others, including teachers and peers, contribute to supporting self-determination (44). The sense of relatedness provides security for young people to be self-determined (17). Hence, supportive relationships encouraged by peer support programs, like peer tutoring, peer counselling, help promote self-determination (44).

Intervention programmes to promote self-determination

Research has shown that the possession of self-determination skills is associated with improved educational outcome in school and with post-school success for youth and adults with disabilities. For example, improved self-determination skills were crucial to academic performance and success, and contributed to increased class participation and post-secondary involvement (45). Self-determination skills lead to improved outcomes in independence and employment as well as in quality of life (46).

Hence, self-determination as a construct becomes an important aspect in education and has been used widely in education programmes for students with disabilities (42). Various models and approaches have been developed to enhance their skills in self-determination (47-53). Most intervention programmes target at teaching skills in decision making, choice making, self-advocacy, self-efficacy, self-awareness and self-evaluation of goals and plans (54).

Field, Hoffman and Posch (55), for example, developed the Steps to Self-determination Curriculum based on the five major components: Know yourself, Value yourself, Plan, Act, Experience Outcome and Learn. The first two components, Know yourself and Value yourself, are about fostering self-knowledge and self-awareness. The components Plan and Act are about acquiring specific skills. Experience Outcome and Learn refer to evaluating of goals and plan and celebrating of success. This curriculum is based on the view that possession of inner knowledge of what one wants and the skills to attain the desired goals are pertinent to self-determination. Individual characteristics such as self-awareness are the building blocks for self-determination, whereas ability to set goals is the outcome of self-determination. Environmental factors, such as opportunities for choice making and the attitudes of others, also contribute to self-determination. This is an example of a comprehensive curriculum that can be used with secondary students with and without disabilities. The self-determination knowledge and skills can be integrated across subject areas to be supported at all levels in school.

The Self-Determined Learning Model of Instruction put forward by Wehmeyer, Palmer, Agran, Mithaug and Martin (56) targets at strengthening the components of self-determination, in which teachers guide students through a three-phase instructional process, namely goal setting, taking action and adjusting the goal or plan. In each phase, students learn to respond to problems by posing and answering a series of four questions critically in a problem-solving process, setting goals to meet their needs, making modifications and application of their self-selected goals, and adjusting actions to complete their plans. Teachers provide a set of objectives for each question and educational support in each phase to facilitate students to be self-directed learners. Hence, students act as active agent in making decisions, choices and taking action. This approach of teaching self-regulated problem solving can be applied across a wide range of content areas for students with and without disabilities. The programme had positive effects on students' self-regulation and achievement of self-selected goals.

Since acquiring self-determination skills facilitates all adolescents, with or without disabilities, to be self-directed learners having personal control of their life, curricula which target at enhancing the components of self-determination mentioned above can be infused into the general curriculum so that all students may benefit. In addition, inclusion of youth with disabilities in mainstream education is a global trend. Deliberate infusion of self-determination instruction and development into the general curriculum will allow students with disabilities to have access to the intervention in the inclusive classrooms (54).

STRATEGIES TO PROMOTING SELF-DETERMINATION

Theoretical approaches like SDT, functional theory and ecological models all consider the social context as an important factor in facilitating or undermining self-determination. School is a significant social context where self-determination of students can be fostered as strength. Promoting self-determination should be a primary educational goal for all students, with or without disabilities (48). SDT posits that students are better able to internalize their motivation and engage in self-regulated learning when their psychological needs for autonomy, competence and relatedness are supported in their school environments. It is pertinent to provide students with opportunities to learn and apply skills to become self-regulated learners.

Ways to facilitate self-determination skills through education programmes

Adolescents, with or without disabilities, will benefit from intentional interventions which promote self-determination (1,47).

Self-determination as a psychological and positive youth development   463

Students can be taught systematically to develop self-determination skills through schools' guidance programmes, life education programmes, or individual learning programmes for students with disabilities and special needs. The curricula which target at enhancing self-determination skills may include activities to develop skills in goal setting, planning, evaluating and monitoring, and choice making.

The curriculum units on self-determination of the Project P.A.T.H.S. are an example of developing self-determination skills systematically through a formal educational curriculum (57).

In addition, learning tasks can be structured to encourage exploration of possibilities, reasonable risk taking, and problem solving. Further, activities which target at enhancing students' self-esteem and self-confidence, appreciation of their strengths and knowledge of their limitations, and promoting self-advocacy will further facilitate students' self-understanding and communication. Through learning the self-regulatory skills of decision making, problem solving and action planning, students' personal control over their learning is likely to increase. They are better able to apply self-determination skills to their personal goals, and become more autonomous learners and self-determined persons (54).

In addition, schools can promote self-determination through integrating the components of self-determination skills into the general curriculum, with emphasis on helping students to apply self-determination skills in identifying personal goals, action planning and evaluating.

Such intentional efforts to promote self-determination is very much in line with the rationale of positive youth development, that is, helping all students to build assets and strengths, leading to the benefits of reduction in at risk behaviour.

Ways to promote autonomous supportive environments

Research studies have shown that students' perceived autonomy support in the classrooms leads to more positive academic outcomes (11). Students who find their learning environment supportive of their needs for competence, autonomy and relatedness will have greater engagement in learning, which exert influence on their psychological adjustment (19). Teachers who are autonomy-supportive also experience a greater personal achievement, psychological needs satisfaction and well-being and less emotional strain (27). A student-directed learning environment where students feel respected and connected with their teachers and peers will lead to a satisfaction of the need for relatedness.

Research studies have demonstrated that the following strategies are important in promoting an autonomous supportive classroom environment, which help nurture students' inner motivational resources (27,54). First, teachers may consider, incorporate and prioritize students' perspectives in learning activities, welcome students' ways of feeling, thinking and acting, and accept that students are capable of autonomous self-regulation and setting personal goals. This will mean that teachers need to find ways to engage students' interests and to introduce tasks that will challenge their competence. Second, it is important to provide explanations and rationales why certain behaviour is worth engaging in so as to facilitate students' internalization and increase their effort to engage. It is also important to make reference to the benefits of self-development (i.e. intrinsic goals) rather than social image, financial success (i.e. extrinsic goals) when asking students to follow their request. Third, provision of a structure and guidance such as classroom expectations, and positive feedback are pertinent in helping students see the association between their behaviour and the outcomes. Fourth, teachers should create conditions in which students learn to take risks, make choices, and evaluate their choices and actions (54). Fifth, patience and trust are necessary in allowing students to learn at their own pace. This will require teachers to listen to students' perspectives, to offer help when students' get stuck, to encourage students' initiatives and to provide time for self-paced learning. Sixth, accepting students' negative emotions and affects, letting students feel that teachers genuinely like, respect, and value them will enhance the students' relationship with teachers, which are critical in satisfying their psychological needs for relatedness as postulated by SDT. Lastly, provision of peer support to help foster supportive relationships and having peers as well as teachers to act as role models is critical for fostering self-determination.

FURTHER DIRECTION FOR RESEARCH AND PRACTICE IN SELF-DETERMINATION

Chamber, Wehmeyer, Saito, Lida, Lee and Singh (42) point to the following four areas which need further research and practice for promoting self-determination. First, in the area of teacher training and support, there is a need to prepare teachers to acquire knowledge and skills in attending to the psychological needs of their students' for competence, relatedness and autonomy, the component skills of self-determination, and the instruction strategies to foster an autonomy-supportive classroom environment and facilitate students to be self-regulated learners. This will have implications for teacher education training at both pre-service and in-service levels. Further research can be directed at examining the needs and competency of teachers in promoting self-determination. Second, there is a need to have systematic implementation strategies in schools. While self-determination skills and components can be taught through specialized programmes, integrating these curriculum packages with the general curriculum has the advantage of providing access to students with or without disabilities. Such curriculum infusion has the benefit of promoting self-determination as a whole-school approach to guidance for the whole-person development of all students (58). Further research may examine the effectiveness of the infusion of self-determination in academic curriculum. Third, parental involvement in promoting self-determination is needed, since an autonomous parental attitude relates to children's adjustment at school (23). Strategies in promoting self-regulated learning and an autonomy-supportive environment can be disseminated to parents via workshops, seminars, and school-home collaboration projects. In addition, component skills in self-determination, such as having children identify goals, action planning and evaluating can be introduced to parents. Research can further examine the effectiveness of this form of family involvement. Lastly, as self-determination is a developmental task, the promotion of self-determination skills needs to begin early in primary schools.

REFERENCES

[1]   Nota L, Soresi S, Ferrari L, Wehmeyer ML. A multivariate analysis of the self-determination of adolescents. J Happiness Stud 2011;12:245-66.

[2]   Deci EL, Ryan RM. The "what" and "why of goal pursuits: human needs and the self-determination of behavior. Psychol Inq 2000;11(4):227-68.

[3]   Chirkov VI. A cross-cultural analysis of autonomy in education: a self-determination theory perspective. Theory Res Educ 2009;7:253-62.

[4]   Deci EL, Ryan RM. Intrinsic motivation and self-determination in human behavior. New York: Plenum, 1985.

[5]   Wehmeyer ML. Self-determination and individuals with severe disabilities: re-examining meanings and misinterpretations. Res Pract Persons Severe Disabl 2005;30:113-20.

[6]   Field S, Martin J, Miller E, Ward M, Wehmeyer M. A practical guide for teaching self-determination. Reston, VA: Council for Exceptional Children, 1998.

[7]   Catalano RF, Berglund ML, Ryan JAM, Lonczak HS, Hawkins JD. Positive youth development in the United States: research findings on evaluations of positive youth development programs. Ann Am Acad Pol Soc Sci 2004;591:98-124.

[8]   Seligman MEP, Csikszentmihalyi M. Positive psychology: an introduction. Am Psychol 2000;55:5-14.

[9]   Soenens B, Vansteenkiste M. Antecedents and outcomes of self-determination in 3 life domains: the role of parents' and teachers' autonomy support. J Youth Adolesc 2005;34(6):589-604.

[10]   Bao XH, Lam SF. Who makes the choice? Rethinking the role of autonomy and relatedness in Chinese children's motivation. Child Dev 2008;79(2):269-83.

[11]   Niemiec CP, Ryan RM. Autonomy, competence, and relatedness in the classroom: applying self-determination theory to educational practice. Theory Res Educ 2009;7:133-44.

[12]   Guay F, Ratelle CF, Chanal J. Optimal learning in optimal contexts: the role of self-determination in education. Can Psychol 2008;49(3):233-40.

[13]   Reeve JM. Self-determination theory applied to educational settings. In: Deci EL, Ryan RM. Handbook of self-determination research. New York, Rochester: University of Rochester Press, 2002:183-203.

[14]   Vansteenkiste M, Zhou M, Lens W, Soenens B. Experiences of autonomy and control among Chinese learners: vitalizing or immobilizing? J Educ Psychol 2005;97(3):468-83.

[15]   Deci EL, Schwartz AJ, Sheinman L, Ryan RM. An instrument to assess adults' orientations toward control versus autonomy with children: reflections on intrinsic motivation and perceived competence. J Educ Psychol 1981;73:642-50.

[16]   Tsai Y, Kunter M, Lüdtke O, Trautwein U, Ryan RM. What makes lessons interesting? The role of situational and individual factors in three school subjects. J Educ Psychol 2008;100:460-72.

[17]   Ryan RM, Deci EL. Self-determination theory and the facilitation of intrinsic motivation, social development, and well-being. Am Psychol 2000;55(1):68-78.

[18]   Vallerand RJ, Bissonnette R. Intrinsic, extrinsic, and amotivational styles as predictors of behavior: a prospective study. J Pers 1992;60:599-620.

[19]   Van Ryzin MJ, Gravely AA, Roseth CJ. Autonomy, belongingness, and engagement in school as contributors to adolescent psychological well-being. J Youth Adolesc 2009;38:1-12.

[20]   Grolnick WS. The psychology of parental control: how well-meant parenting backfires. Mahwah, NJ: Erlbaum, 2002.

[21]   Ryan RM, Deci EL, Grolnick WS. Autonomy relatedness, and the self: their relation to development and psychopathology. In: Cicchetti D, Cohen DJ. Developmental psychopathology Vol.1. theory and methods. Wiley Series on Personality Processes. Oxford: Willey, 1995:618-55.

[22]   Ryan RM, Solky JA. What is supportive about social support? On the psychological needs for autonomy and relatedness. In: Pierce GR, Sarason BR, Sarason IG. Handbook of social support and the family. New York: Plenum, 1996:249-67.

[23]   Joussemet M, Landry R, Koestner R. A self-determination theory perspective on parenting. Can Psychol 2008;49(3):194-200.

[24] Grolnick WS. The role of parents in facilitating autonomous self-regulation for education. Theory Res Educ 2009;7(2):164-73.

[25] d'Ailly H. Children's autonomy and perceived control in learning: a model of motivation and achievement in Taiwan. J Educ Psychol 2003;95:84-96.

[26] Sierens E, Vansteenkiste M, Goossens L, Soenens B, Dochy F. The synergistic relationship of perceived autonomy support and structure in the prediction of self-regulated learning. Br J Educ Psychol 2009;79:57-68.

[27] Reeve JM, Halusic M. How K-12 teachers can put self-determination theory principles into practice. Theory Res Educ 2009;7(2):145-54.

[28] Black AE, Deci EL. The effects of instructors' autonomy support and students' autonomous motivation on learning organic chemistry: a self-determination theory perspective. Sci Educ 2000;84:740-56.

[29] Chirkov VI, Ryan RM, Kim Y, Kaplan U. Differentiating autonomy from individualism and independence: a self-determination theory perspective on internalization of cultural orientations and well-being. J Pers Soc Psychol 2003;84(1):97-110.

[30] Triandis HC. Individualism and collectivism. Boulder, CO: Westview, 1995.

[31] Markus HR, Kitayama S. Cultural and the self: implications for cognition, emotion, and motivation. Psychol Rev 1991;98:224-53.

[32] Cross SE, Gore JS. Cultural models of the self. In: Leary MR, Tangney JP. Handbook of self and identity. New York: The Guilford Press, 2003:536–64.

[33] Iyengar SS, Leeper MR. Rethinking the value of choice: a cultural perspective on intrinsic motivation. J Pers Soc Psychol, 1999;76:349-66.

[34] Hui EKP, Sun RCF, Chow SSY, Chu MHT. Exploring Chinese students' academic motivation: filial piety and self-determination. Educ Psychol 2011;31(3):377-92.

[35] Wehmeyer ML, Abery BH, Zhang D, Ward K, Willis D, Hossain W, et al. Personal self-determination and moderating variables that impact efforts to promote self-determination. Exceptionality 2011;19:19-30.

[36] Abery BH, Stancliffe RJ. The ecology of self-determination. In: Sands DJ, Wehmeyer ML. Self-determination across the life span: independence and choice for people with disabilities. Baltimore, MD: Paul H. Brookes, 1996:111-45.

[37] Carter EW, Lane KL, Pierson MR, Stang KK. Promoting self-determination for transition-age youth: views of high school general and special educators. Except Child 2008;75(1):55-70.

[38] Wehmeyer ML, Palmer SB, Shogren K, Williams-Diehm K, Soukup JH. Establishing a causal relationship between intervention to promote self-determination and enhanced student self-determination. J Spec Educ 2010.

[39] Stancliffe R, Abery B, Smith J. Personal control and the ecology of community living settings: beyond living-unit size and type. Ment Retard 2000;105:431-54.

[40] Wehmeyer ML, Garner NW. The impact of personal characteristics of people with intellectual and developmental disability on self-determination and autonomous functioning. J Appl Res Intellect Disabil 2003;16:255-65.

[41] Lee Y, Wehmeyer ML, Palmer SB, Williams-Diehm K, Davies DK, Stock SE. Examining individual and instruction-related predictors of the self-determination of students with disabilities: multiple regression analyses. Rem Spec Educ 2010;31(6):1-12.

[42] Chambers CR, Wehmeyer ML, Saito Y, Lida KM, Lee Y, Singh V. Self-determination: what do we know? Where do we go? Exceptionality 2007;15(1):3-15.

[43] Field S, Sarver MD, Shaw SF. Self-determination: a key to success in postsecondary education for students with learning disabilities. Rem Spec Educ 2003;24(6):339-49.

[44] Field S, Hoffman A. Preparing youth to exercise self-determination: quality indicators of school environments that promote the acquisition of knowledge, skills, and beliefs related to self-determination. J Disabl Policy Stud 2002;13(114):114-9.

[45] Stang KK, Carter EW, Lane KL, Pierson MR. Perspectives of general and special educators on fostering self-determination in elementary and middle schools. J Spec Educ 2009;43:94-106.

[46] McDougall J, Evans J, Baldwin P. The importance of self-determination to perceived quality of life for youth and young adults with chronic conditions and disabilities. Rem Spec Educ 2010;31:252-60.

[47] Bremer CD, Kachgal M, Schoeller K. Self-determination: supporting successful transition. Res Pract Brief 2003;2(1):1-5.

[48] Eisenman LT, Chamberlin M. Implementing self-determination activities: lessons from schools. Rem Spec Educ 2001;22(3):138-47.

[49] Field S, Hoffman A. Steps to self-determination. Austinl, TX: Prof-Ed, 1996.

[50] Field S, Hoffman A. Lessons learned from implementing the steps to self-determination curriculum. Rem Spec Educ 2002;23(2):90-8.

[51] Karvonen M, Test DW, Wood WM, Brower D, Alzozzine B. Putting self-determination into practice. Except Child 2004;71(1):23-41.

[52] Palmer SB, Wehmeyer ML, Gipson K, Agran M. Promoting access to the general curriculum by teaching self-determination skills. Except Child 2004;70(4):427-39.

[53] Wehmeyer ML. Teaching self-determination to students with disabilities: basic skills for successful transition. Baltimore, MD: Brookes, 1998.

[54] Eisenman LY. Self-determination interventions: building a foundation for school completion. Rem Spec Educ 2007;28:2-8.

[55] Field S, Hoffman A, Posch M. Self-determination during adolescence: a developmental perspective. Rem Spec Educ 1997;18(5):285-93.

[56] Wehmeyer ML, Palmer S, Agran M, Mithaug D, Martin J. Promoting causal agency: the self-determined learning model of instruction. Except Child 2000;66:439-53.

[57] Hui EKP, Tsang SKM. Self-determination as a positive youth construct: conceptual bases and implications for curriculum development. In: Shek DTL, Ma HK, Merrick, J. Positive youth development: development of a pioneering program in a chinese context. Tel Aviv: Freund, 2007:193-200.

[58] Hui EKP. Guiding students for positive development. In: Zhang LF, Biggs J, Watkins D. Learning and development of Asian students: what the 21st century teacher needs to think about. Singapore: Prentice Hall, 2010:221-44.

Submitted: October 05, 2011. *Revised:* November 17, 2011. *Accepted:* December 04, 2011.

In: Alternative Medicine Research Yearbook 2012
Editors: Søren Ventegodt and Joav Merrick

ISBN: 978-1-62808-080-3
© 2013 Nova Science Publishers, Inc.

Chapter 44

POSITIVE IDENTITY AS A POSITIVE YOUTH DEVELOPMENT CONSTRUCT: A CONCEPTUAL REVIEW

Sandra KM Tsang, PhD, FHKPS, CPsych, RSW, RCP (HKPS)[1], Eadaoin KP Hui, PhD, FHKPS, CPsychol (BPS)[2], And Bella CM Law, BSocSc[1]*

[1]Department of Social Work and Social Administration,
The University of Hong Kong, Hong Kong, PRC
[2]Faculty of Education, The University of Hong Kong, Hong Kong, PRC

ABSTRACT

Identity is a core construct in psychology because it refers to how a person addresses issues dealing with who that person is. Important theorists studying the concept of identity, like Erikson, Marcia, and Higgins, assert that identity is organized, learned, and dynamic, and a subjective evaluation of an individual's identity has emotional consequences for that individual. Adolescents who can cultivate a clear and positive identity after their developmental struggles during adolescence often advance more smoothly into adulthood. This paper reviews literature on the nature and structure of identity, and examines its importance on adolescent developmental outcomes. It traces significant determinants of identity and proposes strategies for cultivation of positive identity. Observations on current research gaps in the study of identity and future research directions will also be discussed.

Keywords: Identity formation, identity statuses, dimensions of identity formation, self-esteem

---

* Correspondence: Sandra KM Tsang, PhD, Reg ClinPsy and FHKPS, CPsy (BPS), BSS, RSW, Head, Department of Social Work and Social Administration, The University of Hong Kong, Hong Kong, PRC. E-mail: sandratsang@hku.hk.

INTRODUCTION

Within the field of psychology, the nature and development of identity and related concepts like self and self-identity have attracted voluminous research over many decades. Studies began with Freud's early writings and were popularized by Erikson's theoretical expositions. Since the 1960's, Marcia's empirical operationalization of the concept has led other contemporary theorists like Higgins(1), Berzonsky et al (2), Grotevant (3) to develop it further. According to the PsycInfo database, in the 20 years from 1985 to 2004, there were over 72,000 studies on the topic. Review of such literature suggests that identity is an important social science concept. There are structural and process components in identity. Structurally, identity can be meaningfully organized into general, physical, psychological, social, and spiritual domains. Identity formation also involves dynamic processes as identity evolves along with a person's development throughout their life span. Identity is amenable to extrapersonal influences like environmental changes and life experiences as well as intrapersonal identity processes, including exploration, commitment, and reconsideration. There is also evidence that gender, age and culture patterns at different times affect the development of identity.

Adolescence is a developmental stage characterized by rapid and extensive physical and psychosocial changes which often present developmental crises that challenge the adolescent's coping ability. Successful coping culminates in the formation of a clear and positive identity that can facilitate future development and productive use of personal resources. Problematic coping might make the person vulnerable to emotional and behavioral problems. How adolescents address what they experience in adolescence to formulate their identity has a pivotal impact on their subsequent life journeys.

DEFINITION OF IDENTITY

Identity basically refers to how a person answers the question "Who am I?". Sharma and Sharma (4) said "Identity is an umbrella term used throughout the social sciences to describe an individual's comprehension of him or herself as a discrete, separate entity" (p.119). Psychologists most commonly use the term "identity" to describe "personal identity" or the idiosyncratic things that make a person unique. For example, Grotevant (3) defined identity as the "distinctive combination of personality characteristics and social style by which one defines oneself and by which one is recognized by others" (p.1119). Cognitive psychologists tend to focus on the awareness of self and the capacity for self-regulation, while sociologists examine social identity and role behavior.

Erikson (5) and subsequent researchers (e.g. Ashmore and Jussin (6); Misra (7); Thoits (8)) conceptualized identity as individual versus societal level phenomena. At the individual level, they differentiated amongst "I" (self/identity as knower/subject/process), "Me" (self as known/object/structure) and "Self" ("the self", "selves/identities" and "self-esteem") (8). At the societal level, Misra (7) emphasized the important role of culture in constructing the structure and processes of self. Others (e.g. Hardie et al (9); Thoits and Virshup (10)) also tried to explore the connections between personal identities (similar to self-concept), role/relational identities (definition of self in a particular role in an interactional context) and social/collective identities (identification of self with a social group, culture or category).

Identities have also been conceptualized as blocks that build up the global, unified self-concept that enables a person to function with coherence (11). The development of clear and positive identity/identities involves building self-esteem, facilitating exploration of and commitment to self-definition, reducing self-discrepancies, and fostering role formation and achievement.

THEORIES ON IDENTITY

Following the individual and social concepts of identity, there are theories addressing these two levels, as well as theories defining the structure and dynamics of identity development.

Erikson's identity theory

Erikson (5) is the most prominent theorist to draw attention to the nature and development of identity. He proposed an eight-stage progression of human development over the human life span: infancy, early childhood, childhood, puberty, adolescence, early adulthood, middle adulthood, and late adulthood. Each stage is marked by a psychosocial crisis that involves confronting a fundamental question. The stages are described in terms of alternative traits that are potential outcomes from each crisis. Development is enhanced when a crisis is resolved in favour of the healthy alternative. In the adolescence stage, an identity crisis occurs when adolescents seriously question their essential personal characteristics, their views of themselves, their concerns about how others view them, or their doubts about the meaning and purpose of their existence. The outcome could be either healthy and coherent identity formation or identity confusion. He also postulated that identity can be examined at the ego, personal, and

Erikson's theory established a foundation for research on ego, identity development, and intervention models. Since then, studies on identity have expanded to include a consideration of individual differences; the search for, discovery of, and utilization of innate potentials; critical problem-solving skills; social responsibility; integrity of character; and the impact of social and cultural contexts on identity formation and development (12).

Marcia's identity status theory

Marcia (13,14) popularized Erikson's construct of identity by proposing four identity statuses (identity diffusion, foreclosure, moratorium, and identity achievement) as possible outcomes of identity formation. She also proposed two dimensions, namely exploration and commitment, which influence identity formation. Exploration refers to a process of actively questioning and searching for adult roles and values in the various domains of adolescent life. Commitment refers to firm decisions regarding aspects such as vocation, political ideology, religion, and social roles, and includes specific strategies for achieving personal goals and a

472   *Sandra KM Tsang, Eadaoin KP Hui and Bella CM Law*

desired life path. Identity diffusion is a status in which exploration has not occurred nor has any commitment been made. Foreclosure denotes the status when commitment has been made but is not supported by adequate exploration. Moratorium refers to an active exploration of identity with weak commitment, possibly trying on several different masks at the same time. Identity achievement is the status in which the individual has explored his or her identity potential fruitfully and can now commit to a particular identity. Diffusion is often considered the least adaptive status (15).

Subsequent research (16,17) not only provided strong support for the four-status model, but also allowed exploration to be separated into two types: in-depth exploration and reconsideration. In-depth exploration refers to the extent to which adolescents actively assess the merits of their current choices of commitment, either by themselves or in consultation with significant others. Reconsideration of commitment refers to comparing present commitments with possible alternative commitments. In-depth exploration was found to correlate positively with agreeableness, conscientiousness and openness to experience (16). However, it may also contribute to negative consequences such as having an unclear self-concept, coupled with emotional instability. Reconsideration evokes short term costs as it creates uncertainties and holds up progress, and adolescents stuck in this process might exhibit emotional or behavioral problems. But reconsideration should have a long term positive effect as global contexts are changing rapidly and constant adjustment should be an essential strategy for achievement, or even survival. An example cited by Crocetti (16) involved an Italian college freshman who left his home town for study. He expressed the need to find another best friend in his current context even though he had a very good friend in his home town because he needed social support nearby! This freshman is committed to his existing friendship, but has new needs or even anxieties arising from his new environment, and is thus reconsidering strategic alternatives in order to optimize his condition. Examples like this one clearly illustrate that this additional concept of reconsideration has enriched the identity formation model by taking it from being more linear to being more cyclical.

Higgins's self-discrepancy theory

Instead of centering on the individual, Higgins' self-discrepancy theory (1) focuses on the discrepancies between three self domains and two standpoints on the self. The three self-domains are i) actual self - how a person or others see the attributes that the person possesses; ii) ideal self - the attributes that a person or others would like the person to possess; iii) ought self - the attributes that the person or others think the person should possess. The two standpoints on the self are (i) a person's own and (ii) significant others' (such as parents and teachers) sets of attitudes or values that can be judged. The self-domains and the standpoints on the self can be combined and used to generate six self-state representations: actual/own, actual/other, ideal/own, ideal/other, ought/own, and ought/other. The nature and the scale of the discrepancies between the different types of self-states affect the person's emotional vulnerabilities (18). For example, discrepancies between the actual/own and ideal/own self-states are associated with disappointment and dissatisfaction; discrepancies between the actual/own and ideal/other self-states are associated with shame, embarrassment or feeling downcast; discrepancies between actual/own and ought/other self-states are associated with fear and feeling threatened; and discrepancies between actual/own and ought/own self-states are associated with feelings of moral worthlessness or weakness. However, some discrepancy is inevitable during the search for and the development of identity, and Higgins has proposed strategies to relieve the painful experiences arising from such struggles, such as changing one's actual/own self-concept or self-guides so that they are less discrepant from one another, or changing the accessibility of the discrepancies (1).

Theory of possible selves

The youngest and perhaps most promising member of the so-called "Self Family" in psychological studies aimed at understanding people's behavior is the notion of Possible Selves. Possible Selves represent those elements of the self-concept that individuals could become, would like to become, or are afraid of becoming (19).

The latter is also known as Fear Possible Selves. Empirical research has supported the idea that Possible Selves could be self-regulatory and can serve as road maps for one's behavior. Oyserman and Fryberg (20) reported studies linking increased numbers of positive Possible Selves with a reduced risk of substance use and sexual activity. In addition, Sun and Shek (21) showed that adolescents are less likely to engage in problem behavior when they have a sense of purpose and meaning in life. Exploring Possible Selves among youths in Hong Kong provides researchers, practitioners and policy planners with a helpful way to understand our young people, and sheds light on the development of prevention and intervention programmes that target youths who may be or are affected by drug use and other at risk behaviors.

Identity style theory

The increasing focus on social-cognitive variables generated much interest in studying the role that identity processing styles play in adolescent identity generation. Benzonsky's Identity Style Model postulates that three processing styles can be depicted in adolescent identity formation (22,23). The informational style involves the active searching and evaluation of identity relevant information. The normative style refers to the adherence to conventions, and dependence on the expectations and feedback of significant others when confronted with identity issues. Last but not least, the diffuse-avoidant style denotes a tendency to procrastination in the handling of identity issues. Individual cognitive, social and psychological variables like personality have been found to have an influence on such identity styles (23,24), and the studies have now expanded to examining how significant others like family members (25), teachers and peers affect the establishment and maintenance of such styles.

ASSESSMENT OF IDENTITY

There are at least five aspects of assessing identity: levels and domains of identity, identity statuses, identity dimensions, identity styles, and progressive developmental shifts in identity during its development.

Levels and domains of identity

Identity can be assessed on both a personal level and a social level. Global identity is conceived to be made up of identity in different domains such as physical appearance, athletic competence, scholastic competence, social acceptance, behavioral conduct, and global self-worth (26). Different scales, including culture-specific ones, have been developed to measure specific and global identity. For example, Cheng and Watkins(27) constructed the Chinese Adolescent Self-Esteem Scales (CASES) to assess the self-esteem of Chinese adolescents in terms of seven aspects: social, academic, appearance, moral, family, physical/sport, and general self-esteem.

Identity statuses

According to Meeus (17), identity development can end up in one of four possible identity statuses: diffusion, foreclosure, moratorium, and identity achievement. Each of these statuses can also be examined in connection with other psychosocial outcome correlates, such as psychological well-being, quality of life, identity congruity or discrepancies, strategies and skills in problem-solving and coping, and self-regulation abilities. Quantitative and qualitative methods (like the Identity Status interview) have been devised to assess such statuses (28).

Identity dimensions

In line with the two-dimensional model of identity formation, the Utrecht-Groningen Identity Development Scale (U-GIDS) (17) includes two subscales to assess the two identity dimensions: commitment and in-depth exploration. With emerging evidence of a three-dimensional model of identity, a new exploration scale, reconsideration, was added to form the Utrecht-Management of Identity Commitments Scale (U-MICS) (16).

Identity styles

Based on the Identity Style Model, Berzonsky developed and fine-tuned the Identity Style Inventory, Revised (ISI3) (29), which used 5-point Likert-type items to measure the informational, normative, and diffuse styles. The scales include 11, 9 and 10 items respectively and their internal consistency was around .70.

Developmental shifts in identity

Active attempts were made to capture the dynamic evolutions in identity formation, development, and possible shifts between different identity statuses. Klimstra, Hale III, Raaijmakers, Branje and Meeus(30) conducted a five-wave longitudinal study of 923 early to middle adolescents and 390 middle to late adolescents that provides a comprehensive understanding of change and stability in identity formation in adolescence. Three types of change and stability (mean-level change, rank-order stability, and profile stability) were assessed according to the three-dimension model of identity (commitment, in-depth exploration, and reconsideration). The study is robust in its large sample size, elaborate research design, psychometric specificity and the strength of the measures used, and its sharpness in addressing theoretical postulations. The study has opened up new frontiers in identity assessment and research. It has revealed that there are changes in identity dimensions towards maturity and there is a progressive change in the way that adolescents deal with commitments.

ANTECEDENTS/DETERMINANTS
OF ADOLESCENT IDENTITY

The development of identity is a life-long process, and people at different stages of life have different identities. Stage theories of psychosocial development (e.g. Erikson's psychosocial development theory of 1968 (5), Freud's psychosexual development theory in the 1950s (31)) emphasized that human development proceeds along stages that follow the same sequential order in all people. Each stage is identified by specific developmental characteristics and tasks. Successful achievement of the task in a stage (e.g. feeling securely taken care of during the most vulnerable infancy stage; achieving a clear identity during the identity-searching adolescent stage) will provide adaptive foundational resources for progression into, and successful achievement of, the tasks in the following stages. Conversely, having stumbled in an early stage predicts fewer resources and less chance for success in dealing with the tasks encountered in subsequent stages (e.g. suffering deprivation or abuse in the dependent early childhood years will make a person untrusting of others and difficult to get along with in adulthood). Identity development is particularly vigorous in adolescence (32,33) and the resultant identity status naturally lays the foundation for adulthood development. In identity development, individual factors such as age, gender, physical health and appearance, intelligence, and social skills all cast significant influence on a person's real and perceived identity. Healthy, good looking, intelligent and sociable children can more readily engage support to help them excel in actual performance, self-esteem and even social attractiveness. Regarding the impact of age and maturity on identity, the large-scale five-wave longitudinal study of changes in adolescent identity formation by Klimstra et al (30) found that older adolescents who become more mature with age show decreases in reconsideration, increases in in-depth exploration, and increasingly stable identity dimension profiles. How adolescents deal with commitments has more impact on identity formation than the actual changes in the commitments themselves. Grotevant (3) found that teenagers have more conflicts with their parents in early adolescence and fewer conflicts as they grow into late adolescence because both parents and adolescents understand each other better when the adolescents have a clearer identity.

Studies on gender differences consistently show that in early adolescence girls are normally more mature than boys with respect to identity formation, while boys catch up by late adolescence (30). Gilligan (34,35) pointed out that females define themselves in terms of relationships with other people while males define themselves through achievements (36).

Kling et al (37) found that males had higher self-esteem than females, and that the peak difference was at the ages of 15 to 18 years. In Hong Kong, Watkins, Dong and Xia (38) also found older adolescent girls tend to report significantly lower self-esteem than younger girls and older boys, especially in the areas of physical abilities, reading, mathematics, and general self-concept.

Aside from examining the stages of development and individual characteristics, the Social Development Theory also draws attention to the importance of the risk and protective factors of an individual's significant others in the individual's identity development (39).

There are risk and protective factors in each type of significant others, specifically in the family, school, peers, the community, and the internet in contemporary societies where global information and cyber relationships can be easily accessed. Surveys on Chinese families with adolescents in Hong Kong (40,41) involving samples of over 1,000 adolescent respondents have found that fathers have a stronger influence on the development of their children's self-esteem than mothers, especially in the case of daughters. In Youngblade, Theokas, Schulenberg, Curry, Huang and Novak's large-scale study on the risk and promotive factors of positive youth development in schools, families and communities, it was found that each of these sectors harbour some characteristics conducive to positive youth development (42). Affective and abundant family communication, clear rules about watching television and a healthy parental role model produced healthy youth behavior. Family conflict and aggression posed the risk of causing identity confusion and behavior problems in young people (43). School and community safety were related to higher social competence and decreased externalizing behavior. School violence resulted in a risk of more internalizing and externalizing behavior, poorer academic performance and lower self-esteem. In their attempt to explore the roles personality, identity styles and family functioning play in influencing youth identity, Dunkel, Papini and Berzonsky (25) found that it was personality, instead of family functioning, that accounted more for significant variations in informational and diffuse-avoidant identity style scores. For normative identity style scores, both personality and family functioning were influential.

Regarding cultural determinants of identity, patriarchal societies like most Asian countries still show a more obvious preference for boys, while also harboring higher expectations for boys to achieve, not just for individual merits but also for collective esteem.

Spencer-Rodgers et al (44) found that Chinese and Asian Americans exhibit greater ambivalence towards self-evaluation than do Chinese and Asians from synthesis-oriented cultures. They concluded that identity development varies between Eastern collectivistic cultures and Western individualistic ones. However, with increased globalization and population movement (45), the growth of racial minorities in different societies (16), and handy connections through the internet (46), the continuing validity of this East-West collective-individualistic dichotomy will need to be evaluated.

In addition, with increased attention being paid to multiple intelligences instead of mainly academic achievements, cultural expectations and their impact on identity formation and success has become much more complicated.

ADOLESCENT IDENTITY AND DEVELOPMENTAL OUTCOMES

Meeus has proposed four possible identity outcome statuses, including diffusion, foreclosure, moratorium and identity achievement, with the last being the healthiest of the four statuses (17).

Specifically, an individual's identity profile (strengths and weaknesses across the different identity domains), identity status (including the interplay of exploration and commitment; and the magnitude of discrepancies between real and ideal self) and the ability of that individual to effect necessary improvement to his or her identity development, all have an impact on the immediate positive and negative aspects of the individual's well-being. In addition, it will affect one's long term development into adulthood and the future stages of one's life span.

Positive indicators include self-esteem, life satisfaction, positive affect, quality of life, environmental mastery, positive relations with others like parents (2), teachers and peers, and self-acceptance. Negative indicators include internalizing pathology like stress, depression, and anxiety, as well as externalizing pathological behavior like hostility, aggression, loss of control and disruptive behaviour (4,45). Many such indicators are included as positive youth development constructs in Project P.A.T.H.S., a positive youth development program developed and validated for Chinese adolescents (47).

PROMOTION OF THE DEVELOPMENT OF POSITIVE IDENTITY

The enhancement of positive identity development in young people can be achieved at both the individual and the social levels. Catalano, a researcher on positive youth development programs, conceptualized positive youth identity as "the internal organization of a coherent sense of self" (p.106) (48). He found that "positive identity" was treated as a core construct in nine out of 25 effective positive youth development programs. Specific strategies adopted by these programs to enhance positive identity include:

1. Promoting self-esteem

According to Harter (49), one's evaluation of oneself, often called self-esteem, can influence identity formation and the emotions and performance related to it. Positive self-evaluation typically energizes a person while negative self-evaluation, especially when it is prolonged and hinges upon attributes that cannot be easily changed or acquired, can disturb a person's emotions and performance.

Borba's Esteem Builders curriculum is one of the most comprehensive and widely used skills-based curricula (50). Its theoretical framework is inspired by Branden (51) who defined self-esteem as "the disposition to experience oneself as competent to cope with the basic challenges of life and as worthy of happiness."(p.27).

Borba emphasized five acquired components of authentic self-esteem: (a) security, the feeling of strong assuredness; (b) selfhood, the feeling of self-worth and accurate identity; (c) affiliation, the feeling of belonging and social acceptance; (d) mission, the feeling of purpose; and (e) competence, the feeling of self-empowerment and efficacy. In Hong Kong, the Tung Wah Group of Hospitals indigenized Borba's Esteem Builder curriculum in 1993 and developed programs for use in schools from preschools to secondary schools (52,53).

The Project P.A.T.H.S. developed to enhance positive youth development also built on Borba's model by working on the key components of self-esteem enhancement and identity exploration. The aim is to enhance junior secondary school students' skills in recognizing their self-image, reducing self-discrepancies, and increasing positive self-talk.

The curriculum will also use societal expectations of appropriate gender roles and identity to sharpen gender-sensitive discussions. Skills taught include positive self-evaluation, assertiveness affirmation skills, and understanding and dealing with social expectations and undue negative comments.

2. Fostering exploration and commitment

According to Marcia's identity status theory (13), adolescents have to decide upon their own roles through experiences that expose them to opportunities and situations that challenge how they understand and manage such experiences. Their struggles and exploration through this exposure will promote a more in-depth and multi-angled appraisal of their experience, build up their stress-coping abilities, and advance their problem-solving efficiency and effectiveness. Reconsiderations in the light of new circumstances can also help to refine and clarify their identity. Clarity of identity through such exploration creates the platform for identity commitment(54), and will help the adolescents build the maturity and competence needed to master further life transitions (32,55).

3. Reducing self-discrepancies

During the process of identity search, adolescents often encounter discrepancies between their ideal self, real self, self-perceived self, and their self as perceived by others, or discrepancies between personal and social identities. Such discrepancies will expose adolescents to increased psychosocial risks like emotional and behavioral problems. By identifying the nature and magnitude of such discrepancies, steps can be taken to reduce these disturbing discrepancies, reinforce identity clarity and commitment, and even promote self-esteem (1,32).

Aside from working directly on the individuals themselves, effective management of risk and protective contextual determinants is also important for fostering positive identity.

Traditionally, schools and families are the two most influential developmental contexts for adolescents who normally live at home and study in schools. The physical and psychosocial environments at home and school, the resources of those entities, the opportunities they provide, the support and recognition they give to the youths, together with their rules and values all influence the identity development of the youths.

Schools and families exist in specific cultural and sub-cultural contexts, and the characteristics of such, like gender role expectations, religiosity, and achievement expectations, also release positive or negative energies that influence identity development. In recent decades, penetration of adolescents' daily lives by the media and the internet has enabled young people to access local and global, as well as factual and virtual contexts. In urbanized cities like Hong Kong, young people can command greater information technology than their parents and even their teachers, making it very difficult for adults to provide appropriate guidance to the young(56). The virtual environment enables the manipulation of made-up identities for explorative social interactions. How to keep such "exploration" within functional and adaptive limits is certainly a challenge to information-technology-driven modern life styles. An effective use of such channels should be able to prepare adolescents better to go through their adolescence and be best prepared for adulthood.

RESEARCH GAPS AND FUTURE RESEARCH DIRECTIONS

Since the inception of the concept of identity by fore-runners in psychology, the concept has attracted numerous studies along the following themes:

- The nature and structure of identity, and how to achieve accurate description and assessment.
- Identity formation, including understanding the nature and magnitude of changes in the identity statuses, as well as changes in separate identity dimensions(30).
- Connections between identity, identity dimensions, identity statuses and possible selves, and health, success and well-being.
- Identity management through self, and significant others, and risk and protective contexts

In terms of research methodology, there were formerly limitations to the sample sizes, the duration of research projects, and data collection methods.

In recent years, there has been an expansion from cross-sectional self-report paper-and-pencil quantitative studies to the inclusion of multi-wave longitudinal studies with multi-method data collection in order to test models on how, when and why progressive identity changes take place (e.g. Klimstra et al (30)).

In addition to studies on individual identity, there are also an increasing number of studies on social identity, and useful new themes include (a) symptoms appraisal, (b) health-related norms and behavior, (c) social support, (d) coping, and (e) clinical outcomes (4,57). These help to fill gaps in the research subject areas. There is increased attention given to age, gender and cultural influences. Instead of singling out adolescence as "the" most critical stage in identity development in a life span, there is also an expanded interest in studying emerging adulthood (the lives of people from their late teens to their mid to late 20s in industrialized societies) (58,59).

In view of the increasing geographical and internet-based globalization(46), pressures in changing education systems (60), economic conditions and vocational prospects for young people, it is important that future identity studies be anchored even more firmly on specific reality situations.

Examples include examining whether or not internet-surfing has really created barrier-free access for people with physical disabilities; how people who use fake identities on the internet to create their social networks benefit or suffer from such fluid and real/unreal identities; and identity evolution where people live and work in different places and encounter diverse ethnicities and cultures.

CONCLUSION

Adolescents are the future masters of society. A clear and well-developed identity and favorable self-esteem promises positive development throughout adolescence and even across a whole life span.

As identity is organized, complex, dynamic, and amenable to social influences, it is important to incorporate significant others in the adolescents' ecology in order to provide effective exposure and learning activities and to provide the support necessary (60) for helping adolescents develop a healthy identity.

REFERENCES

[1]   Higgins ET. Self-discrepancy: a theory relating self and affect. Psychol Rev 1987;94(3):319-40.

[2]   Berzonsky MD, Branje SJT, Meeus W. Identity-processing style, psychosocial resources, and adolescents' perceptions of parent-adolescent relations. J Early Adolesc 2007;27(3):324-45.

[3]   Grotevant HD. Adolescent development in family contexts. In: Damon, W, Eisenberg N. Handbook of child psychology Vol. 3. Social, emotional, and personality development. New York: John Wiley, 1998:1097-149.

[4]   Sharma S, Sharma M. Self, social identity and psychological well-being. Psychol Stud 2010;55(2):118-36.

[5]   Erikson EH. Identity, youth, and crisis 1st ed. New York: Norton, 1968.

[6]   Ashmore RD, Jussim L. Towards a second century of the scientific analysis of self and identity. In: Ashmorem RD, Jussim L. Self and identity: fundamental issues Vol. 1. New York: Oxford University Press, 1997:3-19.

[7]   Misra G. Construction of self: a cross-cultural perspective. In: Rao K. Mindscapes. Bangalore: NIMHANS, 2007:32-44.

[8]   Thoits PA. Self, identity, stress and mental health. In: Aneshensel CS, Phelam JC. Handbook of the sociology of mental health. New York: Springer, 1999:345-68.

[9]   Hardie E, Kashima E, Pridmore P. The influence of relational, individual and collective self-aspects on stress, uplifts and health. Self Identity 2005;4:1-24.

[10]   Thoits PA, Virshup LK. Me's and we's: forms and functions of social identities. In: Ashmore RD, Jussim L. Self and identity: fundamental issues Vol. 1. New York: Oxford University Press, 1997: 106-36.

[11]   Stryker S. Symbolic interactionism: a social structure version. CA: Menlo Park, 1980.

[12]   Schwartz SJ. The evolution of Eriksonian and Neo-Eriksonian identity theory and research: a review and integration. Identity: An Int J Theory Res 2001;1(1):7-58.

[13]   Marcia JE. Development and validation of ego-identity status. J Pers Soc Psychol, 1966;3(5):551-8.

[14]   Marcia JE, Waterman AS, Matteson DR, Archer SL, Orlofsky JL. Ego identity: a handbook for psychosocial research. New York: Springer, 1993.

Positive identity as a positive youth development construct

[15] Waterman AS. Identity, the identity statuses, and identity status development: a contemporary statement. Dev Rev 1999;19:591-621.

[16] Crocetti E, Rubini M, Meeus WHJ. Capturing the dynamics of identity formation in various ethnic groups: development and validation of a three-dimensional model. J Adolesc 2008;31:207-22.

[17] Meeus WHJ. Studies on identity development in adolescence: an overview of research and some new data. J Youth Adolesc 1996;25:569-98.

[18] Dweck CS, Higgins ET, Grant-Pillow H. Self-systems give unique meaning to self variables. In: Leary MR, Tangney JP. Handbook of self and identity. New York: Guilford Press, 2003:239-52.

[19] Markus H, Nurius P. Possible selves. Am Psychol, 1986;41(9):954-69.

[20] Oyserman D, Bybee D, Terry K, Hart-Johnson T. Possible selves as roadmaps. J Res Pers 2004;38(2):130-49.

[21] Sun RCF, Shek DTL. Life satisfaction, positive youth development, and problem behavior among Chinese adolescents in Hong Kong. Soc Indic Res 2009;95:455-74.

[22] Berzonsky MD. Self-construction over the life-span: a process perspective on identity formation. In: Neimeyer GJ, Neimeyer RA. Advances in personal construct psychology Vol. 1. CT: Greenwich, 1990:155-86.

[23] Berzonsky MD. Identity processing style, self-construction, and personal epistemic assumptions: a social-cognitive perspective. Eur J Dev Psychol 2004;1:303-15.

[24] Berzonsky MD, Adams GR. Reevaluating the identity status paradigm: still useful after 35 years. Dev Rev 1999;19:557-90.

[25] Dunkel CS, Papini DR, Berzonsky MD. Explaining differences in identity styles: possible roles of personality and family functioning. Identity: An Int J Theory Res 2008;8:349-63.

[26] Harter S. Competence as a dimension of self evaluation: toward a comprehensive model of self-worth. In: Leahy RL. The development of the self. Orlando: Academic Press, 1985:55-121.

[27] Cheng CHK, Watkins D. Age and gender invariance of self-concept factor structure: an investigation of a newly developed Chinese self-concept instrument. Int J Psychol 2000;35(5):186-93.

[28] Marcia JE. Theory and measure: the identity status interview. In: Watzlawik M, Born A. Capturing identity: quantitative and qualitative methods. MD: University Press of America, 2007:1-14.

[29] Berzonsky MD. Identity Style Inventory (ISI3): revised version. Unpublished measure, Cortland: Department of Psychology, State Univ of New York, 1992.

[30] Klimstra TA, Hale III WW, Raaijmakers QAW, Branje SJT, Meeus WHJ. Identity formation in adolescence: change or stability? J Youth Adolesc 2010;39:150-62.

[31] Lerner RM. Concepts and theories of human development, 3rd ed. Mahwah, NJ: Lawrence Erlbaum, 2002.

[32] Finkenauer C, Engels RCME, Meeus W, Oosterwegel A. Self and identity in early adolescence: the pains and gains of knowing who and what you are. In: Brinthaupt TM, Lipka RP. Understanding early adolescent self and identity: applications and interventions. Albany, NY: State Univ New York Press, 2002:25-56.

[33] Kroger J. Identity development: adolescence through adulthood. Thousand Oaks, CA: Sage, 2000.

[34] Gilligan C. In a different voice: psychological theory and women's development. Cambridge, MA: Harvard Univ, 1982.

[35] Gilligan C. In a different voice: psychological theory and women's development. Cambridge, MA: Harvard Univ, 1993.

[36] Josephs RA, Markus HR, Tafarodi RW. Gender and self-esteem. J Pers Soc Psychol 1992;63(3):391-402.

[37] Kling KC, Hyde JS, Showers CJ, Buswell BN. Gender differences in self-esteem: A meta-analysis. Psychol Bull 1999;125(4):470-500.

[38] Watkins D, Dong Q, Xia Y. Age and gender differences in the self-esteem of Chinese children. J Soc Psychol 1997;137(3):374-9.

[39] Hawkins JD, Catalano RF. Investing in your community's youth: an introduction to the communities that care system. 2005. Accessed 2010 May 17. URL:http://download.ncadi.samhsa.gov/Prevl ine/pdfs/ctc/Investing%20in%20Your%20Community's%20Youth.pdf

[40] Tsang SKM. Father-adolescent conflict in Chinese families in Hong Kong. Dissertation. Hong Kong: Univ Hong Kong, 1996.

[41] Shek DTL. Family processes and developmental outcomes in Chinese adolescents. Hong Kong J Pediatr 2004;9:316-24.

[42] Youngblade LM, Theokas C, Schulenberg J, Curry L, Huang I-C, Novak M. Risk and promotive factors in families, schools, and communities: a contextual model of positive youth development in adolescence. Pediatrics 2007;119:S47-53.

[43] Schwartz SJ, Mason CA, Pantin H, Szapocznik J. Effects of family functioning and identity confusion on substance use and sexual behavior in Hispanic Immigrant early adolescents. Identity: An Int J Theory Res, 2008; 8:107-24.

[44] Spencer-Rodgers J, Peng K, Wang L, Hou Y. Dialectical self-esteem and east-west differences in psychological well-being. Pers Soc Psychol Bull 2004;30(11):1416-32.

[45] Jensen LA. Navigating local and global worlds: opportunities and risks for adolescent cultural identity development. Psychol Stud 2011;56(1):62-70.

[46] Beals LM. Content creation in virtual worlds to support adolescent identity development. New Dir Youth Dev 2010;128:45-53.

[47] Shek DTL, Siu AMH, Lee TY, Cheng H, Tsang SKM, Lui J, et al. Development and validation of a positive youth development scale in Hong Kong. Int J Adolesc Med Health 2006;18(3):547-58.

[48] Catalano RF, Berglund ML, Ryan JAM, Lonczak HS, Hawkins JD. Positive youth development in the United States: research findings on evaluations of positive youth development programs. Ann Am Acad Pol Soc Sci 2004;591:98-124.

[49] Harter S. The construction of the self: a developmental perspective. New York: Guilford Press, 1999.

[50] Borba M, Borba C, Reasoner R. A research summary: effectiveness of implementing the esteem builders program school-wide on elementary students' behavior and academic self-concept. 1999. Accessed URL: http://www.micheleborba.com/Pages/PilotStudy.htm

[51] Branden N. The six pillars of self-esteem. New York: Bantam, 1995.

[52] Community Services of Tung Wah Group of Hospitals Promoting Youth. Self-esteem: instructors' manual. Hong Kong: Community Services of Tung Wah Group Hospitals, 1994. (Chinese)

[53] Community Services of Tung Wah Group of Hospitals. Home-school parallel program to promote self-esteem. Hong Kong: Community Services of Tung Wah Group Hospitals, 2000. (Chinese)

[54] Zaff JF, Hair EC. Positive development of the self: self-concept, self-esteem, and identity. In: Bornstein MH, Davidson L, Keyes CLM, Moore KA.Well-being: positive development across the life course. Mahwah, NJ: Lawrence Erlbaum, 2003:235-51.

[55] Clements P, Seidman E. The ecology of middle grades schools and possible selves: theory, research. In: Brinthaupt TM, Lipka RP. Understanding early adolescent self and identity: applications and interventions. Albany, NY: State Univ New York Press, 2002:133-64.

[56] Valkenburg PM, Peter J. Adolescents' identity experiments on the internet: consequences for social competence and self-concept unity. Communic Res 2008;35(2):208-31.

[57] Haslam SA, Jetten J, Postmes T, Haslam C. Social identity, health and well-being: an emerging agenda for applied psychology. Appl Psychol 2009;58:1-23.

[58] Arnett JJ. Emerging adulthood: what is it, and what is it good for? Child Dev Perspect 2007;1(2):68-73.

[59] Nelson LJ, Chen X. Emerging adulthood in China: the role of social and cultural factors. Child Dev Perspect 2007;1(2):86-91.

[60] La Guardia JG. Developing who am I: a self-determination theory approach to the establishment of healthy identities. Educ Psychol 2009;44(2):90-104.

Submitted: October 05, 2011. *Revised:* November 17, 2011. *Accepted:* December 04, 2011.

SECTION FIVE – ACKNOWLEDGMENTS

In: Alternative Medicine Research Yearbook 2012
Editors: Søren Ventegodt and Joav Merrick

ISBN: 978-1-62808-080-3
© 2013 Nova Science Publishers, Inc.

Chapter 45

ABOUT THE EDITOR

Joav Merrick, MD, MMedSci, DMSc, is professor of pediatrics, child health and human development affiliated with Kentucky Children's Hospital, University of Kentucky, Lexington, United States and the Department of Pediatrics, Hebrew University Hadassah Medical Center, Mt Scopus Campus, Jerusalem, Israel, the medical director of the Health Services, Division for Intellectual and Developmental Disabilities, Ministry of Social Affairs and Social Services, Jerusalem, the founder and director of the National Institute of Child Health and Human Development in Israel. Numerous publications in the field of pediatrics, child health and human development, rehabilitation, intellectual disability, disability, health, welfare, abuse, advocacy, quality of life and prevention. Received the Peter Sabroe Child Award for outstanding work on behalf of Danish Children in 1985 and the International LEGO-Prize ("The Children's Nobel Prize") for an extraordinary contribution towards improvement in child welfare and well-being in 1987.

Contact

Office of the Medical Director, Intellectual and Developmental Disabilities, Ministry of Social Affairs and Social Services, POBox 1260, IL-91012 Jerusalem, Israel.
E-mail: jmerrick@zahav.net.il
Home-page: http://jmerrick50.googlepages.com/home

In: Alternative Medicine Research Yearbook 2012
Editors: Søren Ventegodt and Joav Merrick

ISBN: 978-1-62808-080-3
© 2013 Nova Science Publishers, Inc.

Chapter 46

ABOUT THE NATIONAL INSTITUTE OF CHILD HEALTH AND HUMAN DEVELOPMENT IN ISRAEL

The National Institute of Child Health and Human Development (NICHD) in Israel was established in 1998 as a virtual institute under the auspicies of the Medical Director, Ministry of Social Affairs and Social Services in order to function as the research arm for the Office of the Medical Director. In 1998 the National Council for Child Health and Pediatrics, Ministry of Health and in 1999 the Director General and Deputy Director General of the Ministry of Health endorsed the establishment of the NICHD.

MISSION

The mission of a National Institute for Child Health and Human Development in Israel is to provide an academic focal point for the scholarly interdisciplinary study of child life, health, public health, welfare, disability, rehabilitation, intellectual disability and related aspects of human development. This mission includes research, teaching, clinical work, information and public service activities in the field of child health and human development.

SERVICE AND ACADEMIC ACTIVITIES

Over the years many activities became focused in the south of Israel due to collaboration with various professionals at the Faculty of Health Sciences (FOHS) at the Ben Gurion University of the Negev (BGU). Since 2000 an affiliation with the Zusman Child Development Center at the Pediatric Division of Soroka University Medical Center has resulted in collaboration around the establishment of the Down Syndrome Clinic at that center. In 2002 a full course on "Disability" was established at the Recanati School for Allied Professions in the Community, FOHS, BGU and twice a year seminars for specialists in family medicine. In 2005 collaboration was started with the Primary Care Unit of the faculty and disability became part of the master of public health course on "Children and society". In the academic year 2005-2006 a one semester course on "Aging with disability" was started as part of the master of science program in gerontology in our collaboration with the Center for Multidisciplinary Research in Aging.

RESEARCH ACTIVITIES

The affiliated staff has over the years published work from projects and research activities in this national and international collaboration. In the year 2000 the International Journal of Adolescent Medicine and Health and in 2005 the International Journal on Disability and Human development of Freund Publishing House (London and Tel Aviv), in the year 2003 the TSW-Child Health and Human Development and in 2006 the TSW-Holistic Health and Medicine of the Scientific World Journal (New York and Kirkkonummi, Finland), all peer-reviewed international journals were affiliated with the National Institute of Child Health and Human Development. From 2008 also the International Journal of Child Health and Human Development (Nova Science, New York), the International Journal of Child and Adolescent Health (Nova Science) and the Journal of Pain Management (Nova Science) affiliated.

NATIONAL COLLABORATION

Nationally the NICHD works in collaboration with the Faculty of Health Sciences, Ben Gurion University of the Negev; Department of Physical Therapy, Sackler School of Medicine, Tel Aviv University; Autism Center, Assaf HaRofeh Medical Center; National Rett and PKU Centers at Chaim Sheba Medical Center, Tel HaShomer; Department of Physiotherapy, Haifa University; Department of Education, Bar Ilan University, Ramat Gan, Faculty of Social Sciences and Health Sciences; College of Judea and Samaria in Ariel and recently also collaborations has been established with the Department Pediatrics, Hebrew University Hadassah Medical Center, Mt Scopus Campus in Jerusalem.

INTERNATIONAL COLLABORATION

Internationally with the Department of Disability and Human Development, College of Applied Health Sciences, University of Illinois at Chicago; Strong Center for Developmental Disabilities, Golisano Children's Hospital at Strong, University of Rochester School of Medicine and Dentistry, New York; Centre on Intellectual Disabilities, University of Albany, New York; Centre for Chronic Disease Prevention and Control, Health Canada, Ottawa; Chandler Medical Center and Children's Hospital, Kentucky Children's Hospital, Section of Adolescent Medicine, University of Kentucky, Lexington; Chronic Disease Prevention and Control Research Center, Baylor College of Medicine, Houston, Texas; Division of Neuroscience, Department of Psychiatry, Columbia University, New York; Institute for the Study of Disadvantage and Disability, Atlanta; Center for Autism and Related Disorders, Department Psychiatry, Children's Hospital Boston, Boston; Department of Paediatrics, Child Health and Adolescent Medicine, Children's Hospital at Westmead, Westmead, Australia;

International Centre for the Study of Occupational and Mental Health, Düsseldorf, Germany; Centre for Advanced Studies in Nursing, Department of General Practice and Primary Care, University of Aberdeen, Aberdeen, United Kingdom; Quality of Life Research Center, Copenhagen, Denmark; Nordic School of Public Health, Gottenburg, Sweden, Scandinavian Institute of Quality of Working Life, Oslo, Norway; Centre for Quality of Life of the Hong Kong Institute of Asia-Pacific Studies and School of Social Work, Chinese University, Hong Kong.

TARGETS

Our focus is on research, international collaborations, clinical work, teaching and policy in health, disability and human development and to establish the NICHD as a permanent institute at one of the residential care centers for persons with intellectual disability in Israel in order to conduct model research and together with the four university schools of public health/medicine in Israel establish a national master and doctoral program in disability and human development at the institute to secure the next generation of professionals working in this often non-prestigious/low-status field of work. For this project we need your support. We are looking for all kinds of support and eventually an endowment.

CONTACT

Professor Joav Merrick, MD, MMedSci, DMSc
Medical Director, Division for Intellectual and Developmental Disabilities, Ministry of Social Affairs and Social Services, POBox 1260
IL-91012 Jerusalem, Israel
E-mail: jmerrick@zahav.net.il

INDEX

#

20th century, 37, 88, 114, 363
21st century, 22, 467

A

abstraction, 100
abuse, 150, 155, 156, 157, 173, 246, 247, 248, 475, 485
academic learning, 95, 437
academic motivation, 230, 459, 466
academic performance, 230, 415, 418, 422, 428, 433, 440, 444, 445, 446, 447, 449, 450, 457, 461, 476
academic problems, 152
academic success, 410, 415, 436, 437, 457, 459
access, 6, 69, 104, 106, 107, 108, 277, 284, 357, 362, 462, 464, 467, 479, 480
accessibility, 277, 448, 473
acclimatization, 147
accommodation, 381, 417
accounting, 347
accreditation, 108
acetylcholine, 149
acid, 149, 157, 174, 192, 202, 205, 210, 227
acidity, 197, 198
acquaintance, 324, 345
acquisition of knowledge, 466
active transport, 87
activism, 62
activity level, 278
actuality, 372
acupuncture, 16, 38, 119, 140, 164
acute renal failure, 172, 175
AD, 96, 166, 252, 263, 264, 265, 310
adaptability, 118, 436
adaptation(s), 131, 299, 307, 439, 441, 431, 452, 453
adenoids, 161

ADH, 163
ADHD, 145, 146, 147, 148, 151, 152, 154, 155, 157, 161, 165, 173, 435
adjustment, 268, 366, 370, 371, 380, 382, 400, 409, 411, 416, 452, 453, 463, 464, 472
administrators, 232
adolescent adjustment, 397
adolescent behavior, 390
adolescent development, 389, 390, 393, 394, 395, 396, 398, 408, 416, 417, 418, 422, 423, 436, 443, 444, 449, 451, 469
adolescent problem behavior, 401
adult education, 321
adulthood, 154, 164, 259, 275, 277, 278, 281, 282, 283, 285, 310, 313, 314, 315, 316, 318, 319, 320, 324, 347, 348, 349, 415, 423, 434, 456, 469, 471, 475, 477, 479, 481, 482
advancement, 60, 353, 404, 406, 408, 419, 421, 425, 446
adverse effects, 163
adverse event, 82, 83, 249, 291
advertisements, 38
advocacy, 456, 461, 463, 485
aerobic exercise, 174, 279, 282
aesthetic(s), 22, 133, 262, 265, 293, 295
affective disorder, 310
affluence, 344, 345, 362
Africa, 3, 5, 9, 13, 21, 43, 55, 65, 85, 97, 103, 104, 105, 106, 107, 109, 110, 111, 112, 114, 115, 117, 119, 121, 129, 137, 390
African Americans, 235
African-American, 160, 171
agencies, 107
aggregation, 46, 48, 242
aggression, 9, 411, 440, 450, 453, 476, 477
aging population, 22
aging process, 259, 260, 266, 274
aging society, 258
agonist, 151, 175

492   *Index*

agriculture, 41, 55, 58, 59, 60, 61, 62, 213
AIDS, v, 57, 104, 106, 110
airflow obstruction, 160
airways, 161
albuminuria, 179
alcohol abuse, 433
alcohol use, 440
alcoholism, 299
aldosterone, 179
alexithymia, 439
alienation, 309, 353
allergic reaction, 175
allergic rhinitis, 160, 161
allergy, 79, 160
alternative energy, 62
alternative medicine, 13, 21, 65, 74, 82, 83, 85, 97, 103, 111, 117, 121, 129, 137, 249
alternative treatments, 133
alters, 148
amalgam, 14, 86
ambivalence, 476
American Heart Association, 286
American Psychological Association, 413, 414
amine, 300
amino, 192
amnesia, 151
amphetamines, 153, 155
amygdala, 292
amyloidosis, 157
anatomy, 9, 16, 23, 29, 67, 68, 160, 243, 427
ancestors, 294
ancient world, 253
ANCOVAs, 233
anemia, 153, 157, 162
anger, 191, 248, 352
angina, 90, 176
angioedema, 175
angiography, 174
angiotensin converting enzyme, 181
angiotensin II, 175, 180, 181
angiotensin II receptor antagonist, 181
angiotensin receptor blockers, 174, 178
anorexia, 158
ANOVA, 198, 233, 306, 313, 317, 319, 328, 329, 355, 361, 365, 366, 375
anterograde amnesia, 149
antibiotic, 58
anticholinergic, 92, 149
anticholinergic effect, 149
anticonvulsant, 149, 159
antidepressant(s), 146, 149, 156, 161, 164, 274, 277, 282, 285, 287
antidiuretic hormone, 162

antihistamines, 146, 153
antihypertensive agents, 175
antihypertensive drugs, 175, 178, 180
antioxidant, 200
antisocial behavior, 397
anxiety, 92, 96, 106, 129, 133, 146, 147, 148, 149, 155, 157, 163, 164, 230, 267, 274, 282, 290, 291, 295, 296, 298, 299, 300, 323, 325, 326, 327, 328, 330, 331, 370, 411, 414, 433, 437, 447, 449, 453, 458, 477
anxiety disorder, 92, 274, 290
aorta, 170, 173
APA, 385
apnea, 161, 162
appetite, 41, 149, 155
applied psychology, 482
appointments, 373, 375
appraisals, 413
architects, 373
arithmetic, 223
arousal, 118, 150, 161, 164, 265, 311, 434, 437, 447
arrhythmia(s), 163, 231
arsenic, 227
arterial hypertension, 174
arteriosclerosis, 41
arteritis, 173
artery, 172, 173
arthritis, 90, 278, 284
articulation, 381
Asia, 426, 451, 489
Asian Americans, 476
Asian countries, 476
assault, 249
assertiveness, 363, 478
assessment, 18, 27, 107, 137, 138, 154, 170, 240, 272, 273, 280, 283, 293, 294, 299, 302, 304, 310, 324, 352, 358, 364, 411, 414, 427, 433, 434, 439, 444, 445, 446, 448, 451, 475, 479
assessment tools, 433
assets, 262, 393, 423, 463
assimilation, 336, 417
asthma, 38, 173
ataxia, 150, 151, 156
athletic competence, 474
atmosphere, 34, 61, 394
atopy, 161
ATP, 87
atrial fibrillation, 231
attachment, 276, 314, 320, 434, 435, 439, 440, 460
attachment theory, 314, 434, 460
attitudes, 51, 126, 230, 257, 260, 261, 266, 267, 268, 277, 352, 364, 392, 400, 449, 462, 472
attribution, 406, 407, 408, 447

Index

493

audit, 107
auscultation, 170
Austria, xv, 73, 221, 237, 245, 251
authoritarianism, 411
authority(s), 9, 14, 139, 260, 424
autonomic nervous system, 191
autonomy, 258, 259, 277, 304, 346, 366, 393, 423, 425, 455, 456, 457, 458, 459, 461, 462, 463, 464, 465, 466
autosomal dominant, 157
aversion, 291, 297
avoidance, 57, 148, 174, 289, 292, 305
awareness, 29, 48, 52, 118, 119, 130, 132, 185, 186, 188, 189, 190, 192, 345, 383, 394, 412, 430, 431, 433, 460, 461, 470

B

Baars, 243
back pain, 155
bacteria, 124
bacterium, 210
bad habits, 38
banks, 46
barriers, 15, 137, 140, 273, 279, 280, 283, 286
base, 9, 104, 107, 108, 215, 240, 260, 352, 362, 363
basic needs, 272, 353, 354
basic services, 112
BD, 286
Beck Depression Inventory, 282
beef, 196
behavioral change, 296, 452
behavioral problems, 410, 470, 472, 478
behavioral sciences, 349
behaviors, 191, 230, 259, 279, 283, 307, 357, 370, 400, 405, 407, 415, 418, 420, 431, 433, 435, 453, 473
Beijing, 211, 213, 219
beneficial effect, 180, 195, 229, 234, 243, 258, 261, 263, 266, 423
beneficiaries, 362
benefits, 103, 104, 105, 115, 140, 235, 262, 264, 265, 268, 271, 273, 276, 278, 279, 280, 285, 292, 296, 308, 310, 384, 414, 455, 459, 463
benign, 164, 172
benzodiazepine, 152, 165
beverages, 153, 162
BI, 300
bias, 41, 129, 133, 213, 222, 284
Bible, 112
bicarbonate, 174
Big Bang, 24
bing, 437

bioassay, 238, 239
biochemical processes, 88
biochemistry, 23, 28, 30, 58, 67, 90, 94
bioenergy, 86, 87, 94
biofeedback, 164
biological activity, 59
biological rhythms, 48
biological sciences, 23
biological systems, 22, 27, 89, 91, 92, 222, 238, 243, 244
bioluminescence, 243
biosphere, 49, 50
biotechnology, 220
bipolar disorder, 159
birds, 5, 41, 93
birth control, 113
birth rate, 257
birth weight, 182
blame, 408
bleeding, 181
blood, 27, 89, 91, 121, 122, 149, 154, 155, 169, 170, 171, 172, 174, 175, 176, 178, 180, 182, 183, 195, 196, 197, 198, 200, 201, 231, 242, 243, 262, 277
blood flow, 231
blood pressure, 89, 91, 154, 155, 169, 170, 171, 172, 174, 175, 176, 178, 180, 182, 183, 231, 262
blood-brain barrier, 149
blue-collar workers, 373
blueprint, 32
BMI, 171
body image, 259, 423, 426
body mass index, 262, 280
body weight, 196, 197, 273
boils, 60
bonding, 138, 204, 209, 295, 396
bonds, 265, 320
bone(s), 95, 112, 113, 171
bone age, 171
boredom, 395
Botswana, 110
bottom-up, 363
bradycardia, 149, 176
brain, 22, 24, 29, 38, 48, 65, 69, 70, 77, 89, 92, 95, 106, 122, 132, 144, 166, 175, 186, 192, 193, 263, 265, 268, 276, 289, 290, 291, 292, 293, 294, 295, 296, 298, 299, 300
brain activity, 292
brain functioning, 70, 265
brainstem, 175
brainstorming, 4
branching, 241
breakdown, 15, 233
breast cancer, 75, 82

breast feeding, 204
breast milk, 204
breathing, 90, 144, 147, 151, 160, 185, 186, 187, 190, 191, 192, 280
breathlessness, 281
Britain, 8, 15, 321, 430
bronchospasm, 175
bruit, 173
bruxism, 164
Buddhism, 300
building blocks, 68, 87, 461
bullying, 416
burn, 204
bursitis, 231, 235
business strategy, 361, 367
businesses, 212, 213, 218
buyer, 132

C

cables, 239, 240
caffeine, 147, 148, 157
calcium, 178
calcium channel blocker, 178
calibration, 170
CAM, xv, 16, 73, 80, 245, 251
cancer, 26, 27, 75, 79, 85, 86, 91, 93, 94, 95, 120, 133, 134, 298
candidates, 213
capitalism, 52, 364
carbon, 56, 147
carbon dioxide, 147
carbon emissions, 56
cardiac output, 176
cardiac risk, 273
cardinal value, 392
cardiovascular disease(s), 154, 170, 172, 173, 180, 183, 273
cardiovascular function, 180
cardiovascular risk, 172
care model, 34
career development, 127, 320
caregivers, 120, 123, 137, 138, 359, 434
Caribbean, ii
case study(s), 100, 231, 232, 349, 392, 445
cataplexy, 153, 154, 155, 156, 157
catecholamines, 174, 175, 176
categorization, 170, 285
catheter, 197
Caucasians, 171
causal antecedent, 345
causal attribution, 447, 449
causal inference, 345, 418

causal powers, 100
causal relationship, 44, 349, 466
causality, ix, 8, 43, 44, 45, 46, 47, 48, 49, 57, 100, 444
causation, 23, 27, 28
CDC, 273
cell culture, 239
cell differentiation, 89
cell division, 89
cell membranes, 91
cellular calcium, 175
central nervous system (CNS), 109, 151, 153, 156, 159
cerebellum, 239
cerebral cortex, 243, 291
cerebral function, 238
cerebrovascular disease, 170
challenges, ix, xiii, xv, xvi, 5, 9, 16, 18, 40, 55, 74, 99, 109, 129, 133, 182, 271, 272, 279, 292, 304, 314, 348, 383, 408, 409, 418, 428, 437, 444, 447, 449, 452, 455, 457, 477
channel blocker, 177, 179
chaos, 25, 26, 43, 44, 66, 93
chemical(s), 27, 28, 30, 58, 59, 60, 61, 87, 88, 92, 95, 202, 210, 238, 239
chemical reactions, 92, 210, 238
chemotherapy, 91
Chicago, 19, 31, 286, 488
chicken, 130
childhood, 70, 77, 131, 135, 144, 145, 157, 160, 162, 171, 275, 282, 299, 314, 318, 319, 320, 321, 399, 400, 416, 435, 440, 471, 475
China, x, 211, 212, 213, 217, 219, 337, 348, 364, 389, 390, 403, 446, 459, 482
cholesterol, 172, 179, 195, 197, 198, 199, 200
chromatograms, 206
chronic diseases, 56, 57, 58, 95, 173, 273, 278, 283
chronic illness, 144, 272, 273, 278, 283
chronic kidney disease, 180
chronic venous insufficiency, 91
cigarette smoking, 174
circadian rhythm, 144, 151, 152
circumcision, 113
cirrhosis, 140
city(s), 61, 117, 214, 252, 257, 313, 315, 316, 318, 333, 479
citizens, 253, 334, 363
civil society, 114
civilization, 50, 298, 348
clarity, 447, 478
classes, 279, 281
classical mechanics, 45
classification, 166, 169, 170, 181

Index

classroom, 397, 416, 422, 424, 425, 437, 445, 459, 463, 464, 465
classroom environment, 459, 463, 464
clients, 46, 212, 218, 229, 230, 231, 232, 233, 234
climate, 70, 364, 370, 450
clinical application, 399, 400, 440
clinical depression, 282, 286
clinical diagnosis, 18
clinical holistic medicine, 82, 83, 249, 250
clinical psychology, 413, 414
clinical symptoms, 95
clinical trials, 96, 183, 227
close relationships, 371, 398
closure, 348
clothing, 351, 354
cluster analysis, 214, 215
clustering, 214, 238, 240
clusters, 40, 211, 214, 215, 217, 218
CNS, 151, 153, 154, 157, 159, 164, 176
CO_2, 239
coal, 109
coarctation, 170, 174
cognition, 43, 44, 100, 170, 192, 263, 272, 276, 295, 437, 444, 446, 466
cognitive ability(s), 393, 406, 439
cognitive activity, 265, 293
cognitive development, 404, 418, 421, 423, 426, 427
cognitive dysfunction, 161
cognitive function, 105, 106
cognitive impairment, 274
cognitive level, 363
cognitive perspective, 453, 481
cognitive process, 325, 418, 421
cognitive science, 44
cognitive skills, 417, 418, 419, 420, 422
cognitive style, 418
cognitive theory, 280, 363, 428, 450, 452
cognitive therapy, 295
cognitive variables, 452, 473
cognitive-behavioral therapy, 277
coherence, xvi, 47, 48, 76, 78, 94, 95, 244, 302, 359, 385, 471
collaboration, 105, 108, 231, 276, 370, 411, 422, 464, 487, 488
collective unconscious, 47
collectivism, 466
college students, 260, 262, 399, 409, 414, 427, 440, 453
colleges, 390
colon, 278
colon cancer, 278
color, viii
combined effect, 147

commerce, 373
commercial, 103, 104, 196, 373
commodity, 36
common sense, xiii, xvi, 102
communication, 48, 50, 85, 89, 94, 110, 122, 127, 139, 140, 222, 230, 235, 238, 294, 370, 371, 382, 383, 394, 410, 419, 432, 439, 451, 461, 463, 476
communication patterns, 230, 235, 394, 461
communication skills, 139, 140, 382
community service, 353
comorbidity, 172, 274
comparative analysis, 348
compassion, 50, 51, 70, 291, 294, 295, 391, 414
compensation, 113, 331, 354
competition, 18, 132, 296, 361, 364, 367, 410, 453
competitive sport, 132
competitiveness, 219
compilation, 302
complement, 69, 119, 334
complementarity, 45, 46, 222
complex partial seizure, 165
complexity, 4, 22, 25, 27, 31, 40, 42, 43, 44, 68, 69, 70, 74, 93, 123, 310, 380, 430, 435
compliance, 16, 118, 178, 181, 284
complications, 118, 152, 170, 181
composition, 197, 202
compounds, 87
comprehension, 470
compression, 172, 287
compulsive behavior, 158
computer, 198, 213, 296
computer software, 198
conception, 45, 73, 77, 247, 391, 392, 397, 407, 425
conceptualization, 219, 312, 352, 395, 410, 419, 431, 448, 455, 456, 460
concordance, 307, 374
conditioning, 446
conduction, 87, 89
conductors, 373
conference, 3, 4, 6, 10, 14, 56, 210, 367
confidentiality, 247, 305
configuration, 62, 204, 209
conflict, 371, 384, 395, 450, 459, 476, 482
conflict resolution, 371
conformity, 393, 427
Confucius, 261
congestive heart failure, 274
Congress, viii, 95
connective tissue, 231
connectivity, 192, 193
conscientiousness, 345, 472
conscious experiences, 295
consensus, 22, 89, 169, 396

496   *Index*

consent, 305
constipation, 149, 156, 158, 163
constituents, 89, 340
Constitution, 42
construct validity, 439, 445
construction, 316, 320, 348, 370, 380, 417, 418, 421, 447, 481, 482
constructivism, 8, 99, 100
consumers, 59
consumption, 62, 146, 153
contamination, 150
contextual interference, 430
contraceptives, 172
control group, 180, 192, 223, 224, 225, 226, 238, 240, 242
controlled trials, 95, 222, 231, 282
controversial, 151
convergence, 348
conversations, 6, 7, 10, 11, 34, 98, 103, 137, 138, 140, 189
conviction, 46, 189
cooking, 328
cooperation, 451
coordination, 50, 209
Copernican revolution, 15
coping strategies, 370, 374, 434, 435, 436, 437, 458
copyright, viii
coronary heart disease, 75, 82
correlation(s), 59, 172, 265, 277, 304, 313, 317, 340, 349, 353, 357, 375, 376, 377, 411
correlation analysis, 313, 317, 349
cortex, 291, 292
cortical neurons, 237, 238, 239, 242, 243
corticosteroids, 172
cortisol, 262
co-sleeping, 296
cosmos, 50, 96, 391
cost, 37, 56, 80, 82, 92, 105, 120, 139, 178, 248, 279, 280, 284
coughing, 76
counseling, 119, 120, 154, 235, 280, 307, 399, 412, 416
covering, 205, 209, 252
creatinine, 174
creative potential, 124
creative process, 426
creative thinking, 417, 418, 419, 420, 421, 422, 423, 424, 425, 426
creativity, 4, 22, 23, 50, 189, 192, 420, 423, 426, 427, 428, 457
credentials, 349
creep, 132, 157
crises, 74, 78, 314, 444, 470

critical thinking, 417, 418, 419, 420, 421, 422, 423, 424, 425, 426, 427
criticism, 372, 374, 376
crop(s), 41, 58, 59
cross links, 40
cross-cultural comparison, 265
cross-sectional study, 213, 433
crystals, 112
CT, 347, 349, 439, 440, 453, 481
cues, 144, 327
cultivation, 19, 193, 450, 458, 469
cultural beliefs, 397, 400
cultural conditions, 362
cultural differences, 426, 451
cultural imperialism, 114
cultural influence, 219, 479
cultural norms, 433
cultural values, 364, 403, 410, 412, 459
culture, 14, 17, 33, 34, 39, 50, 81, 109, 112, 113, 123, 213, 229, 238, 239, 240, 242, 261, 299, 337, 348, 349, 361, 363, 367, 393, 394, 396, 410, 415, 419, 421, 427, 431, 432, 433, 437, 446, 448, 450, 451, 455, 459, 470, 474
culture conditions, 239
culture medium, 239, 240, 242
cure(s), 37, 75, 76, 82, 99, 105, 132, 137, 138, 196, 246, 253
curricula, 86, 97, 101, 397, 412, 423, 428, 437, 462, 463, 477
curriculum, 75, 131, 280, 399, 413, 424, 425, 427, 437, 438, 452, 461, 462, 463, 464, 467, 477, 478
curriculum development, 399, 413, 427, 438, 452, 467
customers, 212
cycles, 143, 144, 147, 153, 165
cyclical process, 417
cycloplegia, 163
cystourethrogram, 174
cytochrome, 150
cytoplasm, 77

D

daily living, 272, 277, 278, 279
damages, viii
damping, 265
dance, 5, 21, 31, 68, 78, 132
danger, 69, 289, 296, 297, 317, 436
data analysis, 100
data collection, 316, 393, 479
database, 265, 320, 470
DBP, 171
DEA, 149, 151, 154, 157

deaths, 56, 57, 112, 118, 273
decay, 163
deduction, 419
defects, 202
defence, 244
deficiency(s), 41, 59, 154, 157, 196
deficit, 146, 435
degradation, 56, 58, 59
delegates, 7, 134
delinquency, 349
delirium, 150
Delta, 10, 144
delusion(s), 130, 131
dementia, 106, 138, 263, 264, 265, 268, 298, 359
democracy, 334, 346
democratization, 337, 348
demographic characteristics, 381
demographic data, 232
Denmark, xv, 56, 73, 82, 245, 251, 489
Department of Education, 429, 488
dependent variable, 214, 306, 377
depressants, 149, 151, 157, 277
depressive symptomatology, 264, 415
depressive symptoms, 257, 261, 264, 265, 266, 269, 272, 274, 275, 276, 280, 282, 286
deprivation, 334, 347, 475
depth, 74, 120, 187, 204, 260, 262, 472, 474, 475, 478
despair, 275
destiny, 75, 77, 124
destruction, 41, 59, 88, 251, 253
detection, 182, 244
determinism, 45, 49, 446
developed countries, 246, 363
developing countries, 37, 111, 363, 367
developmental disorder, 144
developmental process, 415
developmental theories, 460
deviant behaviour, 440
deviation, 330
diabetes, x, 41, 55, 56, 57, 58, 59, 86, 118, 157, 172, 173, 195, 196, 200, 201, 202, 231, 235, 273, 278, 298, 299
diabetic neuropathy, 157
diabetic patients, 196
diarrhea, 155, 175
diastolic blood pressure, 169, 171, 174, 176
dichotomy, 45, 294, 297, 476
diet, 38, 39, 57, 59, 61, 120, 164, 174, 230
differential diagnosis, 148, 159
diffusion, 87, 472, 474, 477
dignity, 50
diphenhydramine, 146

direct observation, 100
directionality, 436
disability, 35, 39, 80, 257, 264, 266, 274, 275, 276, 277, 283, 286, 290, 299, 466, 485, 487, 489
disability progression, 283
disappointment, 37, 126, 472
disaster, 80
discomfort, 36, 121, 124, 157, 323, 325, 326, 327, 328
discontinuity, 45
discrimination, 119
disease model, 60
disease progression, 120
disease rate, 56, 273
diseases, 17, 22, 24, 27, 30, 35, 39, 56, 58, 59, 75, 85, 86, 94, 112, 114, 121, 123, 125, 172, 173, 174, 196, 252, 278, 290, 298, 299, 300, 363
disequilibrium, 108
disgust, 245, 247
disorder, 26, 40, 70, 107, 120, 146, 147, 148, 151, 152, 153, 154, 156, 157, 162, 165, 166, 169, 181, 196, 282, 435
dispersion, 349
displacement, 162, 348
disposition, 272, 477
dissatisfaction, 16, 25, 472
dissidents, 26
dissonance, 99
distilled water, 205
distress, 56, 150, 262, 290, 371, 385, 436
distribution, 108, 197, 230, 233, 240, 335, 338, 343, 346, 347
distribution of income, 335
diuretic, 163, 175, 179, 180, 181
diuretic medications, 181
divergence, 433
divergent thinking, 418, 420, 422, 426
diversity, 3, 112, 294, 358
dizziness, 149, 150, 155, 156, 158, 163, 175, 176
DNA, 77, 89
doctors, 4, 6, 7, 9, 14, 16, 17, 34, 37, 59, 60, 61, 67, 68, 70, 85, 86, 87, 88, 90, 92, 94, 107, 113, 117, 118, 122, 123, 126, 138, 139, 140, 252, 373
dogs, 195, 196, 197, 198, 199, 200, 201, 202
DOI, 310, 311, 312
domestic labor, 371
dopamine, 158, 297
dopamine agonist, 158
dopaminergic, 154, 157, 158
dosage, 150, 151, 277
dose-response relationship, 282
dosing, 155, 179
Down syndrome, 145, 160, 290, 299

498 *Index*

downward causation, 28
downward comparison, 346
draft, 50
drawing, 392, 449
dream, 67, 130, 144, 155
dreaming, 130, 144
drug addict, 450
drug addiction, 450
drug dependence, 155
drug interaction, 150, 155, 163
drug reactions, 57
drug treatment, x, 57, 203, 205, 209
drugs, 7, 9, 15, 16, 22, 23, 27, 31, 33, 56, 57, 59, 60, 65, 75, 87, 88, 90, 123, 124, 139, 147, 148, 149, 152, 156, 157, 164, 172, 173, 176, 179, 181, 182, 183, 196, 204, 210, 246, 331
drying, 197
dualism, 16
duality, 45, 108, 109
durability, 447
dynamic systems, 209
dyslexia, 452
dyspepsia, 155
dysphoria, 149
dysplasia, 173
dysthymia, 282
dystonia, 158

E

earnings, 338
earthquakes, 252
East Asia, 219, 348
Eastern Europe, 91, 364
eating disorders, 151
ecological systems, 62
ecology, 50, 60, 61, 62, 384, 415, 432, 466, 480, 482
economic behaviour, 48
economic consequences, 104
economic development, 212, 261, 337
economic disadvantage, 394, 397, 400, 416
economic growth, 362, 363
economic incentives, 37
economic indicator, 364
economic performance, 213
economic resources, 258
economic status, 281, 410, 428
economics, 33, 34, 39, 45, 53, 333
edema, 158, 175, 176
education reform, 428
educational aims, 316, 317, 318
educational background, 354
educational objective, 427

educational opportunities, 106
educational settings, 430, 436, 437, 452, 465
educational system, 422
educators, 437, 441, 466
EEA, 298
EEG, 28
egg, 74
egocentrism, 391
EKG, 163
elaboration, 292, 333, 334, 336, 346
elderly population, 274
elders, 272, 286
electric circuits, 96
electric current, 91
electrical tools, 28
electricity, 28, 90, 92
electrocardiogram, 88, 147
electrodes, 92, 292
electroencephalogram, 88, 147
electromagnetic, 26, 28, 30, 70, 85, 86, 87, 89, 91, 92, 94, 95, 238
electromagnetic fields, 28, 30, 91, 95
electromagnetic waves, 89
electromagnetism, 30, 92
electronic circuits, 237
electrophoresis, 206
elementary particle, 48, 93
elementary school, 260, 426
elementary students, 482
e-mail, 88
embryology, 23
EMG, 231
emission, 90, 238
emotion, 215, 287, 294, 405, 409, 423, 430, 431, 432, 433, 434, 435, 436, 437, 438, 439, 440, 441, 445, 466
emotion regulation, 434, 435, 439, 440, 441
emotional distress, 409
emotional experience, 432, 434
emotional health, 57, 125
emotional intelligence, 126, 429, 430, 439, 440
emotional problems, 430, 432, 437
emotional reactions, 308
emotional responses, 353
emotional state, 30, 302, 310, 434, 443
emotional stimuli, 308
emotional well-being, 257, 259, 266, 310, 324, 415, 432
empathy, 363, 370, 440, 453
empirical studies, 308, 421, 435
employees, 50, 51, 213, 361, 362, 363, 364, 365, 366, 367

employment, 212, 218, 324, 331, 337, 362, 363, 373, 461

employment levels, 324

empowerment, 139, 426, 456

encephalitis, 159

encephalopathy, 159, 181

encouragement, 276, 280, 422

end stage renal disease, 170

endocrine, 109, 173, 196, 276, 295

endocrine system, 109

endurance, 279, 362

enemies, 390

energy, ix, 7, 8, 10, 16, 23, 26, 28, 38, 40, 41, 47, 48, 49, 50, 59, 62, 68, 85, 86, 87, 88, 89, 90, 91, 92, 93, 94, 95, 97, 98, 99, 101, 124, 126, 171, 186, 187, 188, 189, 190, 191, 192, 272, 283, 375, 405, 444, 448

engineering, 87

England, 144, 145, 146, 153, 155, 156, 161, 162, 385

enlargement, 29

entrepreneurs, x, 211, 212, 213, 214, 215, 217, 218, 219, 373

entrepreneurship, 212, 219

enuresis, 143, 145, 160, 161, 162, 164, 165, 167

environmental change, 470

environmental control, 448

environmental factors, 214, 295, 410, 460

environmental influences, 410, 446

environmental issues, 57

environmental stimuli, 291, 292, 421

environmental stress(s), 239

environmental sustainability, 57

enzyme(s), 178, 202, 209

epidemic, 103, 104, 105, 106, 108, 110, 118, 165, 362, 363

epidemiologic, 83

epidemiology, 182

epilepsy, 153, 155, 157, 159

epistemology, 100

equality, 334, 335, 336

equilibrium, 23, 30, 49, 192

equipment, 22, 37, 51, 65, 92, 170, 279, 280

equity, 49, 337

erythrocytes, 242

esophagitis, 150

ethanol, 204, 205, 240

ethical standards, 249

ethics, 253, 391, 456

ethnic background, 344

ethnic groups, 171, 481

ethnicity, 273, 410, 445

ethnocentrism, 391

ethylene, 205

etiology, 169, 181, 274

EU, xv, 73, 245, 251

Europe, 16, 73, 91, 103, 105, 321, 347, 348, 359, 367, 370

everyday life, 62, 222, 225, 229, 264, 353, 440

evidence based medicine (EBM), 22

evolution, 14, 17, 27, 31, 32, 42, 48, 49, 77, 103, 105, 109, 192, 289, 290, 291, 292, 294, 295, 297, 480

exaggeration, 340

examinations, 437

excitation, 149, 209

exclusion, 120

executive function(s), 192

exercise, 39, 70, 120, 174, 175, 182, 230, 262, 271, 272, 273, 276, 277, 278, 279, 280, 281, 282, 283, 284, 285, 286, 287, 295, 298, 299, 385, 405, 406, 452, 466

exercise participation, 280, 283, 284

exercise programs, 279, 280, 283, 284

exertion, 265

existential healing, 73, 78, 246

expenditures, 273, 285

experimental design, 221, 225, 226

expertise, 139, 192

exploitation, 57

exports, 212

exposure, 70, 144, 147, 160, 227, 240, 335, 346, 354, 435, 478, 480

expressiveness, 311

expressivity, 434, 437, 440

external environment, 90

external influences, 238

external validity, 231

externalizing behavior, 476

extraction, 205

extraversion, 302, 345

extrovert, 132

eye movement, 144

F

face validity, 214

Facebook, 152

facial expression, 440

facilitators, 4, 268

fainting, 158

fairness, 130

faith, 81, 112, 131, 273, 337, 352, 393, 399, 400

families, 41, 75, 119, 173, 178, 263, 334, 338, 380, 382, 437, 449, 476, 478, 479, 482

family environment, xi, 313, 314, 315, 316, 317, 318, 319

500   *Index*

family factors, 398
family functioning, 394, 476, 481, 482
family history, 153, 157, 160, 164, 171, 172, 173
family income, 264, 334, 336, 337, 338, 339, 340, 341, 342, 343, 344
family life, 262, 318
family members, 230, 354, 473
family physician, ix, 13, 18, 127
family planning, 113
family relationships, 314, 320, 324, 344, 385
family support, 412
famine, 40
farmers, 58, 61
fasting, 174, 196
fat, 59, 197, 198
FDA, 92, 148, 149, 150, 151, 152, 154, 155, 156, 158, 159, 165, 175
fear(s), xvi, 109, 122, 126, 129, 130, 133, 135, 191, 291, 293, 295, 296, 297, 298, 434, 472
feelings, xvi, 7, 33, 89, 122, 123, 126, 157, 186, 247, 289, 290, 291, 292, 293, 294, 295, 296, 297, 305, 335, 338, 352, 353, 356, 357, 359, 362, 364, 411, 412, 416, 425, 430, 432, 434, 439, 473
fertility, 59
fertilizers, 58, 59
fetus, 171, 181
fiber, 239
fibromyalgia, 92, 95, 96
fibrosis, 145, 159, 179
field theory, 22
filial piety, 261, 466
Filipino, 428
filters, 131, 226, 239
filtration, 60
financial, 9, 55, 114, 139, 209, 257, 260, 261, 265, 266, 267, 358, 364, 367, 463
financial incentives, 9
financial planning, 257, 267
financial support, 209
Finland, 313, 416, 488
fires, 307
first generation, 153
fitness, 38, 40, 286, 287, 294
five-factor model, 384
fixation, 240
flame, 188, 189
flavor, 293
flavour, 28, 88
flex, 186
flexibility, 43, 44, 192, 279, 280, 289, 392, 406, 421, 422, 457
flights, 5
flowers, 189

fluctuations, 121, 125
fluid, 162, 163, 176, 209, 231, 438, 480
fluoxetine, 156
fMRI, 300
food, 41, 57, 58, 59, 60, 61, 62, 63, 68, 69, 105, 119, 125, 196, 291, 292, 293, 338, 339, 351, 354
food chain, 60
food industry, 58, 59
food intake, 291
food production, 59
food security, 59
force, 3, 15, 34, 42, 45, 74, 104, 124, 212, 336
forecasting, 66, 69
foreclosure, 471, 474, 477
formal education, 338, 463
formal operational stage, 422
formation, 175, 220, 308, 320, 370, 446, 448, 451, 469, 470, 471, 472, 473, 474, 475, 476, 477, 479, 481
formula, 69
foundations, 37, 232, 310, 452
fractures, 95, 286
France, 21, 65, 85, 323, 327, 452
free radicals, 200
free will, 291
freedom, 119, 362, 457, 459
freedom of choice, 457, 459
frenulum, 162
Freud, 470, 475
friction, 231, 232, 235
friendship, 434, 472
fruits, 81, 174, 191, 220, 273
functional changes, 94
funding, 28, 117, 120
funds, 34, 213
future orientation, 404, 408, 410, 412, 415

G

GABA, 149, 157, 192, 193
Galileo, 15, 22
gambling, 158, 449
gastritis, 150
GDP, 56, 62, 211, 212, 214, 216, 217, 218
gender differences, 234, 381, 394, 410, 436, 437, 475, 481
gender effects, 229, 230, 232, 234
gender gap, 453
gender orientation, 451
gender role, 229, 410, 478, 479
gender-sensitive, 320, 478
gene expression, 209, 210
gene regulation, 89

gene therapy, 8
general intelligence, 430
general practitioner, 15, 16, 282
generalizability, 233, 358, 448
generativity, 275, 281, 320, 444, 445
genes, 77, 290, 291, 293, 298
genetic factors, 171, 182, 435
genetic predisposition, 274
genetics, 70, 86, 272
genome, 65
geography, 102
geometry, 25
Georgia, 281
Germany, 19, 113, 196, 390, 450, 489
germination, 221, 223, 242, 243
gerontology, 258, 261, 269, 488
gifted, 422, 426, 427, 428
gland, 196
glasses, 8, 131
globalization, 337, 348, 361, 367, 433, 451, 476, 479
glomerulonephritis, 172, 173
glucose, 174, 180, 195, 197, 198, 200, 201, 202
glucose oxidase, 197
glue, 126
goal attainment, 404, 405, 406, 407, 408, 410, 447
goal setting, 411, 462, 463
goal-directed behavior, 192, 407
goal-setting, 283, 406, 411
God, 23, 26, 28, 95, 190, 191, 253, 363, 390, 391, 398
governance, 348
governments, 24, 37, 111, 114, 347, 363
grades, 126, 436, 482
grants, 249
grass, 104, 138
grassroots, 63
Greece, 14, 75, 123
greed, 191
Greeks, 40
green revolution, 58, 59
group characteristics, 340
group size, 333, 335, 336, 338, 339, 340, 341, 342, 343, 344, 346
group therapy, 250
group work, 397, 412
growth, x, 27, 53, 56, 58, 62, 74, 89, 101, 173, 176, 185, 193, 210, 219, 221, 222, 223, 225, 226, 227, 238, 239, 240, 247, 249, 261, 271, 273, 304, 337, 362, 363, 393, 396, 401, 404, 407, 408, 423, 431, 440, 444, 447, 456, 476
growth rate, 227
Guangzhou, 213
Guatemala, 53

guessing, 253
guidance, 397, 401, 412, 416, 422, 448, 463, 464, 479
guidelines, 9, 49, 70, 167, 183, 279, 284, 391, 419, 441, 458
guilt, 123, 352
gynecomastia, 179

H

HAART, 110
habituation, 344
hair, 134, 176
half-life, 149, 150, 151, 152, 155, 157, 158
hallucinations, 155, 158, 159
harmony, 37, 48, 74, 93, 324
HE, 166, 285, 438, 440
headache, 150, 151, 155, 156, 158, 175, 176, 179
health care, ix, xvi, 4, 8, 19, 33, 34, 35, 36, 37, 39, 42, 55, 56, 57, 58, 60, 107, 108, 109, 111, 112, 113, 117, 118, 138, 139, 140, 257, 267, 273, 274, 277, 285, 332, 347
health care professionals, 112, 117, 118, 273
health care sector, xvi
health care system, xvi, 58, 112, 113
health condition, 107, 109, 272, 323, 327
health education, 283, 423, 426
health information, 114
health practitioners, 86, 90, 112, 114
health problems, 106, 273, 274, 299
health promotion, 36, 37, 39, 108, 279, 300, 453
health services, 106, 118, 274
health status, xi, 36, 83, 258, 259, 286, 323, 324, 325, 332, 348, 400
heart disease, 41, 55, 56, 58, 86, 231, 278
heart failure, 170, 285, 332
heart rate, 176, 231
heat shock protein, 204
hedonism, 294, 363
height, 169, 171
helplessness, 123, 416
hemolytic anemia, 176
hepatic necrosis, 176
hepatitis, 176
herbicide, 243
heredity, 421
high blood pressure, 169, 181, 182
high school, 305, 311, 373, 409, 426, 428, 440, 453, 466
higher education, 391, 423, 426, 438
higher-order thinking, 424
highly active antiretroviral therapy, 110
hippocampus, 239

502 *Index*

histamine, 149

history, 5, 7, 14, 15, 22, 34, 82, 93, 114, 115, 124, 132, 153, 154, 157, 159, 160, 163, 165, 173, 174, 176, 232, 291, 352, 390

HIV, v, ix, 7, 9, 41, 103, 104, 105, 106, 107, 108, 109, 110, 117, 118, 119, 120

HIV/AIDS, 110, 118, 120

HLA, 154

HM, 348

hobby, 265

holism, 210

holistic medicine, xvi, 81, 82, 249, 250

homeostasis, 23, 85, 90, 94, 118, 292

homes, 267

honesty, 51

Hong Kong, xiii, 140, 333, 336, 337, 338, 343, 345, 347, 348, 389, 397, 399, 400, 401, 403, 409, 415, 416, 417, 423, 426, 427, 428, 429, 441, 443, 446, 450, 452, 455, 460, 469, 473, 475, 476, 478, 479, 481, 482, 489

hopelessness, 392, 396, 411, 412, 416, 436

hormone(s), 65, 89, 148, 163, 243

host, 200

hostility, 477

hotspots, 292, 300

House, 31, 32, 193, 269, 354, 359, 452, 488

housing, 119, 348, 354

human behavior, 192, 299, 398, 414, 444, 452, 465

human body, 30, 35, 48, 62, 90, 91, 97, 98

human brain, 297, 298

human condition, 7

human development, 275, 346, 384, 393, 398, 415, 432, 471, 475, 481, 485, 487, 489

human dimensions, 17

human existence, xiii, xv, 34, 76, 79, 353, 392

human experience, 17, 124, 264

human health, 59, 399

human immunodeficiency virus, 110

human milk, 210

human motivation, 456

human nature, 363, 395

human resources, 109

human right(s), 25, 353, 362

human subjects, 92

human values, 50

humanistic psychology, 460

humidity, 239

humus, 60

Hunter, 440

hunting, 293

husband, 134, 135, 331

hybrid, 58

hydrogen, 67, 204, 209, 210

hydrogen bonds, 209

hygiene, 37, 105, 143, 147, 148, 152, 153, 154, 158, 165

hyperactivity, 146, 192, 296, 435

hypercalcemia, 179

hyperglycemia, 196

hyperkalemia, 175, 179

hyperlipidemia, 171, 273

hypersomnia, 159, 166

hypertension, x, 91, 95, 149, 155, 156, 169, 170, 171, 172, 173, 174, 175, 176, 178, 179, 180, 181, 182, 183, 231, 273, 278

hypertrophy, 160, 161, 172, 178

hypnagogic hallucinations, 153, 156

hypnosis, 164

hypoglycemia, 175, 179

hypokalemia, 179

hyponatremia, 163, 179

hypotension, 149, 158, 174, 176

hypothalamus, 154

hypothesis, 52, 200, 204, 304, 335, 336, 345, 385, 394, 400, 436

hypothyroidism, 153

hypovolemia, 175

hypoxemia, 160

hypoxia, 147

I

iatrogenic, 21, 31, 65, 66

Iceland, 5

ideal(s), 24, 139, 266, 334, 338, 363, 390, 441, 452, 472, 477, 478

identical twins, 27

identification, 100, 174, 211, 212, 214, 215, 218, 334, 335, 357, 391, 471

identity, xii, 24, 28, 56, 67, 308, 335, 337, 353, 370, 374, 393, 394, 397, 418, 423, 426, 427, 452, 460, 466, 469, 470, 471, 472, 473, 474, 475, 476, 477, 478, 479, 480, 481, 482

identity achievement, 471, 474, 477

identity diffusion, 471

ideology, 362, 363, 471

idiosyncratic, 470

illiteracy, 363

illusion(s), 125, 130, 131

image(s), 10, 46, 130, 240, 259, 262, 268

imagery, 82, 130, 280, 447, 452

imagination, 24, 69, 422, 448

immersion, 337

immigrants, 119

immune disorders, 118, 150

immune function, 105

immune system, 109, 118, 121, 124, 200, 296
immunoglobulin(s), 200
impairments, 263, 279
improvements, 56, 105, 120, 231, 279, 354
impulses, 192, 437
impulsivity, 152
impurities, 77, 148
in vitro, 238
incidence, 21, 31, 153, 154, 160, 163, 166, 353, 416
income, xi, 37, 105, 213, 216, 217, 304, 333, 334, 335, 336, 337, 338, 339, 340, 341, 342, 343, 344, 345, 346, 347, 348, 349, 351, 353, 354, 355, 356, 357, 358, 362, 364, 367, 397
income distribution, 335, 339, 340, 343
income inequality, 335, 336, 337, 340, 344, 345, 346
independence, 195, 277, 278, 279, 284, 357, 364, 456, 459, 461, 466
independent variable, 176, 306
indeterminism, 45
India, 193, 203, 210, 230
indigenous knowledge, 18, 57
indirect effect, 375, 379, 380
individual character, 476
individual characteristics, 476
individual development, 380
individual differences, 304, 308, 314, 321, 383, 431, 471
individualism, 337, 466
individuality, 27, 61, 67
individualization, 337
induction, 200, 250, 444
industrialized countries, xvi
industrialized societies, 290, 479
industry(s), 36, 37, 38, 104, 114, 124, 130, 212, 219
inequality, 268, 336, 337, 339, 344, 346, 349, 397
infancy, 108, 144, 182, 258, 320, 434, 438, 471, 475
infants, 147, 164, 170, 181, 192, 235, 296, 298, 440
infection, 58, 104, 105, 106, 110, 120, 162, 204, 210, 298
infectious mononucleosis, 153
inferences, 419, 424
inferiority, 114
infertility, 113
inflammation, 90, 231
information processing, 418, 422, 457
information technology, 60, 366, 446, 479
informed consent, 232
ingredients, 24
inhibition, 144, 175, 192
inhibitor, 180
initiation, 113, 130, 131, 151, 154, 192, 275, 281, 282

injury(s), viii, 35, 90, 92, 140, 152, 164, 172, 173, 204, 278, 299
inner world, 69, 76
insecurity, 265
insomnia, 92, 143, 145, 146, 147, 148, 149, 150, 151, 152, 153, 155, 165, 175
institutions, 363, 461
insulin, x, 171, 172, 195, 196, 197, 198, 200, 201
insulin resistance, 171, 196
integralism, 5
integration, 34, 58, 105, 106, 108, 109, 325, 326, 348, 352, 392, 430, 439, 440, 480
integrative medicine, ix, xiii, xv, 3, 13, 16, 18, 21, 29, 43, 55, 60, 65, 74, 85, 97, 98, 99, 100, 101, 103
integrity, 27, 50, 94, 275, 362, 391, 431, 471
intellect, 291
intellectual disabilities, 461
intelligence, 30, 60, 126, 409, 415, 427, 429, 430, 431, 436, 438, 439, 440, 460, 461, 475
intensive care unit, 170
interaction effect, 233, 336, 340, 356, 357
interaction effects, 340
interdependence, 383, 386
interface, 109
interference, 155, 259
intermediaries, 58, 209
internal clock, 144
internal consistency, 355, 474
internal validity, 222
internalization, 403, 404, 434, 457, 458, 459, 463, 466
internalizing, 409, 476, 477
interpersonal processes, 411
interpersonal relations, 263, 383
interpersonal relationships, 263, 383
interpersonal skills, 50, 211, 213, 214
intervention, 81, 82, 105, 110, 133, 147, 165, 174, 180, 181, 231, 250, 272, 273, 274, 276, 277, 279, 281, 282, 285, 296, 332, 361, 367, 396, 411, 412, 428, 437, 446, 450, 455, 461, 462, 466, 471, 473
intima, 172
intimacy, 75, 82, 320, 324
intoxication, 162
intracranial pressure, 161, 172
intrauterine growth retardation, 170
intrinsic motivation, 450, 452, 457, 458, 465, 466
intrinsic value, 408
introspection, 8
introvert, 132
intrusions, 372
intuition, 9, 24, 29, 69, 132, 133, 134
inventions, 24

504   *Index*

invertebrates, 292
investigative tools, 14
investment, 49, 114, 280, 347, 372, 427, 440
investment model, 440
invitation to participate, 97, 213
ions, 91
Iowa, 310
IQ scores, 460
iron, 140, 157, 159
irradiation, 91
irrigation, 58
irritability, 149, 150, 152, 159
isolation, 27, 86, 105, 276, 353, 357
Israel, ii, xii, xv, 245, 251, 416, 485, 487, 489
issues, 5, 22, 45, 49, 80, 97, 98, 99, 101, 103, 104,
    110, 117, 137, 146, 147, 151, 153, 156, 158, 164,
    172, 235, 258, 261, 275, 290, 299, 310, 370, 390,
    391, 393, 419, 423, 439, 469, 473, 480
Italy, 369, 370, 372, 373, 380, 384

J

Japan, 212, 219, 268, 349
job satisfaction, 361, 366, 367
joint pain, 164
joints, 231
Jordan, 45
justification, 419

K

ketones, 197, 200
kidney(s), 36, 145, 163, 172, 173, 180, 200, 201
knees, 51
knowledge-based economy, 44

L

labor market, 349, 418
laboratory studies, 222, 227
laboratory tests, 174
labour force, 212
lactation, 202
lakes, 61
landscape, 62
languages, 75, 252
lasers, 85, 86, 88, 94
latency, 149, 150, 159
later life, xi, 260, 263, 267, 268, 271, 272, 274, 277,
    278, 281, 284, 285, 314, 319, 320, 346, 349
laws, 22, 65, 66, 419
leaching, 61

lead, 27, 35, 57, 74, 87, 88, 123, 124, 146, 152, 161,
    162, 164, 246, 276, 281, 309, 310, 381, 382, 395,
    411, 412, 461, 463
leadership, 34, 44, 51, 366, 398, 399, 418, 424, 426,
    427, 430
leadership development, 44
Leahy, 481
learners, 423, 462, 463, 464, 465
learning attitudes, 459
learning difficulties, 435
learning disabilities, 466
learning environment, 411, 412, 459, 463
learning process, 212, 424, 433
learning task, 463
legal protection, 370
legislation, 16, 114, 430
legs, 113, 157, 166, 232
leisure, 257, 258, 261, 262, 263, 264, 265, 266, 268,
    269, 273, 275, 278, 279, 286, 324, 370, 410
leisure time, 275, 278, 286
lesions, 201
lesson plan, 428
lethargy, 159
leukotriene modifier, 162
level of education, 373
life changes, 174, 249
life course, 261, 269, 482
life cycle, 281
life expectancy, 106, 257
life experiences, 260, 266, 272, 281, 436, 470
Life Satisfaction Scale, 308, 361, 365
lifestyle changes, 82
lifestyle decisions, 124
lifetime, 70, 77, 154, 272, 274, 299, 300, 310
light, 24, 26, 34, 85, 86, 87, 90, 94, 124, 125, 144,
    148, 152, 202, 212, 223, 227, 238, 239, 261, 266,
    279, 284, 314, 410, 446, 473, 478
Likert scale, 305, 316
lipid metabolism, 180
lipids, 200
lipodystrophy, 118, 120
liquid chromatography, 203
literacy, 362, 426
liver, 140, 145, 150, 163, 200
living arrangements, 267
living conditions, 337, 349, 353, 354
local authorities, 252
local community, 107
locus, 118, 364, 407
logical reasoning, 421
loneliness, 296, 319, 353, 357
longevity, 237, 238, 240, 242, 278, 286

longitudinal study, 284, 320, 383, 394, 415, 426, 433, 438, 474, 475
love, 4, 9, 10, 81, 87, 89, 131, 133, 293, 296, 300, 320, 324, 391, 398
LSD, 249
luminescence, 244
lung cancer, 140, 298
lung function, 231
Luo, xi, 257
lupus, 176
lying, 189, 293
lysine, 239

M

Macedonia, 361, 364, 367
macromolecules, 209
magazines, 265
magnesium, 110
magnetic field(s), 91, 95
magnetism, 85, 90, 94
magnitude, 93, 477, 478, 479
maiming, 41
Mainland China, 337
major depression, 274
major depressive disorder, 287
majority, 57, 59, 334, 338, 343, 358, 371, 372, 376, 381
malaise, 150
malaria, 110
malignancy, 157
malnutrition, 59, 104
maltreatment, 416
mammalian brain, 291, 292
mammals, 291
man, 5, 10, 13, 40, 53, 75, 113, 129, 130, 133, 231, 253, 309, 364
mania, 155, 274
manipulation, 231, 232, 410, 422, 448, 479
manufacturing, 219
manure, 204
mapping, 70
marginal utility, 344
marital partners, 315
marital quality, 394
marital status, 214, 314, 318, 337
market economy, 367
marketing, 151, 347
marriage, 31, 32, 79, 273, 344, 369, 370, 372, 373, 374, 376, 380, 381, 382, 383, 384, 385, 410
married couples, 381, 382, 383
Maryland, 169, 182
mass, 59, 284, 410, 451

mass media, 410, 451
materials, 49, 51, 114, 412, 430
maternal care, 434
mathematical methods, 47
mathematics, 8, 66, 70, 126, 445, 452, 476
matrix, 40
matter, viii, ix, 5, 6, 7, 8, 10, 11, 26, 27, 28, 30, 31, 40, 41, 44, 46, 48, 52, 61, 68, 74, 78, 85, 86, 87, 88, 89, 90, 94, 95, 99, 134, 135, 221, 222, 226, 299, 314, 343, 347, 352, 359, 440
mature economies, 348
MB, 13, 21, 65, 85, 286, 415, 427, 428
measurement(s), 22, 45, 66, 70, 88, 169, 170, 173, 174, 181, 214, 240, 246, 249, 260, 267, 332, 345, 399, 433, 434, 439, 451
media, 38, 172, 239, 273, 394, 397, 423, 426, 479
media messages, 423
mediation, 311, 375, 376, 377, 379
Medicaid, 354
medical care, 57, 258, 261
medical history, 147
medical science, xiii, xvi, 9, 21, 22, 28, 31, 65, 70, 74, 79, 109, 121, 122, 127, 257
medication, 56, 113, 124, 139, 147, 153, 154, 158, 161, 165, 170, 172, 173, 176, 177, 178, 180, 181, 283
melatonin, 143, 144, 146, 148, 150, 151, 165
mellitus, 118, 162, 173, 196, 201
membership, 15, 352, 353, 356
membranes, 209
memory, 48, 149, 161, 192, 302, 310
meninges, 239
mental ability, 431
mental disorder, 82, 123, 274, 290, 297, 300
mental health, 73, 76, 79, 81, 103, 105, 106, 107, 109, 110, 113, 125, 146, 250, 262, 264, 271, 272, 273, 274, 276, 280, 283, 284, 285, 286, 289, 290, 295, 297, 301, 362, 395, 397, 400, 436, 439, 440, 450, 480
mental health professionals, 106
mental illness, 75, 166, 231, 250, 271, 274
mental processes, 418, 422, 452
mental retardation, 440
mental state(s), 7, 126, 192, 232
mentoring, 281, 282
mentorship, 271, 275, 276, 282, 285
mercury, 170
messages, 104, 410, 423, 448
messengers, 89
meta-analysis, 95, 166, 178, 183, 212, 230, 235, 282, 285, 396, 481
metabolic alkalosis, 179
metabolic disorder, 196

506   *Index*

metabolism, 196
metabolites, 150
metabolized, 150
metacognition, 418
metacognitive skills, 425
metals, 119
metaphor, 22, 67
meter, 253
methodology, 6, 82, 100, 182, 320, 325, 327, 328, 332, 479
methylphenidate, 146, 153, 154
microcirculation, 90
micronutrients, 104, 105
microscope, 23, 240, 243
microscopy, 240
midbrain, 175
military, 390
mind-body, 16, 19, 75, 82, 83, 90, 98, 99, 119, 245, 246, 248, 249, 253
Ministry of Education, 267
minority groups, 171
misconceptions, 283, 424
mission, xvi, 51, 114, 122, 363, 390, 478, 487
misunderstanding, 383
misuse, 106, 150, 294, 453
mitochondria, 91
mitosis, 91
mixing, 152
modelling, 214, 311
models, 8, 24, 56, 61, 88, 123, 214, 222, 227, 280, 284, 311, 326, 349, 384, 389, 394, 396, 407, 422, 431, 437, 447, 461, 462, 464, 466, 471, 479
moderates, 229, 232, 436, 440
moderators, 385
modern science, 32
modern society, 121, 124, 349
modernization, 353
modifications, 171, 174, 180, 462
modules, 289, 291, 292, 293, 294, 295, 296, 297, 298, 299
modus operandi, 62
moisture, 60
mold, 114
molecules, 35, 41, 48, 57, 86, 204, 209, 237, 239
monks, 295
mood disorder, 166, 274
morale, 258
morality, 427
moratorium, 471, 474, 477
morbidity, 56, 104, 169, 181, 273, 278, 284, 287, 307
morning stiffness, 91
morphogenesis, 89

morphology, x, 237, 240
mortality, 56, 83, 106, 169, 181, 183, 269, 273, 284, 286, 299, 307
mortality rate, 56
motivation, 192, 219, 272, 283, 363, 366, 367, 403, 404, 405, 406, 407, 408, 413, 414, 416, 424, 445, 447, 452, 455, 456, 457, 458, 459, 462, 465, 466
movement disorders, 164
MR, 110, 182, 183, 300, 321, 347, 428, 452, 466, 481
MRI, 174, 192
multidimensional, 29, 30, 109, 304, 352
multinational corporations, 104
multiple factors, 271
multiple regression, 306, 349, 466
multiple regression analyses, 306, 466
multivariate analysis, 264, 465
mung bean, x, 221, 223, 224, 225, 226
muscle relaxation, 280
muscles, 144, 155, 232, 295
musculoskeletal, 284
museums, 265
music, 78, 135, 152, 263, 295
myocardial infarction, 178
mythology, 131

N

naming, 100, 259
narcolepsy, 143, 153, 154, 155, 156, 157, 159, 165, 166
narratives, 394
national identity, 348
National Institutes of Health, 240
natural disaster(s), 251, 253
Natural Health Products, 5
natural laws, 40
natural resources, 56, 60
natural science, 46
nausea, 155, 156, 158, 175
Nazi Germany, 390
nearsightedness, 298
negative affectivity, 304, 308
negative attitudes, 247, 259
negative consequences, 371, 383, 459, 472
negative effects, 382, 383, 409
negative emotions, 303, 304, 307, 309, 432, 434, 435, 464
negative outcomes, 106, 222, 433
negative relation, 369, 380, 383, 396
negotiation, 50, 348, 439
nematode, 210
nephritis, 172, 173

nephrolithiasis, 179
nephrologist, 181
nephron, 177
nephropathy, 173
nerve, 77, 87, 89, 290, 292, 295, 297
nervous system, 153, 289, 291, 292, 297
nervousness, 151, 155
Netherlands, 347, 349
network theory, 210
neural network(s), 192, 290, 294
neurobiology, 44, 291, 292, 294, 297, 298, 299
neurogenic bladder, 162
neuronal systems, 238
neurons, x, 237, 238, 239, 240, 241, 242
neuroscience, 238, 292, 299, 300
neuroses, 395
neurotransmitter(s), 89, 192, 292, 297, 300
neutral, 291, 302, 303, 365, 430, 431
new paradigm, 3, 5, 8, 9, 10, 13, 14, 21, 24, 25, 31,
    34, 42, 52, 99, 101
New Zealand, 103
Newtonian physics, 14, 67
next generation, 106, 489
NGOs, 62
NHANES, 83
nicotine, 148, 173
Niels Bohr, 86
nightmares, 146, 147, 154, 164, 176
nitrogen, 60, 61, 197
N-N, 332
No Child Left Behind, 430
Nobel Prize, 86, 485
nodes, 62
non-institutionalized, 273
nonsteroidal anti-inflammatory medications, 173
nonverbal cues, 187
norepinephrine, 176
normal distribution, 244
North America, 16
Northern Ireland, 425
Norway, xv, 73, 237, 245, 251, 289, 296, 489
NSAIDs, 172, 173
nucleus, 292
null, 341
nurses, 34, 57, 107, 253, 316, 327, 373
nursing, 204, 323, 332, 399
nursing home, 323
nurturance, 391, 411
nutrient(s), 59
nutrient imbalance, 59
nutrition, 9, 41, 56, 59, 83, 104, 105, 110, 118, 174,
    273, 276, 354
nutritional deficiencies, 59

nutritional status, 70

O

obedience, 51
obesity, 41, 55, 59, 120, 161, 171, 173, 174, 182,
    273, 278, 299
objectification, 67
objective reality, 99, 100
objectivity, 68
obstacles, 406, 407, 414, 426
obstruction, 160, 161, 162, 172
obstructive lung disease, 231, 235
obstructive sleep apnea, 146, 147, 165
occupational therapy, 37
oceans, 61
OH, 160, 161
oil, 56, 61
Oklahoma, 271, 281, 351
old age, 259, 260, 261, 266, 267, 275, 282, 285, 304,
    337
old paradigm, 8, 22
one dimension, 302
openness, 34, 363, 364, 370, 391, 434, 472
openness to experience, 363, 472
operant conditioning, 164
operations, 213
opioids, 158, 297, 300
opportunities, 51, 118, 212, 213, 218, 271, 282, 285,
    289, 292, 337, 347, 362, 412, 422, 423, 424, 461,
    462, 478, 482
Oppositional Defiant Disorder, 145
oppression, 252
optimal performance, 304
optimism, 261, 391, 393, 403, 404, 407, 408, 409,
    410, 411, 412, 413, 414, 415, 416, 447, 449, 451
optimists, 407, 409, 414, 415
oral presentations, 445
organ(s), 34, 35, 88, 89, 90, 122, 135, 150, 170, 172,
    174, 176, 178, 180, 298
organic matter, 59, 60
organism, 33, 57, 59, 60, 85, 88, 89, 91, 94, 204,
    209, 238, 239
organizational culture, 364
organize, 417, 444, 456
originality, 317, 420, 421, 422
orthostatic hypotension, 175, 176
oscillation, 209, 238
osmosis, 87
osteoarthritis, 95, 284
outpatient(s), 170, 332
outreach, 119
outreach programs, 119

overlap, 274, 275
overpopulation, 40, 41
overweight, 58, 171
overweight adults, 58
ownership, 348
oxalate, 197
oxygen, 67, 90, 91, 161
oxyhemoglobin, 147

P

P.A.T.H.S., 397, 401, 416, 427, 463, 477, 478
Pacific, 427, 489
pain, 36, 75, 90, 91, 92, 96, 123, 134, 146, 165, 229, 231, 232, 233, 234, 250, 275, 276, 284, 290, 293, 296, 297, 299, 300, 310, 323, 325, 326, 327, 328, 330, 332
pain management, 92
palliative, 396, 400
pancreas, 200, 201
paradigm shift, 5, 10, 14, 15, 24, 52, 60, 61
parallel, 60, 101, 114, 327, 330, 340, 420, 482
parallelism, 325, 327, 330
parasite, 204
parental control, 465
parental influence, 400
parental involvement, 412, 452, 458, 464
parental support, 395, 411
parenting, 394, 398, 411, 455, 465
paroxetine, 146
participants, 4, 6, 9, 34, 82, 98, 117, 211, 233, 245, 246, 247, 248, 259, 263, 280, 305, 309, 316, 318, 319, 323, 324, 325, 328, 329, 354, 358, 369, 372, 373, 374, 375, 376, 377, 381, 382, 396, 397, 434
patents, 212
path analysis, 268, 427
pathogenesis, 204
pathogens, 204
pathology, 88, 118, 243, 282, 477
pathophysiology, 160
pathways, 65, 108, 403, 404, 405, 406, 407, 410, 412, 416, 439
peace, 124, 189, 391, 392, 396, 439
pedagogy, 425
peer group, 318
peer influence, 389, 426
peer relationship, 394, 400, 440, 458
peer review, 90, 222
peer support, 312, 461, 464
peer tutoring, 461
pelvic floor, 82
perceived control, 466
perceived health, 277, 315, 321

perceived self-efficacy, 445, 453
percentile, 169, 170, 171, 180
pericardial effusion, 176
permission, viii, 113, 144, 145, 146, 153, 155, 156, 161, 162, 165, 181, 238, 303
perseverance, 406, 447
personal accounts, 260
personal consciousness, xvi
personal contact, 392
personal control, 282, 405, 410, 457, 458, 460, 462, 463
personal development, 74, 447
personal goals, 400, 404, 456, 457, 459, 463, 471
personal history, 173
personal identity, 470
personal life, 365
personal problems, 112
personal qualities, 436
personal relations, 397, 461
personal relationship, 397, 461
personal stories, 5
personality, 131, 212, 213, 235, 268, 272, 305, 307, 308, 310, 312, 349, 363, 370, 383, 384, 407, 409, 414, 415, 431, 434, 439, 470, 473, 476, 480, 481
personality characteristics, 370, 470
personality disorder, 310
personality traits, 212, 213, 268, 414, 431
persuasion, 443, 448
pessimism, 408, 413, 414
pessimists, 409, 414, 415
pH, 197, 198, 205
pharmaceutical(s), 28, 57, 60, 81, 82, 83, 85, 88, 94, 114, 124, 151, 196, 249
pharmacological treatment, 282
pharmacology, 23, 86, 137, 138
pharmacotherapy, 276, 287
phenotype, 182
Philadelphia, 182, 399
phosphate, 240
phosphorus, 61
photons, 47, 48, 89, 90, 238, 239
photosensitivity, 179
physical abuse, 94, 249
physical activity, xi, 189, 263, 271, 273, 275, 277, 278, 279, 280, 284, 285, 286, 287, 296
physical attractiveness, 234
physical characteristics, 260
physical exercise, 41, 252, 265, 273, 279, 286, 310
physical fitness, 262, 278
physical health, 73, 106, 109, 110, 125, 144, 246, 257, 261, 262, 264, 266, 271, 272, 274, 280, 285, 396, 400, 409, 416, 475
physical inactivity, 287

physical phenomena, 45
physical sciences, 23
physical stressors, 109
physical structure, 28
physical therapy, 82
physical well-being, 268, 407, 414
physicians, xvi, 14, 15, 16, 67, 73, 79, 123, 124, 157, 252, 316, 327
physics, 8, 22, 23, 28, 29, 44, 45, 46, 47, 49, 53, 86, 87, 88, 93, 95, 126, 222, 238, 239, 244
Physiological, 448
physiological mechanisms, 22
physiology, 7, 16, 17, 23, 67, 91, 243
pilot study, x, 193, 221, 235, 238, 242, 243, 250
pineal gland, 148
pioglitazone, 202
PISA, 452
placebo, 26, 67, 81, 87, 91, 95, 231
plants, 57, 60, 99, 108, 113, 119, 203, 204, 205, 206, 207, 208, 209, 210, 222, 225, 246, 264
plasma membrane, 204
plasticity, 38
platform, 436, 478
Plato, 123, 127
plausibility, 227
playing, 152, 264
pleasure, 5, 293, 299, 300, 304, 309, 310, 347, 352, 358, 362
PM, 155, 287, 359, 400, 428, 482
pneumonia, 57
poetry, 131
Poincaré, 44
polar, 47
polarity, 92
policy, xiii, 4, 49, 267, 346, 348, 361, 367, 473, 489
policy making, 4
political participation, 357
political parties, 363
politics, 4, 33, 34, 39, 138
pollution, 30, 56, 57, 70, 337
polymers, 204
polythene, 203, 204
polyunsaturated fat, 200
polyunsaturated fatty acids, 200
pools, 284
population, 37, 49, 56, 62, 96, 99, 104, 106, 178, 196, 258, 260, 264, 265, 271, 273, 275, 284, 290, 296, 300, 305, 332, 337, 347, 348, 381, 382, 399, 415, 446, 476
population size, 265
porphyria, 150
positive attitudes, 234, 257, 258, 259, 260, 261, 266
positive correlation, 340

positive emotions, 301, 302, 304, 307, 310, 311
positive feedback, 7, 277, 463
positive mental health, 396, 414
positive mood, 262, 433
positive relationship, 371, 395, 458, 460
positivism, 99, 100
postural hypotension, 158
potassium, 27, 91, 174, 177, 179
potassium sparing diuretics, 177
potato, 244
poverty, 22, 104, 118, 337, 338, 341, 349, 351, 353, 354, 356, 358, 362, 363
Prader-Willi syndrome, 145, 160
prayer, 87, 93, 96, 391
PRC, 333, 349, 389, 403, 417, 429, 443, 455, 469
precedents, 45
predictor variables, 375
prefrontal cortex, 192
pregnancy, 157, 175, 178, 181, 183, 413
prejudice, 108
preparation, viii, 122, 209, 222, 374, 375, 376, 380, 392, 411, 412, 448
preschool, 439
preschool children, 439
preschoolers, 321
prescription drugs, 92
president, 139
prestige, 261, 266
preterm delivery, 171
preventative care, 137, 140
prevention, xvi, 36, 37, 39, 56, 57, 85, 94, 108, 119, 127, 178, 182, 183, 271, 272, 274, 275, 276, 278, 285, 298, 300, 384, 413, 428, 453, 473, 485
priapism, 149
primary function, 36, 292
primary school, 130, 316, 373, 416, 425, 427, 464
principles, 17, 34, 39, 49, 53, 55, 69, 118, 232, 239, 393, 466
prior knowledge, 424
prisons, 9
private practice, 4
private sector, 104, 114
privatization, 361, 364, 366
probability, 47, 217, 405, 419
problem behavior(s), 397, 400, 416, 418, 473, 481
problem solving, 212, 218, 383, 424, 434, 462, 463
problem-based learning, 424
problem-solving, 409, 415, 417, 418, 420, 421, 422, 424, 425, 445, 447, 462, 471, 474, 478
problem-solving skills, 424, 471
professionals, 3, 7, 29, 36, 61, 91, 103, 106, 123, 316, 396, 487, 489
profit, 58, 122

510   *Index*

programming, 170
project, 117, 118, 119, 120, 222, 225, 246, 316, 391,
    425, 426, 427, 450, 489
proliferation, 139
propaganda, 131, 132
proposition, 226
prosocial behavior, 397
prosperity, 257
protease inhibitors, 205
protection, 139, 276, 370
protective factors, 261, 383, 396, 415, 476
proteins, 195, 197, 198, 199, 200, 203, 204, 205,
    206, 207, 208, 209, 210
proteinuria, 180, 197
Prozac, 124
psychiatric disorders, 144, 148, 165, 193
psychiatric hospitals, 282
psychiatrist, 124, 129
psychiatry, 82, 107, 300
psychoanalysis, 234
psychological development, 314, 427
psychological distress, 371, 398, 401
psychological health, 106, 143, 165, 259, 287, 353,
    357
psychological phenomena, 29
psychological problems, 328, 396
psychological processes, 445, 446, 447, 448
psychological resources, 302
psychological states, 118
psychological stress, 118
psychological variables, 347, 357, 473
psychological well-being, 258, 261, 301, 304, 310,
    311, 393, 397, 400, 409, 412, 416, 450, 453, 457,
    465, 474, 480, 482
psychology, 8, 15, 35, 47, 60, 82, 285, 289, 298, 299,
    304, 310, 311, 314, 351, 352, 356, 367, 368, 399,
    404, 413, 414, 415, 416, 432, 433, 451, 452, 456,
    460, 465, 469, 470, 479, 480, 481
psychometric properties, 433, 434, 445, 446
psychopathology, 166, 310, 395, 465
psychopharmacology, 166
psychosocial development, 314, 393, 418, 423, 426,
    475
psychosocial factors, 261
psychosocial support, 231
psychostimulants, 154, 159, 165
psychotherapy, 127, 131, 232, 234, 235, 246, 249,
    250, 283
puberty, 148, 152, 418, 471
public health, 4, 19, 55, 56, 105, 108, 150, 271, 274,
    286, 487, 489
public policy, 284
public resources, 344

public service, 487
publishing, xvi
pumps, 122
punishment, 289, 291, 292, 293, 297, 299
purpura, 172

Q

qualitative research, 260, 392
quantitative concept, 46
quantum mechanics, 23, 44, 45, 53, 100
quantum phenomena, 45
quantum state, 45
quantum theory, 28, 88
Queensland, 33
questioning, 56, 427, 471
questionnaire, 214, 232, 248, 313, 316, 338, 340,
    354, 355, 369, 373, 374

R

race, 109, 119, 130, 234, 354
racial minorities, 476
radiation, 87, 89, 94
radio, 152, 264
radiography, 37
radiotherapy, 23
rainforest, 57
random assignment, 235
rape, x, 245, 246, 247, 248, 250
rash, 175, 179
rationality, 420, 427
RCP, 416, 443, 455, 469
RE, 166, 285, 299, 349, 358, 439, 440
reaction time, 161
reactions, 121, 125, 155, 156, 176, 179, 230, 391,
    392
reactivity, 308
readership, 359
reading, 8, 10, 79, 138, 192, 263, 264, 265, 452, 476
real estate, 213
realism, 100, 102
reality, 8, 24, 31, 43, 44, 46, 49, 50, 66, 67, 70, 77,
    80, 86, 93, 96, 100, 186, 187, 189, 226, 391, 405,
    480
reasoning, 100, 294, 395, 404, 406, 418, 419, 422,
    424, 425
reasoning skills, 424
recall, 164, 302, 451
recalling, 421
receptors, 149, 150, 157, 175, 176, 178
reciprocity, 382, 444, 448

Index 511

recognition, 9, 13, 15, 24, 51, 86, 104, 106, 107, 108, 124, 169, 181, 210, 212, 234, 274, 275, 397, 478
recommendations, viii, 104, 158, 169
reconstruction, 427
recovery, 276, 282, 372
recreation, 38, 39
recreational, 284
recurrence, 178
red blood cells, 242
red wine, 133
redevelopment, 348
reductionism, 21, 22, 57
reflexes, 289, 292, 297
reflux nephropathy, 174
reform, 428
refugees, 119
regression, 214, 217, 264, 340, 341, 342, 343, 375, 376, 379, 380
regression analysis, 264, 340, 341
regression model, 340, 342, 343, 379, 380
regulations, 62
rehabilitation, 36, 37, 75, 396, 452, 485, 487
rejection, 114, 300
relational dimension, 19
relationship quality, 314
relatives, 153, 258, 264, 265, 372
relativity, 8, 44
relaxation, 138, 209, 210, 233, 234, 262, 263, 264, 265
relevance, 35, 299, 359, 395
reliability, 214, 222, 260, 268, 308, 338, 355, 361, 365, 392, 434, 445
relief, 92, 133, 134, 139, 140, 229, 233, 234
religion, 31, 32, 81, 112, 338, 347, 390, 391, 395, 396, 399, 400, 401, 471
religiosity, 390, 392, 393, 395, 398, 400, 479
religious beliefs, 393
religiousness, 391, 398
REM, 144, 147, 149, 153, 154, 156, 159, 161, 164, 165
remission, 26, 279, 280, 282, 286
renal artery stenosis, 174, 175
renal failure, 157, 170, 172, 173
renin, 171, 175
repetitions, 240
replication, 96, 222, 308, 397
reproductive age, 178
requirements, 139
research efforts, xvi, 258, 261
researchers, xiii, xv, xvi, 34, 43, 44, 56, 61, 77, 92, 100, 171, 212, 221, 231, 239, 253, 258, 259, 260, 301, 302, 308, 352, 370, 373, 391, 392, 410, 430, 434, 438, 445, 456, 459, 470, 473

resettlement, 380
resilience, 363, 393, 396, 409, 412, 416, 435, 436
resistance, 59, 160, 175, 176, 202, 269, 279, 282, 286
resolution, 159, 162, 172
resources, xvi, 49, 56, 59, 62, 78, 108, 109, 139, 218, 248, 269, 281, 344, 345, 357, 361, 367, 370, 372, 383, 397, 447, 448, 450, 459, 463, 470, 475, 478, 480
response format, 355
responsiveness, 235
restless legs syndrome, 143, 146, 165, 166
restoration, 55, 56, 60, 91, 292, 392, 396
restructuring, 348, 380
retail, 213
retinopathy, 170, 172
retirement, 262
retirement age, 262
revenue, 284
rewards, 289, 292, 294, 295, 296, 297, 299, 320
RH, 269, 385, 427
rhabdomyolysis, 149
rheumatoid arthritis, 95
rhinitis, 155
rhythm, 89, 91, 95, 148, 154, 174, 235
rights, viii, 140, 253
rings, 252
risk factors, 160, 170, 182, 202, 259, 264, 265, 275, 299, 371, 383, 426
RNA, 89
ROI, 240
role playing, 448
romantic relationship, 314, 371, 382, 418
root(s), ix, 55, 57, 99, 104, 129, 130, 133, 319, 352
routes, 406
rules, 6, 325, 331, 419, 420, 450, 476, 478
rural areas, 265
rural people, 15
Russia, 90, 92, 347

S

sadness, 126, 129, 133, 352
safety, 80, 260, 279, 280, 296, 324, 356, 408, 476
SAS, 198
saturation, 98
scar tissue, 231
school achievement, 313
school adjustment, 397, 400, 411, 416, 458
school climate, 415
school learning, 412, 424
school success, 316, 317, 436, 453, 461
school support, 452

Index

Schrödinger equation, 45
scientific method, 66
scientific papers, 69, 75
scientific progress, 14, 37
scope, 274, 308, 310, 390
second language, 445
Second World, 35
secondary education, 416, 423, 460
secondary school students, 427, 445, 446, 452, 478
secondary schools, 423, 449, 455, 478
secondary students, 462
secretion, 89
security, 257, 261, 265, 267, 314, 320, 337, 358, 408, 434, 457, 461, 478
sedative, 143, 149, 151, 165
sedative medication, 143, 165
seed, 60, 61, 204
seedlings, x, 221, 223, 224, 225, 226, 242
seizure, 150
selective attention, 346
selenium, 110
self esteem, 347
self-actualization, xvi, 393, 460
self-awareness, 73, 80, 81, 82, 291, 430, 457, 461
self-concept, 309, 311, 447, 449, 470, 471, 472, 473, 476, 481, 482
self-conception, 309
self-confidence, 346, 353, 403, 404, 408, 452, 463
self-control, 219
self-definition, 258, 259, 267, 471
self-discipline, 191
self-discrepancy, 472
self-doubt, 445
self-employed, 122
self-empowerment, 478
self-esteem, 76, 230, 250, 283, 284, 308, 353, 397, 409, 411, 415, 416, 423, 428, 457, 463, 469, 470, 471, 474, 475, 476, 477, 478, 480, 481, 482
self-evaluations, 259, 266
self-expression, xvi
self-identity, 444, 455, 470
self-image, 478
self-knowledge, 461
self-paced learning, 464
self-perceptions, 260
self-regulation, 192, 210, 305, 311, 408, 414, 416, 418, 425, 447, 452, 457, 458, 462, 463, 466, 470, 474
self-reports, 308, 340, 445
self-sufficiency, 258, 283
self-understanding, 189, 412, 463
self-worth, 258, 409, 411, 474, 478, 481
seller, 132

semantic association, 192
seminars, 464, 487
sensation(s), 132, 157, 158, 292, 294, 296, 299
senses, 125, 155, 308
sensitivity, 225, 301, 302, 308, 437, 451
sensors, 60
sensory experience, 293
sequencing, 192
serotonin, 297
sertraline, 165
serum, 157, 175, 197
serum ferritin, 157
service organizations, 361, 365, 366, 367
services, viii, 15, 46, 107, 108, 139, 213, 361, 363, 366, 367, 391
SES, 216, 217, 277, 316, 317
sewage, 61
sex, 75, 109, 169, 171, 230, 235, 245, 247, 265, 278, 334
sex hormones, 171
sexology, 82, 246
sexual abuse, 164, 245, 246, 247, 248
sexual activity, 473
sexual behavior, 482
sexual health, 80, 165, 181
sexual violence, 246, 247, 248
sexuality, 75, 79, 159, 247
sexually transmitted diseases, 108
sham, 95
shamanism, 221
shame, 246, 247, 472
shape, 6, 89, 126, 212, 240, 394, 395, 397
shared emotional connection, 352, 357
shelter, 351, 354
shock, x, 50, 92, 203, 204, 205, 208, 209, 210
shock therapy, 92
shortage, 139
showing, 43, 44, 66, 104, 120, 205, 222, 259, 266, 294, 307, 357, 390, 394, 396, 408, 425, 435, 438, 446, 449, 458
side effects, 82, 83, 91, 92, 146, 149, 150, 152, 154, 156, 157, 179, 180, 249
signalling, 89, 243
signals, 38, 48, 89, 90
significance level, 198
signs, 30, 59, 66, 182
silver, 286
Singapore, 243, 467
sinusitis, 61
skills training, 448
skin, 62, 113, 155, 296
slaves, 253
sleep apnea, 160, 162, 165, 166

sleep deprivation, 165
sleep disorders, xiii, 143, 144, 147, 165, 166
sleep disturbance, 166, 275
sleep habits, 147
sleep latency, 149, 152, 157
sleep medicine, 143, 144
sleep paralysis, 153, 155, 156
sleep stage, 144, 148, 163
sleep terrors, 164, 165
sleep walking, 147, 164
smoking, 41, 70, 140, 273, 284, 298, 317, 449, 450, 453
smooth muscle, 176
smooth muscle cells, 176
snoring, 147, 160
soccer, 132, 444, 450, 452
sociability, 263, 264, 268
social acceptance, 416, 474, 478
social activities, 39, 261
social adjustment, 440
social capital, 348, 349, 448
social care, 107, 108
social circle, 418
social class, 83, 212, 319
social cognition, 332, 451
social comparison, 333, 334, 335, 336, 337, 340, 341, 343, 344, 345, 346, 347, 349, 411
social comparison theory, 333, 334, 335, 336, 343, 344, 347, 349
social competence, 396, 439, 476, 482
social construct, 425
social context, 382, 410, 433, 435, 436, 458, 462
social desirability, 434
social development, 465
social environment, 271, 296, 434, 447, 456
social exclusion, 300
social fabric, 52
social gerontology, 258, 259
social group, 394, 471
social hierarchy, 253
social identity, 470, 479, 480
social image, 463
social indicator, 362, 363
social influence(s), 480
social information processing, 436
social integration, 257, 262, 266, 267
social interactions, 49, 276, 422, 431, 432, 435, 437, 479
social learning, 394
social life, 325, 435
social network, 263, 268, 284, 296, 299, 347, 480
social norms, 456, 457
social organization, 263, 268

social participation, 260, 264
social phenomena, 44
social policy, 348, 349, 363
social problems, 418
social psychology, 268, 348, 349
social relations, 277, 295, 296, 300, 353, 362, 366
social relationships, 277, 362, 366
social resources, 261, 267
social responsibility, 471
social roles, 418, 471
social sciences, 45, 289, 470
social services, 358, 446
social situations, 297
social skills, 430, 434, 436, 475
social status, 392
social stress, 35
social structure, 282, 480
social support, 257, 258, 261, 262, 263, 264, 266, 268, 269, 276, 277, 281, 283, 286, 320, 353, 409, 412, 416, 450, 453, 465, 472, 479
social transition, 361, 363, 364
social workers, 35, 412
socialism, 349, 364
socialization, 230, 263, 400, 432, 437, 438
sociocultural contexts, 415
socioeconomic status, 218, 277, 279, 286, 314, 316, 421
sociology, 35, 314, 480
sodium, 27, 91, 156, 174, 177, 179
software, 213, 240
solidarity, 50, 124
solution, 46, 132, 421
South Africa, x, 3, 5, 8, 9, 13, 14, 21, 23, 33, 34, 43, 55, 58, 63, 65, 85, 97, 99, 101, 103, 104, 105, 108, 110, 111, 112, 114, 117, 118, 119, 121, 129, 132, 137, 138, 245, 246
Southeast Asia, 348
Soviet Union, 364
SP, 210, 399, 427
space-time, 44, 45, 186
Spain, 332, 367
special education, 451, 456, 460
specialists, 4, 112, 113, 133, 487
specialization, 373
species, 49, 74, 196, 200, 209, 290
spectroscopy, 192, 209, 210, 227
speculation, 232, 433
speech, 91, 186, 422
speed of light, 47
spending, 55, 67, 263, 273, 285, 318, 338
spinal cord, 162, 272
spinal cord injury, 272
spinal cord tumor, 162

514 Index

spine, 131, 231
spiritual care, 396
spirituality, xvi, 109, 249, 311, 389, 390, 391, 392, 393, 394, 395, 396, 397, 398, 399, 400
Spring, 127
SS, 166, 182, 202, 286, 332, 384, 414, 439, 466
stability, 277, 302, 320, 321, 337, 371, 382, 383, 437, 474, 481
stabilization, 430
stakeholders, 50
standard deviation, 215, 224, 240, 338, 339, 374
standard error, 214, 216, 217, 240
standardization, 148
stars, 112
statistics, 47, 66, 69, 70, 372
stenosis, 173
stereotypes, 259, 266, 410, 412
sterile, 204, 205, 207, 239
steroids, 150, 162, 173
stigma, 108
stimulant, 146, 148, 151, 154
stimulation, 86, 92, 96, 263, 292, 299, 393
stimulus, 192, 203, 209, 265, 293, 302
stomach, 134, 231
storage, 223
storytelling, 98
stratification, 100, 347
strength training, 279
stressful events, 109, 371, 382
stressful life events, 276, 371, 435
stressors, 68, 290, 436, 447, 450, 453
stretching, 41, 279, 280, 419, 420
structural equation modeling, 100, 392
structure, 19, 31, 41, 45, 48, 86, 204, 209, 210, 214, 266, 331, 337, 364, 414, 434, 458, 463, 466, 469, 470, 471, 479, 481
structuring, 262
style(s), 4, 171, 180, 230, 258, 264, 265, 362, 363, 408, 415, 420, 423, 426, 428, 434, 435, 450, 451, 455, 458, 470, 473, 476, 480, 481
subgroups, 223, 313, 315, 316, 320, 449
subjective experience, xvi, 14, 261, 263, 264, 359
subjective well-being, 263, 289, 291, 299, 310, 311, 321, 332, 344, 347, 349, 352, 353, 354, 357, 358, 359, 364, 371, 398, 435, 436, 439
subjectivity, 283
sub-Saharan Africa, 120
substance abuse, 153, 310
substance use, 423, 426, 473, 482
successful aging, 258, 261, 263, 264, 269, 285
sucrose, 205
suicidal ideation, 412, 416, 436
suicide, 123, 140, 274

suicide rate, 274
Sun, x, xi, xii, 42, 211, 311, 401, 403, 404, 413, 416, 417, 419, 427, 459, 466, 473, 481
superimposition, 114
supervision, 181, 239, 265
supervisor, 51, 232
supplementation, 91, 105, 110, 157, 158
supplier, 372
suppression, 114, 149, 156, 434
suprachiasmatic nucleus, 144, 148, 150
surgical intervention, 108, 109
surgical technique, 29, 65
surplus, 296
survival, 73, 76, 77, 80, 82, 83, 239, 278, 289, 290, 293, 294, 296, 297, 353, 472
survival rate, 278
susceptibility, 201, 310, 448
sustainability, 4, 7, 49, 55, 56, 63
sustainable development, 56
Sweden, 268, 301, 305, 489
swelling, 90, 91
Switzerland, 202, 221, 239, 240, 349
symptomatic treatment, 57, 94
symptoms, 23, 28, 30, 36, 57, 58, 60, 108, 123, 154, 155, 157, 158, 175, 235, 252, 264, 265, 271, 272, 274, 275, 276, 277, 281, 282, 283, 396, 409, 447, 479
synapse, 238, 242
synchronize, 89
syndrome, 137, 138, 145, 153, 157, 159, 162, 166, 170, 172, 173, 174, 176
synthesis, 17, 27, 31, 86, 95, 476
systematic desensitization, 448
systolic blood pressure, 171

T

tachycardia, 149, 163, 164, 175, 176
Taiwan, xi, 257, 258, 259, 260, 261, 262, 263, 264, 265, 266, 267, 268, 269, 409, 453, 466
talent, 431
target, 170, 174, 176, 178, 279, 281, 284, 295, 430, 456, 461, 462, 463, 473
task demands, 450
task performance, 418, 422, 447, 449
taxation, 212
taxonomy, 427
teacher training, 464
teachers, 154, 305, 373, 397, 411, 412, 424, 425, 429, 434, 437, 438, 444, 447, 448, 449, 450, 451, 452, 457, 458, 461, 462, 463, 464, 465, 466, 472, 473, 477, 479
team members, 46

Index

teams, 49, 139, 140

techniques, 21, 22, 23, 26, 31, 37, 47, 70, 99, 120, 137, 138, 185, 186, 231, 232, 280, 325, 392, 438, 458

technology(s), 16, 33, 34, 37, 38, 39, 50, 62, 66, 68, 86, 90, 91, 92, 95, 257, 361, 367, 479

teens, 181, 479

teeth, 164

teleological, 28, 88

telephone, 280, 338, 349

telephone numbers, 338

tellers, 113

temperament, 302, 303, 306, 308, 310, 311, 435

temperature, 223, 239

temporal lobe, 159, 165

temporal lobe epilepsy, 159, 165

tendon(s), 91

tension, 28, 90, 231, 235, 369, 370, 372, 374, 375, 376, 377, 378, 379, 381, 382, 383

tension headache, 231, 235

tensions, 40, 121, 125, 381

territorial, 352, 359

territory, 70

tertiary education, 450

testing, 119, 174, 198, 282, 313, 317, 439, 444

test-retest reliability, 308

tetrad, 47

textbook(s), 82 90

therapeutic agents, 176, 180

therapeutic benefits, 235

therapeutic effects, 96

therapeutic encounter, 124, 230

therapeutic goal, 245, 247, 248

therapeutic practice, 246

therapeutic process, 230

therapeutic relationship, 229, 230, 235

therapeutic touch, 246, 247

therapist, 229, 230, 232, 233, 234, 235

therapy, x, 38, 57, 82, 86, 90, 92, 95, 96, 147, 148, 158, 164, 180, 183, 186, 193, 196, 229, 230, 231, 232, 233, 234, 235, 237, 238, 239, 240, 242, 246, 247, 248, 249, 252, 275, 277, 286, 295, 413

think critically, 427

thinking styles, 418, 420, 426, 428

Thomas Kuhn, 14, 22, 23

thoughts, 5, 13, 14, 97, 125, 126, 129, 130, 133, 186, 191, 192, 230, 291, 307, 391, 403, 404, 405, 406, 407, 408, 413, 417, 419, 422, 424, 430, 438

threats, 246, 290, 447

three-dimensional model, 474, 481

three-way interaction, 330

thrombosis, 172

time constraints, 373

time periods, 152, 313, 316, 317

time use, 262

tissue, 88, 89, 90, 205, 231, 239

tobacco, 146, 173, 273, 440

tonsils, 147, 161

tooth, 163

top-down, 363

touch therapy, 252

toxic effect, 30, 200

toxicity, 170, 196, 200

toxin, 70

tracheostomy, 161

tracks, 411

trade, 213, 361, 367

traditional authorities, 364

traditions, 28, 77, 109, 125, 193, 311

trainees, 232

training, 15, 18, 38, 57, 60, 88, 107, 108, 113, 114, 119, 123, 192, 212, 218, 232, 279, 282, 286, 295, 383, 384, 397, 422, 424, 426, 435, 447, 464

training programs, 383

trait anxiety, 396

traits, 93, 212, 259, 268, 302, 308, 431, 471

trajectory, 62, 404, 411

transactions, 432, 441

transcendence, 391

transformation(s), 6, 17, 18, 19, 50, 118, 175, 185, 191, 298

translation, 93, 187, 188, 284, 286

transmission, 90, 95, 110, 209, 243

transportation, 276, 279, 280

trauma, 35, 70, 118, 153, 159, 172, 246, 248, 249, 250

traumatic events, 247, 411

tremor, 156

trial, 95, 96, 107, 110, 160, 165, 197, 198, 199, 200, 221, 223, 224, 225, 226, 235, 279, 280, 282, 286, 287

triangulation, 100

tricyclic antidepressant(s), 149, 156, 159, 165

triggers, 124, 276

triglycerides, 175, 179, 197

Trinidad, 440

tuberculosis, 104, 110

Tukey HSD, 224

tumor, 153, 172, 173

turbulence, 66, 93

tutoring, 428

twist, 129, 133

type 1 diabetes, 202

U

UK, 53, 103, 166, 193, 347, 348, 349, 426, 427, 430, 440, 452
ultrasonography, 182
ultrasound, 71, 86, 174
UN, 35
underlying mechanisms, 109, 157
unforeseen circumstances, 8
unhappiness, 56, 78, 79, 303, 305
uniform, 27, 259
unions, 95
United, 15, 16, 19, 35, 56, 103, 105, 110, 143, 165, 169, 171, 182, 185, 229, 271, 273, 285, 351, 354, 356, 358, 367, 390, 393, 400, 409, 413, 428, 430, 439, 450, 453, 465, 482, 485, 489
United Kingdom, 103, 105, 110, 171, 409, 430, 489
United Nations, 35, 56
United States, 15, 16, 19, 143, 165, 169, 171, 182, 185, 229, 271, 273, 285, 351, 354, 356, 358, 367, 390, 393, 400, 409, 413, 428, 430, 439, 450, 453, 465, 482, 485
universe, 7, 22, 32, 40, 48, 65, 74, 77, 86, 99, 253
universities, 15, 86, 390
university education, 138, 316
urban, 41, 59, 214, 218, 260, 315, 317, 348, 440
urban areas, 260, 315, 317
urban population, 218
uric acid, 27, 174, 179
uric acid levels, 179
urinalysis, 174
urinary retention, 149, 156, 163
urinary tract, 172, 173, 174
urinary tract infection, 174
urine, 175, 197, 200
USA, 57, 240, 300, 321, 367
USSR, 349
UV, 87, 205

V

vacuum, 395, 398
vaginal acupressure, 250
Valencia, 368
validation, 299, 310, 311, 400, 414, 415, 438, 439, 452, 480, 481, 482
valuation, 421
vanadium, 202
variables, 27, 100, 211, 213, 214, 217, 233, 234, 267, 277, 318, 329, 347, 357, 367, 375, 376, 396, 433, 448, 466, 481

variations, 61, 86, 87, 99, 197, 198, 199, 201, 320, 419, 435, 445, 451, 476
varicose veins, 91
varieties, 61, 86, 114
vasculitis, 172
vasoconstriction, 175
vegetables, 104, 174, 273
vein, 62, 172, 197, 409
velocity, 93
venlafaxine, 156
verbal persuasion, 448
vertigo, 176
vessels, 175, 176
Viagra, 124
victimization, 310
victims, 245, 246, 247, 248, 249, 416, 453
video games, 152
videos, 263
Viking, 63
violence, 9, 40, 41, 138, 246, 318, 319, 411, 416, 476
viral infection, 106
viruses, 48, 124
vision(s), xvi, 3, 9, 10, 23, 34, 46, 57, 117, 118, 119, 129, 163
visualization, 44
vitamin A, 105
vitamin B3, 200
vitamin C, 157, 200
vitamin D, 27, 59, 87
vitamin D deficiency, 59
vitamins, 105, 110, 202
vocabulary, 55, 432, 450
vocalizations, 164
voiding, 164, 174
vote, 353
vulnerability, 124, 310, 448
Vygotsky, 422, 426, 427

W

waking, 144, 147, 148, 155
walking, 36, 40, 43, 164, 189, 252, 264, 279, 327, 328
wants and needs, 363, 364
Washington, 385, 413, 414, 450
waste, 26, 55
water, x, 38, 56, 67, 105, 162, 203, 204, 205, 206, 207, 208, 209, 210, 223, 279, 282
water structure, 203, 204, 209
water supplies, 105
waterways, 57
weakness, 160, 473
wealth, 49, 75, 347, 359, 392, 410

Index 517

web, 10, 31, 40, 41, 42, 86, 90, 95, 160, 238
weeping, 134, 135
weight gain, 156, 163
welfare, 344, 349, 485, 487
welfare state, 349
wellness, 19, 37, 38, 104, 229, 232, 399, 412
western culture, 76, 77
wetting, 164
White House, 396
white matter, 239
white-collar workers, 373
WHO, 35
WIC, 354
wilderness, 196
wires, 237
witchcraft, 108, 114
withdrawal, 149, 150, 151, 152, 154, 164, 175
withdrawal symptoms, 150, 151, 152
Women, Infants, and Children, 354
wool, 40
work ethic, 364
workers, 39, 51, 106, 107, 112, 117, 118, 119, 260, 268, 316, 373
workforce, 103, 104, 110
working conditions, 315
working memory, 192
workload, 366
workplace, 41, 51, 104, 352, 438
World Health Organisation, 35, 42
World Health Organization, 42, 107, 108

world-machine, 22
worldview, 14, 15, 98, 391
worldwide, 55, 56, 58, 112, 166
worms, 291, 292
worry, 352, 357
wound healing, 120
writing tasks, 450

X

X-factor, 132

Y

Yale University, 440
yes/no, 264
yield, 58, 169, 181, 239, 446
young adults, 171, 313, 314, 315, 316, 321, 331, 381, 394, 399, 400, 467
young people, 260, 324, 390, 427, 428, 430, 435, 446, 447, 448, 449, 455, 456, 458, 460, 461, 473, 476, 477, 479, 480

Z

zinc, 105, 110
zygote, 77